# *Obstetrics and Gynecology*

SIXTH EDITION

# *Obstetrics and Gynecology*

## SIXTH EDITION

American College of Obstetrics and Gynecology (ACOG)

*with*

### Charles R. B. Beckmann, MD, MHPE

Professor of Obstetrics and Gynecology, Offices of Ambulatory Care and OBGYN Academic Affairs, Department of Obstetrics and Gynecology, Albert Einstein Medical Center/Thomas Jefferson University College of Medicine, Philadelphia, PA

### Frank W. Ling, MD

Clinical Professor, Department of Obstetrics and Gynecology, Vanderbilt University School of Medicine, Nashville, TN; Partner, Women's Health Specialists, PLLC, Germantown, TN

### Barbara M. Barzansky, PhD, MHPE

Director, Division of Undergraduate Medical Education, American Medical Association

### William N. P. Herbert, MD

Professor and Chair, Department of Obstetrics and Gynecology, University of Virginia, Charlottesville, VA

### Douglas W. Laube, MD, MEd

Professor, Department of Obstetrics and Gynecology, University of Wisconsin Medical School, Madison, WI

### Roger P. Smith, MD

Professor, Department of Obstetrics and Gynecology, University of Missouri at Kansas City, Kansas City, MO

Wolters Kluwer | Lippincott Williams & Wilkins
Health

Philadelphia · Baltimore · New York · London
Buenos Aires · Hong Kong · Sydney · Tokyo

*Acquisitions Editor: Susan Rhyner*
*Developmental Editor: Kathleen H. Scogna*
*Managing Editors: Jessica Heise and Jennifer Verbiar*
*Editorial Assistant: Catherine Noonan*
*Marketing Manager: Jennifer Kuklinski*
*Project Manager: Paula C. Williams*
*Designer: Stephen Druding*
*Production Services: Circle Graphics*

Sixth Edition

Copyright © 2010, 2006, 2002, 1998, 1995, 1992 by Lippincott Williams & Wilkins, a Wolters Kluwer business.

351 West Camden Street          530 Walnut Street
Baltimore, MD 21201             Philadelphia, PA 19106

Printed in China

9 8 7 6 5 4 3 2

**Library of Congress Cataloging-in-Publication Data**

Obstetrics and gynecology.—6th ed. / Douglas W. Laube . . . [et al.].
    p. ; cm.
Includes bibliographical references and index.
ISBN 978-0-7817-8807-6
1. Gynecology. 2. Obstetrics. I. Laube, Douglas W.
[DNLM: 1. Genital Diseases, Female. 2. Pregnancy. WP 140 O14 2010]
RG101.O24 2010
618—dc22
                    2009000502

## DISCLAIMER

Care has been taken to confirm the accuracy of the information present and to describe generally accepted practices. However, the authors, editors, and publisher are not responsible for errors or omissions or for any consequences from application of the information in this book and make no warranty, expressed or implied, with respect to the currency, completeness, or accuracy of the contents of the publication. Application of this information in a particular situation remains the professional responsibility of the practitioner; the clinical treatments described and recommended may not be considered absolute and universal recommendations.

The authors, editors, and publisher have exerted every effort to ensure that drug selection and dosage set forth in this text are in accordance with the current recommendations and practice at the time of publication. However, in view of ongoing research, changes in government regulations, and the constant flow of information relating to drug therapy and drug reactions, the reader is urged to check the package insert for each drug for any change in indications and dosage and for added warnings and precautions. This is particularly important when the recommended agent is a new or infrequently employed drug.

Some drugs and medical devices presented in this publication have Food and Drug Administration (FDA) clearance for limited use in restricted research settings. It is the responsibility of the health care provider to ascertain the FDA status of each drug or device planned for use in their clinical practice.

To purchase additional copies of this book, call our customer service department at **(800) 638-3030** or fax orders to **(301) 223-2320.** International customers should call **(301) 223-2300.**

Visit Lippincott Williams & Wilkins on the Internet: http://www.lww.com. Lippincott Williams & Wilkins customer service representatives are available from 8:30 am to 6:00 pm, EST.

# FOREWORD

The fifth edition of this excellent text has been the most widely used student text in obstetrics and gynecology. The same educators and authors have prepared the new sixth edition of this popular book with many improvements, including updated information and new features. They have made this valuable text even better than the previous editions.

Each chapter has been reviewed and revised to focus on the "core" material students need to learn in the obstetrics/gynecology clerkship. A pool of questions, now available in an online question-bank format, makes it easier for students to perform self-testing and self-evaluation. The online format allows students to create custom tests and track their scoring progress. The educational impact of the book is further enhanced by revised figures and tables that make for better organization of important information. Most important,

the superb educational material is based on the latest edition of APGO objectives and includes significant educational material provided by ACOG.

All the authors and editorial advisers are to be congratulated on the production of a medical text based on sound educational principles. This new edition will undoubtedly be the number one text for students on the obstetrics and gynecology clerkship. I strongly recommend it, not only for students, but also for residents, faculty, and other individuals interested in education.

**Martin L. Stone, M.D.**
*Past president, ACOG*
*Founding member and past vice-president, APGO*
*Professor and Chairman (Emeritus)*
*Department of Obstetrics and Gynecology*
*SUNY at Stony Brook, New York*

The primary goal of this book is to provide the basic information about obstetrics and gynecology that medical students need to complete an obstetrics and gynecology clerkship successfully and to pass national standardized examinations in this content area. Practitioners may also find this book helpful in that it provides practical information in obstetrics, gynecology, and women's health necessary for physicians and advanced practice nurses in other medical specialties. Family physicians will find this book especially useful in their certification examinations. Nurse-midwives will likewise find this book helpful for many practice issues.

In publication now for 17 years, *Obstetrics and Gynecology* is proud to welcome the American College of Obstetricians and Gynecologists (ACOG)—the leading group of professionals providing health care to women—as a partner in authorship. With over 52,000 members, ACOG maintains the highest clinical standards for women's health care by publishing practice guidelines, technology assessments, and opinions emanating from its various committees on a variety of clinical, ethical, and technologic issues. These guidelines and opinions were used extensively as evidence-based clinical information in the writing of each chapter. In addition, each chapter in the sixth edition was co-authored by a member of the Junior Fellow College Advisory Council (JFCAC) of ACOG and other junior fellows in practice. The junior fellows are on the cutting edge of obstetric and gynecologic practice and education, yet retain an understanding of the concepts necessary for medical students to master.

The senior editors of this edition supervised and directed every aspect of this revision. All leaders in medical education, the senior authors were sole original authors and are obstetrician–gynecologists with additional degrees in education and experience as clerkship and residency program directors, chairs of university departments, national leadership positions in academic obstetrics and gynecology, and involvement in the preparation of standardized examinations for medical students. The partnership of a senior editor with an ACOG junior fellow in the revision of each chapter has resulted in a unique clinical and educational focus that no other clerkship textbook on the market offers.

The book has undergone a comprehensive revision. Key features of this edition include:

- Correlation of chapters with the **Medical Student Educational Objectives** published by the Association of Professors of Gynecology and Obstetrics (APGO).

In 2004, the Undergraduate Medical Education Committee of APGO revised the APGO *Medical Student Educational Objectives* to reflect current medical information, and include expected competence levels to be achieved by students, as well as best methods of evaluating the achievement of each objective. The 8th edition of the objectives provides an organized and understandable set of objectives for all medical students, regardless of future specialty choice. The Educational Topic numbers and titles employed in this text are used with permission of the Association of Professors of Gynecology and Obstetrics, and coincide with those in the APGO *Medical Student Educational Objectives*, 8th edition. Although APGO did not participate in the authorship of this text, we extend our gratitude to them for the provision of the Educational Objectives, which have proved so valuable to educators and students alike. For the complete version of the APGO *Medical Student Educational Objectives*, visit their website at www.apgo.org.

- Each chapter has been rewritten referencing ACOG Practice Guidelines, Committee Opinions, and Technology Assessments. These references are given in each chapter for the student who wishes to pursue independent study on a particular topic.

- The artwork in the book has been rendered in full color and in an anatomical style familiar to today's medical students. Great care has been taken to construct illustrations that teach crucial concepts. New photos have been chosen to illustrate key clinical features, such as those associated with sexually transmitted diseases. Other photos provide examples of the newest imaging techniques used in obstetrics and gynecology.

- Integration of the latest information and guidelines regarding several key topics, including the 2006 Consensus Guidelines for the Management of Women with Abnormal Cervical Screening Tests published by the American Society for Colposcopy and Cervical Pathology and the 2008 National Institute of Child Health and Human Development Workshop Report on Electronic Fetal Monitoring.

- Appendices include ACOG's Woman's Health Record form, Periodic Assessment recommendations, and Antepartum Record form.

- An extensive package of study questions written by the senior authors and ACOG Junior Fellows is available in an online format at Lippincott Williams & Wilkins student Web site.

Within each chapter are several features that will assist the medical student in reading, studying, and retaining key information:

- Chapters are concise and focused on key clinical aspects.
- Shaded boxes throughout the text provide critical clinical "pearls" for specific issues encountered in gynecologic and obstetric practice.
- An abundance of lists, boxes, and tables provides rapid access to crucial points.
- Italicized type emphasizes the "take-home message" that students should know about a particular topic.

We are justifiably enthusiastic about the significant changes that have been made to this edition, and we believe that they will be of tremendous benefit to medical students and other readers who need core information for the primary and obstetric–gynecologic care of women. As a new generation enters the health care profession and the dynamics of providing health care continue to change, women's health care remains central to the promotion of our society's health and well-being. *Obstetrics and Gynecology* intends to be at the forefront of medical education for this new generation of health care providers and will continue its commitment to providing the most reliable evidence-based medical information to students and practitioners.

# ACKNOWLEDGMENTS

We extend our appreciation to Susan Rhyner, Jessica Heise, Jennifer Kuklinski, Catherine Noonan, Paula Williams, Jennifer Verbiar, and Stephen Druding at Lippincott Williams & Wilkins for their seemingly tireless help and encouragement during the arduous preparation of *Obstetrics and Gynecology*, 6th edition. Likewise, we acknowledge the many contributions from the staff at the American College of Obstetricians and Gynecologists, including Kathleen Scogna and Rebecca Rinehart, former Director of Publications, and the wise counsel and support of Dr. Ralph Hale, Executive Vice President of the College. We continue to be grateful for the innovative art provided by Rob Duckwall and Dragonfly studios for this edition and Joyce Lavery in previous editions, and for the thoughtful indexing of Barbara Hodgson, which adds to the usefulness of the book for new learners. We again extend our traditional special thanks to Carol-Lynn Brown, our first editor, for her foresight and support in the early development of this book.

# CONTENTS

# The Woman's Health Examination

This chapter deals primarily with APGO Educational Topics:

Topic 1:   History

Topic 2:   Examination

Topic 3:   Pap Smear and Cultures

Topic 4:   Diagnosis and Management Plan

Topic 5:   Personal Interaction and Communication Skills

Students should be able to explain the components of the woman's health history and physical examination, including routine specimens that are collected. They should be able to conduct a thorough history, perform an appropriate examination, including obtaining tissue for cultures and the Pap smear as indicated, and generate a problem list, leading to a management plan. When seeing patients, students should be able to interact with them in a cooperative, nonjudgmental, and supportive fashion, recognizing the importance of protecting the patients' interests.

Obstetrics was originally a separate branch of medicine, and **gynecology** was a division of surgery. Knowledge of the pathophysiology of the female reproductive tract led to a natural integration of these two areas, and obstetrics and gynecology merged into a single specialty. Obstetricians can now undergo further training in maternal fetal medicine, which deals with high-risk pregnancies and prenatal diagnosis. *Likewise, gynecology now includes general gynecology (which deals with nonmalignant disorders of the reproductive tract and associated organ systems, family planning, and preconception care), gynecologic oncology, reproductive endocrinology–infertility, and pelvic reconstructive surgery and urogynecology.* These areas constitute the majority of the requisite knowledge and skills expected of the fully trained **obstetrician–gynecologist** specialist.

Currently, many obstetrician–gynecologists also provide complete care for women throughout their lives. Obstetrician–gynecologists should have additional knowledge and skills in primary and preventive health care needs of women, and be able to identify situations in which to refer patients to specialists. Obstetrician–gynecologists must be able to establish a professional relationship with patients and be able to perform a general and woman's health history, review of systems, and physical examination. Finally, as with all physicians, obstetrician–gynecologists

must fully understand the concepts of evidence-based medicine and incorporate them into their scholarship and practice in the context of a well-established pattern of lifelong learning and self-evaluation.

The demographics of women in the United States are undergoing profound change. A woman born today will live 81 or more years, experiencing menopause at 51 to 52 years of age. *Unlike previous generations, they will spend more than one-third of their lives in menopause.* The absolute number and the proportion of all women over the age of 65 are projected to increase steadily through 2040 (Fig. 1.1). These women will expect to remain healthy (physically, intellectually, and sexually) throughout menopause. Health care providers must keep the needs of this changing population in mind in their practice of medicine, especially in the provision of primary and preventive care.

## THE DOCTOR–PATIENT RELATIONSHIP

Starting with the first interaction with the patient, the physician strives to establish and develop a professional relationship of mutual trust and respect. At the same time, the patient usually decides if the physician is knowledgeable and trustworthy and whether she will accept recommendations that are made.

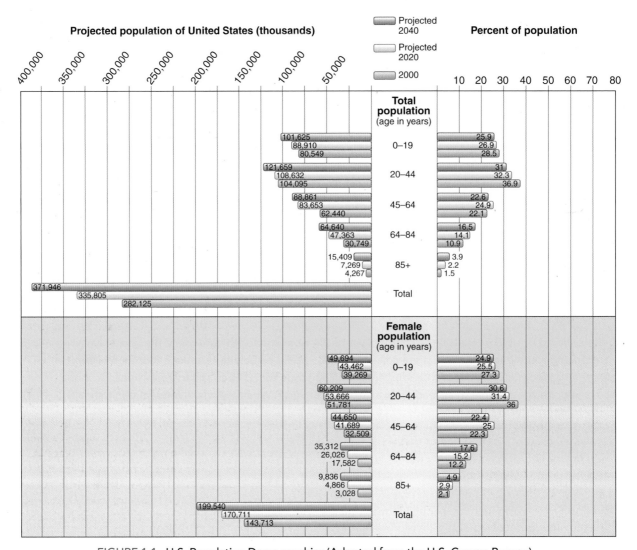

FIGURE 1.1. U.S. Population Demographics (Adapted from the U.S. Census Bureau).

The process begins with an appropriate greeting, which may or may not include a handshake. Surnames should generally be used, because the patient–physician relationship, although friendly, is professional. "What brought you to the office today?" or "How may I help you today?" are neutral opening questions that allow the patient to frame a response that includes her problems, concerns, and reasons for the visit.

In the past, practitioners focused on finding the patient's problems and fixing them "for her." *Modern health care of women involves the patient to a much greater extent in the care process.* This cooperative model is based on the following principles:

- **Engagement** involves forming or strengthening the physician–patient relationship during medical encounters. Engagement is achieved by using a pleasant, consistent tone of voice and building rapport with the patient. The goal of engagement is to form a partnership between patient and physician.

- **Empathy** occurs when a patient feels that she is being seen, heard, and accepted for who she is. Empathy is being able to view the situation or the encounter truly from the patient's perspective.

- **Educating** a patient about her health care and treatment options permits her to make decisions based on informed consent. It also helps the patient understand the necessity of treatment interventions, which may increase compliance.

- **Enlistment** is an invitation from the physician to the patient to collaborate in care, including in the decision-making process, which may also improve compliance.

## HEALTH EVALUATION: HISTORY AND PHYSICAL EXAMINATION

Routine health care involves a detailed history and physical examination. *Routine visits are also a good time to counsel patients about issues that affect health care and to perform routine screening tests based on age and risk factors.* Screening and primary and secondary care are discussed in Chapter 2. This chapter focuses on the initial physical examination and history-taking that forms the basis of a patient's health care.

A comprehensive medical record should be kept and maintained for each patient and updated periodically. This record includes a medical history, physical examination, and laboratory and radiology results. Information from referrals and other medical services outside the purview of the obstetrician–gynecologist should be integrated into the medical record. The American College of Obstetricians and Gynecologists (ACOG) offers a form called the **ACOG Women's Health Record** to assist health care providers in their daily practice (Appendix A). It also includes screening recommendations and coding information.

## Medical History

Information contained in the medical history includes discussion of the chief complaint, history of present illness, review of systems, and a medical history that includes a gynecologic history, obstetric history, health history, and social history.

- **Chief complaint** is a concise statement describing the symptom, problem, condition, diagnosis, physician-recommended return, or other factor that is the reason for the encounter. A chief complaint may not be present if the patient is seeing the obstetrician–gynecologist for preventive care. History of present illness is a chronologic description of the development of the patient's present illness.
- **Review of systems** is an inventory of body systems, obtained through a series of questions, which seeks to identify signs and symptoms that the patient has experienced or is experiencing.
- **Past, family,** and **social history** consists of a review of general medical, obstetric, and gynecologic history; family health history; allergies; current medications; and sexual and social history.

### GYNECOLOGIC HISTORY

The gynecologic history focuses on the menstrual history, which begins with **menarche,** the age at which menses began. The basic menstrual history includes:

- Last menstrual period (LMP)
- Length of periods (number of days of bleeding)
- Number of days between periods
- Any recent changes in periods

Episodes of bleeding that are "light, but on time" should be noted as such, because they may have diagnostic significance. Estimation of the amount of menstrual flow can be made by asking whether the patient uses pads or tampons, how many are used during the heavy days of her flow, and whether they are soaked or just soiled when they are changed. It is normal for women to pass clots during menstruation, but normally they should not be larger than the size of a dime. Specific inquiry should be made about **irregular bleeding** (bleeding with no set pattern or duration), **intermenstrual bleeding** (bleeding between menses), or **postcoital bleeding** (bleeding during or immediately after coitus).

The menstrual history may include **perimenstrual symptoms** such as anxiety, fluid retention, nervousness, mood fluctuations, food cravings, variations in sexual feelings, and difficulty sleeping. Cramps and discomfort during the menses are common, but abnormal when they interfere with daily activities of living (ADLs) or when they require more analgesia than provided by non-narcotic analgesia. Menstrual pain is mediated through prostaglandins and should be responsive to nonsteroidal anti-inflammatory drugs (NSAIDs). Inquiry about duration (both how long the patient has noted this pain and how long each episode of pain lasts), quality, radiation of the pain to areas outside the pelvis, and association with body position or daily activities, completes the pain history.

*The term* **menopause** *refers to the cessation of menses for greater than 1 year.* **Perimenopause** *is the time of transition from menstrual to non-menstrual life when ovarian function begins to wane,* often lasting 1 to 2 years. Significant and disruptive perimenopausal symptoms require treatment. The perimenopausal period often begins with increasing menstrual irregularity and varying or decreased flow, associated with hot flushes, nervousness, mood changes, and decreased vaginal lubrication with sexual activity and altered libido (see Chapter 37, Menopause).

The gynecologic history also includes a sexual history. *Taking a sexual history is facilitated by behaviors, attitudes, and direct statements by the physician that project a nonjudgmental manner of acceptance and respect for the patient's lifestyle.* A good opening question is, "Please tell me about your sexual partner or partners." This question is gender-neutral, leaves the issue of number of partners open, and also gives the patient considerable latitude for response. However, these questions must be individualized to each patient.

Data that should be elicited in the sexual history include whether the patient is currently or ever has been sexually active, the lifetime number of sexual partners, the partners' gender/s, and the patient's current and past methods of contraception. A patient's contraceptive history should include the method currently used, when it was begun, any problems or complications, and the patient's and her partner's satisfaction with the method. Previous contraceptive methods and the reasons they were discontinued may prove relevant. If no contraceptive actions are being taken, inquiry should be made as to why, which may include the desire for conception or concerns about contraceptive options as understood by the patient. Finally, patients should be asked about behaviors that put them at high risk for the acquisition of human immunodeficiency virus (HIV), hepatitis, or other sexually transmitted infections.

## OBSTETRIC HISTORY

The basic obstetric history includes the patient's **gravidity,** or number of pregnancies (Box 1.1). A pregnancy can be a live birth, miscarriage, premature birth (less than 37 weeks of gestation), or an abortion. Details about each live birth are noted, including birthweight of the infant, sex, number of weeks at delivery, and type of delivery. The patient should be asked about any pregnancy complications, such as diabetes, hypertension, and preeclampsia, and whether she has a history of depression, either before or after a pregnancy. A breastfeeding history is also useful information.

If a patient has a history of **infertility** (generally defined as failure to conceive for 1 year with sufficiently frequent sexual encounters), questions concerning both partners should cover previous diseases or surgery that may affect fertility, previous fertility (previous children with the same or other partners), duration that pregnancy has been attempted, and the frequency and timing of sexual intercourse.

## PAST HISTORY

Past history includes information about any gynecologic disease and/or treatment that the patient has had, including the diagnosis, the medical and/or surgical treatment, and the results. Questions about previous gynecologic surgery should include the name of the procedure; indication; when, where, and by whom the surgery was performed; and the results. Operative notes may contain useful information, for example, regarding pelvic adhesions, and should be obtained, if possible. The patient should be asked specifically about a history of sexually transmitted diseases (STDs), such as gonorrhea, herpes, chlamydia, genital warts (condylomata), hepatitis, acquired immune deficiency syndrome (AIDS), herpes, and syphilis. *To the extent possible, the patient's immunization history should be documented.*

## FAMILY HISTORY

The **family history** should list illnesses occurring in first-degree relatives, such as diabetes, cancer, osteoporosis, and heart diseases. *Information gained from the family history may indicate a genetic predisposition for a hereditary disease.* This information may guide selection of specific tests or other interventions for the surveillance of the patient and perhaps other family members. Preconceptional counseling also may be offered.

## SOCIAL HISTORY

Patients should be asked about behaviors and lifestyle issues that may potentially affect their health and increase their risk. *The outcome of this discussion provides a meaningful basis for counseling and interventions.* All patients should be asked about the following issues:

- Tobacco use
- Alcohol use: amount and type
- Use of illegal drugs and misuse of prescription drugs
- Intimate-partner violence
- Sexual abuse
- Health hazards at work and at home; seatbelt use
- Nutrition, diet, and exercise, including folic acid and calcium intake
- Caffeine intake

Questions can also be asked about whether the patient has an advance directive and whether she is interested in organ donation.

## REVIEW OF SYSTEMS

Following the medical history, an overall assessment of a patient's health history on a system-by-system basis should be conducted. This assessment provides an opportunity for a more focused evaluation of the patient. This review should encompass all body systems (Box 1.2).

---

**BOX 1.1**
**Common Terms Used to Describe Parity**

| | |
|---|---|
| Gravida | A woman who is or has been pregnant |
| Primigravida | A woman who is in or who has experienced her first pregnancy |
| Multigravida | A woman who has been pregnant more than once |
| Nulligravida | A woman who has never been pregnant and is not now pregnant |
| Primipara | A woman who is pregnant for the first time or who has given birth to only one child |
| Multipara | A woman who has given birth two or more times |
| Nullipara | A woman who has never given birth or who has never had a pregnancy progress beyond the gestational age of an abortion |

## BOX 1.2
## Review of Systems

### REVIEW OF SYSTEMS (ROS)

| 1. CONSTITUTIONAL | ☐ NEGATIVE <br> ☐ FEVER | ☐ WEIGHT LOSS <br> ☐ FATIGUE | ☐ WEIGHT GAIN <br> ☐ OTHER | TALLEST HEIGHT_____ |
|---|---|---|---|---|
| 2. EYES | ☐ NEGATIVE <br> ☐ OTHER | ☐ VISION CHANGE | ☐ GLASSES/CONTACTS | |
| 3. EAR, NOSE, AND THROAT | ☐ NEGATIVE <br> ☐ HEADACHE | ☐ ULCERS <br> ☐ HEARING LOSS | ☐ SINUSITIS <br> ☐ OTHER | |
| 4. CARDIOVASCULAR | ☐ NEGATIVE <br> ☐ EDEMA | ☐ ORTHOPNEA <br> ☐ PALPITATION | ☐ CHEST PAIN <br> ☐ OTHER | ☐ DIFFICULTY BREATHING ON EXERTION |
| 5. RESPIRATORY | ☐ NEGATIVE <br> ☐ SHORTNESS OF BREATH | ☐ WHEEZING | ☐ HEMOPTYSIS <br> ☐ COUGH | ☐ OTHER |
| 6. GASTROINTESTINAL | ☐ NEGATIVE <br> ☐ CONSTIPATION | ☐ DIARRHEA <br> ☐ FLATULENCE | ☐ BLOODY STOOL <br> ☐ PAIN | ☐ NAUSEA/VOMITING/INDIGESTION <br> ☐ FECAL INCONTINENCE   ☐ OTHER |
| 7. GENITOURINARY | ☐ NEGATIVE <br> ☐ FREQUENCY <br> ☐ DYSPAREUNIA <br> ☐ ABNORMAL VAGINAL BLEEDING | ☐ HEMATURIA <br> ☐ INCOMPLETE EMPTYING <br> ☐ ABNORMAL OR PAINFUL PERIODS | ☐ DYSURIA <br><br><br> ☐ ABNORMALVAGINAL DISCHARGE | ☐ URGENCY <br> ☐ INCONTINENCE <br> ☐ PMS <br> ☐ OTHER |
| 8. MUSCULOSKELETAL | ☐ NEGATIVE <br> ☐ MUSCLE OR JOINT PAIN | ☐ MUSCLE WEAKNESS | ☐ OTHER | |
| 9a. SKIN | ☐ NEGATIVE <br> ☐ DRY SKIN | ☐ RASH <br> ☐ PIGMENTED LESIONS | ☐ ULCERS <br> ☐ OTHER | |
| 9b. BREAST | ☐ NEGATIVE <br> ☐ DISCHARGE | ☐ MASTALGIA <br> ☐ MASSES | ☐ OTHER | |
| 10. NEUROLOGIC | ☐ NEGATIVE <br> ☐ TROUBLE WALKING | ☐ SYNCOPE <br> ☐ SEVERE MEMORY PROBLEMS | ☐ SEIZURES | ☐ NUMBNESS <br> ☐ OTHER |
| 11. PSYCHIATRIC | ☐ NEGATIVE <br> ☐ SEVERE ANXIETY | ☐ DEPRESSION <br> ☐ OTHER | ☐ CRYING | |
| 12. ENDOCRINE | ☐ NEGATIVE <br> ☐ HOT FLASHES | ☐ DIABETES <br> ☐ HAIR LOSS | ☐ HYPOTHYROID <br> ☐ HEAT/COLD INTOLERANCE | ☐ HYPERTHYROID <br> ☐ OTHER |
| 13. HEMATOLOGIC/LYMPHATIC | ☐ NEGATIVE <br> ☐ BLEEDING | ☐ BRUISES <br> ☐ ADENOPATHY | ☐ OTHER | |
| 14. ALLERGIC/IMMUNOLOGIC | (SEEFIRST PAGE) | | | |

## Physical Examination

The physical examination encompasses an evaluation of a patient's overall health as well as a breast and gynecologic examination. *The general physical examination serves to detect abnormalities suggested by the medical history as well as unsuspected problems.* Specific information the patient gives during the history should guide the practitioner to areas of physical examination that may not be surveyed in a routine screening. The extent of the examination is based on the practitioner's clinical relationship with the patient, what is being medically managed by other clinicians, and what is medically indicated. Areas that are included in this general examination are listed in Box 1.3.

## Breast Examination

The **breast examination** by a physician remains the best means of early detection of breast cancer when combined with appropriately scheduled mammography and regular breast self-examination (BSE). The results of the breast examination may be expressed by description or diagram, or both, usually with reference to the quadrants and tail region of the breast or by allusion to the breast as a clock face with the nipple at the center (Fig. 1.2).

The breasts are first examined by **inspection,** with the patient's arms at her sides, and then with her hands pressed against her hips, and/or with her arms raised over her head (Fig. 1.3). If the patient's breasts are especially large and pendulous, she may be asked to lean forward so

## BOX 1.3
## Physical Examination

### PHYSICAL EXAMINATION

| PATIENT NAME: | BIRTH DATE:  /  / | ID NO.: | DATE:  /  / |
|---|---|---|---|

**CONSTITUTIONAL**

• VITAL SIGNS (RECORD ≥ 3 VITAL SIGNS):

HEIGHT: _____ WEIGHT: _____ BMI: _____ BLOOD PRESSURE (SITTING): _____ TEMPERATURE: _____ PULSE: _____ RESPIRATION: _____

• GENERAL APPEARANCE (NOTE ALL THAT APPLY):

☐ WELL-DEVELOPED  ☐ OTHER        ☐ NO DEFORMITIES  ☐ OTHER
☐ WELL-NOURISHED  ☐ OTHER        ☐ WELL-GROOMED    ☐ OTHER
☐ NORMAL HABITUS  ☐ OBESE  ☐ OTHER

**NECK**

• NECK      ☐ NORMAL  ☐ ABNORMAL _____
• THYROID   ☐ NORMAL  ☐ ABNORMAL _____

**RESPIRATORY**

• RESPIRATORY EFFORT  ☐ NORMAL  ☐ ABNORMAL _____
• AUSCULTATED LUNGS   ☐ NORMAL  ☐ ABNORMAL _____

**CARDIOVASCULAR**

• AUSCULTATED HEART
   SOUNDS   ☐ NORMAL  ☐ ABNORMAL _____
   MURMURS  ☐ NORMAL  ☐ ABNORMAL _____
• PERIPHERAL VASCULAR  ☐ NORMAL  ☐ ABNORMAL _____

**GASTROINTESTINAL**

• ABDOMEN  ☐ NORMAL  ☐ ABNORMAL _____
• HERNIA   ☐ NONE  ☐ PRESENT _____
• LIVER/SPLEEN
   LIVER   ☐ NORMAL  ☐ ABNORMAL _____
   SPLEEN  ☐ NORMAL  ☐ ABNORMAL _____
• STOOL GUAIAC, IF INDICATED  ☐ POSITIVE  ☐ NEGATIVE

**LYMPHATIC**

• PALPATION OF NODES (CHOOSE ALL THAT ARE APPLICABLE)
   NECK   ☐ NORMAL  ☐ ABNORMAL _____
   AXILLA ☐ NORMAL  ☐ ABNORMAL _____
   GROIN  ☐ NORMAL  ☐ ABNORMAL _____
   OTHER SITE ☐ NORMAL  ☐ ABNORMAL _____

**SKIN**

• INSPECTED/PALPATED  ☐ NORMAL  ☐ ABNORMAL _____

**NEUROLOGIC/PSYCHIATRIC**

• ORIENTATION  ☐ TIME  ☐ PLACE  ☐ PERSON  ☐ COMMENTS
• MOOD AND AFFECT  ☐ NORMAL  ☐ DEPRESSED  ☐ ANXIOUS  ☐ AGITATED  ☐ OTHER

**GYNECOLOGIC (AT LEAST 7)**

• BREASTS             ☐ NORMAL  ☐ ABNORMAL _____
• EXTERNAL GENITALIA  ☐ NORMAL  ☐ ABNORMAL _____
• URETHRAL MEATUS     ☐ NORMAL  ☐ ABNORMAL _____
• URETHRA             ☐ NORMAL  ☐ ABNORMAL _____
• BLADDER             ☐ NORMAL  ☐ ABNORMAL _____
• VAGINA/PELVIC SUPPORT ☐ NORMAL  ☐ ABNORMAL _____
• CERVIX              ☐ NORMAL  ☐ ABNORMAL _____
• UTERUS              ☐ NORMAL  ☐ ABNORMAL _____
• ADNEXA/PARAMETRIA   ☐ NORMAL  ☐ ABNORMAL _____
• ANUS/PERINEUM       ☐ NORMAL  ☐ ABNORMAL _____
• RECTAL              ☐ NORMAL  ☐ ABNORMAL _____

(SEE ALSO "STOOL GUAIAC" ABOVE)

• TOTAL NUMBER OF BULLETED (•) ELEMENTS EXAMINED: _____

American College of Obstetricians and Gynecologists

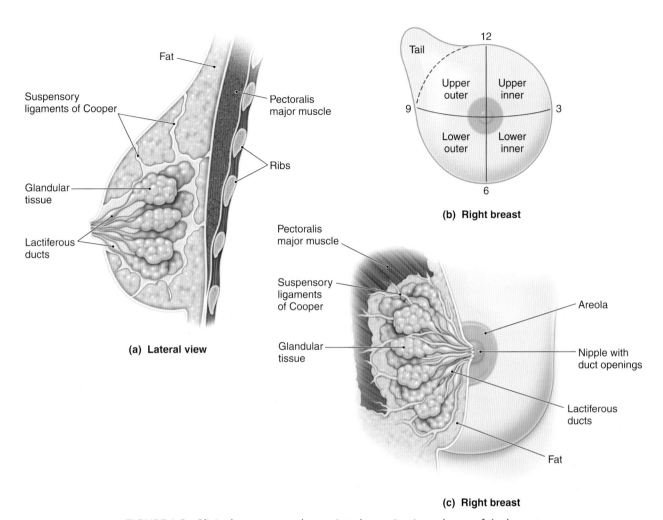

FIGURE 1.2. Clinical anatomy and associated examination schema of the breast.

that the breasts hang free of the chest, facilitating inspection. Tumors often distort the relations of these tissues, causing disruption of the shape, contour, or symmetry of the breast or position of the nipple. Some asymmetry of the breasts is common, but marked differences or recent changes deserve further evaluation.

Discolorations or ulcerations of the skin of the breast, areola, or nipple, or edema of the lymphatics that causes a leathery puckered appearance of the skin (referred to as *peau d'orange*, or like the skin of an orange), are abnormal. A clear or milky breast discharge is usually bilateral and associated with stimulation or elevated prolactin levels (**galactorrhea**). Bloody discharge from the breast is abnormal and usually unilateral; it usually does not represent carcinoma, but rather inflammation of a breast structure. Evaluation is necessary to exclude malignancy. Pus usually indicates infection, although an underlying tumor may be encountered.

Very large breasts may pull forward and downward, causing upper back pain and stooped shoulders. Disabling pain and posture is usually considered sufficient for use of insurance coverage for breast reduction.

**Palpation** follows inspection, first with the patient's arms at her sides and then with the arms raised over her head. This part of the examination is usually done with the patient in the supine position. The patient may also be seated, with her arm resting on the examiner's shoulder or over her head, for examination of the most lateral aspects of the axilla. Palpation should be done with slow, careful maneuvers using the flat part of the fingers and not the tips. The fingers are moved up and down in a wavelike motion, moving the tissues under them back and forth, so that any breast masses that are present can be more easily felt. The examiner should cover the entire breast in a spiral or radial pattern, including the axillary tail. If masses are found, their size, shape, consistency (soft, hard, firm, cystic), and mobility, as well as their position, should be determined. Women with large breasts may have a firm ridge of tissue located transversely along the lower edge of the breast. This is the inframammary ridge, and is a normal finding.

The examination is concluded with gentle pressure inward and then upward at the sides of the areola to ex-

**Inspection**

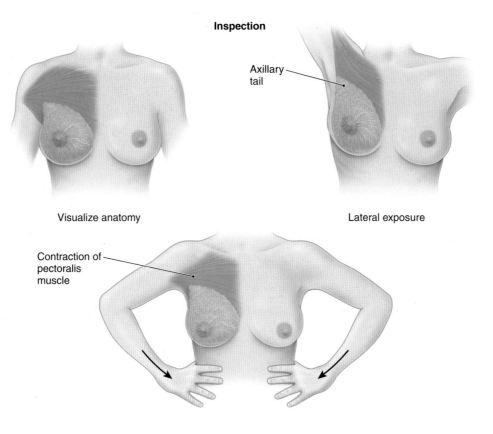

Visualize anatomy                    Lateral exposure

**Breast palpation techniques**

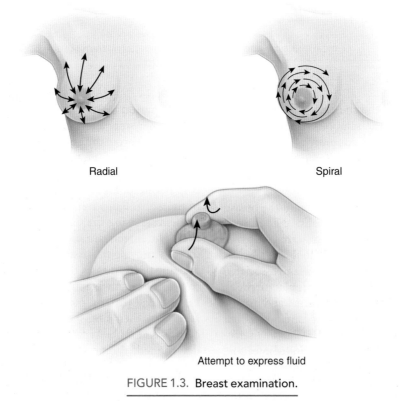

Radial                    Spiral

Attempt to express fluid

FIGURE 1.3.  Breast examination.

press fluid. If fluid is noted on inspection or is expressed, it should be sent for culture and sensitivity and cytopathology (fixed in the same manner as for a slide-technique Pap test).

## Pelvic Examination

Preparation for the pelvic examination begins with the patient emptying her bladder. Everything that is going to happen should be explained before it occurs. Following the precept "Talk before you touch" avoids anything unexpected.

Abdominal and pelvic examinations require relaxation of the muscles. Techniques that help the patient to relax include encouraging the patient to breathe in through her nose and out through her mouth, gently and regularly, rather than holding her breath, and helping the patient to identify specific muscle groups (such as the abdominal wall or the pelvic floor) that need to be made more loose.

Communication with the patient during the examination is important. An abrupt or stern command, such as "Relax now; I'm not going to hurt you," may raise the patient's fears, whereas a statement such as, "Try to relax as much as you can, although I know that it's a lot easier for me to say than for you to do" sends two messages: (1) that the patient needs to relax, and (2) that you recognize that it is difficult, both of which demonstrate patience and understanding. Saying something such as, "Let me know if anything is uncomfortable, and I will stop and then we will try to do it differently" tells the patient that there might be discomfort, but that she has control and can stop the examination if discomfort occurs. Likewise, stating, "I am going to touch you now" is helpful in alleviating surprises. Using these statements demonstrates that the examination is a cooperative effort, further empowering the patient in facilitating care.

### POSITION OF THE PATIENT AND EXAMINER

The patient is asked to sit at the edge of the examination table and an opened draping sheet is placed over the patient's knees. If a patient requests that a drape not be used, the request should be honored.

Positioning the patient for examination begins with the elevation of the head of the examining table to approximately 30 degrees from horizontal. The physician or an assistant should help the patient assume the **lithotomy position** (Fig. 1.4). The patient should be asked to lie back, place her heels in the stirrups, and then slide down to the end of the table until her buttocks are flush with the edge of the table. After the patient is in the lithotomy position, the drape is adjusted so that it does not obscure the clinician's view of the perineum or obscure eye contact between patient and physician.

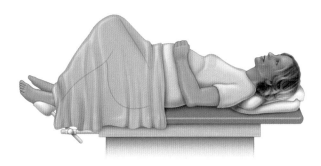

FIGURE 1.4. Lithotomy position during a pelvic position.

The physician should sit at the foot of the examining table, with the examination lamp adjusted to shine on the perineum. The lamp is optimally positioned in front of the physician's chest a few inches below the level of the chin, at approximately an arm's length distance from the perineum. The physician should glove both hands. After contact with the patient, there should be minimal contact with equipment such as the lamp. Removing the speculum from the drawer prior to touching the patient will help to prevent contamination of other speculums and equipment (e.g., table, drawers, and lamp).

### INSPECTION AND EXAMINATION OF THE EXTERNAL GENITALIA

*The pelvic examination begins with the inspection and examination of the external genitalia.* Inspection should include the mons pubis, labia majora and labia minora, perineum, and perianal area. Inspection continues as palpation is performed in an orderly sequence, starting with the clitoral hood, which may be pulled back to inspect the glans proper. The labia are spread laterally to allow inspection of the introitus and outer vagina. The urethral meatus and the areas of the urethra and Skene glands should be inspected. The forefinger is placed an inch or so into the vagina to gently milk the urethra. A culture should be taken of any discharge from the urethral opening. The forefinger is then rotated posteriorly to palpate the area of the Bartholin glands between that finger and the thumb (Fig. 1.5).

### SPECULUM EXAMINATION

*The next step is the **speculum examination**.* The parts of the speculum are shown in Figure 1.6. There are two types of specula in common use for the examination of adults. The **Pederson speculum** has flat and narrow blades that barely curve on the sides. The Pederson speculum works well for most nulliparous women and for postmenopausal women

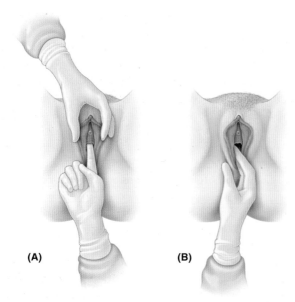

FIGURE 1.5. Palpation of the Bartholin, urethral, and Skene glands. (A) Palpation of urethral and Skene glands and "milking" of urethra. (B) Palpation of Bartholin glands.

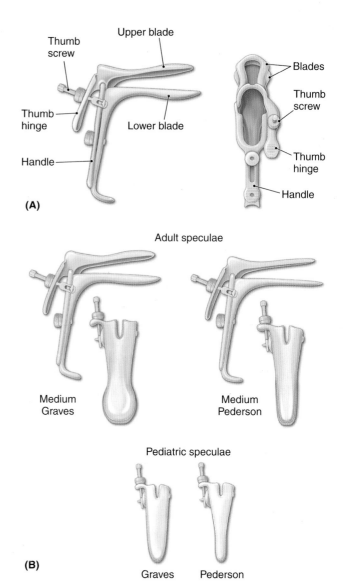

FIGURE 1.6. The vaginal speculum. (A) Parts of the vaginal speculum. (B) Types of vaginal specula.

with atrophic, narrowed vaginas. **The Graves speculum** has blades that are wider, higher, and curved on the sides; it is more appropriate for most parous women. Its wider, curved blades keep the looser vaginal walls of multiparous women separated for visualization. A Pederson speculum with extra narrow blades may be used for visualizing the cervix in pubertal girls.

The speculum should be warmed either with warm water or by holding it in the examiner's hand. Warming the speculum is done for the comfort of the patient and to aid with insertion.

*Insertion of the speculum should take into account the normal anatomic relations*, as illustrated in Figure 1.7. By inserting the speculum along the axis of the vagina, minimal force is needed and comfort is maximized. Until recently, use of lubricants was avoided because of interference with cytologic interpretation, although this is less of a concern with liquid-based Pap test techniques. Situations that may require lubricant use are encountered infrequently and include some prepubertal girls, some postmenopausal women, and patients with irritation or lesions of the vagina.

Most physicians find that control of pressure and movement of the speculum are facilitated by holding the speculum with the dominant hand. The speculum is held by the handle with the blades completely closed. The first two fingers of the opposite hand are placed on the perineum laterally and just below the introitus; pressure is applied downward and slightly inward until the introitus is opened slightly. If the patient is sufficiently relaxed, this downward pressure on the perineum causes

the introitus to open, into which the speculum may be easily inserted. *The speculum is initially inserted in a horizontal plane with the width of the blades oblique to the vertical axis of the introitus. The speculum is then directed posteriorly at an approximately 45-degree angle from horizontal; the angle is adjusted as the speculum is inserted, so that the speculum slides into the vagina with minimal resistance.* If the patient is not relaxed, posterior pressure from a finger inserted in the vagina sometimes relaxes the perineal musculature.

*As the speculum is inserted, a slight continuous downward pressure is exerted so that distension of the perineum is used to create space into which the speculum may advance.* Taking advantage of the distensibility of the perineum and vagina posterior to the introitus is a crucial concept for the effi-

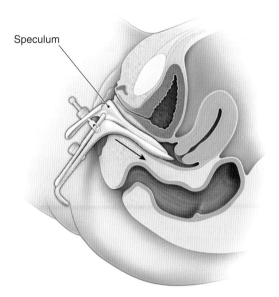

Speculum

FIGURE 1.7. Speculum insertion.

cient and comfortable manipulation of the speculum examination (and later for the bimanual and rectovaginal examination). Pressure superiorly causes pain in the sensitive area of the urethra and clitoris. The speculum is inserted as far as it will go, which in most women means insertion of the entire speculum length. The speculum is then opened in a smooth and deliberate fashion. With slight tilting of the speculum, the cervix slides into view between the blades of the speculum. The speculum is then locked into the open position using the thumbscrew. *Failure to find the cervix most commonly results from not having the speculum inserted far enough.* Keeping the speculum fully inserted while opening the speculum does not result in discomfort.

When the speculum is locked into position, it usually stays in place without being held. For most patients,

the speculum is opened sufficiently by use of the upper thumbscrew. In some cases, however, more space is required. This may be obtained by gently expanding the vertical distance between the speculum blades by use of the screw on the handle of the speculum. With the speculum in place, the cervix and the deep lateral vaginal vault may be inspected and specimens obtained. Before obtaining tissue samples for the Pap test, the patient should be told that she may feel a slight "scraping" sensation, but no pain. Specimens are collected to fully evaluate the transformation zone, where cervical intraepithelial neoplasia is more likely to be encountered. *Specimens are obtained from the exocervix and endocervix and either plated on slides which are immediately fixed with a preservative spray or placed in a liquid collection medium* (Fig. 1.8).

*Speculum withdrawal also allows for inspection of the vaginal walls.* After telling the patient that the speculum is to be removed, the blades of the speculum are opened slightly by putting pressure on the thumb hinge, and the thumbscrew is completely loosened. Opening the speculum blades slightly before starting to withdraw the speculum avoids pinching the cervix between the blades. The speculum is withdrawn approximately 1 inch before pressure on the thumb hinge is slowly released. The speculum is withdrawn slowly enough to allow inspection of the vaginal walls. The blades of the speculum are naturally brought together by vaginal wall pressure. *As the end of the speculum blades approaches the introitus, there should be no pressure on the thumb hinge, otherwise the anterior blade can flip up, hitting the sensitive vaginal, urethral, and clitoral tissues.*

## BIMANUAL EXAMINATION

*The **bimanual examination** uses both a "vaginal" hand and an "abdominal" hand to entrap and palpate the pelvic organs.*

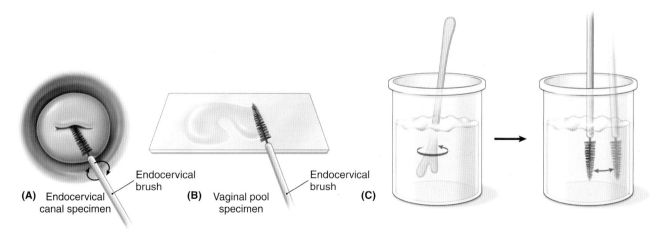

**(A)** Endocervical canal specimen — Endocervical brush    **(B)** Vaginal pool specimen — Endocervical brush    **(C)**

FIGURE 1.8. Pap smear collection. (A) Obtaining endocervical portion of Pap smear. (B) Spread specimen before fixation within 10 seconds. (C) Placement of specimens in liquid collection medium.

The bimanual examination begins by exerting gentle pressure on the abdomen approximately halfway between the umbilicus and the pubic hair line with the abdominal hand, while inserting the index and middle fingers of the vaginal hand into the vagina to approximately 2 inches and gently pushing downward, distending the vaginal canal. The patient is asked to feel the muscles being pushed on and to relax them as much as possible. Then both the index and middle fingers are inserted into the vagina until they rest at the limit of the vaginal vault in the posterior fornix behind and below the cervix. A great deal of space may be created by posterior distension of the perineum. Occasionally, only the index finger of the vaginal hand can be comfortably inserted.

During the bimanual examination, the pelvic structures are "caught" and palpated between the abdominal and vaginal hands. Whether to use the dominant hand as the abdominal or vaginal hand is a question of personal preference. *A common error in this part of the pelvic examination is failure to make effective use of the abdominal hand.* Pressure should be applied with the flat part of the fingers, not the fingertips, starting midway between the umbilicus and the hairline, moving downward in conjunction with upward movements of the vaginal hand. The bimanual examination continues with the circumferential examination of the cervix for its size, shape, position, mobility, and the presence or absence of tenderness or mass lesions (Fig. 1.9).

**Bimanual examination of the uterus** is accomplished by lifting the uterus up toward the abdominal fingers so that it may be palpated between the vaginal and abdominal hands. The uterus is evaluated for its size, shape, consistency, configuration, and mobility; for masses or tenderness; and for position. The uterus may tilt on its long axis (from cervix to fundus, **version**) yielding three positions (**anteverted, midposition,** and **retroverted**). It may also tilt on a shorter axis (from just above or at the area of the lower uterine segment, **flexion**) yielding two positions (**anteflexed** and **retroflexed**) (see Fig. 4-12). The retroverted, retroflexed uterus has three particular clinical associations: (1) it is especially difficult to estimate gestational age by bimanual examination, (2) it is associated with dyspareunia and dysmenorrhea, and (3) its position behind and below the sacral promontory may lead to the obstetric complication of uterine inculcation. *Cervical position is often related to uterine position. A posterior cervix is often associated with an anteverted or midposition uterus, whereas an anterior cervix is often associated with a retroverted uterus.* Sharp flexion of the uterus, however, may alter these relations.

*The bimanual examination technique varies somewhat with the position of the uterus.* Examination of the anterior and midposition uterus is facilitated with the vaginal fingers lateral and deep to the cervix in the posterior fornix. The uterus is gently lifted upward to the abdominal fingers and a gentle side-to-side "searching" motion of the vaginal fingers is combined with steady pressure and palpation by the abdominal hand to determine the characteristics of the uterus.

Examination of the retroverted uterus may be more difficult. In some cases, the vaginal fingers may be slowly pushed below or at the level of the uterine fundus, after which gentle pressure exerted inward and upward causes the uterus to antevert, or at least to move "upward," somewhat facilitating palpation. Then palpation is accomplished as in the normally anteverted uterus. If this cannot be done, a waving motion with the vaginal fingers in the posterior fornix must be combined with an extensive rectovaginal examination to assess the retroverted uterus.

**Bimanual examination of the adnexa** to assess the ovaries, fallopian tubes, and support structures begins by placing the vaginal fingers to the side of the cervix, deep in the lateral fornix. The abdominal hand is moved to the same side, just inside the flare of the sacral arch and above the pubic hairline. Pressure is then applied downward and toward the symphysis with the abdominal hand, at the same time lifting upward with the vaginal fingers. The same movements of the fingers of both hands used to assess the uterus are used to assess the adnexal structures, which are brought between the fingers by these maneuvers to evaluate their size, shape, consistency, configuration, mobility, and tenderness, as well as to palpate for masses. *Special care must be taken when examining the ovaries, which are sensitive even in the absence of pathology. The ovaries are palpable in normal menstrual women approximately half of the time, whereas palpation of ovaries in postmenopausal women is less common.*

## RECTOVAGINAL EXAMINATION

When indicated, a **rectovaginal examination** forms part of the complete pelvic examination on initial and annual examination, as well as at interval examinations whenever clinically indicated.

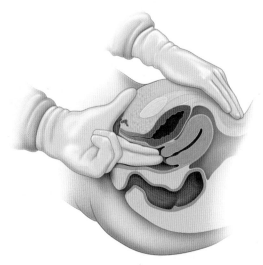

FIGURE 1.9. Bimanual examination of the uterus and adnexa.

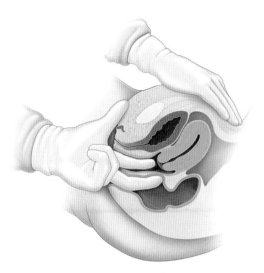

FIGURE 1.10. **Rectovaginal examination.**

The rectovaginal examination is begun by changing the glove on the vaginal hand and using a liberal supply of lubricant. *The examination may be comfortably performed if the natural inclination of the rectal canal is followed: upward at a 45-degree angle for approximately 1 to 2 cm, then downward* (Fig. 1.10). This is accomplished by positioning the fingers of the vaginal hand as for the bimanual examination, except that the index finger is also flexed. The middle finger is then gently inserted through the rectal opening and inserted to the "bend" where the angle turns downward. The index (vaginal) finger is inserted into the vagina, and both fingers are inserted until the vaginal finger rests in the posterior fornix below the cervix, and the rectal finger rests as far as it can go into the rectal canal. Asking the patient to bear down as the rectal finger is inserted is not necessary, and may add to the tension of the patient. Palpation of the pelvic structures is then accomplished, as in their vaginal palpation. The uterosacral ligaments are also palpated to determine if they are symmetrical, smooth, and nontender (as normally), or if they are nodular, slack, or thickened. The rectal canal is evaluated, as are the integrity and function of the rectal sphincter. After palpation is complete, the fingers are rapidly but steadily removed in a reversal of the sequence of movements used on insertion. Care should be taken to avoid contamination of the vagina with fecal matter. A guaiac determination is routinely made from fecal material collected on the rectal finger in patients 40 years or older.

At the conclusion of the pelvic examination, the patient is asked to move back up on the table and, thereafter, to sit up.

## FOLLOW-UP AND CONTINUITY OF CARE

Depending on the reason for the patient's visit—either for a specific medical problem or for a preventive examination, further assessments and a management plan can be established. If the patient has consulted the physician for a specific problem, a differential diagnosis may be formulated. Interventions can take the form of behavior modification, additional monitoring, treatment, or referral. If the patient has had a preventive health care examination, issues that arise during the history and physical examination and a long-term plan for addressing these issues should be discussed. Screening tests and immunizations that are appropriate for the patient should also be administered (see Chapter 2, The Obstetrician–Gynecologist's Role in Screening and Preventive Care).

## SUGGESTED READINGS

American College of Obstetricians and Gynecologists. *Guidelines for Women's Health Care: A Resource Manual.* 3rd ed. Washington, D.C.: ACOG; 2007.
American College of Obstetricians and Gynecologists. Primary and preventive care: periodic assessments, Committee Opinion No. 357. *Obstet Gynecol.* 2006;108(6):1615–1622.

# The Obstetrician–Gynecologist's Role in Screening and Preventive Care

As the population ages, the health care needs of women will change, and thus the provision of primary and preventive care in the obstetric and gynecologic setting must evolve to meet these needs. The obstetrician–gynecologist is in a unique position to provide screening, preventive care, and counseling to women that can have a positive impact on morbidity and mortality.

**Preventive care** is beneficial and cost-effective over time. Preventive medicine encompasses both primary and second prevention. In **primary prevention,** an attempt is made to eliminate risk factors for disease and thus prevent its occurrence. Primary prevention may include health education and behavioral interventions to promote a healthier lifestyle, including fitness and nutrition, hygiene, smoking cessation, personal safety, and sexuality. It also includes immunizations. **Secondary prevention** focuses on **screening tests** for diseases that are performed at an early and usually asymptomatic stage, allowing prompt intervention that reduces morbidity and mortality. Screening tests are performed as part of periodic health assessments that afford an opportunity to evaluate and counsel patients based on their age and risk factors.

## IMMUNIZATIONS

In the United States, vaccination programs that focus on infants and children have decreased the occurrence of many childhood diseases. However, many adolescents and adults are affected by vaccine-preventable diseases, such as influenza, varicella, hepatitis A, hepatitis B, measles, rubella, and pneumococcal pneumonia. Each year it is estimated that pneumococcal infection, influenza, and hepatitis B cause as many as 45,000 deaths in adults. Obstetrician–gynecologists and other clinicians who provide general well-woman examinations and preconception care have opportunities in which to counsel women on the need for immunizations and can provide immunizations or referrals to vaccination clinics or services.

It may be helpful to ask new patients to provide previous vaccination records. The clinician should attempt to gather a complete immunization history from each patient, including risk factors indicating the need for immunization. If there are doubts about past immunizations, it is safest to assume that a patient has not been immunized and initiate the appropriate vaccination series. The recommended vaccinations for women are listed in Box 2.1. Immunization recommendations change quickly; the most current recommendations can be accessed at the CDC's National Immunization Program Web page (www.cdc.gov/vaccines).

The HPV vaccine is discussed in detail in Chapter 43, Cervical Neoplasia and Carcinoma. The American College of Obstetricians and Gynecologists recommends the initial vaccination for girls aged 11–12 years. Although obstetrician–gynecologists are not likely to care for many girls in this age group, they are critical to the widespread use of the vaccine for females aged 13–26. During a health care visit with a girl or woman in the age range for vaccination, an assessment of the patient's HPV vaccine status should be conducted and documented in the patient record. The quadrivalent HPV vaccine is most effective when given before any exposure to HPV infection, but sexually active women can receive and benefit from the quadrivalent vaccine.

## SECONDARY PREVENTION: PERIODIC ASSESSMENT AND SCREENING

Periodic assessments conducted at regular intervals (e.g., annually) are an integral part of preventive health care and include screening, evaluation, and counseling. Recommendations for periodic health assessments and screening are segregated by age group and are based on risk factors (Appendix B). Assessment should include a thorough medical history, physical examination, and laboratory testing.

---

**BOX 2.1**
**Recommended Vaccinations for Women**

---

Age: 13 to 18 Years
**DTaP**
Booster (once between ages 11 and 16)
**Hepatitis B**
One series if not previously immunized
**HPV**
One series for those not previously immunized
**Meningococcal**
Before entry into high school for individuals not
　　previously immunized
**Influenza**
Annually

For High-Risk Groups:
**Hepatitis A**
One series if not already immunized
**Pneumococcal pneumonia**
Once if not already immunized*
**MMR**
One series if not already immunized
**Varicella**
One series if not already immunized

Age 19 to 39 Years
**DTaP booster**
Once every 10 years
**HPV**
For women age 26 and younger± not previously
　　immunized. Given at 0, 2, and 6 months.
**Influenza**
Annually

For High-Risk Groups:
**MMR**
Once
**Varicella**
One series
**Hepatitis A**
One series
**Hepatitis B**
One series
**Pneumococcal pneumonia**
Once*
**Meningococcal**
Once

Age 40 to 64 Years
**DTaP booster**
Every 10 years
**Herpes zoster**
Once for women aged 60 years and older if not
　　already immunized
**Influenza**
Annually

For High-Risk Groups:
**MMR**
Once
**Varicella**
One series
**Hepatitis A**
One series
**Hepatitis B**
One series
**Pneumococcal vaccine**
Once*
**Meningococcal vaccine**
Once

Age 65 Years and Older
**DTaP booster** (every 10 years)
**Herpes zoster**
Once if not already immunized
**Influenza**
Annually
**Pneumococcal pneumonia**
Once*

For High-Risk Groups:
**Hepatitis A**
One series
**Hepatitis B**
One series
**Pneumococcal vaccine**
Once*
**Meningococcal vaccine**
Once

---

DTaP = diphtheria, tetanus, pertussis; HPV = human papillomavirus; MMR = measles, mumps rubella.
*Based on risk factors, some women may need to have the vaccination repeated after 5 years.
±The "26" in "26 and younger" stems from the research population used to create the data in the first FDA application which was approved; its upper limit was 26 years. It is anticipated that the age for use will increase above 26 as more studies are reported with more robust study populations and that the vaccination of males will also be approved.
Modified from American College of Obstetricians and Gynecologists. *Immunizations for Adolescents and Adults.* Patient Education Pamphlet 117. Washington, DC: ACOG; 2008.

*The findings elicited from the history and physical examination and results of laboratory tests help guide interventions and counseling and may reveal additional risks that require targeted screening or evaluation.*

The recommendations presented in Appendix B have been selected from many sources. A variety of factors have been considered in recommending the assessments and screening tests, such as the leading causes of morbidity and mortality in each age group. Other factors are chronic health conditions that limit activity of working-age adults in the United States, such as arthritis or other musculoskeletal disorders, and circulatory disorders that become more prevalent as women age.

## Characteristics of Screening Tests

The principle behind routine screening is to detect the presence of disease in asymptomatic individuals without specific risk factors. The diseases screened for should be prevalent in the population and amenable to early intervention. Screening tests are currently available for a variety of cancers, metabolic disorders, and sexually transmitted diseases. Examples of screening tests are the Pap test and mammography

Not every disease can be detected by screening, and screening is not cost-effective or feasible for every disease. The concepts of **sensitivity** and **specificity** are used to describe the efficacy of screening tests in detecting a disorder. The sensitivity of a test is the proportion of affected individuals that test positive on the screening test. The specificity is the proportion of unaffected individuals that test negative on the screening test. *An effective screening test should be both sensitive (it has a high detection rate) and specific (it has a low false-positive rate).* Other criteria for effective screening tests pertain to the population being tested and the disease itself (Box 2.2).

## Cancer Screening

Tests are available to detect some, but not all, cancers. There is no screening test with the requisite sensitivity and specificity to detect ovarian cancer. Women should be educated about the early signs and symptoms of ovarian cancer that may aid in earlier diagnosis (see Chapter 46, Ovarian and Adnexal Disease). Likewise, screening tests are not available for endometrial, vaginal, or vulvar cancers. Endometrial cancer can often be diagnosed at an early stage based on symptoms (see Chapter 45, Cancer of the Uterine Corpus).

*Endometrial, vulvar, and vaginal biopsies are not screening tests.*

### BREAST CANCER

Breast cancer is the most common cancer among women in the United States, after skin cancer. It has a lifetime risk

---

> **BOX 2.2**
> **Criteria for Screening Tests**
>
> **Criteria for the Disease**
> • Asymptomatic period long enough to allow detection
> • Prevalent enough to justify screening
> • Treatable; treatment in an asymptomatic stage (preferably a superior treatment)
> • Sufficient effect on quality and/or length of life
>
> **Criteria for the Test**
> • Sensitive
> • Specific
> • Safe
> • Affordable
> • Acceptable to patients
>
> **Criteria for the Population to Be Tested**
> • High disease prevalence
> • Accessible
> • Compliant with testing and treatment

of 12.5%, and it is the second leading cause of cancer-related death in women. It is important that clinicians assess each patient's breast cancer risk by taking a thorough history, because the recommendations for screening differ based on risk factors. A computer program called the Breast Cancer Risk Assessment Tool is available to estimate a patient's risk of developing breast cancer (see Chapter 31, Disorders of the Breast).

For women at average risk, there are two major screening examinations for breast cancer: **clinical breast examination** and **screening mammography.** The American College of Obstetricians and Gynecologists (ACOG) recommends:

• An annual clinical breast examination for all women
• Screening mammography every 1 to 2 years starting at age 40, and yearly at age 50, for women at average risk.

The American Cancer Society (ACS) recommends:

• Clinical breast examinations every 3 years for women between the ages of 20 and 39 years at average risk.
• Annual clinical breast examination and screening mammography starting at age 40 for women at average risk.

Despite a lack of definitive data supporting or negating the efficacy of **breast self-examination (BSE),** BSE has the potential to detect palpable breast cancer and can be recommended.

Ultrasound and magnetic resonance imaging (MRI) have no current role in screening women at average risk. These imaging modalities are used for the assessment of palpable masses. *MRI is also recommended, in addition to yearly mammography, for women at very high risk (greater than 20% lifetime risk).*

## CERVICAL CANCER

**Cervical intraepithelial neoplasia (CIN)** is the precursor lesion to cervical cancer. CIN may regress spontaneously, but, in some cases, CIN 2 and CIN 3 progresses to cancer over time. *Exfoliative cytology, specifically the* **Pap test** *(either slide or liquid-based) with or without type-specific HPV identification, allow early diagnosis in most cases.* The reduction in mortality from cervical cancer since the Pap test was introduced in the 1940s is testimony to the success of this screening program.

The following are recommendations for cervical cancer screening for women:

- Annual cervical cytology screening should begin approximately 3 years after initiation of sexual intercourse, but no later than age 21 years. Women younger than 30 years should undergo annual cervical cytology screening.
- Women who have had 3 consecutive negative annual Pap test results may be screened every 2 to 3 years if they are age 30 or older with no history of CIN 2 or 3, immunosuppression, HIV infection, or diethylstilbestrol (DES) exposure in utero. Annual cervical cytology is another option for women 30 years and older. The use of combination cervical cytology and human papillomavirus (HPV) DNA screening is appropriate for women 30 years and older. Women who receive negative results on both tests should be rescreened no more frequently than every 3 years.
- Women who have had a total hysterectomy (removal of the uterus and cervix) for reasons other than cervical cancer no longer need to be screened for cervical cancer. Women who have had a supracervical hysterectomy should continue to be screened. Women who have undergone hysterectomy with removal of the cervix and have a history of CIN 2 or CIN 3 should continue to be screened annually until three consecutive negative vaginal cytology test results are achieved.

## COLORECTAL CARCINOMA

With over 75,000 new cases of **colorectal cancer** annually in women and over 25,000 deaths, colorectal cancer is the third leading cause of cancer death in women, after lung cancer and breast cancer. Because early detection (preinvasive or early invasive stage) allows effective management for most patients, screening is appropriate and recommended.

*Screening for colorectal cancer is recommended for all women at average risk, starting at the age of 50.* The preferred method is **colonoscopy,** performed every 10 years.

Other acceptable screening tests include:

- Annual **fecal occult blood testing (FOBT) or fecal immunochemical testing (FIT)**
- Flexible sigmoidoscopy every 5 years. This test will miss right-sided lesions, which may account for up to 65% of advanced colorectal cancers in women.
- Combination of annual fecal occult blood testing and flexible sigmoidoscopy
- Double contrast barium enema every 5 years

Both FOBT and FIT require two or three samples of stool collected by the patient at home and returned for analysis. Screening by FOBT of a single stool sample from a rectal examination by the physician is not adequate for the detection of colorectal cancer and is not recommended. Different recommendations apply to women at increased risk and at high risk.

## Sexually Transmitted Diseases

Appropriate STD screening in nonpregnant women depends on the age of the patient and the assessment of risk factors (Box 2.3). Because of the risk that STDs pose in pregnancy, pregnant women are routinely screened for syphilis, HIV, chlamydia, and gonorrhea.

### HUMAN IMMUNODEFICIENCY VIRUS

The demographic of the HIV epidemic has changed over the last 2 decades. Prevalence has increased among adolescents, women, persons who reside outside metropolitan areas, and heterosexual men and women. Many are not aware that they are infected.

*HIV testing is recommended for all women, and targeted testing is recommended for women with risk factors.* Although women of reproductive age should be tested at least once in their lifetime, there is no consensus regarding repeat

---

**BOX 2.3**
**Risk Factors for Sexually Transmitted Diseases**

- History of multiple sex partners
- Sexual partner with multiple sexual contacts
- Sexual contact with individuals with culture-proved STD
- History of repeated STDs
- Attendance at clinics for STDs
- Presence of a developmental disability

American College of Obstetricians and Gynecologists. Primary and preventive care: periodic assessments, ACOG Committee Opinion No. 357. *Obstet Gynecol.* 2006;108:1615–1622.

testing. Obstetrician–gynecologists should review their patient's risk factors annually and assess the need for retesting. Repeat HIV testing should be offered at least annually to women who:

- Are injection-drug users
- Have sex partners who are injection-drug users or are HIV-infected
- Exchange sex for drugs or money
- Have been diagnosed with another sexually transmitted disease in the last year
- Have had more than one sex partner since their most recent HIV test

Obstetrician–gynecologists should also encourage women and their prospective sex partners to be tested prior to initiating a new sexual relationship. Periodic retesting could be considered even in the absence of risk factors, depending on clinical judgment and the patient's wishes.

The most common screening test is the **enzyme-linked immunosorbent assay (ELISA),** which is performed on a blood sample. There are also ELISA tests that use saliva or urine. A positive (reactive) ELISA must be confirmed by a supplemental test, such as the Western blot, to make a positive diagnosis.

### CHLAMYDIA INFECTION

Infection caused by ***Chlamydia trachomatis*** is the most commonly reported bacterial STD in the United States. Over one million cases were reported to the CDC in 2006, and it is estimated that another 1.7 million cases go undiagnosed. If untreated, chlamydia can cause significant long-term complications, including infertility, ectopic pregnancy, and chronic pelvic pain. Diagnosing chlamydia promptly is necessary to prevent these complications. *Sexually active women 25 years of age and younger should receive annual screening for chlamydia. Asymptomatic women aged 26 and older who are at high risk for infection should be routinely screened.* Nucleic acid amplification tests (NAATs) of endocervical swab specimens can identify infection in asymptomatic women with high specificity and sensitivity. NAATs of vaginal swabs and urine samples have comparable sensitivity and specificity.

## Gonorrhea Infection

Of the estimated 700,000 new cases of **gonorrhea** annually, less than half are reported. Infection can be symptomatic with cervicitis and vaginal discharge, or it may be asymptomatic. Gonorrhea may lead to pelvic inflammatory disease, which is associated with long-term morbidity due to chronic pelvic pain, ectopic pregnancy, and infertility.

ACOG recommends screening of women based on risk factors. *Asymptomatic women aged 26 and older should receive*

*routine screening if they are at high risk for infection.* All sexually active adolescents should also be routinely screened. Screening can be done by cervical cultures or by newer techniques such as NAATs and nucleic acid hybridization tests that have better sensitivity with comparable specificity (see Chapter 27, Sexually Transmitted Diseases).

## Syphilis

**Syphilis** is not a common disease in the United States, but the rate has increased over the last few years. Almost 10,000 cases were diagnosed in 2006, which translates into a rate of 1 case of primary or secondary syphilis per 100,000 women.

Syphilis is a systemic disease caused by the bacteria *Treponema pallidum.* If untreated, syphilis may progress from a primary infection characterized by a painless ulcer (chancre), to secondary and tertiary infections. Signs and symptoms of secondary infection include skin manifestations and lymphadenopathy; tertiary infection may cause cardiac or ophthalmic manifestations, auditory abnormalities, or gummatous lesions. Serologic tests may be negative in the early stages of infection.

*ACOG recommends annual syphilis screening for women at increased risk* (see Box 2.3). All pregnant women should be serologically screened as early as possible in pregnancy and again at delivery. Due to the possibility of a false-negative result in early stages of infection, patients who are considered at high risk or who are from areas of high prevalence should be retested at the beginning of the third trimester.

Screening includes initially nontreponemal tests such as VDRL (Venereal Disease Research Laboratory) or rapid plasma reagin (RPR). These tests are followed by confirmatory treponemal tests such as *T. pallidum* particle agglutination (TP-PA). The specificity of the nontreponemal tests may be reduced in the presence of other conditions such as pregnancy, collagen vascular disease, advanced cancer, tuberculosis, malaria, or rickettsial diseases.

## METABOLIC AND CARDIOVASCULAR DISORDERS

Routine screening can also be applied to noninfectious and noncancerous diseases, such as metabolic disorders and cardiovascular disease. Women should be evaluated for lifestyle issues and risks based on a history and physical examination. In many cases, early identification of risk factors and appropriate interventions are key components of disease prevention.

### OSTEOPOROSIS

**Osteoporosis** affects approximately 13% to 18% of American women aged 50 years and older, and another 37%

to 50% have **osteopenia,** or low bone mineral density. Osteoporosis-associated fracture, especially of the hip and spine, are leading causes of morbidity and mortality, increasing in proportion to age. Osteoporosis is a largely preventable complication of menopause. Screening strategies and pharmacologic interventions are available to prevent and treat osteoporosis.

**Bone mineral density (BMD)** is an indirect measure of bone fragility. BMD is measured using dual-energy x-ray absorptiometry (DXA) of the hip or the lumbar spine. The results are expressed in standard deviations compared with a reference population stratified by age, sex, and race. The **T-score** is expressed as the standard deviation from the mean peak bone mineral density of a normal, young-adult population; and the **Z-score** is expressed as the standard deviation from the mean bone mineral density of a reference population of the same sex, race, and age as the patient. Z- and T-scores are used for hip and spine measurements. The World Health Organization (WHO) defines a normal BMD T-score as ≥–1. Osteopenia (low bone mass) is defined as a T-score between –1 and –2.5. Osteoporosis is defined as a T-score ≤–2.5. Because of variance in the measurements obtained by the different commercial devices and at different sites, T- and Z-scores cannot be used as true screening tests, but they are good predictors of the risk of fracture. This information can be used to guide decisions about interventions including lifestyle changes and medical therapy to prevent or slow bone loss.

*ACOG recommends bone mineral density testing for all postmenopausal women starting at age 65. Bone mineral density testing should also be performed in younger postmenopausal women who have at least one risk factor for osteoporosis* (Box 2.4). In addition, postmenopausal women who experience a fracture should have bone mineral density testing to ascertain if they are osteoporotic; if so, treatment for osteoporosis is added to the therapy for the fracture. Certain diseases or medical conditions (e.g., Cushing disease, hyperparathyroidism, hypophosphatasia, inflammatory bowel disease, lymphoma, and leukemia) and certain drugs (e.g., phenobarbital, phenytoin, corticosteroids, lithium, and tamoxifen) are associated with bone loss. Women with these conditions or taking these drugs may need to be tested more frequently.

Women should be counseled on the risks of osteoporosis and related fractures and the following preventive measures:

- Adequate calcium consumption (at least 1000 to 1500 mg/d) using dietary supplements if dietary sources are not adequate
- Adequate vitamin D consumption (400 to 800 international units daily) and exposure to the natural sources of this nutrient
- Regular weight-bearing and muscle-strengthening exercises to reduce falls and prevent fractures
- Smoking cessation
- Moderation of alcohol intake
- Fall prevention strategies

---

**BOX 2.4**
**Risk Factors for Osteoporotic Fracture in Postmenopausal Women**

- History of prior fracture
- Family history of osteoporosis
- Caucasian race
- Dementia
- Poor nutrition
- Smoking
- Low weight and body mass index
- Estrogen deficiency*
  - Early menopause (age younger than 45 years) or bilateral oophorectomy
  - Prolonged premenopausal amenorrhea (>1 year)
- Long-term low calcium intake
- Alcoholism
- Impaired eyesight despite adequate correction
- History of falls
- Inadequate physical activity

*A patient's current use of hormone therapy does not preclude estrogen deficiency.
Data from Osteoporosis prevention, diagnosis, and therapy. NIH Consensus Statement 2000;17(1):1–45.

---

## Diabetes Mellitus

**Diabetes mellitus** is a group of disorders that share hyperglycemia as a common feature. Even when symptoms are not present, the disease can cause long-term complications. Ideally, it should be detected and treated in its early stages. *A screening fasting blood glucose test is recommended for women beginning at age 45 and every 3 years thereafter.* Screening should begin at a younger age or more frequently in individuals with risk factors, which include being overweight (body mass index ≥25), a family history of diabetes mellitus, habitual physical inactivity, having given birth to a newborn weighing more than 9 pounds, history of gestational diabetes, and hypertension.

## Thyroid Disease

**Thyroid disease** is often asymptomatic and if untreated can lead to serious medical conditions. *Thyroid-stimulating hormone levels should be tested every 5 years starting at the age of 50.*

## Hypertension

It is estimated that approximately 30% of adults aged 20 and older have **hypertension,** which is defined as a systolic blood pressure of ≥140 mm Hg or a diastolic blood pressure of ≥90 mm Hg. Hypertension is one of the most important risk factors for heart disease and cerebrovascular accidents (CVAs), two of the three leading causes for mortality among women. Hypertension is also a leading cause of mortality. About a third of those with hypertension do not know they have it. *Screening for hypertension is recommended for women and girls 13 years of age and older. Screening may be repeated every 2 years in persons with normal blood pressure or annually with higher levels.*

### Lipid Disorders

Coronary heart disease (CHD) is a leading cause of death for both men and women in the United States and accounts for approximately 500,000 deaths each year. Abnormal cholesterol levels have been linked to atherosclerosis and cardiovascular and cerebrovascular disease. Clinical trials have shown that a 1% reduction in serum cholesterol levels results in a 2% reduction in CHD rates. Lipid levels are assessed with regard to **low-density lipoprotein (LDL), high-density lipoprotein (HDL),** and **triglycerides.** About one in five adult Americans has a high total cholesterol level (≥240 mg/dL).

*Current guidelines recommend that women without risk factors have a lipid profile assessment every 5 years, beginning at age 45 years.* Earlier screening may be appropriate in women with risk factors. Risk factors for high cholesterol are a family history of familial hyperlipidemia, family histology of premature (age younger than 50 years for men and younger than 60 years for women) cardiovascular disease, diabetes mellitus, and multiple coronary heart disease risk factors (e.g., tobacco use, hypertension).

### Obesity

**Obesity** is associated with increased risk for heart disease, type 2 diabetes, hypertension, some types of cancer (endometrial, colon, breast), sleep apnea, osteoarthritis, gallbladder disease, and depression. *Measurement of height and weight and the calculation of a BMI are recommended as part of the periodic assessment* (Box 2.5). Obese people with a body mass index (BMI) of 30 or more have up to twofold increased risk of death.

### PREVENTIVE CARE

*Because screening is not available for all conditions, risks for some conditions can be decreased through lifestyle changes.* Examples include smoking cessation to decrease the risk of lung cancer; exercise and dietary changes to decrease cardiovascular disease, obesity, type 2 diabetes, and osteoporosis; avoidance of risk factors for STDs; and moderation of alcohol intake to reduce certain cancer risks.

---

> **BOX 2.5**
> **Body Mass Index**
>
> - BMI  <18.5 = underweight
> - BMI  18.5–24.9 = normal weight
> - BMI  25–29.9 = overweight
> - BMI  30–34.9 = obesity (Class I)
> - BMI  35–39.9 = obesity (Class II)
> - BMI  ≥40 = extreme obesity
>
> National Heart, Lung, and Blood Institute and North American Association for the Study of Obesity. *The Practical Guide: Identification, Evaluation, and Treatment of Overweight and Obesity in Adults.* Bethesda, MD: National Institutes of Health; 2000.

### SUGGESTED READINGS

American College of Obstetricians and Gynecologists. Breast cancer screening, ACOG Practice Bulletin No. 42. *Obstet Gynecol.* 2003; 101:821–832.

American College of Obstetricians and Gynecologists. Cervical cancer screening in adolescents, ACOG Committee Opinion No. 300. *Obstet Gynecol.* 2004;104:885–889.

American College of Obstetricians and Gynecologists. Cervical cytology screening, ACOG Practice Bulletin No. 45. *Obstet Gynecol.* 2003;102:417–427.

American College of Obstetricians and Gynecologists. Evaluation and management of abnormal cervical cytology and histology in the adolescent, ACOG Committee Opinion No. 330. *Obstet Gynecol.* 2006;107:963–968.

American College of Obstetricians and Gynecologists. *Guidelines for Women's Health Care: A Resource Manual.* 3rd ed. Washington, D.C.: ACOG; 2007:294–353.

American College of Obstetricians and Gynecologists. Human papillomavirus vaccination, ACOG Committee Opinion No. 344. *Obstet Gynecol.* 2006;108:699–705.

American College of Obstetricians and Gynecologists. *Immunizations for Adolescents and Adults.* ACOG Patient Education Pamphlet No. 117. Washington, DC: ACOG; 2007.

American College of Obstetricians and Gynecologists. Osteoporosis, ACOG Practice Bulletin No. 50. *Obstet Gynecol.* 2004;103:203–216.

American College of Obstetricians and Gynecologists. Primary and preventive care: periodic assessments, ACOG Committee Opinion No. 357. *Obstet Gynecol.* 2006;108:1615–1622.

American College of Obstetricians and Gynecologists. Role of the obstetrician–gynecologist in the screening and diagnosis of breast masses, ACOG Committee Opinion No. 334. *Obstet Gynecol.* 2005; 106:1141–1142.

American College of Obstetricians and Gynecologists. Routine cancer screening, ACOG Committee Opinion No. 356. *Obstet Gynecol.* 2006;108:1611–1613.

American College of Obstetricians and Gynecologists. The role of the generalist obstetrician–gynecologist in the early detection of ovarian cancer. ACOG Committee Opinion No. 280. *Obstet Gynecol.* 2002;100:1413–1416.

American College of Obstetricians and Gynecologists. The role of the obstetrician–gynecologist in the assessment and management of obesity, ACOG Committee Opinion No. 319. *Obstet Gynecol.* 2005;106:895–899.

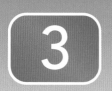

CHAPTER

3

# Ethics in Obstetrics and Gynecology

## CREATING AN ETHICAL FRAMEWORK FOR PRACTICE AND PROFESSIONAL LIFE

Physicians often encounter ethical dilemmas in the context of their dealings with patients. *The use of an organized ethical framework in such situations is valuable in ensuring that evaluating situations and making decisions can be done in a systematic manner, rather than based on the physician's emotions, personal bias, or social pressures.* Physicians, in training or practice, are expected as professionals to be able to exemplify ethical virtues in their practice and professional life. For medicine, the organization of ethical principles into codes of conduct and useful frameworks began 2500 years ago with the Hippocratic Oath. Currently, principles have evolved into a code of professional ethics developed to guide physicians in physician–patient relationships, conduct, and practice.

Several methods for ethical decision making in medicine exist. Each of these methods has both merits and limitations. When put into practice, they can promote understanding of common ethical practices regarding informed consent, honesty, and confidentiality.

### Principle-Based Ethics

*In recent decades, medical decision making has been dominated by principle-based ethics.* In this framework, four principles are used to identify, analyze, and address ethic dilemmas:

- **Respect for patient autonomy** acknowledges an individual's right to hold views, make choices, and take actions based on his or her beliefs or values. Respect for autonomy provides a strong moral foundation for informed consent, in which a patient, adequately informed about her medical condition and available therapies, freely chooses specific treatments or nontreatment.

- **Beneficence** is the obligation to promote the well-being of others, and **nonmaleficence** obliges an individual to avoid doing harm. Both beneficence and nonmaleficence are fundamental to the ethical practice of medicine. The application of these principles consists of balancing benefits and harms, both intentional harms and those than can be anticipated to arise despite the best intentions (e.g., unwanted adverse effects of medication or complications of surgical treatment). In balancing beneficence with respect for autonomy, the clinician should define the patient's best interests as objectively as possible. Attempting to override patient autonomy to promote what the clinician perceives as a patient's best interests is called paternalism.

- **Justice** is the principle of rendering what is due to others. It is the most complex of the ethical principles, because it deals not only with the physician's obligation to render to a patient what is owed, but also with the physician's role in the allocation of limited resources in the broader community. In addition, various criteria such as need, effort, contribution, and merit are important in determining what is owed and to whom it is owed. Justice is the obligation to treat equally those who are alike or similar according to whatever criteria are selected. Individuals should receive equal treatment, unless scientific and clinical evidence establishes that they differ in ways that are relevant to the treatments in question. Determination of the criteria on which these judgments are based is a highly complex moral process, as exemplified by the ethical controversies about providing or withholding renal dialysis and organ transplantation.

### Other Ethical Frameworks

In addition to principle-based ethics, several alternative approaches have been promoted, including virtue-based ethics, the ethic of care, feminist ethics, communitarian ethics, and case-based approaches.

- **Virtue-based ethics** relies on healthcare professionals possessing qualities of character that dispose them to make choices and decisions that achieve the well-being of others. These qualities of character include trustworthiness, prudence, fairness, fortitude, temperance, integrity, self-effacement, and compassion. Virtues complement rather than replace principles, because they are necessary to interpret and apply methods in medical ethics with moral sensitivity and judgment.
- **Ethic of care** is concerned primarily with responsibilities that arise from attachment to others, rather than with the impartiality that traditional ethics demands. The moral foundations underlying the ethic of care are not rights and duties, but commitment, empathy, compassion, caring, and love.
- **Feminist ethics** calls attention to the way that gender distorts traditional analyses. Ethical decisions about women's healthcare may be biased by attitudes and traditions about gender roles that are embedded in our culture. Feminist ethics challenges these presuppositions and their consequences.
- **Communitarian ethics** challenges the primacy often attributed to respect for autonomy in principle-based ethics. It emphasizes shared values, ideals, and goals of the community.
- **Case-based reasoning** is ethical decision making based on precedents set in specific cases, analogous to the role of case law in jurisprudence. An accumulated body of influential cases and their interpretation provide moral guidance. Case-based reasoning asserts the priority of practice over theory, rejects the primacy of principles, and recognizes the emergence of principles from a process of generalization from analysis of cases.

## ETHICAL FOUNDATIONS

Obstetrician-gynecologists, as members of the medical profession, have ethical responsibilities not only to patients, but also to society, to other health professionals, and to themselves. The ethical foundations discussed in this section are based on the five ethical principles of autonomy, beneficence, nonmaleficence, veracity, and justice.

### Patient–Physician Relationship

*The welfare of the patient should be central to all considerations in the patient–physician relationship.* The right of individual patients to make their own decisions about their healthcare is fundamental (autonomy). Physicians and other healthcare providers are charged with strict avoidance of discrimination on the basis of race, color, religion, national origin, or any other factor.

### Physician Conduct and Practice

Obstetrician-gynecologists must deal honestly with patients and colleagues at all times (veracity). This includes avoiding misrepresentation of themselves through any form of communication and maintaining medical competence through study, application, and enhancement of skills. *Any behavior that diminishes a physician's capability to practice, such as substance abuse, must be immediately addressed.* The physician should modify his or her practice until the diminished capacity has been restored to an acceptable standard to avoid harm to patients (nonmaleficence). Physicians are obligated to respond to evidence of questionable conduct or unethical behavior by other physicians through appropriate procedures established by the relevant organization.

### Avoiding Conflicts of Interest

If potential conflicts of interest arise, physicians are expected to recognize these situations and deal with them through public exposure. *Conflicts of interest should be resolved in accordance with the best interest of the patient, respecting a woman's autonomy to make healthcare decisions.* The physician should function as an advocate for the patient.

### Professional Relations

*The obstetrician–gynecologist's relationships with other physicians, nurses, and healthcare professionals should reflect fairness, honesty, and integrity, sharing a mutual respect and concern for the patient.* The physician should consult, refer, or cooperate with other physicians, healthcare professionals, and institutions to the extent necessary to serve the best interest of the patient.

### Societal Responsibilities

*The obstetrician–gynecologist has a continuing responsibility to society as a whole and should support and participate in activities that enhance the community.* As a member of society, the obstetrician–gynecologist should respect the laws of that society. As professionals and members of medical societies, physicians are required to uphold the dignity and honor of the profession.

### Informed Consent

The primary purpose of the consent process is to protect patient autonomy. By encouraging an ongoing and open communication of relevant information (adequate disclosure), the physician enables the patient to exercise personal choice. This sort of communication is central to a satisfactory physician–patient relationship. Discussions for the purpose of educating and informing patients about their healthcare options are never completely free of the informant's bias. Practitioners should seek to uncover their own biases and endeavor to maintain objectivity in the face of those biases while disclosing to the patient any personal biases that could influence the practitioner's recommendations. *A patient's right to make her own decisions about medical issues extends to the right to refuse recommended medical treatment.* The freedom to accept or refuse recommended medical treatment has legal as well as ethical foundations.

*In order to give informed consent, a patient must be able to understand the nature of her condition and the benefits and risks of the treatment that is recommended as well as those of the alternative treatments.* A patient's capacity to understand depends on her maturity, state of consciousness, mental acuity, education, cultural background, native language, the opportunity and willingness to ask questions, and the way in which the information is presented. Diminished capacity to understand is not necessarily the same as legal incompetence. Critical to the process of informing the patient is the physician's integrity in choosing the information that is given to the patient and respectfulness in presenting it in a comprehensible way. The point is not merely to disclose information, but to ensure patient comprehension of relevant information. Voluntariness—the patient's freedom to choose among alternatives—is also an important element of informed consent, which should be free from coercion, pressure, or undue influence.

## ETHICAL CONSIDERATIONS IN OBSTETRICS AND GYNECOLOGY

Issues surrounding maternal and fetal rights are uniquely central to obstetrics and gynecology. The primary concern of physicians is to provide the best care to their patients. However, recent legal actions and policies aimed at protecting the fetus as an entity separate from the woman have challenged the rights of pregnant women to make decisions about medical interventions and have criminalized maternal behavior that is believed to be associated with fetal harm or adverse perinatal outcomes. *Threats and incarceration have been proved to be ineffective in reducing the incidence of alcohol or drug abuse, and removing children from the home may only subject them to worse risks in the foster-care system.* ACOG and medical ethicists have consistently maintained that the rights of the mother in considerations of medical care or the therapeutic alliance of physician and patient take precedence over those of the fetus.

Conflicts between maternal and fetal rights arise when a pregnant woman engages in behaviors, such as illicit drug use, that may put her fetus at risk. *According to the principle of autonomy, obstetrician–gynecologists are obligated to respect the mother's prerogative to make choices and take action based on her beliefs or values, even if these choices and actions are harmful to herself and her child.* However, the physician is also obligated under the principle of benefi-

cence to promote the well-being of others. In situations in which a pregnant woman is putting her fetus at risk through harmful behaviors, the obstetrician–gynecologist should provide accurate and clear information regarding the consequences of the harmful behaviors. The patient should also be referred to an appropriate treatment program. Treatment is both more effective and less expensive than restrictive policies.

The ethical principle of justice governs access to care and fair distribution of resources. Therefore, implementation of universal screening for risky behaviors is an important step in equalizing access to care and in assessing the resources that are needed for particular patients. Psychosocial screening of all women seeking pregnancy evaluation or prenatal care should be performed regardless of social status, educational level, or race and ethnicity. Because risks may not be evident at the first prenatal visit, screening should be repeated at least once a trimester. There is evidence that women who are screened for psychosocial issues once each trimester are half as likely as women who are not screened to have a low–birth-weight or preterm baby. Screening consists of questions designed to elicit information regarding current and past alcohol and drug use, ability to access prenatal care, and safety at home. Screening questions are now included in the ACOG Obstetric Medical History form (Appendix C).

Another maternal–fetal conflict may arise if a pregnant woman rejects medical advice or interventions that are necessary to avert fetal complications or death. Again, the pregnant woman's autonomous decisions should be respected as long as she is competent to make informed medical decisions. *The obstetrician's response to a patient's unwillingness to cooperate with medical advice should be to convey clearly the reasons for the recommendations to the pregnant woman, examine the barriers to change along with her, and encourage the development of health-promoting behavior.* When conveying this information, the obstetrician must keep in mind that medical knowledge has limitations and medical judgment is fallible. He or she should make every effort to present a balanced evaluation of expected outcomes for both the woman and the fetus. Even if a woman's autonomous decision seems not to promote beneficence-based obligations (of the woman or the physician) to the fetus, the obstetrician must respect the patient's autonomy, continue to care for the pregnant woman, and not intervene against the patient's wishes, regardless of the consequences (Box 3.1).

## GUIDELINES FOR ETHICAL DECISION MAKING

It is important for the individual physician to find or develop guidelines for decision making that can be applied consistently in facing ethical dilemmas. Guidelines consisting of several logical steps can aid the practitioner in analyzing and resolving an ethical problem. The approach

## BOX 3.1
## One Case Study: Five Approaches

Although several approaches to ethical decision making may all produce the same answer in a situation that requires a decision, they focus on different, though related, aspects of the situation and decision. Consider, for instance, how they might address interventions for fetal well-being if a pregnant woman rejects medical recommendations or engages in actions that put the fetus at risk.*

A *principle-based approach* would seek to identify the principles and rules pertinent to the case. These might include beneficence–nonmaleficence to both the pregnant woman and her fetus, justice to both parties, and respect for the pregnant woman's autonomous choices. These principles cannot be applied mechanically. After all, it may be unclear whether the pregnant woman is making an autonomous decision, and there may be debates about the balance of probable benefits and risks of interventions to all the stakeholders, as well as about which principle should take priority in this conflict. Professional codes and commentaries may offer some guidance about how to resolve such conflicts.

A *virtue-based approach* would focus on the courses of action to which different virtues would and should dispose the obstetrician–gynecologist. For instance, which course of action would follow from compassion? From respectfulness? And so forth. In addition, the obstetrician–gynecologist may find it helpful to ask more broadly: Which course of action would best express the character of a good physician?

An *ethic of care* would concentrate on the implications of the virtue of caring in the obstetrician–gynecologist's special relationship with the pregnant woman and with the fetus. In the process of deliberation, individuals using this approach generally would resist viewing the relationship between the pregnant woman and her fetus as adversarial, acknowledging that most of the time women are paradigmatically invested in their fetus' well-being and that maternal and fetal interests usually are aligned.* If, however, a real conflict does exist, the obstetrician–gynecologist should resist feeling the need to take one side or the other. Instead, he or she should seek a solution in identifying and balancing his or her duties in these special relationships, situating these duties in the context of a pregnant woman's values and concerns, instead of specifying and balancing abstract principles or rights.

A *feminist* ethics approach would attend to the social structures and factors that limit and control the pregnant woman's options and decisions in this situation, and would seek to alter any that can be changed.* It also would consider the implications any intervention might have for further control of women's choices and actions—for instance, by reducing a pregnant woman, in extreme cases, to the status of "fetal container" or "incubator."

Finally, a *case-based approach* would consider whether there are any relevantly similar cases that constitute precedents for the current one. For instance, an obstetrician–gynecologist may wonder whether to seek a court order for a cesarean delivery that he or she believes would increase the chances of survival for the child-to-be, but that the pregnant woman continues to reject. In considering what to do, the physician may ask, as some courts have asked, whether there is a helpful precedent in the settled consensus of not subjecting a nonconsenting person to a surgical procedure to benefit a third party, for instance, by removing an organ for transplantation.†

*Harris LH. Rethinking maternal-fetal conflict: gender and equality in perinatal ethics. *Obstet Gynecol.* 2000;96(5):786–791.
† In re: A. C., 572 A.2d 1235 (D.C. Ct. App. 1990).
Adapted from American College of Obstetricians and Gynecologists. Ethical decision making in obstetrics and gynecology. ACOG Committee Opinion no. 390. *Obstet Gynecol.* 2007;110(6):1479–1487.

that follows incorporates elements of several proposed schemes and is affirmed by ACOG.

1. *Identify the decision makers.* The first step in addressing any problem is to answer the question, "Whose decision is it?" Generally, the patient is presumed to have the authority and capacity to choose among medically acceptable alternatives or to refuse treatment. An individual's capacity to make a decision depends on that individual's ability to understand information and appreciate the implications of that information when making a personal decision. If a patient is thought to be incapable of making a decision or has been found legally incompetent, a surrogate decision maker must be identified. In the absence of a durable power of attorney, family members have been called on to render proxy decisions. In some situations, the court may be called on to appoint a guardian. A surrogate decision maker should make the

decision that the patient would have wanted or, if the patient's wishes are not known, that will promote the best interests of the patient. The physician has an obligation to assist the patient's representatives in examining the issues and reaching a resolution.

2. *Collect data, establish facts.* It is important to be as objective as possible when collecting the information on which to base a decision. Consultants may be called upon to ensure that all available information about the diagnosis, treatment, and prognosis has been obtained.

3. *Identify all medically appropriate options.* Using consultation as necessary, identify all of the options available, including those raised by the patient or other concerned parties.

4. *Evaluate options according to the values and principles involved.* Start by gathering information about the values of the involved parties, the primary stakeholders, and try to get a sense of the perspective each is bringing to the discussion. The values of the patient generally will be the most important consideration as decision making proceeds. Then, determine whether any of the options violates ethical principles that all agree are important. Eliminate those options that, after analysis, are found to be morally unacceptable by all parties. Finally, reexamine the remaining options according to the interests and values of each party. Some alternatives may be combined successfully.

5. *Identify ethical conflicts and set priorities.* Try to define the problem in terms of the ethical principles involved (e.g., beneficence versus respect for autonomy), and weigh the principles underlying each of the arguments made. Studying a similar case may be helpful. In doing so, the physician should look for important differences and similarities between this and other cases.

6. *Select the option that can be best justified.* Try to arrive at a rational resolution to the problem, one that can be justified to others in terms of widely recognized ethical principles.

7. *Reevaluate the decision after it is acted on.* Repeat the evaluation of the major options in light of information gained during the implementation of the decision. Was the best possible decision made? What lessons can be learned from the discussion and resolution of the problem?

## SUGGESTED READINGS

American College of Obstetricians and Gynecologists. Ethical decision making in obstetrics and gynecology. ACOG Committee Opinion No. 390. *Obstet Gynecol.* 2007;110(6):1479–1487.

American College of Obstetricians and Gynecologists. Innovative practice: ethical guidelines. ACOG Committee Opinion No. 352. *Obstet Gynecol.* 2006;108(6):1589–1595.

American College of Obstetricians and Gynecologists. Maternal decision making, ethics, and the law. ACOG Committee Opinion No. 321. *Obstet Gynecol.* 2005;106(5):1127–1137.

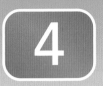

# Embryology and Anatomy

An understanding of reproductive anatomy and its developmental precursors is important for learners in their ability to apply basic diagnostic and therapeutic principles in patient care.

K nowledge of the embryology and anatomy of the female genital system is helpful in understanding both normal anatomy and the congenital anomalies that occur. Embryology may be useful in many areas of gynecologic and obstetric practice. For example, in gynecologic oncology, embryology can assist clinicians in predicting the growth and routes of spread of gynecologic cancers; in urogynecology and pelvic reconstructive surgery, it can enhance a surgeon's comprehension of the components of pelvic support and possible defects. It can also play a key role in understanding and diagnosing various aspects of sexual dysfunction.

The ovaries, fallopian tubes, uterus, and upper portion of the vagina are derived from the intermediate mesoderm, while the external genitalia develop from genital swellings in the pelvic region. Beginning in the 4th week (postfertilization) of development, the intermediate mesoderm forms the **urogenital ridges** along the posterior body wall. As their name implies, these ridges contribute to the formation of the urinary and genital systems (Fig. 4.1).

*The gonads, genital ducts, and external genitalia all pass through an* **indifferent** *(undifferentiated) stage in which it is not possible to determine sex based on the appearance of these structures.* The genetic sex of an embryo is determined by the sex chromosome (X or Y) carried by the sperm that fertilizes the oocyte. The Y chromosome contains a gene called *SRY* (**sex-determining region on Y**) that encodes a protein called **testis-determining factor (TDF).** When this protein is present, the embryo develops male sex characteristics. The ovary-determining gene is *WNT4;* when this gene is present and *SRY* is absent, the embryo develops female characteristics. *Gonads become structurally male or female by the 7th week of development, and external genitalia become differentiated by the 12th week.* The influence of androgens is crucial in the normal development of the external genitalia. Any condition that increases the level of androgen production in a female embryo will cause developmen-

tal anomalies. For example, the genetic disease **congenital adrenal hyperplasia (CAH)** causes a decreased production of cortisol that results in a compensatory increase in androgens. The genitalia of female fetuses with CAH are ambiguous, that is, neither normal female nor normal male.

## Development of the Ovary

Ovaries are homologous to the testes in the male. *Both types of gonads begin development as* **gonadal** *or* **genital ridges** *that form during the 5th week of gestation from the urogenital ridges.* Fingerlike bands of epithelial cells project from the surface of the gonad into each gonadal ridge, forming irregularly shaped **primary sex cords.** Growth of these cords into the gonadal ridge results in the creation of an outer cortex and an inner medulla in the indifferent gonad.

**Primordial germ cells** that give rise to gametes appear in the wall of the yolk sac (now called the umbilical vesicle) during the 3rd week of development (see Fig. 4.1). From this location, primordial germ cells migrate along the allantois in the connecting stalk to the dorsal mesentery of the hindgut and then into the gonadal ridges, where they become associated with the primary sex cords by the 6th week. In the female, the primordial germ cells become **oogonia,** which divide by mitosis during fetal life; no oogonia are formed after birth. If the primordial germ cells fail to migrate to the genital ridges, the ovary does not develop.

By approximately the 10th week of development, the undifferentiated gonad has developed into an identifiable ovary. Primary sex cords degenerate, and secondary sex cords or **cortical cords** appear. These cords extend from the surface epithelium into the underlying mesenchyme (Fig. 4.2, right column of figure). By approximately 16 weeks

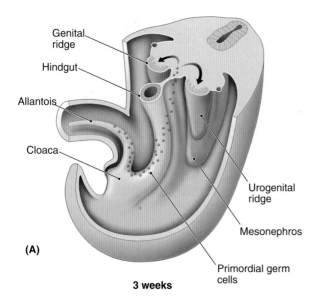

**(A)**

- Genital ridge
- Hindgut
- Allantois
- Cloaca
- Urogenital ridge
- Mesonephros
- Primordial germ cells

**3 weeks**

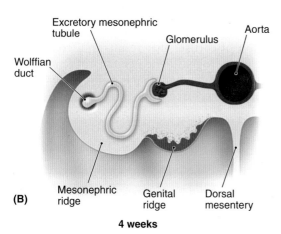

**(B)**

- Excretory mesonephric tubule
- Glomerulus
- Aorta
- Wolffian duct
- Mesonephric ridge
- Genital ridge
- Dorsal mesentery

**4 weeks**

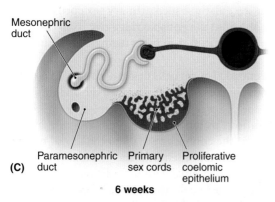

**(C)**

- Mesonephric duct
- Paramesonephric duct
- Primary sex cords
- Proliferative coelomic epithelium

**6 weeks**

FIGURE 4.1. Early development of the urogenital system. (A) Beginning at approximately 3 weeks of gestation, urogenital ridges arise along the posterior wall of the coelomic cavity. Primordial germ cells migrate across the allantois into the genital ridges. (B) and (C) These transverse sections through the lumbar region of the human embryo show development of the indifferent gonad from the genital ridges at 4 weeks and 6 weeks of gestation. (Modified from Sadler TW. *Langman's Medical Embryology.* 10th ed. Baltimore, MD: Lippincott Williams & Wilkins; 2006:240–241.

of gestation, cortical cords in the ovary organize into **primordial follicles.** Each follicle eventually consists of an oogonium, derived from a primary germ cell, surrounded by a single layer of squamous follicular cells, derived from the cortical cords. Follicular maturation begins when the oogonia enter the first stage of meiotic division (at which point they are called **primary oocytes**). *Oocyte development is then arrested until puberty, when one or more follicles are stimulated to continue development each month* (see Chapter 34, Puberty).

In male embryos, the primary sex cords do not degenerate; instead, they develop into **seminiferous** (or **testis**) **cords** that eventually give rise to the rete testis and seminiferous tubules (see Fig. 4.2, left column of figure). A layer of dense connective tissue (the **tunica albuginea**) separates the seminiferous cords from the surface epithelium, which eventually becomes the testis. Cortical cords do not form in the male embryo.

As they develop, gonads descend from their starting point high up in the primitive body cavity, where they are attached to a mesenchymal condensation called the **gubernaculum.** Ovaries move caudally to a location just below the rim of the true pelvis immediately adjacent to the fimbriated end of the fallopian tubes. The testis, on the other hand, continues to descend, eventually migrating through the anterior abdominal wall just superior to the inguinal ligament. The gubernaculum in the female fetus eventually forms the ovarian and round ligaments (see Fig. 4.2 and Fig. 4.3).

## Development of the Genital Ducts

In both male and female embryos, two pairs of ducts develop—the **mesonephric (wolffian)** and **paramesonephric (müllerian) ducts.** *As with the gonad, these ducts pass through an indifferent stage in which both pairs of ducts are present in both the male and the female embryo.* Differentiation of the female ductal system is not dependent on development of the ovaries (Fig. 4.4).

In the male embryo, the mesonephric ducts, which drain the embryonic mesonephric kidneys, eventually form the epididymis, ductus deferens, and ejaculatory ducts. *In the female embryo, the mesonephric ducts disappear. The paramesonephric ducts persist to form major parts of the female reproductive tract (the fallopian tubes, uterus, and upper portion of the vagina).* Paramesonephric ducts begin as invaginations of the epithelium covering the urogenital ridges, eventually forming longitudinally oriented tubes. The cranial end of each duct opens into the body (future peritoneal) cavity. The ducts grow caudally until the two caudal ends contact the posterior wall of the urogenital sinus. This contact induces the posterior wall to proliferate and form the **vaginal plate** that eventually gives rise to the lower portion of the vagina. Meanwhile, the lower ends of the paramesonephric ducts fuse to form the upper portion

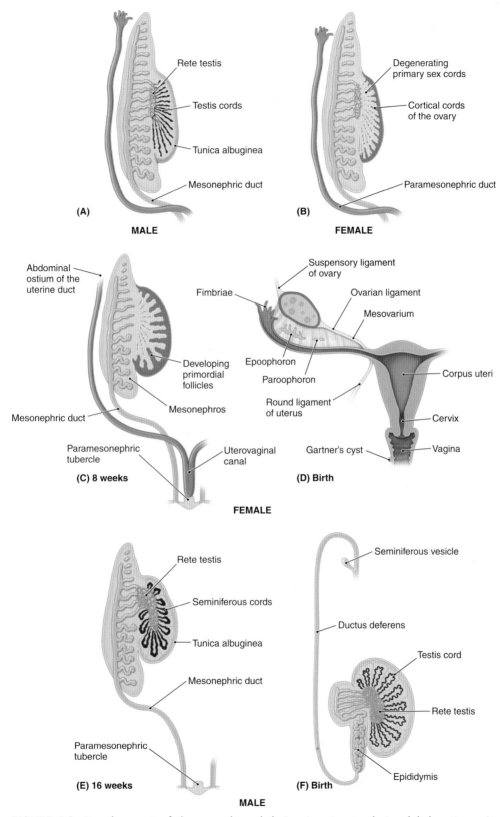

FIGURE 4.2. Development of the gonads and their migration to their adult locations. At approximately 6 weeks of gestation, the gonads have differentiated into either male or female (A and B). In female embryos, the paramesonephric ducts develop into the uterus, uterine tubes, and part of the vagina (C and D). In male embryos, the mesonephric ducts develop into the main genital tracts (ductus deferens) (E and F). (Modified from Sadler TW. *Langman's Medical Embryology*. 10th ed. Baltimore, MD: Lippincott Williams & Wilkins; 2006:243 and 245.)

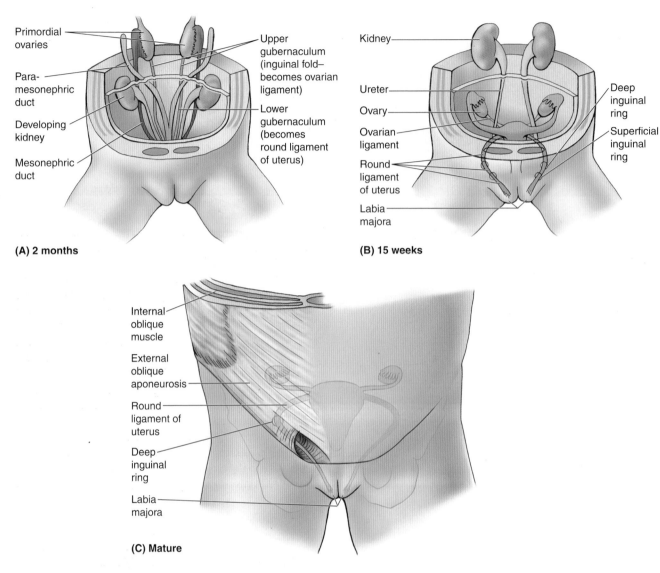

Primordial ovaries
Para-mesonephric duct
Developing kidney
Mesonephric duct
Upper gubernaculum (inguinal fold— becomes ovarian ligament)
Lower gubernaculum (becomes round ligament of uterus)

**(A) 2 months**

Kidney
Ureter
Ovary
Ovarian ligament
Round ligament of uterus
Labia majora
Deep inguinal ring
Superficial inguinal ring

**(B) 15 weeks**

Internal oblique muscle
External oblique aponeurosis
Round ligament of uterus
Deep inguinal ring
Labia majora

**(C) Mature**

**Anterior views**

FIGURE 4.3.  Route of the migrating gonads in a female embryo. (A) At 2 months, the early gonads are located high up in the coelomic cavity attached to the gubernaculum. (B) The gubernaculum migrates through the anterior abdominal wall just above the inguinal ligament; this process also takes place in the male embryo. (C) The ovaries arrest their descent in the ovarian fossa, immediately subjacent to the uterus on either side. (From Moore KL, Dalley AF. *Clinically Oriented Anatomy*. 5th ed. Baltimore, MD: Lippincott Williams & Wilkins; 2006:Fig. 2.14.)

of the vagina, cervix, and uterus. The cranial portion of each duct remains separated and forms the fallopian tube on each side. As the ducts move toward fusion in the midline, they carry a fold of peritoneum with them that becomes the **broad ligament.**

## Development of the External Genitalia

The **cloaca** is formed from a dilatation of the caudal end of the hindgut and is covered exteriorly by the cloacal membrane. Eventually, the cloaca is separated into the urogeni-

tal sinus anteriorly and the anorectal canal posteriorly by the **urorectal septum.** This septum forms from a collection of mesoderm in the pelvic floor that grows downward during the 5th to the 8th weeks of gestation to reach the **cloacal membrane.** At the same time, the **genital tubercle** develops at the cranial end of the cloacal membrane, while **labioscrotal swellings** and **urogenital folds** appear on each side (Fig. 4.5A). The genital tubercle enlarges in both the male and the female (Fig. 4.5B). In the presence of estrogens and the absence of androgens, external genitalia are feminized. The genital tubercle develops into the cli-

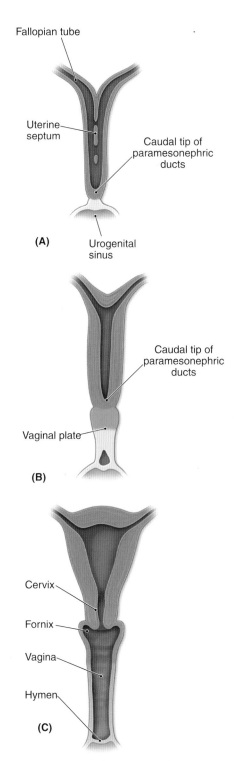

**(A)**

Fallopian tube

Uterine septum

Caudal tip of paramesonephric ducts

Urogenital sinus

**(B)**

Caudal tip of paramesonephric ducts

Vaginal plate

**(C)**

Cervix

Fornix

Vagina

Hymen

FIGURE 4.4. Development of the internal reproductive organs from the müllerian ducts in the female embryo. (A) Initially, the ducts are separate structures that begin to fuse lengthwise at their caudal ends. (B) This fusion creates the lumen of the uterus. Simultaneously, the vagina develops where the urogenital sinus meets the müllerian ducts, the vaginal plate. (C) Eventually, the uterus, cervix and vagina are formed. (Modified from Sadler TW. *Langman's Medical Embryology.* 10th ed. Baltimore, MD: Lippincott Williams & Wilkins; 2006:246.)

toris (Fig. 4.5C). The unfused urogenital folds form the labia minora, and the labioscrotal swellings become the labia majora (Fig. 4.5D).

*At approximately 15 weeks of gestation, transverse ultra-sonography can distinguish between the two sexes, although it is not definitive.*

## ANATOMY

### Bony Pelvis

The bony **pelvis** is composed of the paired innominate bones and the sacrum. The innominate bones are joined anteriorly to form the **symphysis pubis,** and each is articulated posteriorly with the sacrum through the sacroiliac joint (Fig. 4.6). The **sacrum** is composed of five or six sacral vertebrae, which are fused in adulthood. The sacrum articulates with the coccyx inferiorly and with the fifth lumbar vertebra superiorly.

The pelvis is divided into the **greater pelvis (false pelvis)** and the **lesser pelvis (true pelvis),** which are separated by the linea terminalis. The greater pelvis distributes the weight of the abdominal organs and supports the pregnant uterus at term. The greater pelvis is bounded by the lumbar vertebrae posteriorly, an iliac fossa bilaterally, and the abdominal wall anteriorly. The true pelvis contains the pelvic viscera including the uterus, vagina, bladder, fallopian tubes, ovaries, and the distal rectum and anus. It is formed by the sacrum and coccyx posteriorly and by the ischium and pubis laterally and anteriorly.

*In obstetrics, it is important to assess the size of the pelvis to determine whether it is of adequate capacity for vaginal birth.* This evaluation is based on the diameters of the pelvic outlet, pelvic inlet, and midpelvis. Measurement of these diameters is called **pelvimetry** and can be made radiographically, with computed tomography (the most accurate method), or during a pelvic examination. One of the most important measurements is that of the **obstetrical conjugate** (Fig. 4.7), which is the narrowest fixed distance through which the fetal head must pass during a vaginal delivery.

*The obstetric conjugate cannot be measured directly due to the presence of the bladder.*

It is calculated indirectly by measuring the **diagonal conjugate,** which is the distance between the lower border of the pubis anteriorly to the lower sacrum at the level of the ischial spines. The obstetric conjugate is 1.5 to 2 cm shorter. In general, it should be 11.0 cm or greater to accommodate a fetal head of normal size. Other measurements include the **interspinous diameter** (the distance between the ischial spines) and **transverse diameter** (the distance measured at the greatest width of the superior aperture).

FIGURE 4.5. Comparison of the development of male and female external genitalia. (A) Early in gestation, the genital tubercle develops along with labioscrotal swellings and urogenital folds. (B) Shortly thereafter, the genital tubercle enlarges in both the male and female embryo. (C) The posterior commissure forms, effectively dividing genitals from anus. (D) Without the influence of a Y chromosome, the phallus regresses in relative size to form the clitoris.

FEMALE                                                     MALE

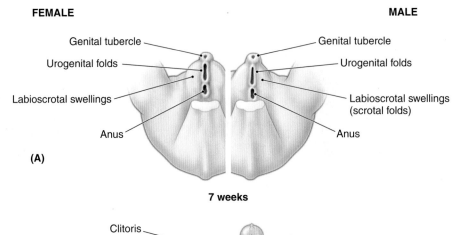

**(A)**

**7 weeks**

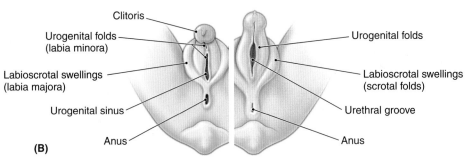

**(B)**

**10 weeks**

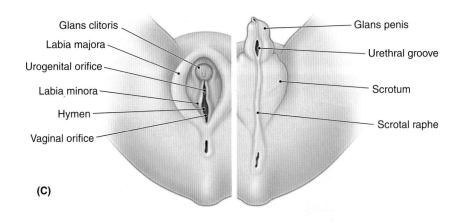

**(C)**

**12 weeks**

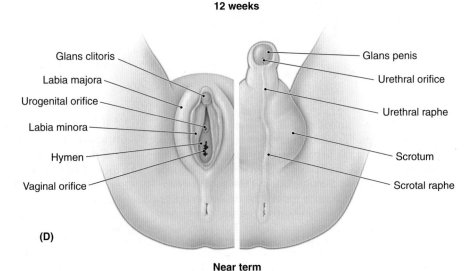

**(D)**

**Near term**

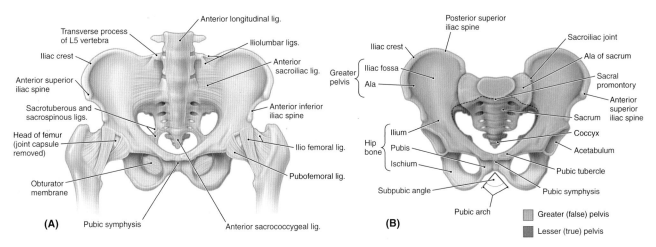

FIGURE 4.6. The bony pelvis. (A) Anterior view of the pelvis; the greater and lesser pelves are color-coded. (B) The pelvic ligaments shown in detail. (From Moore, KL and Dalley AF. *Clinically Oriented Anatomy.* 5th ed. Baltimore, MD: Lippincott Williams & Wilkins; 2006: Figs. 3.3B and 3.2A.)

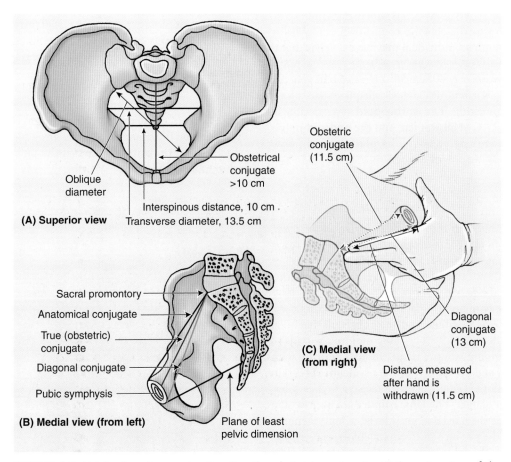

FIGURE 4.7. Pelvic diameters and estimating the obstetric conjugate. (A) Superior view of the pelvis showing the diameters that are measured in pelvimetry. (B) Medial view of the pelvis demonstrating the diagonal conjugate and the obstetrical conjugate. (C) Measurement of the obstetrical conjugate. The examiner palpates the sacral promontory with the tip of the *middle finger.* The distance between the tip of the *index finger,* which is 1.5 cm shorter than the middle finger, and the place on the hand where the pubic symphysis is felt is measured to yield the obstetrical conjugate, which should be at least 11 cm. (From Moore KL, Dalley AF. *Clinically Oriented Anatomy.* 5th ed. Baltimore, MD: Lippincott Williams & Wilkins; 2006: Fig. B3.2.)

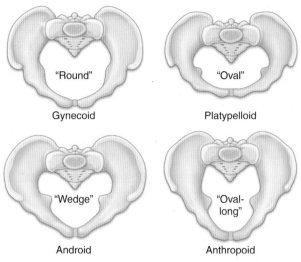

FIGURE 4.8. Caldwell-Moloy pelvic types.

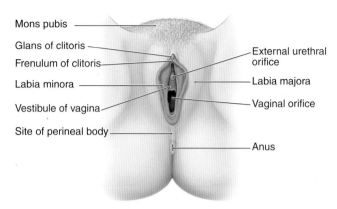

FIGURE 4.9. External female genitalia.

The female pelvis may be classified into four basic types, according to the scheme of Caldwell and Moloy (Fig. 4.8), although an individual may have a pelvis that is a mixture of types. *The most common type is the **gynecoid** pelvis, occurring in approximately 40% to 50% of women.* In general, this pelvic shape is cylindrical and has adequate space along its length and breadth. The **anthropoid** type occurs in approximately 25% of all women, and the **android** pelvis occurs in approximately 20%. The **platypelloid** pelvis occurs in only 2% to 5% of women.

## Vulva and Perineum

*The **perineum** comprises the area of the surface of the trunk between the thighs and the buttocks, extending from the coccyx to the pubis.* Anatomists also use the term "perineum" to refer to the shallow *compartment* that lies deep to this area and inferior to the pelvic diaphragm.

The **vulva** contains the labia majora, labia minora, mons pubis, clitoris, vestibule, and ducts of glands that open into the vestibule (Fig. 4.9). The **labia majora** are folds of skin with underlying adipose tissue, fused anteriorly with the mons pubis and posteriorly at the perineum. The skin of the labia majora contains hair follicles as well as sebaceous and sweat glands. The **labia minora** are narrow skin folds lying inside the labia majora. The labia minora merge anteriorly with the prepuce and frenulum of the clitoris, and posteriorly with the labia majora and the perineum. The labia minora contain sebaceous and sweat glands, but no hair follicles, and there is no underlying adipose tissue. The **clitoris,** which is located anterior to the labia minora, is the embryologic homolog of the penis. It consists of two crura (corresponding to the corpora cavernosa in the male) and the glans, which is found superior to the point of fusion of the crura. On the ventral surface of the glans is the **frenulum,** the fused junction of the labia minora. The vestibule

lies between the labia minora and is bounded anteriorly by the clitoris and posteriorly by the perineum. The urethra and the vagina open into the vestibule in the midline. The **ducts of Skene (paraurethral) glands** and **Bartholin glands** also empty into the vestibule. Secretions from the Bartholin glands are responsible for sexually stimulated vaginal lubrication.

The muscles of the vulva (superficial transverse perineal, bulbocavernosus, and ischiocavernosus) lie superficial to the fascia of the **urogenital diaphragm** (Fig. 4.10). The vulva rests on the triangular-shaped urogenital diaphragm, which lies in the anterior part of the pelvis between the ischiopubic rami.

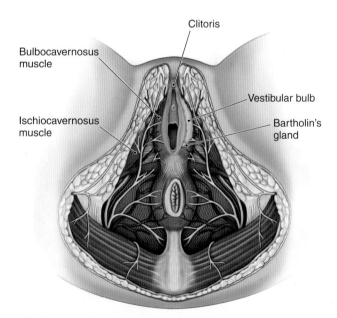

FIGURE 4.10. The urogenital diaphragm with the skin and subcutaneous fat cut away. The musculature, blood supply, and nerve supply constitute the external part of the pelvic floor.

## The Vagina

The lumen of the **vagina** is lined by a stratified squamous epithelium and surrounded by three layers of smooth muscle. Beneath the smooth muscle layers is a submucosal layer of connective tissue containing a rich supply of veins and lymphatic vessels. In children and young women, the anterior and poster walls of the vagina are in contact due to the presence of submucosal rugae. *Because the vagina is collapsed, it appears H-shaped in cross section.* The underlying rugae connect to the tendinous arch of the pelvic fascia, which is the major support of the walls of the vagina and help maintain its normal architecture. With age and childbirth, the connection between the vaginal walls and the muscular pelvis may weaken or deteriorate, weakening the pelvic floor and causing the surrounding structures (bladder, rectum, urethra, and uterus) to become less stable.

The **cervix** joins the vagina at an angle between 45° and 90°. The area around the cervix, the fornix, is divided into four regions: the anterior fornix, two lateral fornices, and the posterior fornix. The posterior fornix is in close proximity to the peritoneum that forms the floor of the posterior pelvic **cul-de-sac** (pouch of Douglas). The cervical opening to the vagina, the **external os,** is round to oval in women who have not had children, but is often a transverse slit after childbirth. The portion of the cervix that projects into the vagina is covered with stratified squamous epithelium, which resembles the vaginal epithelium. The squamous epithelium changes to a simple columnar epithelium in the **transition (transformation) zone.** This zone is found at about the level of the external cervical os, although it is found higher in the endocervical canal in postmenopausal women (the histology of the cervix is discussed in more detail in Chapter 43, Cervical Neoplasia and Carcinoma).

At its lower end, the vagina traverses the urogenital diaphragm and is then surrounded by the two bulbocavernosus muscles of the vulva. These muscles act as a sphincter. The **hymen,** a fold of mucosal-covered connective tissue, somewhat obscures the external vaginal orifice. The hymen is fragmented into irregular remnants with sexual activity and childbearing. The major blood supply to the vagina is from the **vaginal artery,** a branch of the hypogastric artery, also known as the internal iliac and parallel veins.

## Uterus and Pelvic Support

The **uterus** lies between the **rectum** and the **bladder** (Fig. 4.11). Various pelvic ligaments help support the uterus and other pelvic organs. The **broad ligament** overlies the structures and connective tissue immediately adjacent to the uterus. Because it contains the uterine arteries and veins and the ureters, it is important to identify the broad ligament during surgery. The **infundibulopelvic ligament** connects the ovary to the posterior abdominal wall and is composed mainly of the ovarian vessels. The **uterosacral ligament** connects the uterus at the level of the cervix to the sacrum and is therefore its primary support. The **cardinal ligament** is attached to the side of the uterus immediately inferior to the **uterine artery.** The **sacrospinous ligament** connects the sacrum to the iliac spine and is not attached to the uterus. This ligament is frequently used surgically to support the pelvic viscera.

The two major portions of the uterus are the cervix and the **body (corpus),** which are separated by a narrower isthmus. The length of the cervix is established at puberty. Before puberty, the relative lengths of the body of the uterus and cervix are approximately equal; after puberty, under the influence of increased estrogen levels, the ratio of the body to the cervix changes to between 2:1 and 3:1. The part of the body where the two uterine tubes enter it is called the **cornu.** The part of the corpus above the cornu is referred to as the fundus. In a woman who has had no children, the uterus is approximately 7 to 8 cm long and 4 to 5 cm wide at the widest part. The cervix is relatively cylindrical in shape and is 2 to 3 cm long. The body is generally pear-shaped, with the anterior surface flat and the posterior surface convex. In cross section, the lumen of the uterine body is triangular.

The wall of the uterus consists of three layers:

(1) The inner mucosa, or **endometrium,** consists of simple columnar epithelium with underlying connective tissue, which changes in structure during the menstrual cycle.
(2) The middle layer, or **myometrium,** consists of smooth muscle. This layer becomes greatly distensible during pregnancy; during labor, the smooth muscle in this layer contracts in response to hormonal stimulation.
(3) The outermost layer, or **perimetrium,** consists of a thin layer of connective tissue. It is distinct from the **parametrium,** a subserous extension of the uterus between the layers of the broad ligament.

The position of the uterus can vary depending on the relationship of a straight axis that extends from the cervix to the uterine fundus to the horizontal. When a woman is in the dorsal lithotomy position, the uterus may be bent forward (**anteversion, AV**), slightly forward but functionally straight (**mid-position, MP**), or bent backward (**retroversion, RV**). The top of the uterus can also fold forward (**anteflexion, AF**) or backward (**retroflexion, RF**). Five combinations of these configurations are possible (Fig. 4.12). The position of the uterus is clinically important. For example, estimation of gestational age in the late part of the first trimester may be difficult when the uterus is in the RVRF or RV positions. Risk of uterine perforation during procedures such as dilatation & curettage or insertion of an intrauterine device is increased in a woman with a retroflexed or anteflexed uterus. Applying traction on the cervix to pull the uterine canal into a straight line can greatly reduce this risk.

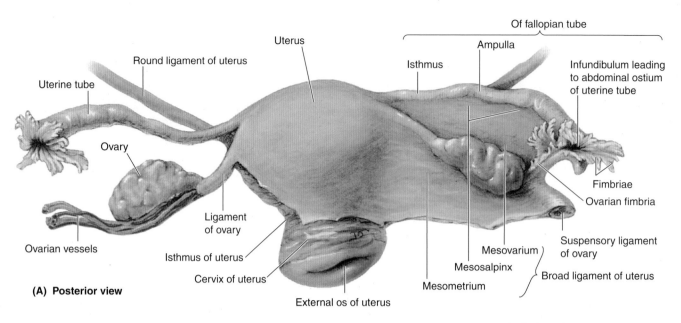

Uterus

Round ligament of uterus

Uterine tube

Ovary

Ovarian vessels

Ligament of ovary

Isthmus of uterus

Cervix of uterus

External os of uterus

Of fallopian tube

Ampulla

Isthmus

Infundibulum leading to abdominal ostium of uterine tube

Fimbriae

Ovarian fimbria

Suspensory ligament of ovary

Mesovarium

Mesosalpinx

Mesometrium

Broad ligament of uterus

**(A) Posterior view**

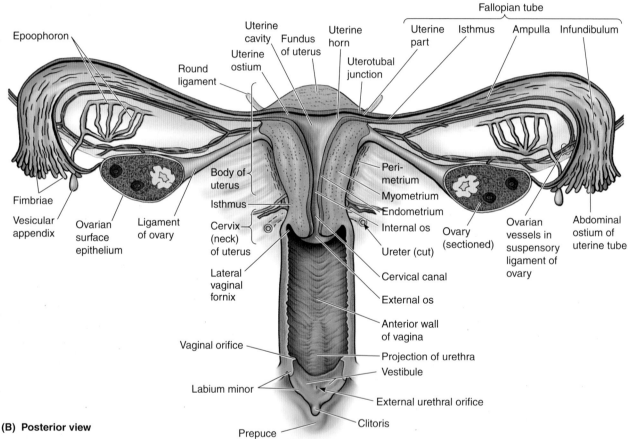

Epoophoron

Round ligament

Uterine cavity

Uterine ostium

Fundus of uterus

Uterine horn

Uterotubal junction

Fallopian tube

Uterine part

Isthmus

Ampulla

Infundibulum

Fimbriae

Vesicular appendix

Ovarian surface epithelium

Ligament of ovary

Body of uterus

Isthmus

Cervix (neck) of uterus

Lateral vaginal fornix

Vaginal orifice

Labium minor

Prepuce

Clitoris

Peri-metrium

Myometrium

Endometrium

Internal os

Ureter (cut)

Cervical canal

External os

Anterior wall of vagina

Projection of urethra

Vestibule

External urethral orifice

Ovary (sectioned)

Ovarian vessels in suspensory ligament of ovary

Abdominal ostium of uterine tube

**(B) Posterior view**

FIGURE 4.11.  Internal female reproductive organs. (From Moore KL, Dalley AF. *Clinically Oriented Anatomy.* 5th ed. Baltimore, MD: Lippincott Williams & Wilkins; 2006: Fig. 3.39A&B.)

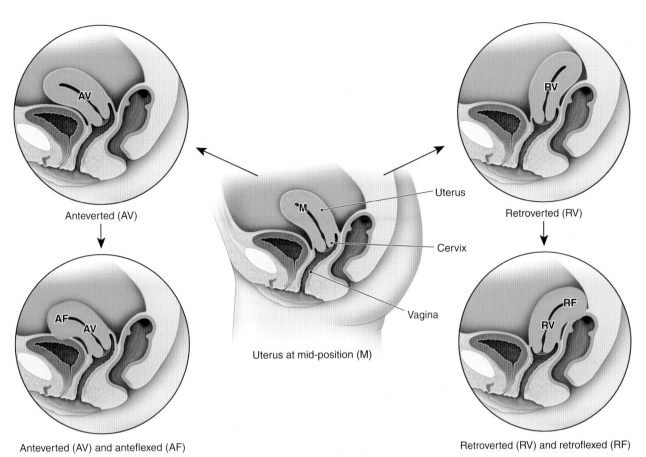

Anteverted (AV)

Uterus at mid-position (M)

Retroverted (RV)

Anteverted (AV) and anteflexed (AF)

Retroverted (RV) and retroflexed (RF)

FIGURE 4.12. Positions of the uterus within the pelvis. (From Moore KL, Dalley AF. *Clinically Oriented Anatomy.* 5th ed. Baltimore, MD: Lippincott Williams & Wilkins; 2006:B3.17A-D)

The blood supply to the uterus comes primarily from the uterine arteries, with a contribution from the ovarian arteries, whereas the venous plexus drains through the uterine vein.

*Of particular importance in pelvic surgery is the relative position of the uterine artery to the ureter.*

The arteries travel in a lateral to medial direction at the level of the internal os of the cervix. At the point where they meet the uterus, they overlie the ureter. This proximity can cause inadvertent injury during pelvic surgery. The ureters lie between 1.5 cm and 3 cm from the uterine sidewall at this point (Fig. 4.13).

## Uterine Tubes

The **fallopian (uterine) tubes (oviducts)** are approximately 7 to 14 cm in length, and are divided into three portions: a narrow and straight isthmus, which adjoins the opening into the uterus; the **ampulla,** or central portion; and the **infundibulum,** which is fringed by the

finger-shaped fimbriae. The fallopian tubes surround the ovary and collect the oocyte at the time of ovulation. The fallopian tubes are supplied by the ovarian and uterine arteries. The epithelial lining of the fallopian tube is ciliated columnar; the cilia beat toward the uterus, assisting in oocyte transport.

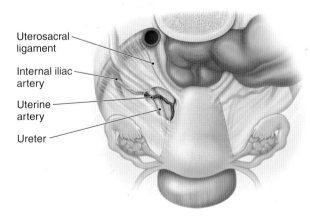

FIGURE 4.13. Relative locations of the ureter and uterine artery. During pelvic surgery, it is important to correctly identify the ureter in order to avoid injury to the uterine artery.

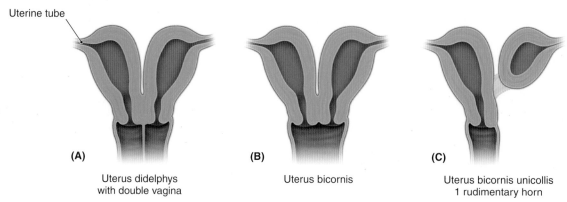

Uterine tube

(A)

Uterus didelphys
with double vagina

(B)

Uterus bicornis

(C)

Uterus bicornis unicollis
1 rudimentary horn

FIGURE 4.14. Uterine and vaginal anomalies. These anomalies result from abnormal or incomplete fusion of the paramesonephric ducts.

## Ovaries

Each ovary is approximately 3 to 5 cm long, 2 to 3 cm wide, and 1 to 3 cm thick in the menstrual years. The size decreases by approximately two-thirds after menopause, when follicular development ceases. The ovary is attached to the broad ligament by the **mesovarium,** to the uterus by the ovarian ligament, and to the side of the pelvis by the suspensory ligament of the ovary (infundibulopelvic ligament), which is the lateral margin of the broad ligament. The outer ovarian cortex consists of follicles embedded in a connective tissue stroma. Embryologically, this stroma is the medulla that originated as the gonadal ridge, while the cortex originated as coelomic epithelium. The medulla contains smooth muscle fibers, blood vessels, nerves, and lymphatics.

The ovaries are mainly supplied by the ovarian arteries, which are direct branches of the abdominal aorta, but there also is a blood supply from the uterine artery, a branch of the hypogastric artery (or internal iliac artery). Venous return via the right ovarian vein is directly into the inferior vena cava, and from the left ovary into the left renal vein.

## ANOMALIES OF THE FEMALE REPRODUCTIVE SYSTEM

Anatomic anomalies are infrequent and arise from defects during embryologic development. **Ovarian dysgenesis** or congenital absence is rare except in cases of chromosomally abnormalities. In Turner syndrome (45XO), there are streaks of abnormal ovarian tissues in the pelvis. In the anatomically female patient with a male chromosome compliment (46XY), the gonads only partially descend and can usually be found in the pelvis or even in the inguinal canal.

*Much more common are müllerian (paramesonephric) abnormalities, most of which stem from incomplete or anomalous fusion of the müllerian ducts.* Absence of the uterus occurs when the müllerian ducts degenerate, a condition called **müllerian agenesis** (Fig. 4.14). This condition is

associated with vaginal anomalies (such as absence of the vagina), because vaginal development is stimulated by the developing uterovaginal primordium. Since the vulva and the external portion of the vagina develop from the invagination of the urogenital sinus, the external genitalia can appear normal in these women. A double uterus (**uterus didelphys**) occurs when the inferior parts of the müllerian ducts do not fuse; this condition may be associated with a double or a single vagina. A **bicornuate uterus** results when lack of fusion is limited to the superior portion of the uterine body. If one of the ducts is poorly developed and fusion with the other duct does not occur, the result is a bicornuate uterus with a rudimentary **horn.** This horn may or may not communicate with the uterine cavity.

The mesonephric ducts normally degenerate in the female embryo during development of the reproductive tract. However, remnants of the mesonephric ducts can persist, which can manifest as Gartner cysts (Fig. 4.15).

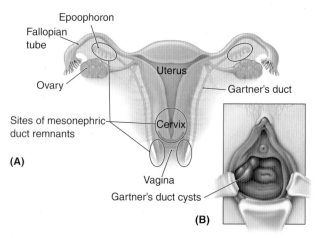

Epoophoron

Fallopian tube

Ovary

Uterus

Gartner's duct

Sites of mesonephric duct remnants

Cervix

(A)

Vagina

Gartner's duct cysts

(B)

FIGURE 4.15. Gartner cysts. (A) These cysts are remnants of the mesonephric ducts that are not completely resorbed during development. (B) Gartner cysts are located along the sidewall of the vagina and can be identified during a pelvic examination.

These cysts are located along the vaginal wall or within the broad ligament of the uterus.

Since the paramesonephric system develops alongside the renal system, frequently when one system is abnormally formed, an abnormality in the other is frequently present. For example, in a woman with renal agenesis on one side, an abnormal fallopian tube is often found. Conversely, despite the functional connection between the ovaries and fallopian tubes, a lack of one does not indicate a probable lack of the other.

## SUGGESTED READING

Butler WJ, Price TM. Sexual development and puberty. In: *Precis: Reproductive Endocrinology*. 3rd ed. Washington, DC: American College of Obstetricians and Gynecologists; 2007:31–68.

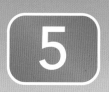
# 5 Maternal–Fetal Physiology

This chapter deals primarily with APGO Educational Topic:

Topic 8:   Maternal–Fetal Physiology

Knowledge of the maternal anatomic and physiologic changes associated with pregnancy and the physiology of the placenta and fetus will allow the student to distinguish between normal and abnormal conditions in the pregnant patient.

The maternal physiologic changes that occur during pregnancy are directly linked to the specific metabolic demands of the fetus. The numerous physiologic adaptations of pregnancy are not the result of a single factor or event; rather, they are the culmination of the biochemical interactions that occur between three distinct interacting systems: maternal, fetal, and placental.

## MATERNAL PHYSIOLOGY

### Cardiovascular System

*The earliest and most dramatic changes in maternal physiology are cardiovascular.* These changes improve fetal oxygenation and nutrition.

#### ANATOMIC CHANGES

During pregnancy, the heart is displaced upward and to the left and assumes a more horizontal position as its apex is moved laterally (Fig. 5.1). These position changes are the result of diaphragmatic elevation caused by displacement of abdominal viscera by the enlarging uterus. In addition, ventricular muscle mass increases and both the left ventricle and atrium increase in size parallel with an increase in circulating blood volume.

#### FUNCTIONAL CHANGES

*The primary functional change in the cardiovascular system in pregnancy is a marked increase in **cardiac output**.*

Overall, cardiac output increases 30% to 50%, with 50% of that increase occurring by 8 weeks' gestation. In the first half of pregnancy, cardiac output rises as a result of increased stroke volume, and in the latter half of pregnancy, as a result of increased maternal heart rate while the stroke volume returns to near-normal, nonpregnant levels. These changes in stroke volume are due to alterations in circulating blood volume and systemic vascular resistance. Circulating blood volume begins increasing by 6 to 8 weeks' gestation and reaches a peak increase of 45% by 32 weeks' gestation. Systemic vascular resistance decreases because of a combination of the smooth muscle-relaxing effect of progesterone, increased production of vasodilatory substances (prostaglandins, nitric oxide, atrial natriuretic peptide), and arteriovenous shunting to the uteroplacental circulation.

However, late in pregnancy, cardiac output may decrease when venous return to the heart is impeded because of vena caval obstruction by the enlarging gravid uterus. At times, in term pregnancy, nearly complete occlusion of the inferior vena cava occurs, especially in the supine position, with venous return from the lower extremities shunted primarily through the dilated paravertebral collateral circulation.

The distribution of the enhanced cardiac output varies during pregnancy. The uterus receives about 2% of the cardiac output in the first trimester, increasing to up to 20% at term, mainly by means of a relative reduction of the fraction of cardiac output that goes to the splanchnic bed and skeletal muscle. However, the absolute blood flow to these areas does not change, because of the increase in cardiac output that occurs in late pregnancy.

During pregnancy, arterial blood pressure follows a typical pattern. When measured in the sitting or standing position, diastolic blood pressure decreases beginning in the 7th week of gestation and reaches a maximal decline of 10 mm Hg from 24 to 32 weeks. Blood pressure then gradually returns to nonpregnant values by term. Resting maternal pulse increases as pregnancy progresses, increasing by 10–18 beats per minute over the nonpregnant value by term.

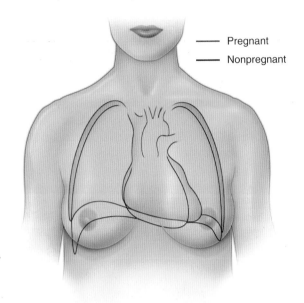

FIGURE 5.1. Changes in the outline of the heart, lungs, and thoracic cage. Adapted from Bonica JJ, McDonald JS, eds. *Principles and Practice of Obstetric Analgesia and Anesthesia.* 2nd ed, Baltimore, MD: Williams & Wilkins; 1995:47,Fig 2.

During labor, at the time of uterine contraction, cardiac output increases approximately 40% above that in late pregnancy, and mean arterial pressure increases by approximately 10 mm Hg. A decline in these parameters following administration of an epidural anesthetic suggests that many of these changes are the result of pain and apprehension. Cardiac output increases significantly immediately after delivery, because venous return to the heart is no longer blocked by the gravid uterus impinging on the vena cava and because extracellular fluid is quickly mobilized.

### Symptoms

Although most women do not become overtly hypotensive when lying supine, perhaps one in 10 have symptoms that include **dizziness, light-headedness,** and **syncope.** These symptoms, often termed the inferior vena cava syndrome, may be related to ineffective shunting via the paravertebral circulation when the gravid uterus occludes the inferior vena cava.

### Physical Findings

The cardiovascular system is in a hyperdynamic state during pregnancy. *Normal physical findings on cardiovascular examination include an* **increased second heart sound split with inspiration, distended neck veins,** *and* **low-grade systolic ejection murmurs,** *which are presumably associated with increased blood flow across the aortic and pulmonic valves.* Many normal pregnant women have an S$_3$ gallop, or third heart

sound, after midpregnancy. Diastolic murmurs should not be considered normal in pregnancy.

### Diagnostic Tests

*Serial blood pressure assessment is an essential component of each prenatal care visit.*

Blood pressure recordings during pregnancy are influenced by maternal position; therefore, a consistent position should be used during prenatal care, facilitating the recognition of trends in blood pressure during pregnancy and their documentation. *Measured blood pressure is highest when a pregnant woman is seated, somewhat lower when supine, and lowest while lying on the side.* In the lateral recumbent position, the measured pressure in the superior arm is about 10 mm Hg lower than that simultaneously measured in the inferior arm. Blood pressures higher than the nonpregnant values for a particular patient should be presumed abnormal pending evaluation.

The normal anatomic changes of the maternal heart in pregnancy can produce subtle, but insignificant, changes in chest radiographs and electrocardiograms. In chest radiographs, the cardiac silhouette can appear enlarged, causing a misinterpretation of cardiomegaly. In electrocardiograms, a slight left axis deviation may be apparent.

## Respiratory System

The changes that occur in the respiratory system during pregnancy are necessitated by the increased oxygen demand of the mother and fetus. These changes are primarily mediated by progesterone.

### Anatomic Changes

*The maternal thorax undergoes several morphologic changes due to pregnancy.* The diaphragm is elevated approximately 4 cm by late pregnancy due to the enlarging uterus. Additionally, the subcostal angle widens as the chest diameter and circumference increase slightly (see Figure 5.1).

### Functional Changes

*Pregnancy is associated with an increase in total body oxygen consumption of approximately 50 mL O$_2$/min, which is 20% greater than nonpregnant levels.* Approximately 50% of this increase is consumed by the gravid uterus and its contents, 30% by the heart and kidneys, 18% by the respiratory muscles, and the remainder by the mammary tissues.

Functional adaptations in the pulmonary system enhance oxygen delivery to the lungs. Figure 5.2 lists respiratory volumes and capacities associated with pregnancy. The consequence of diaphragmatic elevation is a 20% reduction in the residual volume and functional residual capacity plus a 5% reduction in total lung volume. Although

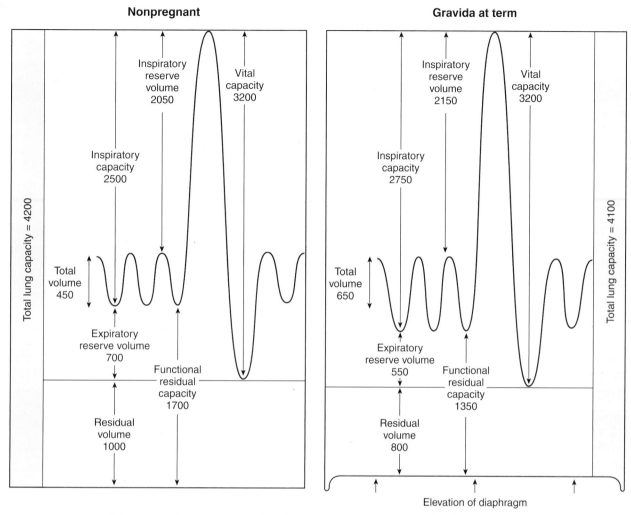

**Nonpregnant**

**Gravida at term**

FIGURE 5.2. Pulmonary volumes and capacities in the nonpregnant state and in the gravida at term. Adapted from Bonica JJ, McDonald JS, eds. *Principles and Practice of Obstetric Analgesia and Anesthesia*. 2nd ed, Baltimore, MD: Williams & Wilkins; 1995:49,Figs 2–4.

the maternal respiratory rate is essentially unchanged, there is a 30% to 40% increase in tidal volume due to a 5% increase in inspiratory capacity, resulting in a 30% to 40% increase in minute ventilation.

This significant increase in minute ventilation during pregnancy is associated with important changes in the acid–base equilibrium. Progesterone causes increased central chemoreceptor sensitivity to $CO_2$, which results in increased ventilation and a reduction in arterial $P_{CO_2}$. The respiratory alkalosis that results from a decreased arterial $P_{CO_2}$ in pregnancy is compensated by increased renal excretion of bicarbonate, yielding normal pregnancy bicarbonate levels, which means that maternal arterial pH is normal.

## SYMPTOMS

Although airway conductance and total pulmonary resistance are reduced in pregnancy, **dyspnea** is common in pregnant women. Dyspnea of pregnancy is believed to be a physiologic response to a low arterial $P_{CO_2}$. Allergy-like symptoms or chronic colds are also common. Mucosal hyperemia associated with pregnancy results in marked nasal stuffiness and an increased amount of nasal secretions.

## PHYSICAL FINDINGS

Despite the anatomic and functional changes in the respiratory system during pregnancy, no significant changes in the pulmonary examination are apparent.

## DIAGNOSTIC TESTS

*Arterial blood gas assessment during pregnancy normally shows a compensated respiratory alkalosis.*

Arterial $P_{CO_2}$ levels of 27 to 32 mm Hg and bicarbonate levels of 18 to 31 mEq/L should be considered normal.

Maternal arterial pH is maintained at normal levels of 7.40 to 7.45 (see Table 5.1).

During normal pregnancy, chest radiography may demonstrate prominent pulmonary vasculature due to the increased circulating blood volume.

## Hematologic System

The physiologic adaptations in the maternal hematologic system maximize the oxygen-carrying capacity of the mother to enhance oxygen delivery to the fetus. In

| TABLE 5.1 Common Laboratory Values in Each Trimester of Pregnancy | First Trimester | Second Trimester | Third Trimester |
|---|---|---|---|
| **Respiratory System** | | | |
| pH | 7.40–7.46 | — | — |
| $PaO_2$ (mm Hg) | 75–105 | — | — |
| $PaCO_2$ (mm Hg) | 26–32 | — | — |
| $HCO^{-3}$ (mEq/L) | 18–26 | — | — |
| **Hematologic System** | | | |
| Hemoglobin (g/dL) | 108–140 | 100–132 | 104–140 |
| Hematocrit (%) | 31.2–41.2 | 30.1–38.5 | 31.7–40.9 |
| Platelet count ($\times 10^9$/L) | 149–357 | 135–375 | 121–373 |
| Leukocyte count ($\times 10^9$/L) | 3.9–11.9 | 5.0–12.6 | 5.3–12.9 |
| Fibrinogen (g/L) | — | — | 3.13–5.53 |
| **Renal System** | | | |
| Sodium (mmol/L) | 131–139 | 133–139 | 133–139 |
| Potassium (mmol/L) | 3.4–4.8 | 3.5–4.7 | 3.7–4.7 |
| Creatinine (µmol/L) | 25–79 | 25–74 | 23–93 |
| Urea nitrogen (mmol/L) | — | 6.1–12.1 | 5.4–15.8 |
| Uric acid (µmol/L) | 75–251 | 118–250 | 144–360 |
| **Gastrointestinal System** | | | |
| Albumin, total (g/L) | 33–43 | 29–37 | 28–36 |
| Protein, total (g/L) | 58–72 | 56–64 | 52–65 |
| Alkaline phosphatase, total (U/L) | 22–91 | 33–97 | 73–267 |
| Alanine transaminase (ALT) | 4–28 | 4–28 | 0–28 |
| Aspartate transaminase (AST) | 4–30 | 1–32 | 2–37 |
| Amylase | 11–97 | 19–92 | 22–97 |
| Lactate dehydrogenase | 217–506 | 213–525 | 227–622 |
| **Endocrine System** | | | |
| Thyroxine ($T_4$), total (nmol/L) | 61–153 | 78–150 | 59–147 |
| Triiodothyronine ($T_3$), total (nmol/L) | 1.1–2.7 | 1.4–3.0 | 1.6–2.8 |
| Free $T_4$ (pmol/L) | 8.8–16.8 | 4.8–15.2 | 3.5–12.7 |
| Thyrotropin (TSH) (mU/L) | 0–4.4 | 0–5.0 | 0–4.2 |
| Cortisol (nmol/L) | 205–632 | 391–1407 | 543–1663 |
| Calcium, ionized (mmol/L) | 1.13–1.33 | 1.13–1.29 | 1.14–1.38 |

Adapted from Gronowski AM. *Handbook of Clinical Laboratory Testing During Pregnancy.* Totowa (NJ): Humana Press; 2004.

addition, they minimize the effects of impaired venous return and blood loss associated with labor and delivery.

## ANATOMIC CHANGES

*The primary anatomic adaptation of the maternal hematologic system is a marked increase in plasma volume, red cell volume, and coagulation factors.* Maternal plasma volume begins to increase as early as the sixth week of pregnancy and reaches a maximum at 30 to 34 weeks' gestation, after which it stabilizes. The mean increase in plasma volume is approximately 50% in singleton gestations and greater in multiple gestations. Red cell volume also increases during pregnancy, although to a lesser extent than plasma volume, averaging about 450 mL. *Maternal blood volume increases 35% by term.*

Adequate iron availability is essential to the increase in maternal red cell volume during pregnancy. The normal pregnant patient requires a total of 1000 mg of additional iron: 500 mg is used to increase maternal red cell mass, 300 mg is transported to the fetus, and 200 mg is used to compensate for normal iron loss. Because iron is actively transported to the fetus, fetal hemoglobin levels are maintained regardless of maternal iron stores. Supplemental iron use in pregnancy is intended to prevent iron deficiency in the mother, not to prevent either iron deficiency in the fetus or to maintain maternal hemoglobin concentration.

*To meet maternal iron needs in a woman who is not anemic, 60 mg of elemental iron is recommended daily.*

Iron from dietary sources may not be sufficient, and the National Academy of Sciences recommends an iron supplement of 27 mg (present in most prenatal vitamins). In the form of ferrous sulfate, 60 mg of iron is a dosage of 300 mg. Patients who are anemic should receive 60–120 mg of iron. Leukocyte count and platelet counts may vary during pregnancy. White blood cell counts typically increase slightly in pregnancy, returning to nonpregnant levels during the puerperium. During labor, the white blood cell count may further increase, primarily from increased granulocytes, presumably linked with stress-associated demargination rather than a true disease-associated inflammatory response. Platelet counts may decline slightly, but remain within the normal, nonpregnant range.

The concentration of numerous clotting factors is increased during pregnancy. Fibrinogen (factor I) increases by 50%, as do fibrin split products and factors VII, VIII, IX, and X. Prothrombin (factor II) and factors V and XII remain unchanged. In contrast, the concentration of key inhibitors of coagulation, activated protein C and protein S, both decrease.

## FUNCTIONAL CHANGES

During pregnancy, functional adaptations in maternal erythrocytes enable enhanced oxygen uptake in the lungs, allowing increased oxygen delivery to the fetus and promoting $CO_2$ exchange from fetus to mother. *The increase in oxygen delivery to the lungs and the amount of hemoglobin in the blood result in a significant increase in the total oxygen-carrying capacity.* In addition, the compensated respiratory alkalosis of pregnancy causes a shift in the maternal oxygen dissociation curve to the left, via the Bohr effect. In the maternal lungs, hemoglobin affinity for oxygen increases, whereas in the placenta, the $CO_2$ gradient between fetus and mother is increased, which facilitates transfer of $CO_2$ from fetus to mother. See p. 54 for further discussion.

*Pregnancy is considered a* **hypercoagulable state** *with an increased risk of venous thromboembolism, both during pregnancy and the puerperium.*

The risk of thromboembolism doubles during pregnancy and increases to 5.5 times the normal risk during the puerperium.

## SYMPTOMS AND PHYSICAL FINDINGS

Some **edema** is normal in pregnancy, and swelling of the hands, face, legs, ankles, and feet may occur. This tends to be worse late in pregnancy and during the summer.

## DIAGNOSTIC TESTS

Pregnancy results in alterations in the normal ranges of several hematologic indices. The disproportionate increase in plasma volume, compared with red cell volume, results in a decrease in hemoglobin concentration and hematocrit during pregnancy, often referred to as a **physiologic anemia**. At term, the average hemoglobin concentration is 12.5 g/dL, compared with approximately 14 g/dL in the nonpregnant state. Values less than 11.0 g/dL are usually due to iron deficiency, but such values should prompt investigation for other kinds of anemia that may occur simultaneously with iron-deficiency anemia. Treatment of any anemia should be administered. The leukocyte count can range from 5000 to 12,000/L, and may increase to as much as 30,000/L during labor and the puerperium. (Neither of these higher values is associated with infection.)

The most notable alteration in the coagulation system is increased concentration of fibrinogen, which ranges from 300 to 600 mg/dL in pregnancy, compared with 200 to 400 mg/dL in the nonpregnant state. Despite the prothrombotic state of pregnancy, in vitro clotting times do not change.

## Renal System

The renal system is the site of increased functional activity during pregnancy to maintain fluid, solute, and acid–base balance in response to the marked activity of the cardio-respiratory systems.

## ANATOMIC CHANGES

*The primary anatomic change of the renal system is enlargement and dilation of the kidneys and urinary collecting system.* The kidneys lengthen by approximately 1 cm during pregnancy as a result of greater interstitial volume as well as distended renal vasculature. The renal calyces, pelves, and ureters dilate during pregnancy because of mechanical and hormonal factors. Mechanical compression of the ureters occurs as the uterus enlarges and rests on the pelvic brim. The right ureter is usually more dilated than the left, possibly due to dextrorotation of the uterus and compression from the enlarged right ovarian venous plexus. Progesterone causes relaxation of the smooth muscle of the ureters, which also results in dilation. In addition, because progesterone also decreases bladder tone, residual volume is increased. As the uterus enlarges as pregnancy progresses, bladder capacity decreases.

## FUNCTIONAL CHANGES

*The majority of pregnancy-associated functional changes in the renal system are a result of an increase in renal plasma flow.* Early in the first trimester, renal plasma flow begins to increase, and, at term, it may be 75% greater than nonpregnant levels. Similarly, the glomerular filtration rate (GFR) increases to 50% over the nonpregnant state. This increase in GFR results in an increased load of various solutes presented to the renal system. Urinary glucose excretion increases in virtually all pregnant patients; a trace of glucose on routine prenatal colorimetric "dipstick" evaluation is normal and is usually not associated with glycemic pathology. Amino acids and water-soluble vitamins, such as vitamin $B_{12}$ and folate, are also excreted to a greater extent compared with the nonpregnant state. However, there is no significant increase in urinary protein loss, which means that any proteinuria that occurs during pregnancy should engender consideration of illness. In addition, sodium metabolism remains unchanged. The potential loss of this electrolyte caused by an increased GFR is compensated for by an increase in renal tubule reabsorption of sodium.

All components of the renin-angiotensin-aldosterone system increase during pregnancy. Plasma renin activity is up to 10 times that of the nonpregnant state and renin substrate (angiotensinogen) and angiotensin increase approximately fivefold. Normal pregnant women are relatively resistant to the hypertensive effects of the increased levels of renin-angiotensin-aldosterone, whereas women with hypertensive disease and hypertensive disease of pregnancy are not.

## SYMPTOMS

The anatomic changes in the renal system result in a few common symptomatic complaints during pregnancy.

Compression of the bladder by the enlarged uterus results in **urinary frequency** that is not associated with urinary tract or bladder infection. In addition, 20% of women experience **stress urinary incontinence,** and loss of urine should be considered in the differential diagnosis when rupture of membranes is suspected. Finally, urinary stasis throughout the renal collecting system predisposes to an increased incidence of pyelonephritis in patients with asymptomatic bacteriuria.

## PHYSICAL FINDINGS

As pregnancy advances, pressure from the presenting part on the maternal bladder can cause edema and protrusion of the bladder base into the anterior vagina. No significant changes in the renal examination are apparent during pregnancy.

## DIAGNOSTIC TESTS

The pregnancy-associated functional changes in the renal system result in a number of alterations in common tests of renal function. *Serum levels of creatinine and blood-urea-nitrogen (BUN) decrease in normal pregnancy.* Serum creatinine values fall from a nonpregnant level of 0.8 mg/dL to pregnancy levels of 0.5 to 0.6 mg/dL by term. Creatinine clearance increases 30% above the nonpregnant norms of 100 to 115 mL/min. BUN also falls about 25% to levels of 8 to 10 mg/dL at the end of the first trimester, and is maintained at these levels for the remainder of the pregnancy. Because glucosuria is common during pregnancy, quantitative urine glucose measurements are often elevated, but may not signify an abnormal blood sugar. By comparison, renal protein excretion is unchanged during pregnancy, and the nonpregnant range of 100 to 300 mg per 24 hours remains valid.

If imaging of the renal system is performed during pregnancy, normal dilation of the renal collecting system resembling hydronephrosis is noted on ultrasound or intravenous pyelogram.

## Gastrointestinal System

The anatomic and functional changes in the gastrointestinal system that occur during pregnancy are due to the combined effect of the enlarging uterus and the hormonal action of pregnancy. These changes produce a number of pregnancy-related symptoms that can range from mild discomfort to severe disability.

## ANATOMIC CHANGES

The primary anatomic change related to pregnancy is the displacement of the stomach and intestines due to the enlarging uterus. Although the stomach and intestines change in position, they do not change in size. The liver and biliary tract also does not change in size, but the portal vein enlarges due to increased blood flow.

## FUNCTIONAL CHANGES

Functional changes in the gastrointestinal system are the result of the hormonal action of progesterone and estrogen. *Generalized smooth muscle relaxation mediated by progesterone produces lower esophageal sphincter tone, decreased gastrointestinal motility, and impaired gallbladder contractility.* As a result, transit time in the stomach and small bowel increases significantly—15% to 30% in the second and third trimesters, and more during labor. Additionally, the imbalance between the lower intraesophageal pressures and increased intragastric pressures, combined with the lower esophageal sphincter tone, leads to gastroesophageal reflux. Reduced gallbladder contractility, in combination with estrogen-mediated inhibition of intraductal transportation of bile acids, leads to an increased prevalence of gallstones and cholestasis of bile salts. Estrogen also stimulates hepatic biosynthesis of proteins such as fibrinogen, ceruloplasmin, and the binding proteins for corticosteroids, sex steroids, thyroid hormones, and vitamin D.

## SYMPTOMS

Some of the earliest and most obvious symptoms of pregnancy are noted in the gastrointestinal system. Although energy requirements vary from person to person, most women increase their caloric intake by about 200 kcal/day. **Nausea and vomiting of pregnancy (NVP),** or **"morning sickness,"** typically begins between 4 and 8 weeks of gestation, and abates by the middle of the second trimester, usually by 14 to 16 weeks. The cause of this nausea is unknown, although it appears to be related to elevated levels of progesterone, human chorionic gonadotropin, and relaxation of the smooth muscle of the stomach. Severe NVP, which is known as **hyperemesis gravidarum,** can result in weight loss, ketonemia, or electrolyte imbalance.

Many patients report **dietary cravings** during pregnancy. Some may be the result of the patient's perception that a particular food may help with nausea. Pica is an especially intense craving for substances such as ice, starch, or clay. Other patients develop dietary or olfactory aversions during pregnancy. Ptyalism is perceived by the patient to be the excessive production of saliva, but probably represents the inability of a nauseated woman to swallow the normal amounts of saliva that are produced.

Symptoms of **gastroesophageal reflux** typically become more pronounced as pregnancy advances and intra-abdominal pressure increases. **Constipation** is common in pregnancy and is associated with mechanical obstruction of the colon by the enlarging bowel, reduced motility as elsewhere in the gastrointestinal tract, and increased water absorption during pregnancy. Generalized **pruritus** may result from intrahepatic cholestasis and increased serum bile acid concentrations.

## PHYSICAL FINDINGS

The two most notable gastrointestinal pregnancy-related physical findings are **gingival disease** and **hemorrhoids.** Although the incidence of dental caries does not change with pregnancy, the gums become more edematous and soft during pregnancy, and bleed easily with vigorous brushing. On occasion, violaceous pedunculated lesions, called epulis gravidarum, appear at the gum line. These lesions, which are actually pyogenic granulomas, sometimes bleed very easily, but usually regress within 2 months of delivery. Rarely, excessive bleeding may occur, requiring excision of the granuloma. Hemorrhoids are common in pregnancy and are caused by both constipation and elevated venous pressures resulting from increased pelvic blood flow and the effects of the enlarging uterus.

## DIAGNOSTIC TESTS

Some markers of hepatic function may be altered during pregnancy. Total serum alkaline phosphatase concentration is doubled, mainly due to increased placental production. Serum cholesterol levels increase during pregnancy. Although total albumin increases, serum levels of albumin are lower during pregnancy, primarily due to hemodilution. Levels of aspartate transaminase, alanine transaminase, $\gamma$-glutamyl transferase, and bilirubin are largely unchanged or slightly lower. Serum amylase and lipase concentrations are also unchanged.

## Endocrine System

Pregnancy influences the production of several endocrine hormones that control the physiologic adaptations in other organ systems.

## THYROID FUNCTION

*Pregnancy produces an overall **euthyroid** state, despite several changes in thyroid regulation.* The thyroid gland enlarges moderately during pregnancy, but does not produce thyromegaly or goiter. In the first trimester, human chorionic gonadotropin (hCG), which has thyrotropin-like activity, stimulates maternal thyroxine ($T_4$) secretion and produces a transient rise in the free $T_4$ concentration (Fig. 5.3). The decline in placental hCG production following the first trimester results in normalization of free $T_4$ concentrations. Beginning early in pregnancy, estrogen induces hepatic synthesis of thyroxine-binding globulin (TBG), resulting in an increase in total $T_4$ and total triiodothyronine ($T_3$) levels. Levels of free $T_4$ and free $T_3$, the active hormones, are unchanged from the normal range for nonpregnant patients.

## ADRENAL FUNCTION

*Although pregnancy does not alter the size or morphology of the adrenal gland, it does influence hormone synthesis.* As with TBG, estrogen induces hepatic synthesis of cortisol-binding globulin, resulting in elevated levels of serum cortisol. The concentration of free plasma cortisol progressively

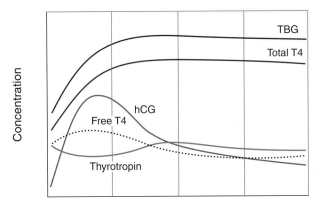

FIGURE 5.3. Changes in maternal thyroid function during pregnancy. The effects of pregnancy on the mother include a marked and early increase in hepatic production of thyroxine-binding globulin (TBG) and placental production of human chorionic gonadotropin (hCG). The increase in serum TBG, in turn, increases serum thyroxine ($T_4$) concentrations; hCG has thyrotropin-like activity and stimulates maternal $T_4$ secretion. The transient hCG-induced increase in the serum free $T_4$ level inhibits maternal secretion of thyrotropin. Adapted from Burrow GN, Fisher DA, Larsen R. Maternal and fetal thyroid function. *N Engl J Med.* 1994;331(16):1072–1078.

increases from the first trimester until term. Levels of corticotropin (ACTH) rise in conjunction with serum cortisol. Levels of aldosterone increase markedly due to enhanced adrenal synthesis. Maternal levels of deoxycorticosterone increase as the result of estrogen stimulation of renal synthesis, rather than increased adrenal production. Maternal levels of dehydroepiandrosterone sulfate decrease due to increased hepatic uptake and conversion to estrogen.

## Metabolism

### CARBOHYDRATE METABOLISM

*Pregnancy has a diabetogenic effect on maternal carbohydrate metabolism, characterized by reduced tissue response to insulin, hyperinsulinemia, and hyperglycemia.* Insulin resistance is primarily due to the action of human placental lactogen (hPL), which increases the resistance of peripheral tissues to the effects of insulin. The hormone hPL is secreted in proportion to placental mass, resulting in increased insulin resistance as pregnancy progresses. Progesterone and estrogen may also contribute to insulin resistance. Hepatic glycogen synthesis and storage is increased, and gluconeogenesis is inhibited.

*The net effect of these changes is that the maternal response to a glucose load is blunted, producing postprandial hyperglycemia.*

Additionally, the fetoplacental unit serves as a constant drain on maternal glucose levels. Glucose is the primary fuel for the placenta and fetus and, thus, delivery of glucose from the mother to the fetus occurs by facilitated diffusion. As a result, maternal hypoglycemia develops during periods of fasting.

### LIPID METABOLISM

*Pregnancy causes an increase in circulating concentrations of all lipids, lipoproteins, and apolipoproteins.* During early pregnancy, fat storage in central tissues predominates. Later in pregnancy, lipolysis predominates, possibly triggered by maternal fasting hypoglycemia. In the absence of glucose, increased plasma concentrations of free fatty acids, triglycerides, and cholesterol provide energy for the mother; this has been characterized as **accelerated starvation.** Following delivery, the concentrations of all lipids return to nonpregnancy levels, a process accelerated by breastfeeding.

### PROTEIN METABOLISM

Pregnancy is characterized by the intake and utilization of approximately 1 kg of protein above the normal nonpregnant state. At term, 50% of the additional protein is utilized by the fetus and placenta, and the remainder is shared by the uterus, breasts, maternal hemoglobin, and plasma proteins.

## Other Maternal Systems

### MUSCULOSKELETAL

As pregnancy advances, a compensatory **lumbar lordosis** (anterior convexity of the lumbar spine) is apparent. This change is functionally useful, because it helps keep the woman's center of gravity over the legs; otherwise, the enlarging uterus would shift it anteriorly. However, as a result of this change in posture, virtually all women complain of low back pain during pregnancy. Increasing pressure caused by intra-abdominal growth of the uterus may result in an exacerbation of hernia defects, most commonly seen at the umbilicus and in the abdominal wall (diastasis recti, a physiologic separation of the rectus abdominus muscles). Beginning early in pregnancy, the effects of relaxin and progesterone result in a relative laxity of the ligaments. The pubic symphysis separates at approximately 28 to 30 weeks. Patients often complain of an unsteady gait and may fall more commonly during pregnancy than during the nonpregnant state, as a result of both these changes and an altered center of gravity.

To provide for adequate calcium supplies to the fetal skeleton, calcium stores are mobilized. Maternal serum ionized calcium is unchanged from the nonpregnant state, but maternal total serum calcium decreases. There is a significant increase in maternal parathyroid hormone, which maintains serum calcium levels by increasing absorption from the intestine and decreasing the loss of calcium through the kidney. The skeleton is well-maintained despite these elevated levels of parathyroid hormones. This may be because of the effect of calcitonin. Although the rate of bone turnover increases, there is no loss of bone density during a normal pregnancy if adequate nutrition is supplied.

## SKIN

*Pregnancy induces several characteristic changes in the appearance of the maternal skin.* Although the exact etiology of these changes has not been established, hormonal influences appear to predominate.

**Vascular spiders (spider angiomata)** are most common on the upper torso, face, and arms. **Palmar erythema** occurs in more than 50% of patients. Both are associated with increased levels of circulating estrogen and regress after delivery. **Striae gravidarum** occur in more than half of pregnant women and appear on the lower abdomen, breasts, and thighs. Initially, striae can be either purple or pink; eventually, they become white or silvery. These striae are not related to weight gain, but are solely the result of the stretching of normal skin. There is no effective therapy to prevent these "stretch marks," and once they appear, they cannot be eliminated.

Pregnancy may produce characteristic **hyperpigmentation,** which is believed to be the result of elevated levels of estrogen and a **melanocyte-stimulating hormone** and a cross-reaction with the structurally similar hCG. Hyperpigmentation commonly affects the umbilicus and perineum, although it may affect any skin surface. The lower abdomen **linea alba** darkens to become the **linea nigra.** The "mask of pregnancy," or **chloasma (melasma),** is also common and may never disappear completely. **Skin nevi** can increase in size and pigmentation, but resolve after pregnancy; however, removal of rapidly changing nevi is recommended during pregnancy, because of the risk of malignancy. **Eccrine sweating** and **sebum production** increase during normal pregnancy, with many patients complaining of acne.

Hair growth during pregnancy is maintained, although there are more follicles in the **anagen (growth)** phase and fewer in the **telogen (resting)** phase. Late in pregnancy, the number of hairs in telogen is approximately half of the normal 20%, so that postpartum, the number of hairs entering telogen increases; thus, there is significant hair loss 2 to 4 months after pregnancy. Hair growth typically returns to normal 6 to 12 months after delivery. Patients are often concerned about this "hair loss," until they are reassured that it is transient and that hair growth will renew.

## REPRODUCTIVE TRACT

The effects of pregnancy on the vulva are similar to the effects on other skin. Because of an increase in vascularity, vulvar varicosities are common and usually regress after delivery. An increase in vaginal transudation as well as stimulation of the vaginal epithelium results in a thick, profuse vaginal discharge, called **leukorrhea of pregnancy.** The epithelium of the endocervix everts onto the ectocervix, which is associated with a mucous plug.

During pregnancy, the uterus undergoes an enormous increase in weight from the 70-g nonpregnant size to approximately 1100 g at term, primarily through hypertrophy of existing myometrial cells. After pregnancy, the uterus returns to an only slightly increased size as the actual number of cells comprising it are minimally increased. Similarly, the uterine cavity enlarges to a volume of up to as much as 5 liters, compared to less than 10 mL in the nongravid state.

## BREASTS

*The breasts increase in size during pregnancy, rapidly in the first 8 weeks and steadily thereafter.* In most cases, the total enlargement is 25% to 50%. The nipples become larger and more mobile and the areola larger and more deeply pigmented, with enlargement of the Montgomery glands. Blood flow to the breasts increases as they change to support lactation. Some patients may complain of breast or nipple tenderness and a tingling sensation. Estrogen stimulation also results in ductal growth, with alveolar hypertrophy being a result of progesterone stimulation. During the latter portion of pregnancy, a thick, yellow fluid can be expressed from the nipples. This is **colostrum,** more common in parous women. Ultimately, lactation depends on synergistic actions of estrogen, progesterone, prolactin, human placental lactogen, cortisol, and insulin.

## OPHTHALMIC

The most common visual complaint during pregnancy is blurred vision. This visual change is primarily caused by increased thickness of the cornea associated with fluid retention and decreased intraocular pressure. These changes are manifest in the first trimester and regress within the first 6 to 8 weeks postpartum. Therefore, changes in corrective lens prescriptions should not be encouraged during pregnancy.

# FETAL AND PLACENTAL PHYSIOLOGY

## Placenta

The placenta is an essential and unique "organ of pregnancy," with key functions in respiratory and metabolite exchange and in hormone synthesis and regulation. It is the crucial point of connection between the mother and fetus. The placenta allows the fetus to live and grow until it is mature and able to survive in the outside world.

All gases involved in fetal respiration cross the placenta by simple diffusion. Fetal uptake of $O_2$ and excretion of $CO_2$ depend on the blood-carrying capacities of the mother and fetus for these gases and on the associated uterine and umbilical blood flows.

*The single primary metabolic substrate for placental metabolism is glucose.* It is estimated that as much as 70% of the glucose transferred from the mother is used by the placenta. The glucose that crosses the placenta does so by facilitated diffusion. Other solutes that are transferred from the mother to the fetus depend on the concentration gradient as well as on their degree of ionization, size, and lipid solubility. There is active transport of amino acids, resulting in levels that are higher in the fetus than in the mother. Free fatty acids have very limited placental transfer, resulting in levels that are lower in the fetus than in the mother.

The placenta also produces estrogen, progesterone, hCG, and hPL. These hormones are important for the maintenance of pregnancy, for labor and delivery, and for lactation.

## Fetal Circulation

*Oxygenation of fetal blood occurs in the placenta rather than in the fetal lungs.* This oxygenated blood (80% saturated) is carried from the placenta to the fetus through the umbilical vein, which enters the portal system of the fetus and branches off to the left lobe of the liver (Fig. 5.4). The umbilical vein then becomes the origin of the ductus venosus. Another branch joins the blood flow from the portal vein to the right lobe of the liver. Fifty percent of the umbilical blood supply goes through the ductus venosus. The blood flow from the left hepatic vein is mixed with the blood in the inferior vena cava and is directed toward the foramen ovale. Consequently, the well-oxygenated umbilical vein blood enters the left ventricle. Less-oxygenated blood in the right hepatic vein enters the inferior vena cava and then flows through the tricuspid valve into the right ventricle. Blood from the superior vena cava also preferentially flows through the tricuspid valve to the right ventricle. Blood from the pulmonary artery primarily flows through the ductus arteriosus into the aorta.

The fetal ventricles work in a parallel circuit, with blood flow from the right and left unequally distributed to the pulmonary and systemic vascular beds. Within a fetal heart rate range of 120 to 180 bpm, the fetal cardiac output remains relatively constant. Overall, less than 10% of right ventricular cardiac output goes to the fetal lungs. The remainder of the right ventricular cardiac output is shunted through the ductus arteriosus to the descending aorta. Output from the left ventricle into the proximal aorta supplies highly saturated blood (65% saturated) to the brain and upper body. Once joined by the ductus arteriosus, the descending aorta then supplies blood to the lower portion of the fetal body, with a major portion of this blood being delivered to the umbilical arteries, which carry deoxygenated blood to the placenta.

The umbilical blood flow represents about 40% of the combined output of both fetal ventricles. In the last half of pregnancy, this flow is proportional to fetal growth (approximately 300 mL/mg per minute), so that umbilical blood flow is relatively constant, normalized to fetal weight. This relationship allows measurement of fetal blood flow to be used as an indirect measure of fetal growth and fetal well-being.

## Hemoglobin and Oxygenation

Fetal hemoglobin, like adult hemoglobin, is a tetramer composed of two copies of two different peptide chains. But unlike adult **hemoglobin A (Hgb A),** which is composed of α and β chains, fetal hemoglobin is composed of a series of different pairings of peptide chains that change as embryonic and fetal development progresses. In late fetal life, **hemoglobin F (Hgb F),** composed of 2 α chains and 2 β chains, predominates. *The key physiologic difference between adult Hgb A and fetal Hgb F is that, at any given oxygen tension, Hgb F has higher oxygen affinity and oxygen saturation than Hgb A.* The main reason for this functional difference is that Hgb A binds 2,3-DPG (diphosphoglycerate) more avidly than Hgb F.

The Bohr effect modulates the oxygen-binding capacity of hemoglobin and plays an important role in exchange of $O_2$ and $CO_2$ between the maternal and fetal circulations. As maternal blood enters the placenta, the maternal respiratory alkalosis facilitates transfer of $CO_2$ from the fetal circulation to the maternal circulation. Loss of $CO_2$ from the fetal circulation causes a rise in the fetal blood pH, shifting the fetal oxygen dissociation curve to the left and resulting in increased oxygen-binding affinity (Fig. 5.5). Conversely, as the maternal circulation takes up $CO_2$, the blood pH decreases, resulting in a shift in the maternal oxygen dissociation curve to the left, reducing oxygen affinity. Hence, a favorable gradient is created, facilitating diffusion of $O_2$ from the maternal to the fetal circulation. Therefore, although the partial pressure of oxygen in fetal arterial blood is only 20 to 25 mm Hg, the fetus is adequately oxygenated.

## Kidney

The fetal kidney becomes functional in the 2nd trimester, producing dilute, hypotonic urine. The rate of fetal urine production varies with fetal size and ranges from 400 to 1200 mL/day. Fetal urine becomes the primary source of the amniotic fluid by the middle of the 2nd trimester.

## Liver

The fetal liver is slow to mature. The fetal liver capacity for glycogen synthesis and bilirubin conjugation increases

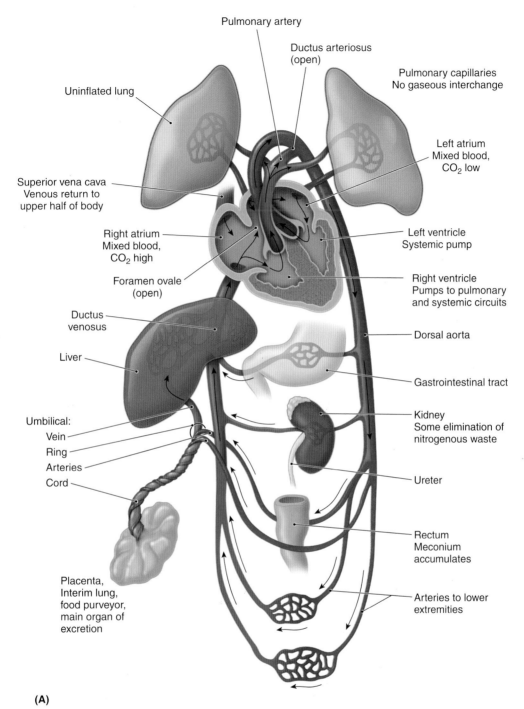

Pulmonary artery

Ductus arteriosus
(open)

Pulmonary capillaries
No gaseous interchange

Uninflated lung

Left atrium
Mixed blood,
$CO_2$ low

Superior vena cava
Venous return to
upper half of body

Right atrium
Mixed blood,
$CO_2$ high

Left ventricle
Systemic pump

Foramen ovale
(open)

Right ventricle
Pumps to pulmonary
and systemic circuits

Ductus
venosus

Dorsal aorta

Liver

Gastrointestinal tract

Umbilical:

Kidney
Some elimination of
nitrogenous waste

Vein

Ring

Arteries

Cord

Ureter

Rectum
Meconium
accumulates

Placenta,
Interim lung,
food purveyor,
main organ of
excretion

Arteries to lower
extremities

**(A)**

FIGURE 5.4. Fetal circulation at term (A) and after delivery (B). Note the changes in function of the ductus venosus, foramen ovale, and ductus arteriosus in the transition from intrauterine to extrauterine existence. Blue, deoxygenated blood; red, oxygenated blood. *(continued on next page)*

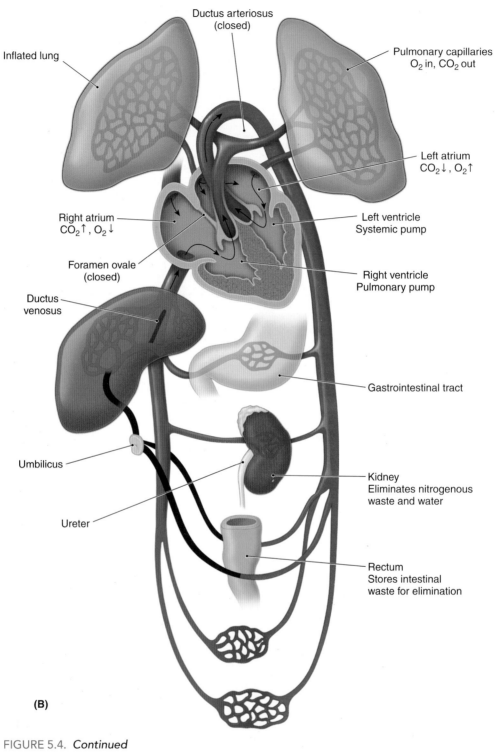

**(B)**

FIGURE 5.4. *Continued*

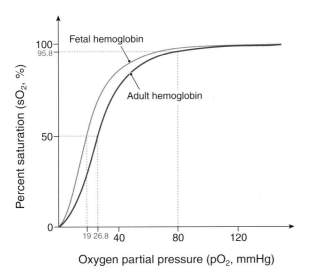

FIGURE 5.5. HgbA vs. HgbF oxygen saturation curve. The oxygen saturation curve for fetal hemoglobin (blue) appears left-shifted when compared with adult hemoglobin (red), because fetal hemoglobin has a greater affinity for oxygen.

with gestational age. As a consequence, during fetal life, bilirubin is primarily eliminated through the placenta. Hepatic production of coagulation factors is deficient and may be attenuated in newborn life due to vitamin K deficiency. Routine neonatal administration of vitamin K prevents newborn hemorrhagic disorders.

## Thyroid Gland

The fetal thyroid gland develops without direct influence from the mother, becoming functional by the end of the first trimester, so that, thereafter, levels of fetal $T_3$, $T_4$, and TBG increase throughout the rest of gestation. *The placenta does not transport the thyroid-stimulating hormone, and only moderate amounts of $T_3$ and $T_4$ cross the placenta.* The mother is the primary source of the thyroid hormone for the fetus prior to 24–28 weeks of gestation.

## Gonads

The primordial germ cells migrate during the eighth week of gestation from the endoderm of the yolk sac to the genital ridge. At this point, the gonads are undifferentiated. Differentiation into the testes occurs 6 weeks after conception, if the embryo is 46, XY. This testicular differentiation appears to depend on the presence of the H–Y antigen and the Y chromosome. If the Y chromosome is absent, however, an ovary develops from the undifferentiated gonad. Development of the fetal ovary begins at

approximately 7 weeks. The development of other genital organs depends on the presence or absence of specific hormones and is independent of gonadal differentiation. If the fetal testes are present, testosterone and the müllerian inhibitory factor inhibit the development of female external genitalia. If these two hormones are not present, the female genitalia develop, with regression of the wolffian ducts.

## IMMUNOLOGY OF PREGNANCY

Although the maternal immune system is not altered in pregnancy, the antigenically dissimilar fetus is able to survive in the uterus without being rejected. The key to this successful fetal allograft appears to be the placenta. The placenta serves as an effective interface between the maternal and fetal vascular compartments by keeping the fetus from direct contact with the maternal immune system. The placenta also produces estrogen, progesterone, hCG, and hPL, all of which may contribute to suppression of maternal immune responses on a local level. In addition, the placenta is the site of origin for blocking antibodies and masking antibodies, which alter the immune response.

The mother's systemic immune system remains intact, as evidenced by leukocyte count, B and T cell count and function, and immunoglobulin (Ig) levels. *Because IgG is the only immunoglobulin that can cross the placenta, maternal IgG comprises a major proportion of fetal immunoglobulin, both in utero and in the early neonatal period.* In this fashion, **passive immunity** is transferred to the fetus.

In this environment, the fetal immune system is afforded the opportunity to gradually develop and mature by term. Fetal lymphocyte production begins as early as 6 weeks of gestation. By 12 weeks of gestation, IgG, IgM, IgD, and IgE are present and are produced in progressively increasing amounts throughout pregnancy. At birth, the newborn fetus is equipped with both passive immunity and a mature immunologic system to defend against infectious diseases.

## SUGGESTED READINGS

American Academy of Pediatrics; American College of Obstetricians and Gynecologists. *Guidelines for Perinatal Care.* 6th ed. Elk Grove Village, IL: American Academy of Pediatrics; 2007.

American College of Obstetricians and Gynecologists. Thromboembolism in pregnancy. ACOG Practice Bulletin No. 19. *Obstet Gynecol.* 2000;96(2):1–10.

American College of Obstetricians and Gynecologists. Thyroid disease in pregnancy. ACOG Practice Bulletin No. 37. *Obstet Gynecol.* 2002;100(2):387–396.

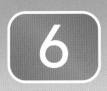

CHAPTER

# 6 Preconception and Antepartum Care

The student should recognize the relationship between good health, both prior to and during pregnancy, and reduced maternal and fetal morbidity/mortality and optimal pregnancy outcomes. Ongoing fetal assessment and early identification of fetal complications are the cornerstones of comprehensive obstetric care and allow for effective intervention.

## PRECONCEPTION COUNSELING AND CARE

Preconception counseling and care is intended to optimize a woman's health for pregnancy, ideally commencing before conception, with a preconception visit. During this visit a thorough family and medical history of both parents is obtained, as well as a physical examination of the prospective mother. The goal of this visit is to minimize adverse health effects for the mother and fetus and to promote a healthy pregnancy. Preexisting conditions that may affect conception, pregnancy, or both are identified and addressed. For example, neural tube defects (NTDs) are associated with folic acid deficiency. Discussion about folic acid supplementation is an essential component of preconception. In addition, women with conditions such as maternal phenylketonuria or diabetes can reduce the risks of adverse fetal effects by establishing strict metabolic control before conception and continuing it throughout the pregnancy. Establishing metabolic control of these conditions during pregnancy is believed to be of lesser benefit.

All health encounters during a woman's reproductive years, particularly those that are a part of preconception care, should include counseling about appropriate medical care and behaviors to optimize pregnancy outcomes. The following maternal assessments may serve as the basis for this counseling:

- Family planning and pregnancy spacing
- Family history
- Genetic history
- Medical, surgical, psychiatric, and neurologic histories
- Current medications
- Substance use
- Domestic abuse and violence
- Nutrition
- Environmental and occupational exposures
- Immunity and immunization status
- Risk factors for sexually transmitted diseases

- Obstetric and gynecologic history
- Physical examination
- Assessment of socioeconomic, education, and culture context

Vaccinations should be offered to women found to be at risk for or susceptible to rubella, varicella, and hepatitis B. All pregnant women should be tested for HIV infection, unless they decline the test. A number of other tests can be performed for specific indications:

- Screening for sexually transmitted diseases
- Testing for maternal diseases based on medical or reproductive history
- Mantoux test with purified protein derivative for tuberculosis
- Screening for genetic disorders based on racial and ethnic background:
  - Sickle hemoglobinopathies (African Americans)
  - Beta-thalassemia (individuals of Mediterranean and Southeast Asian descent; African Americans)
  - Alpha-thalassemia (individuals of Southeast Asian and Mediterranean descent; African Americans)
  - Tay-Sachs disease (Ashkenazi Jews, French Canadians, and Cajuns)
  - Canavan disease and familial dysautonomia (Ashkenazi Jews)
  - Cystic fibrosis (while carrier frequency is higher among Caucasians of European and Ashkenazi descent, carrier screening should be made available to all couples)
  - Screening for other genetic disorders on the basis of family history

Patients should be counseled regarding the benefits of the following activities:

- Exercise
- Reducing weight before pregnancy, if obese; increasing weight, if underweight

- Avoiding food faddism
- Avoiding pregnancy within one month of receiving a live attenuated vaccine (e.g., rubella)
- Preventing HIV infection
- Determining the time of conception by an accurate menstrual history
- Abstaining from tobacco, alcohol, and illicit drug use before and during pregnancy
- Taking 0.4 mg of folic acid daily while attempting pregnancy and during the first trimester of pregnancy for prevention of NTDs; women who have had a prior NTD-affected pregnancy should consume 4 mg of folic acid per day in the preconception period. This amount can be achieved by adding a separate supplement to a single multivitamin tablet to provide a total of 4 mg of folic acid while avoiding excessive intake of fat-soluble vitamins, which may have adverse fetal effects if taken in high doses.
- Maintaining good control of any preexisting medical conditions (e.g., diabetes, hypertension, asthma, systemic lupus erythematosus, seizures, thyroid disorders, inflammatory bowel disease).

## ANTEPARTUM CARE

Women who receive early and regular antepartum care are more likely to have healthier infants. The goals of obstetric care are to (1) provide easy access to care, (2) promote patient involvement, and (3) provide a team approach to ongoing surveillance and education for the patient and about her fetus. High-risk conditions can be identified and a management plan established for any complications that may arise. Routine antepartum care provides an opportunity for screening, periodic assessments, and patient education.

Antepartum surveillance begins with the first prenatal visit. At this time, the health care provider begins to compile an obstetric database of information. Appendix C contains a format for documenting information. Complete antepartum care includes the following:

- Diagnosing pregnancy and determining gestational age
- Monitoring the progress of the pregnancy with periodic examinations and appropriate screening tests
- Assessing the well-being of the woman and her fetus
- Providing patient education that addresses all aspects of pregnancy
- Preparing the patient and her family for her management during labor, delivery, and the postpartum interval.
- Detecting medical and psychosocial complications and instituting indicated interventions

An important aspect of prenatal/antepartum care is to educate the mother and her family about the value of screening for and managing the unexpected complications that may develop. Specific conditions to which poor maternal and neonatal outcomes are often attributed include preterm labor and preterm delivery, preterm infection, intrauterine growth restriction, hypertension and preeclampsia, diabetes mellitus, birth defects, multiple gestation, and abnormal placentation.

## DIAGNOSIS OF PREGNANCY

For a woman with regular menstrual cycles, a history of one or more missed periods following a time of sexual activity without effective contraception strongly suggests early pregnancy. Fatigue, nausea/vomiting, and breast tenderness are often associated symptoms.

On physical examination, softening and enlargement of the pregnant uterus becomes apparent 6 or more weeks after the last normal menstrual period. At approximately 12 weeks of gestation (12 weeks from the onset of the last menstrual period), the uterus is generally enlarged sufficiently to be palpable in the lower abdomen. Other genital tract findings early in pregnancy include congestion and a bluish discoloration of the vagina (**Chadwick sign**) and softening of the cervix (**Hegar sign**). Increased pigmentation of the skin and the appearance of circumlinear striae on the abdominal wall occur later in pregnancy and are associated with progesterone effects and physical stretching of the dermis. Palpation of fetal parts and the appreciation of fetal movement and fetal heart tones are diagnostic of pregnancy, but at a more advanced gestational age. The patient's initial perception of fetal movement (called "quickening") is not usually reported before 16 to 18 weeks of gestation, and often as late as 20 weeks in first-time mothers.

Pregnancy cannot be diagnosed only on the basis of symptoms and subjective physical findings. A **pregnancy test** is needed to confirm the diagnosis. Once a positive pregnancy test is identified and before fetal heart activity (beating fetal heart) is seen on ultrasound, the physician and patient must be aware of signs and symptoms of an abnormal pregnancy, including those associated with spontaneous abortion, ectopic pregnancy, and trophoblastic disease. Several types of urine pregnancy tests are available that measure **human chorionic gonadotropin (hCG)** produced in the syncytiotrophoblast of the growing placenta. Because hCG shares an $\alpha$-subunit with luteinizing hormone (LH), interpretation of any test that does not differentiate LH from hCG must take into account this overlap in structure. The concentration of hCG necessary to evoke a positive test result must therefore be high enough to avoid a false-positive diagnosis of pregnancy. Standard laboratory urine pregnancy tests become positive approximately 4 weeks following the first day of the last menstrual period (i.e., around the time of the missed period). Home urine pregnancy tests have a low false-positive rate but a high false-negative rate (the test result is negative even though the patient is pregnant). *All urine pregnancy tests are best performed on early-morning urine specimens, which contain the highest concentration of hCG.*

**Serum pregnancy tests** are more specific and sensitive because they test for the unique β-subunit of hCG, allowing detection of pregnancy very early in gestation, often before the patient has missed a period. During the first few weeks, the status of a pregnancy may be evaluated by following serial quantitative hCG levels and comparing them to the expected rise derived from normative data for proven normal intrauterine pregnancies. Such serial studies often allow differentiation of normal and abnormal pregnancy, or indicate that further testing of other kinds is needed for the same purpose.

**Ultrasound examination** can detect pregnancy early in gestation. With an abdominal ultrasound, the ultrasound transducer is placed on the maternal abdomen, allowing visualization of a normal pregnancy gestational sac 5 to 6 weeks after the beginning of the last normal menstrual period (corresponding to β-hCG concentrations of 5000 to 6000 mIU/mL) **Transvaginal ultrasound** often detects pregnancy at 3 to 4 weeks of gestation (corresponding to β-hCG concentrations of 1000 to 2000 mIU/mL) because the probe is placed in the posterior fornix of the vagina only a few centimeters from the uterine cavity, compared to the relatively longer distance from the abdominal wall to the same location. If the β-hCG concentration is >4000 mIU/mL, the embryo should be visualized and cardiac activity detected by all ultrasound techniques.

**Detection of fetal heart activity ("fetal heart tones")** is also almost always evidence of a viable intrauterine pregnancy. With a traditional, nonelectronic, acoustic fetoscope, auscultation of fetal heart tones is possible at or beyond 18 to 20 weeks of gestational age. The commonly used electronic Doppler devices can detect fetal heart tones at approximately 12 weeks of gestation.

## THE INITIAL PRENATAL VISIT

At the initial prenatal appointment, a comprehensive history is taken, focusing on past pregnancies, gynecologic history, medical history with attention to chronic medical issues and infections, information pertinent to genetic screening, and information about the course of the current pregnancy. A complete physical examination is performed, including breast and pelvic examinations, as well as routine first trimester laboratory studies (Table 6.1). Other studies may be performed as indicated. The patient is given instructions concerning routine prenatal care, warning signs of complications, whom to contact with questions or problems, and nutritional and social service information.

The initial obstetric pelvic examination also includes a description of the various diameters of the bony pelvis (see Chapter 4, Embryology and Anatomy), assessment of the cervix (including cervical length, consistency, dilation, and effacement), and size (usually expressed in weeks), shape, consistency (firm to soft), and mobility. When the uterus grows in size so that it exits the pelvis, the fundal height in

centimeters represents the gestational age of the fetus from that time to about 36 weeks.

## Risk Assessment

Risk assessment is an important part of the initial antenatal evaluation. *Questions about history and chronic medical conditions are important in order to identify the pregnant woman who is at risk for complications and to initiate a management plan at the appropriate time.* In addition to understanding the medical risks, it is important to understand each woman's social circumstances, some of which may place her at risk for both physical and emotional complications. Patients should be questioned about the following aspects of their lifestyle that could pose a risk and receive appropriate counseling, if indicated:

- Nutrition and weight-gain counseling
- Sexual activity
- Exercise
- Smoking
- Environmental and work hazards
- Tobacco
- Alcohol
- Illicit/recreational drugs
- Domestic violence
- Seat belt use

## Initial Assessment of Gestational Age: Estimated Date of Delivery

*Gestational age is the number of weeks that have elapsed between the first day of the last menstrual period (not the presumed time of conception) and the date of delivery.* Establishing an accurate estimated gestational age and **estimated date of delivery (EDD)** is an important part of the initial antepartum visit. Issues such as prematurity and postterm pregnancy and their subsequent management, as well as the timing of screening tests (i.e., maternal serum screening for trisomy 21 and NTDs, assessment of fetal maturity) are affected by the accuracy of gestational age.

**Naegele's rule** is an easy way to calculate the EDD: add 7 days to the first day of the last normal menstrual flow and subtract 3 months. In a patient with an idealized 28-day menstrual cycle, ovulation occurs on day 14; therefore, the conception age of the pregnancy is actually 38 weeks. The use of the first day of the last menstrual period as a starting point for gestational age is standard, and gestational, not conceptional, age is used. "Normal" pregnancy lasts 40 ±2 weeks, calculated from the first day of the last normal menses (menstrual or gestational age).

To establish an accurate gestational age, *the date of onset of the last normal menses is crucial.* A light bleeding episode should not be mistaken for a normal menstrual period. A history of irregular periods or taking medications that alter

## TABLE
## 6.1    Laboratory Tests

**LABORATORY AND EDUCATION**

| INITIAL LABS | DATE | RESULT | REVIEWED |
|---|---|---|---|
| BLOOD TYPE | / / | A      B      AB      O | |
| D (Rh) TYPE | / / | | |
| ANTIBODY SCREEN | / / | | |
| HCT/HGB/MCV | / / | _____ % _____ g/dL | |
| PAP TEST | / / | NORMAL/ABNORMAL/_____ | |
| VARICELLA | / / | | |
| RUBELLA | / / | | |
| VDRL | / / | | |
| URINE CULTURE/SCREEN | / / | | |
| HBsAg | / / | | |
| HIV COUNSELING/TESTING* | / / | POS.      NEG.      DECLINED | |

| OPTIONAL LABS | DATE | RESULT | |
|---|---|---|---|
| HEMOGLOBIN ELECTROPHORESIS | / / | AA  AS  SS  AC  SC  AF  ↑A$_2$<br>POS.      NEG.      DECLINED | |
| PPD | / / | | |
| CHLAMYDIA | / / | | |
| GONORRHEA | / / | | |
| CYSTIC FIBROSIS | / / | POS.      NEG.      DECLINED | |
| TAY-SACHS | / / | POS.      NEG.      DECLINED | |
| FAMILIAL DYSAUTONOMIA | / / | POS.      NEG.      DECLINED | |
| HEMOGLOBIN | | | |
| GENETIC SCREENING TESTS (SEE FORM B) | / / | | |
| OTHER | | | |

| 8–20-WEEK LABS (WHEN INDICATED/ELECTED) | DATE | RESULT | |
|---|---|---|---|
| ULTRASOUND | / / | | |
| 1ST TRIMESTER ANEUPLOIDY RISK ASSESSMENT | / / | POS.      NEG.      DECLINED | |
| MSAFP/MULTIPLE MARKERS | / / | POS.      NEG.      DECLINED | |
| 2ND TRIMESTER SERUM SCREENING | / / | POS.      NEG.      DECLINED | |
| AMNIO/CVS | / / | | |
| KARYOTYPE | / / | 46,XX  OR  46,XY/OTHER_____ | |
| AMNIOTIC FLUID (AFP) | / / | NORMAL_____  ABNORMAL_____ | |
| ANTI-D IMMUNE GLOBULIN (RHIG) | / / | | |

**COMMENTS/ADDITIONAL LABS**

*Check state requirements before recording results.

*(CONTINUED)*

PROVIDER SIGNATURE (AS REQUIRED)_____

ACOG ANTEPARTUM RECORD (FORM D)

| TABLE 6.1 | Laboratory Tests (Continued) |
|---|---|

Patient Addressograph

**LABORATORY AND EDUCATION** *(continued)*

| 24–28-WEEK LABS (WHEN INDICATED) | DATE | RESULT | | COMMENTS/ADDITIONAL LABS |
|---|---|---|---|---|
| HCT/HGB/MCV | / / | _____ % _____ g/dL | | |
| DIABETES SCREEN | / / | 1 HOUR_____ | | |
| GTT (IF SCREEN ABNORMAL) | / / | ____FBS ____1 HOUR ____2 HOUR ____3 HOUR | | |
| D (Rh) ANTIBODY SCREEN | / / | | | |
| ANTI-D IMMUNE GLOBULIN (RhIG) GIVEN (28 WKS OR GREATER) | / / | SIGNATURE _____ | | |

| 32–36-WEEK LABS | DATE | RESULT | | |
|---|---|---|---|---|
| HCT/HGB | / / | _____ % _____ g/dL | | |
| ULTRASOUND (WHEN INDICATED) | / / | | | |
| HIV (WHEN INDICATED)* | | | | |
| VDRL (WHEN INDICATED) | / / | | | |
| GONORRHEA (WHEN INDICATED) | / / | | | |
| CHLAMYDIA (WHEN INDICATED) | / / | | | |
| GROUP B STREP | / / | | | |

*Check state requirements before recording results.

**COMMENTS**

PROVIDER SIGNATURE (AS REQUIRED)_____

ACOG ANTEPARTUM RECORD (FORM D, *continued*)

cycle length (e.g., oral contraceptives, other hormonal preparations, and psychoactive medications) can confuse the menstrual history. If sexual intercourse is infrequent or timed for conception based on assisted reproductive techniques (ARTs), a patient may know when conception is most likely to have occurred, thus facilitating an accurate calculation of gestational age.

Obstetric ultrasound examination is the most accurate measurement available in the determination of gestational age. Pelvic examination by an experienced examiner is accurate, within 1 to 2 weeks, in determining gestational age until about 14 to 16 weeks, at which time the lower uterine segment begins to form, thereby making clinical estimation of gestational age less accurate. In addition, in women with a retroverted uterus, estimation of gestational age is less accurate than in women with other positions of the uterus.

## SUBSEQUENT ANTENATAL VISITS

Regular monitoring of the mother and fetus is essential for identifying complications that may arise during pregnancy and to provide assurance and support for mother and family, especially for first pregnancies or when previous pregnancies have been complicated or had unfortunate outcomes. For a patient with a normal pregnancy, periodic antepartum visits at 4-week intervals are usually scheduled until 28 weeks, at 2- to 3-week intervals between 28 and 36 weeks, and weekly thereafter. Patients with high-risk pregnancies or those with ongoing complications usually are seen more frequently, depending on the clinical circumstances. At each visit, patients are asked about how they are feeling and if they are having any problems, such as vaginal bleeding, nausea and vomiting, dysuria, or vaginal discharge. After quickening, patients are asked if they continue to feel fetal movement, and if it is the same or less since the last antepartum visit. Decreased fetal movement after the time of fetal viability is a warning sign requiring further evaluation of fetal well-being.

Every prenatal assessment includes the following assessments:

- Blood pressure
- Weight
- Urinalysis for albumin and glucose

It is important to determine baseline blood pressure and urine protein levels at the first antepartum visit. Blood pressure generally declines at the end of the first trimester and rises again in the third trimester. After 20 weeks of gestation, an increase in the systolic pressure of more than 30 mm Hg or an increase in the diastolic pressure of more than 15 mm Hg above the baseline level suggests (but alone does not diagnose) **gestational hypertension** (see Chapter 16, Hypertension in Pregnancy). Comparison with baseline levels is necessary in order to accurately distinguish preexisting hypertension from hypertension associated with pregnancy.

Maternal weight is another important parameter to follow through pregnancy, as weight gain recommendations differ for women of differing prepregnancy **body mass index (BMI).** A total weight gain of 25 to 35 lb is only appropriate for a woman of normal BMI (see Table 6.2). The obese pregnant woman with a pregravid BMI ≥30 is at risk for multiple complications during pregnancy, including preeclampsia, gestational diabetes, and need for cesarean delivery. Between monthly visits, a 3- to 4-lb weight gain is generally appropriate for a woman of normal BMI. Significant deviation from this trend may require nutritional assessment and further evaluation.

Obstetric physical findings made at each visit include fundal height measurement, documentation of the presence and rate of fetal heart tones, and determination of the presentation of the fetus. Until 18 to 20 weeks, the uterine size is generally stated as weeks' size, such as "12 weeks' size." After 20 weeks of gestation (when the fundus is palpable at or near the umbilicus in a woman of normal body habitus and a singleton pregnancy in the vertex presentation), the uterine size can be assessed with the use of a tape measure, which is the **fundal height measurement.** In this procedure, the top of the uterine fundus is identified and the zero end of the tape measure is placed at this uppermost part of the uterus. The tape is then carried anteriorly across the abdomen to the level of the symphysis pubis. From 16 to 18 weeks of gestation until 36 weeks of gestation, the fundal height in centimeters (measured from the symphysis to the top of the uterine fundus) is roughly equal to the number of weeks of gestational age in normal singleton pregnancies in the cephalic presentation within an anatomically normal uterus (Fig. 6.1). Until 36 weeks in the normal singleton pregnancy, the number of weeks of gestation approximates the fundal height in centimeters. Thereafter, the fetus moves downward into the pelvis beneath the symphysis pubis ("lightening," or engagement of the head into the true pelvis), so that the fundal height measurement is increasingly unreliable.

**Fetal heart rate** should be verified at every visit, by direct auscultation or by the use of a fetal Doppler ultra-

| TABLE 6.2 | Institute of Medicine Guidelines for Total Weight Gain During Pregnancy, Based on Prepregnancy Body Mass Index (BMI) |
|---|---|
| **Prepregnancy BMI (lb)** | **Recommended Total Weight Gain (lb)** |
| Less than 19.8 | 28–40 |
| 19.8–26.0 | 25–35 |
| 26.1–29.0 | 15–25 |
| More than 29.0 | At least 15 |

From American College of Obstetrics and Gynecology. *Guidelines for Perinatal Care.* 6th ed. Washington, DC: American College of Obstetrics and Gynecology; 2007:86.

Figure 9.7, p. 112). In the first maneuver, breech presentation can be appreciated by outlining the fundus and determining what part is present. The head is hard and well-defined by ballottement, especially when the head is freely mobile in the fluid-filled uterus; the breech is softer, less round, and, therefore, more difficult to outline. In the second and third maneuvers, the examiner's palms are placed on either side of the maternal abdomen to determine the location of the fetal back and small parts. In the fourth maneuver, the presenting part is identified by exerting pressure over the pubic symphysis. If a breech presentation persists at 36 and 38 weeks, the option of **external cephalic version (ECV)** should be discussed with the patient. This procedure involves turning the fetus from the breech presentation to a vertex presentation to allow vaginal rather than cesarean delivery. It is contraindicated in the presence of multifetal gestation, fetal compromise, uterine anomalies, and problems of placentation.

## ULTRASOUND

In the United States, approximately 65% of pregnant women have at least one ultrasound examination. *The optimal timing for a single ultrasound examination in the absence of specific indications for a first-trimester examination is at 16–20 weeks of gestation.* Ultrasonography in the first trimester may be performed either transabdominally or transvaginally. If a transabdominal examination is not definitive, a transvaginal or transperineal examination should be performed whenever possible. First trimester ultrasonography is used to confirm the presence of an intrauterine pregnancy, estimate gestational age, diagnose and evaluate multiple gestations, confirm cardiac activity, and evaluate pelvic masses or uterine abnormalities (as an adjunct to chorionic villus sampling, embryo transfer, or localization and removal of intrauterine contraceptives). It is also useful for evaluating vaginal bleeding, suspected **ectopic pregnancy,** and pelvic pain.

An ultrasound examination may be targeted to help diagnose chromosomal abnormalities in the first trimester. One such examination is measurement of **nuchal transparency (NT),** the lucent area behind the head in the **nuchal region.** Use of standardized techniques for measuring nuchal translucency has resulted in higher detection rates for Down syndrome, trisomy 18, trisomy 13, and Turner syndrome.

*Recent studies demonstrate improved detection of Down syndrome at lower false-positive rates when nuchal translucency measurement is combined with biochemical markers (see "Screening Tests" below).*

*Various types of ultrasound examinations performed during the second or third trimester can be categorized as "standard," "limited," or "specialized." A standard examination is performed during the second or third trimester of pregnancy.*

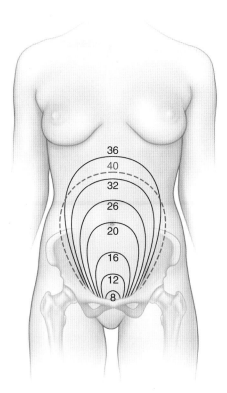

FIGURE 6.1. Fundal height. In a normal singleton pregnancy in the vertex presentation, fundal height roughly corresponds to gestational age between 16 and 36 weeks of gestation. A convenient guideline is 20 weeks equals 20 cm equals fundus at umbilicus in a woman with a normal body habitus. After 36 weeks, the fundal height either grows more slowly, or actually decreases as the uterus changes shape and/or the fetal head engages in the pelvis.

sound device. The normal fetal heart rate is 110 to 160 bpm, with higher rates found in early pregnancy. The maternal pulse may also be detected with the Doppler device, so simultaneous palpation of maternal pulse and auscultation of fetal pulse may be necessary to differentiate the two. Deviation from the normal rate or occasional arrhythmias must be evaluated carefully.

Several determinations concerning the fetus can be made by **palpation of the pregnant uterus,** such as identifying the presentation, or "presenting part" of the fetus; that is, what part of the fetus is entering the pelvis first. Before 34 weeks of gestation, breech, oblique, or transverse presentations are not uncommon. The presentation of the fetus may also vary from day to day. At term, more than 95% of fetuses are in the cephalic presentation (head down). Approximately 3.5% are breech (bottom first), and 1% are shoulder first. Unless the fetus is in a transverse lie (the long axis of the fetus is not parallel with the mother's long axis), the presenting part will be either the head (vertex, cephalic) or the breech (buttocks).

The presentation of the fetus can be appreciated on clinical exam with the use of **Leopold maneuvers** (see

It includes an evaluation of fetal presentation, amniotic fluid volume, cardiac activity, placental position, fetal biometry, and an anatomic survey. If technically feasible, the uterus and adnexa also are examined. A limited examination is performed when a specific question requires investigation. In an emergency, for example, a limited examination can be performed to evaluate heart activity in a bleeding patient. A detailed or targeted anatomic specialized examination is performed when an anomaly is suspected on the basis of history, biochemical abnormalities or clinical evaluation, or suspicious results from either the limited or standard ultrasound examination. Other specialized examinations might include fetal Doppler, biophysical profile, fetal echocardiography, or additional biometric studies.

*Evaluation of placental and cervical abnormalities may be accomplished with ultrasonography.* Placental abruption can be identified by ultrasonography in approximately half of all patients who present with bleeding and do not have placenta previa. Color-flow Doppler ultrasound assessment is used to identify placenta accreta. Transvaginal ultrasound examination most accurately can visualize the cervix, and also can be employed to detect or rule out placenta previa as well as an abnormally shortened cervix, which has been correlated with an increased risk of preterm delivery when measured at 26–30 weeks of gestation.

## SCREENING TESTS

In addition to the routine laboratory tests performed at the initial antepartum visit, additional tests are performed at specific intervals throughout the pregnancy to screen for birth defects and other conditions. The specific tests and intervals for each are indicated on the Antepartum Record (see Appendix C). Additional laboratory testing, such as testing for sexually transmitted diseases or tuberculosis, are recommended or offered on the basis of the patient's history, physical examination, parental desire, or in response to public health guidelines.

There are several options for screening for fetal aneuploidy (abnormal number of chromosomes) such as trisomy 18 and 21 (see also Chapter 7, Assessment of Genetic Disorders in Obstetrics and Gynecology, for a detailed discussion of each of these markers). Options for screening include:

- **First trimester screening** (10–13 weeks of gestation), which includes serum screening for pregnancy-associated plasma protein A (PPA) and beta-hCG, and an ultrasound assessment of nuchal transparency.
- **Second trimester screening** (15–20 weeks of gestation) consisting of **triple** (maternal serum α-fetal protein [MSAFP], estriol, and hCG) or **quadruple ("quad")** (MSAFP, hCG, estriol, and inhibin) screening tests.
- **Integrated first-and-second trimester screening,** which includes all of the first trimester screening tests

listed in addition to a PAPP-A test and a quad screen, with or without an ultrasound examination for neural tube defects, in the second trimester.

A **glucose challenge test (GCT)** is a screening test performed for gestational diabetes in the third trimester, unless the pregnant patient is obese or at high risk for developing diabetes. In these cases, the test should be performed at the first visit. If the test result is abnormal, a **glucose tolerance test (GTT)** is performed to confirm diabetes. Universal screening for **group B streptococcus (GBS)** is performed at 32 to 36 weeks' gestation, and treatment is based on culture results. In addition, measurement of hemoglobin and hematocrit levels is repeated in the third trimester.

## SPECIFIC TECHNIQUES OF FETAL ASSESSMENT

*Continued evaluation of the fetus includes techniques for assessment of fetal (1) growth, (2) well-being, and (3) maturity.* These tests must be interpreted in light of the clinical context and provide a basis for management decisions.

### Assessment of Fetal Growth

Fetal growth can be assessed by fundal height measurement, as the initial measure, and ultrasonography. The increase in fundal height through pregnancy is predictable. If the fundal height measurement is significantly greater than expected (i.e., **large for gestational age [LGA]**), possible considerations include incorrect assessment of gestational age, multiple pregnancy, macrosomia (large fetus), hydatidiform mole, or excess accumulation of amniotic fluid (polyhydramnios). A fundal height measurement less than expected, or **small for gestational age (SGA),** suggests the possibility of incorrect assessment of gestational age, hydatidiform mole, fetal growth restriction, inadequate amniotic fluid accumulation (oligohydramnios), or even intrauterine fetal demise. Deviation in fundal height measurement should be closely evaluated.

Ultrasound is the most valuable tool in assessing fetal growth. *Ultrasound has many potential uses for both fetal dating and identifying any fetal anomalies.* In early pregnancy, determination of the gestational-sac diameter and the crown-to-rump length correlates closely with gestational age. Later in pregnancy, measurement of the biparietal diameter of the skull, the abdominal circumference, the femur length, and the cerebellar diameter can be used to assess gestational age and, using various formulas, to estimate fetal weight.

### Assessment of Fetal Well-Being

Assessment of **fetal well-being** includes subjective maternal perception of fetal activity and several objective tests using electronic fetal monitoring and ultrasonography. Tests of fetal well-being have a wide range of use, including the assessment of fetal status at a particular time and prediction of future well-being for varying time intervals, depending on the test and the clinical situation.

*Evaluation of **fetal activity** is a common indirect measure of fetal well-being.* A variety of methods can be used to quantify fetal activity, including the time necessary to achieve a certain number of movements each day, or counting the number of movements (**"kick counts"**) in a given hour. This type of testing is easily performed and involves the patient in her own care. If the mother notices less movement, further evaluation may be needed.

Fetal monitoring tests can provide more objective information about fetal well-being. These tests include the nonstress test (NST), contraction stress test (CST) (called the oxytocin challenge test [OCT] if oxytocin is used), biophysical profile (BPP), and ultrasonography of umbilical artery blood flow velocity. Although there is no optimal time to initiate fetal testing, there are several maternal and pregnancy-related indications (Box 6.1).

## NONSTRESS TEST

*The **nonstress test** measures the fetal heart rate, which is monitored with an external transducer for at least 20 minutes.* The patient is asked to note fetal movement, usually accomplished by pressing a button on the fetal monitor, which causes a notation on the monitor strip. The tracing is observed for fetal heart rate accelerations (Fig. 6.2). The results are considered reactive (or reassuring) if two or more fetal heart rate accelerations occur in a 20-minute period, with or without fetal movement discernible by the mother. A nonreactive (nonreassuring) tracing is one without sufficient heart rate accelerations in a 40-minute period. *A nonreactive NST should be followed with further fetal assessment.*

---

**BOX 6.1**
## Indications for Fetal Testing

Maternal conditions:
- Antiphospholipid syndrome
- Hyperthyroidism (poorly controlled)
- Hemoglobinopathies (hemoglobin SS, SC, or S-thalassemia)
- Significant heart disease
- Systemic lupus erythematosus
- Chronic renal disease
- Insulin-treated diabetes mellitus
- Hypertensive disorders

Pregnancy-related conditions:
- Pregnancy-induced hypertension
- Decreased fetal movement
- Oligohydramnios
- Polyhydramnios
- Intrauterine growth restriction
- Postterm pregnancy
- Isoimmunization (moderate to severe)
- Previous fetal demise
- Multiple gestation (with significant growth discrepancy)

From American College of Obstetrics and Gynecology. *Guidelines for Perinatal Care.* 6th ed. Washington, DC: American College of Obstetrics and Gynecology; 2007:112.

---

## CONTRACTION STRESS TEST

*Whereas the NST evaluates the fetal heart rate response to fetal activity, the **contraction stress test** measures the response of the fetal heart rate to the stress of a uterine contraction.* During a uterine contraction, uteroplacental blood flow is temporar-

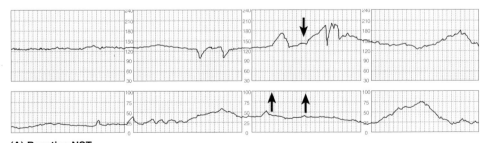

**(A) Reactive NST**

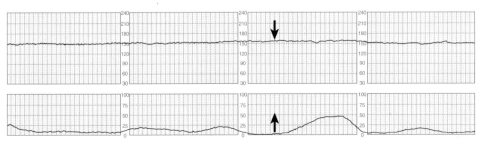

**(B) Nonreactive NST**

FIGURE 6.2. Nonstress testing. (A) Reactive nonstress test (NST); note fetal heart rate acceleration in response to fetal movement. (B) Nonreactive NST; note lack of fetal heart rate acceleration in response to fetal movement.

ily reduced by the contracting myometrium. A healthy fetus is able to compensate for this intermittent decreased blood flow, whereas a fetus that is compromised may be unable to do so. To perform a CST, a tocodynamometer is placed on the maternal abdomen along with a fetal heart rate transducer for a baseline tracing for 10 to 20 minutes. If there are no contractions, they are induced by nipple self-stimulation or oxytocin (this test is called an OCT). A negative (normal) result is indicated if there is no change from the baseline fetal heart rate and no fetal heart rate decelerations. *If decelerations occur, the results can be considered positive, equivocal, or unsatisfactory, depending on the pattern, frequency, and strength of the deceleration.*

These tests of fetal well-being have a significant incidence of false-positive results (i.e., results suggesting that the fetus is in jeopardy, though the fetus is actually healthy). *For this reason, the results of these tests must be interpreted collectively, and the tests themselves repeated to verify the results.* When multiple test results are reassuring, they tend to rule out a problem. When all results are nonreassuring, they tend to signify the presence of a problem.

## BIOPHYSICAL PROFILE

If an OCT is positive, evidence to support fetal well-being, such as that provided by a **biophysical profile (BPP),** is sought. The BPP is a series of five assessments of fetal well-being, each of which is given a score of 0 (absent) or 2 (present) [Table 6.3]. The parameters include a reactive NST, the presence of fetal breathing movements, the presence of fetal movement of the body or limbs, the finding of fetal tone (flexed extremities as opposed to a flaccid posture), and an adequate amount of amniotic fluid volume. A total score of 8 to 10 is considered reassuring. A total score of

6 is equivocal and generally should lead to delivery if the patient is at term. If the patient is preterm, retesting within 12 to 24 hours may be appropriate. A score of 4 or less is nonreassuring and warrants further evaluation and consideration of delivery. Irrespective of the score, more frequent BPP testing or consideration of delivery may be warranted when oligohydramnios is present.[1(p116)] Management based on the BPP depends not only on the score itself, but also on the gestational age of the fetus.

*Modified BPP combines use of an NST and assessment of an amniotic fluid index (AFI). The AFI is a semiquantitative, four-quadrant assessment of amniotic fluid depth.* The importance of adequate **amniotic fluid volume** is well-established. Diminished amniotic fluid is thought to represent decreased fetal urinary output caused by chronic stress and shunting of blood flow away from the kidneys. The decreased amniotic fluid provides less support for the umbilical cord, which may be more compressed, reducing blood flow. *The modified BPP is less cumbersome than the BPP and appears to be as predictive of fetal well-being.*

## DOPPLER ULTRASOUND OF UMBILICAL ARTERY

**Umbilical Artery Doppler flow ultrasonography** is a noninvasive technique to assess resistance to blood flow in the placenta. It can be used in conjunction with other biophysical tests in high-risk pregnancies associated with suspected intrauterine growth restriction. Umbilical cord Doppler flow velocimetry is based on the characteristics of the systolic blood flow and the diastolic blood flow. The most commonly used index to quantify the flow velocity waveform is the systolic/diastolic ratio. As peripheral resistance increases, diastolic flow decreases and may become

| TABLE 6.3 | Components of the Biophysical Profile |
|---|---|
| **Biophysical Variable** | **Normal Result** |
| NST | Because the probability of fetal well-being is identical with scores of 10 out of 10 and 8 out of 10, the NST may be excluded if all other parameters of the BPP are reassuring in more than 97% of cases without adverse consequences. |
| Fetal breathing movements | One of more episodes of rhythmic fetal breathing movements of 30 seconds or more within 30 minutes |
| Fetal movement | Three or more discrete body or limb movements within 30 minutes |
| Fetal tone | One or more episodes of fetal extremity extension with return to flexion, or opening and closing of hand within 30 minutes |
| Quantification of amniotic fluid volume | A pocket of amniotic fluid that measures at least 2 cm in two planes perpendicular to each other |

From American College of Obstetrics and Gynecology. *Guidelines for Perinatal Care.* 6th ed. Washington, DC: American College of Obstetrics and Gynecology; 2007:116.

absent or reserve, and the systolic/diastolic ratio increases. Reversed end-systolic flow can be seen with severe cases of intrauterine growth restriction secondary to uteroplacental insufficiency and may suggest impending fetal demise.

## Assessment of Fetal Maturity

Fetal maturity should always be taken into consideration when delivering a fetus electively or preterm in high-risk pregnancies. Several tests are available to assess fetal maturity (Box 6.2). Because the respiratory system is the last fetal system to mature functionally, many of the tests available to assess fetal maturity focus on this organ system. Several phospholipids, collectively known as **surfactant,** enter the amniotic fluid where they can be obtained by amniocentesis and measured. Surfactant is necessary for normal lung function, as it maintains the patency of the alveolar sacs. The ratio of two phospholipids, **lecithin and sphingomyelin,** called the **L/S ratio,** has been used to determine fetal lung maturity, but other tests are rapidly replacing use of this ratio. Another important phospholipid contained in the surfactant complex is **phosphatidylglycerol (PG),** a marker of complete pulmonary maturation that is present after 35 weeks of gestation.

Neonates delivered before their lungs have matured are at risk of **respiratory distress syndrome (RDS),** a serious and life-threatening condition caused by lack of surfactant. RDS in newborns is manifest by signs of respiratory failure—grunting, chest retractions, nasal flaring, and hypoxia—possibly leading to acidosis and death. Management consists of skillful support of ventilation and correction of associated metabolic disturbances until the neonate can ventilate without assistance. Administration of synthetic or semi-synthetic surfactant to the neonate has resulted in improved outcomes for infants with RDS.

Results of pulmonary function tests that indicate immaturity do not have a high predictive value for RDS. Because no test indicating maturity can completely eliminate the risk of RDS or other neonatal complications, the risk of adverse fetal outcome following delivery must be weighed against the potential risk of allowing the pregnancy to continue.

## ANTEPARTUM PATIENT EDUCATION

Plans for the antepartum, intrapartum, and postpartum periods provide an opportunity for patient education and interaction. The Antepartum Record in Appendix C provides a list of the issues to be discussed during antepartum care.

## Employment

A woman with an uncomplicated pregnancy can usually continue to work until the onset of labor. In a normal pregnancy, there are few restrictions concerning work, although it is beneficial to allow moderate activity and to allow for periods of rest. Strenuous work (standing or repetitive, strenuous, physical lifting) is best avoided.

A period of 4 to 6 weeks generally is required for a woman's physical condition to return to normal. However, the patient's individual circumstances may be a factor in determining when she returns to work. The length of a woman's leave from work can depend on whether there are pregnancy or delivery complications, the work involved, the employer attitude, the rules of the health care system under which the patient receives care, and the wishes of the patient. The Federal Family and Medical Leave Act and state laws should be consulted to determine the family and medical leave that is available.[1(p118)]

## Exercise

In the absence of either medical or obstetric complications, up to 30 minutes of moderate exercise per day on most if not all days of the week is acceptable (Box 6.3). Each sport should be reviewed for its potential risk, and activities with a high risk for falling or for abdominal trauma should be avoided.

Overly strenuous exercise, especially for prolonged periods, should be avoided. Patients unaccustomed to regular exercise should not undertake vigorous new programs during pregnancy. **Supine exercises** should be discontinued after the first trimester to minimize circulatory changes brought on by pressure of the uterus on the vena cava. Any activity should be discontinued if discomfort, significant shortness of breath, or pain in the chest or abdomen appears (Box 6.4). Changes in body contour and balance will alter the advised types of activities; abdominal trauma should be avoided.

Sitting in a hot tub or sauna after exercise is of concern to pregnant women. Possible hyperthermia may be teratogenic. Pregnant women might reasonably be advised to remain in saunas for no more than 15 minutes,

---

**BOX 6.2**
**Tests To Assess For Fetal Maturity**

Surfactant/albumen ratio (fetal lung maturity index)
Lecithin/sphingomyelin ratio
Phosphatidylglycerol
Foam stability index
Fluorescence polarization
Optical density at 650 nm
Lamellar body counts
Saturated phosphatidylcholine

> ## BOX 6.3
> ### Contraindications to Aerobic Exercise During Pregnancy
>
> **Absolute**
> - Hemodynamically significant heart disease
> - Restrictive lung disease
> - Incompetent cervix/cerclage
> - Multiple gestation at risk for premature labor
> - Persistent second-trimester or third-trimester bleeding
> - Placenta previa after 26 weeks of gestation
> - Premature labor during the current pregnancy
> - Ruptured membranes
> - Preeclampsia/pregnancy-induced hypertension
>
> **Relative**
> - Severe anemia
> - Unevaluated maternal cardiac arrhythmia
> - Chronic bronchitis
> - Poorly controlled type 1 diabetes
> - Extreme morbid obesity
> - Extreme underweight (BMI <12)
> - History of extremely sedentary lifestyle
> - Intrauterine growth restriction in current pregnancy
> - Poorly controlled hypertension
> - Orthopedic limitations
> - Poorly controlled seizure disorder
> - Poorly controlled hyperthyroidism
> - Heavy smoker
>
> From American College of Obstetrics and Gynecologists. Exercise during pregnancy and the postpartum period. ACOG Committee Opinion No. 267. *Obstet Gynecol.* 2002;99(1):171–173.

> ## BOX 6.4
> ### Warning Signs to Terminate Exercise While Pregnant
>
> Vaginal bleeding
> Dyspnea prior to exertion
> Dizziness
> Headache
> Chest pain
> Muscle weakness
> Calf pain or swelling (need to rule out thrombophlebitis)
> Preterm labor
> Decreased fetal movement
> Amniotic fluid leakage
>
> From American College of Obstetrics and Gynecologists. American College of Obstetricians and Gynecologists. Exercise during pregnancy and the postpartum period. ACOG Committee Opinion No. 267. *Obstet Gynecol.* 2002;99(1):171–173.

and in hot tubs for no more than 10 minutes. In a hot tub, if a woman's head, arms, shoulders, and upper chest are not submerged, there is less surface area to absorb heat.

## Nutrition and Weight Gain

Concerns about adequate nutrition and weight gain during pregnancy are common. Poor nutrition, obesity, and food faddism are associated with poor perinatal outcome. **Pica,** or an inclination for nonnutritional substances such as ice, food starch, or clay or dirt, is often associated with anemia.

A complete nutritional assessment is an important part of the initial antepartum assessment, including history of dietary habits, special dietary issues or concerns, and weight trends. Anorexia and bulimia increase risks for associated problems such as cardiac arrhythmias, gastrointestinal pathology, and electrolyte disturbances. Calculation of BMI is useful because it relates weight to height, allowing for a better indirect measurement of body fat distribution than is obtained with weight alone. Further, because of the "personalized nature" of an individual's BMI, it is often more useful in teaching a patient about diet and weight issues than an abstract table.

Recommendations for total weight gain during pregnancy and the rate of weight gain per month appropriate to achieve it may be made based on a body mass index calculated for the prepregnancy weight (see Table 6.3). The components that make up the average weight gain in a normal singleton pregnancy are listed in Table 6.4. The maternal component of this weight gain starts in the first trimester and increases linearly after the second trimester. Fetal growth is most rapid in the second half of pregnancy, with the normal fetus tripling its weight in the last 12 weeks.

Published **recommended daily allowances** (RDAs) for protein, minerals, and vitamins are useful approximations. It should be kept in mind, however, that the RDAs are a combination of estimates and are values adjusted near the top of the normal ranges to encompass the estimated needs of most women. Thus, many women have an adequate diet for their individual needs, even though it does not supply all the RDAs. Vitamin supplementation is appropriate for specific therapeutic indications, such as a patient's inability or unwillingness to eat a balanced, adequate diet, or clinical demonstration of a specific nutritional risk. Except for iron, mineral supplementation is likewise not required in otherwise healthy women; the National Academy of science recommends 27 mg of iron supplementation.

| TABLE 6.4 | Components of Average Weight Gain in a Normal Singleton Pregnancy Weight | |
|---|---|---|
| **Organ, Tissue, Fluid** | **(kg)** | **(lb)** |
| Maternal | | |
| Uterus | 1.0 | 2.2 |
| Breasts | 0.4 | 0.9 |
| Blood | 1.2 | 2.6 |
| Water | 1.7 | 3.7 |
| Fat | 3.3 | 7.3 |
| Subtotal | 7.6 | 16.7 |
| Fetal | | |
| Fetus | 3.4 | 7.5 |
| Placenta | 0.6 | 1.3 |
| Amniotic fluid | 0.8 | 1.8 |
| Subtotal | 4.8 | 10.6 |
| Total | 12.4 | 27.3 |

Financial problems, the inability to get to a grocery store, and foodstuffs unique to a patient's social group that differ in substantial quantitative ways with respect to important nutrients, may prevent some women from obtaining adequate nutrition, even if the volume of foodstuffs seems sufficient. The WIC Federal Supplemental food program, food stamp programs, and Aid for Families with Dependent Children are resources that may help in these situations.

## Breastfeeding

The benefits of **breastfeeding** include, for the newborn, excellent nutrition and provision of immunologic protection; and, for the mother, more rapid uterine involution, economy, maternal–child bonding, to some extent natural contraception, and, often, more rapid weight loss associated with extra calorie expenditure. Contraindications to breastfeeding include certain maternal infections and use of medications. It is important to support a woman who chooses not to breastfeed. The use of breast pumps and milk storage may allow a mother to continue breastfeeding while continuing to work.

## Sexual Activity

Sexual intercourse is not restricted during a normal pregnancy, although advice about more comfortable positions in later pregnancy may be appreciated—for example, side-to-side or the female-superior position. Sexual activity may be restricted or prohibited under certain high-risk circumstances, such as known placenta previa, premature rupture of membranes, or actual or history of preterm labor (or delivery). Education of the patient (and partner) about safe sex practices is as important in antepartum as in regular gynecologic care.

## Travel

Up to 36 weeks of gestation, women can safely fly. Air travel is not recommended for women who have medical or obstetric complications, such as hypertension, poorly controlled diabetes mellitus, or sickle cell disease. This recommendation is not due to substantial risk to either mother or fetus, but because of the likelihood that labor may ensue away from home and customary health care providers. If a long trip near term is planned, it is useful for the patient to carry a copy of her obstetric record in case she requires obstetric care. When traveling, patients are advised to avoid long periods of inactivity, such as sitting. Walking every 1 to 2 hours, even for short periods, promotes circulation, especially in the lower legs, and decreases the risk of venous stasis and possible thromboembolism. Additionally, preventive antiemetic medicine should be considered for pregnant women with increased nausea. Education about the regular use of a seat belt is especially important, with the seat belt worn low on the hip bones, between the protuberant abdomen and the pelvis.

## Teratogens

Many patient inquiries concern the teratogenic potential of environmental exposures. Major **birth defects** are apparent at birth in 2% to 3% of the general population, and the possible occurrence of fetal malformations or mental retardation is a frequent cause of anxiety among pregnant women. Of these, about 5% may be a result of maternal exposure to drugs or environmental chemicals, and only approximately 1% can be attributed to pharmaceutical agents. The most important determinants of the developmental toxicity of an agent are timing, dose, and fetal susceptibility. Many agents have teratogenic effects only if taken while the susceptible fetal organ system is forming.

The health care provider may wish to consult with or refer such patients to health care professionals with special knowledge or experience in teratology and birth defects. The Organization of Teratology Information Services provides information on teratology issues and exposures in pregnancy (www.otispregnancy.org).

## MEDICATIONS

Very few medications have been proven to be true human teratogens (Box 6.5). Most commonly prescribed medications are relatively safe in pregnancy. The Food and Drug Administration assigns medications a pregnancy risk factor

## BOX 6.5
### Drugs or Substances Suspected or Proven to Be Human Teratogens

| | |
|---|---|
| ACE inhibitors[a] | Kanamycin |
| Aminopterin | Lithium |
| Androgens | Methimazole |
| A-11 antagonists[b] | Methotrexate |
| Busulfan | Misoprostol |
| Carbamazrepine | Penicillamine |
| Chlorbiphenyls | Phenytoin |
| Cocaine | Radioactive iodine |
| Coumarins | Streptomycin |
| Cyclophosphamide | Tamoxifen |
| Danazol | Tetracycline |
| Diethylstilbestrol (DES) | Thalidomide |
| Ethanol | Tretinoin |
| Etretinate | Trimethadione |
| Isotretinoin | Valproic acid |

[a]Angiotensin-converting enzyme inhibitors.
[b]Angiotensin II receptor antagonists.
Adapted from Briggs GG, Freeman RK, Yaffe SJ. *Drugs in Pregnancy and Lactation: A Reference Guide to Fetal and Neonatal Risk.* 8th ed. Philadelphia, PA: Lippincott Williams & Wilkins 2008.
From Cunningham GF, Leveno KJ, Bloom SL, Hauth JC, Gilstrap LC, Wenstom KD, eds. *Williams Obstetrics.* 22nd ed. New York: McGraw Hill Professional; 2005:T14–1.

based on information about the medication and its risk–benefit ratio. These pregnancy risk factors help guide the appropriate use of medications in pregnancy (see Table 6.5). Table 6.6 provides a summary of the teratogenicity of many common medications.

## IONIZING RADIATION

Ionizing radiation exposure is universal; most radiation originates from beyond the earth's atmosphere, from the land, and from endogenous radionuclides. The total radiation exposure from these sources is approximately 125 mrads per year. Although radiation exposure has the potential to cause gene mutations, growth impairment, chromosome damage and malignancy, or fetal death, large doses are required to produce discernible fetal effects. Large doses (10 rads) during the first two weeks after fertilization are required to produce a deleterious effect. In the first trimester, 25 rads are required to produce detectable damage, and 100 rads are required later in pregnancy. Diagnostic radiation usually exposes the fetus to much less than 5 rads, depending on the number of radiographs taken and the maternal site examined (Table 6.7).

## METHYL MERCURY

Industrial pollution is the major source of mercury entry in our ecosystem. Large fish, such as tuna, shark, and king mackerel, retain higher levels of mercury from the smaller fish and organisms they consume. Hence, women who eat these fish are storing high levels of mercury.

The FDA recommends that pregnant women limit their ingestion of albacore tuna to 6 ounces per week or to 12 ounces per week of fish and shellfish varieties thought to be low in mercury.

## HERBAL REMEDIES

Herbal remedies are not regulated as prescription or over-the-counter drugs, the identity and quantity of their ingredients are unknown, and there are virtually no studies of their teratogenic potential. Because it is not possible to assess their safety, pregnant women should be counseled to avoid these substances. Remedies containing substances with pharmaceutical properties that could theoretically have adverse fetal affects include the following:

- Echinacea—causes fragmentation of hamster sperm at high concentrations
- Black cohosh—contains a chemical that acts like an estrogen
- Garlic and willow barks—have anticoagulant properties
- Ginkgo—can interfere with effects of monamine oxidase inhibitors; has anticoagulant effects
- Real licorice—has hypertensive and potassium-wasting effects
- Valerian—intensifies the effects of prescription sleep aids
- Ginseng—interferes with the effects of monamine oxidase inhibitors
- Blue cohosh and pennyroyal—stimulate uterine musculature; pennyroyal also can cause liver damage, renal failure, disseminated intravascular coagulation, and maternal death

## ALCOHOL

Alcohol is the most common teratogen to which a fetus is exposed, and alcohol consumption during pregnancy is a leading preventable cause of mental retardation, developmental delay, and birth defects in the fetus. There is substantial evidence that fetal toxicity is dose-related and that the exposure time of greatest risk is the first trimester. There is no established safe level of alcohol use during pregnancy. Women who are pregnant or who are at risk for pregnancy should not drink alcohol. Although consumption of small amounts of alcohol early in pregnancy is unlikely to cause serious fetal problems, patients are best advised to refrain from alcohol entirely.

| | |
|---|---|
| **TABLE 6.5** | Medications in Pregnancy and Breastfeeding: FDA Classification |

| Risk Factor Category | Description |
|---|---|
| A | Controlled human studies demonstrate no evidence of risk in pregnancy in any trimester, and the possibility of fetal harm appears remote. |
| B | Animal studies have revealed no evidence of harm to the fetus; however, there are no adequate and well-controlled studies in pregnant women.<br>OR<br>Animal studies have shown an adverse effect, but adequate and well-controlled studies in pregnant women have failed to demonstrate a risk to the fetus in any trimester. |
| C | Animal studies have shown an adverse effect and there are no adequate and well-controlled studies in pregnant women.<br>OR<br>No animal studies have been conducted and there are no adequate and well-controlled studies in pregnant women. |
| D | Adequate well-controlled or observational studies in pregnant women have demonstrated a risk to the fetus.<br>However, the benefits of therapy may outweigh the potential risk. For example, the drug may be acceptable if needed in a life-threatening situation or serious disease for which safer drugs cannot be used or are ineffective. |
| X | Adequate well-controlled or observational studies in animals or pregnant women have demonstrated positive evidence of fetal abnormalities or risks.<br>*The use of the product is contraindicated in women who are or may become pregnant.* |

| | |
|---|---|
| **TABLE 6.6** | Summary of Teratogenicity of Various Medications |

| Drug | Effect |
|---|---|
| Tetracyclines | Yellow-brown discoloration of deciduous teeth has been associated with the use of medications such as doxycycline and minocycline. |
| Sulfonamides | Avoid near delivery due to the risk of hyperbilirubinemia through the displacement of bilirubin from protein-binding sites. |
| Nitrofurantoin | Rare theoretic risk of hemolytic anemia in women with a G6-phosphate dehydrogenase deficiency. For infants under 1 month of age and those with a known G-6-PD deficiency, nitrofurantoin is contraindicated because of potential hemolysis. |
| Quinolones | Associated with irreversible arthropathies and cartilage erosion in animal studies. No teratogenic effects have been demonstrated in animal studies. |
| Metronidazole | Not teratogenic to fetuses exposed in the first trimester |
| Warfarin | Highly teratogenic due to their ability to easily cross the placental barrier. If exposed between weeks 6 and 9, the fetus is at risk of developing a warfarin embryopathy—nasal and midface hypoplasia with stippled vertebral and femoral epiphyses. Later exposure is associated with hemorrhage-related fetal abnormalities, such as hydrocephalus. |
| Heparin and low-molecular weight heparins | Anticoagulant of choice for use in pregnancy. The large, polar molecules do not cross the placenta and, hence, are not teratogenic. The newer low-molecular weight heparins are not associated with fetal malformations. |
| Phenytoin | May produce abnormal facies, cleft lip or palate, microcephaly, growth deficiency, and hypoplastic nails and distal phalanges in as many as 10% of exposed offspring. |
| Valproic acid and carbamazepine | Exposure during embryogenesis is associated with a 1% to 2% risk of spina bifida and neural tube defects. |

*(continued)*

| TABLE 6.6 | Summary of Teratogenicity of Various Medications *(Continued)* |
|---|---|
| **Drug** | **Effect** |
| SSRIs | Paroxetine: Increased risk of ventral and atrial septal cardiac defects<br>All SSRIs: Exposure late in pregnancy associated with a neonatal behavioral syndrome (increased muscle tone, irritability, jitteriness, and respiratory distress) |
| ACE inhibitors | Associated with numerous fetal anomalies, including growth restriction, limb contractures, and abnormalities in cavarum development |
| Diuretics | Thiazide diuretics: When given near delivery, the fetus may experience thrombocytopenia with associated bleeding and electrolyte disturbances<br>All: May interfere with breast milk production |
| Beta blockers | Reported associations with fetal growth restriction and neonatal hypoglycemia; neonates may experience transient mild hypotension with symptomatic beta-blockade |
| Calcium channel Blockers | Generally considered safe during pregnancy |
| Methyldopa and hydralazine | Generally considered safe during pregnancy |
| Alkylating agents | Cyclophosphamide: Associated with missing or hypoplastic digits of the hands and feet when the fetus is exposed in the first trimester; second semester exposure is not associated with defects |
| Methotrexate | Alters normal folic acid metabolism; high doses can lead to growth restriction, severe limb abnormalities, posteriorly rotated ears, micrognathia, and hypoplastic supraorbital ridges |
| Androgens | Exposure to exogenous androgens between 7 and 12 weeks can cause full masculinization, with later exposure causing partial masculinization. |
| Testosterone and anabolic steroids | Can result in varying degrees of virilization, including labioscrotal fusion and phallic enlargement, depending on the timing and extent of exposure |
| Danazol | Dose-related patterns of clitorimegaly, urogenital sinus malformation, and labioscrotal fusion |
| Aspirin and acetaminophen | Aspirin: Theoretical risk of premature closure of the ductus arteriosus<br>Acetaminophen: Not associated with an increased risk of defect |
| NSAIDs | In general, not teratogenic and can be used short-term in the third trimester, with reversible fetal effects<br>Indomethacin: Used as a tocolytic agent; constriction of the fetal ductus arteriosus and neonatal pulmonary hypertension have been associated with the use of indomethacin near delivery |
| Pseudoephedrine | Retrospective study found an increased risk of gastroschisis (a congenital defect of the anterior abdominal wall characterized by an opening beside the umbilical cord that allows bowel to protrude); should be avoided in the first trimester. |
| Benzodiazepines | Teratogenicity is not clearly defined; exposed neonates should be monitored for transient withdrawal symptoms. |
| Lithium | Associated with an increase in cardiovascular malformations, although evidence for a significant increase has been challenged; limiting exposure until after 8 weeks' gestation to allow the cardiac structures to complete organogenesis is reasonable. |
| Vitamin A | Extremely high doses of Vitamin A are associated with congenital anomalies, but categorization is limited by the small number of confirmed cases. |
| Isotretinoin | A potent teratogen; associated with significant fetal loss and malformations with first-trimester use |
| Tretinoin | Topical retinoid gel; information about teratogenicity is lacking; women should avoid during pregnancy |

| TABLE 6.7 | Estimated Fetal Exposure From Some Common Radiologic Procedures | |
|---|---|
| **Procedure** | **Fetal Exposure** |
| CT scan of abdomen and lumbar spine | 3.5 rad |
| Barium enema or small bowel series | 2–4 rad |
| Intravenous pyelography | ≥1 rad |
| CT scan of head or chest | <1 rad |
| CT pelvimetry | 250 rad |
| Hip film (single view) | 200 rad |
| Abdominal film (single view) | 100 cGy |
| Mammography | 7–20 rad |
| Chest x-ray (2 views) | 0.02–0.07 rad |
| Dental x-ray | <0.01 rad |
| Magnetic resonance imaging | 0 |

(Modified from American College of Obstetricians and Gynecologists. *Precis: Obstetrics.* 3rd ed. Washington, DC: American College of Obstetricians and Gynecologists; 2005:14.)

**Fetal alcohol syndrome (FAS)** is a congenital syndrome characterized by alcohol use during pregnancy and by three findings:

1. Growth restriction (which may occur in the prenatal period, the postnatal period, or both)
2. Facial abnormalities, including shortened palpebral fissures, low-set ears, midfacial hypoplasia, a smooth philtrum, and a thin upper lip
3. Central nervous system dysfunction, including microcephaly; mental retardation; and behavioral disorders, such as attention deficit disorder

The exact risk incurred by maternal alcohol use is difficult to establish, because the complex pattern of symptoms associated with FAS can make diagnosis difficult. Consumption of 8 or more drinks daily throughout pregnancy confers a 30% to 50% risk of having a child with FAS. However, even low levels of alcohol consumption (two or fewer drinks per week) have been associated with increased aggressive behavior in children.

## Tobacco Use

The risks of **smoking** during pregnancy have been well-established and include risks to the fetus such as intrauterine growth restriction, low birth weight, and fetal mortality. It is important for the obstetrician to take advantage of the prenatal visits to educate patients about the risks of smoking for both themselves and their newborns and to coordinate appropriate resources to help patients quit. Counseling programs are available to help patients quit smoking. Nicotine replacement products may be considered, although their safety in pregnancy has not been documented.

## Substance Abuse

The use of illicit substances by women of childbearing age has led to an increased number of neonates having had in utero exposure and subsequent risk of adverse effects from a variety of drugs. Fetal drug exposure often is unrecognized because of the lack of overt symptoms or structural anomaly following birth.

Illicit drugs may reach the fetus via placental transfer or may reach the newborn through breast milk. The specific effect on the fetus and newborn varies with the respective substances. An opiate-exposed fetus may experience withdrawal symptoms in utero if the woman stops or when the woman goes through withdrawal, either voluntarily or under supervision, or after birth when the delivery by way of the placenta ceases.

Universal screening, using biologic specimens, of women and newborns for substance abuse is not recommended. However, all pregnant women should be asked at their first prenatal visit about past and present use of alcohol, nicotine, and other drugs, including recreational use of prescription and over-the-counter medications. Use of specific screening questionnaires may improve detection rates. A woman who acknowledges use of these substances should be counseled about the perinatal implications of their use during pregnancy, and offered referral to an appropriate drug-treatment program if chemical dependence is suspected. Careful follow-up during the postpartum period is also recommended.

## COMMON SYMPTOMS

### Headaches

Headaches are common in early pregnancy and may be severe. The etiology of such headaches is not known. Treatment with acetaminophen in usual doses is recommended and is generally adequate. A persistent headache unrelieved by acetaminophen should be further evaluated.

### Edema

The presence of significant **edema** in the lower extremities (dependent edema) and/or hands is very common in pregnancy and, by itself, is not abnormal. Fluid retention can be associated with hypertension, however, so that blood pressure as well as weight gain and edema must be evaluated in a clinical context before the findings are presumed to be innocuous.

### Nausea and Vomiting

The majority of pregnant women experience some degree of upper gastrointestinal symptoms in the first trimester of pregnancy. Classically, these symptoms are worse in the morning (the so-called **morning sickness**). However, patients may experience symptoms at other times or even throughout the day. Most mild cases of nausea and vomiting can be resolved with lifestyle and dietary changes, including consuming more protein, vitamin B$_6$, or vitamin B$_6$ with doxylamine. Usually, nausea and vomiting improve significantly by the end of the first trimester. Effective and safe treatments for more serious cases include *antihistamine H1-receptor blockers and phenothiazines.* The most severe form of pregnancy-associated nausea and vomiting is **hyperemesis gravidum,** which occurs in less than 2% of pregnancies. This condition may require hospitalization, with fluid and electrolyte therapy and medications.

## Heartburn

**Heartburn** (gastric reflux) is common, especially postprandially, and is often associated with eating large meals or spicy or fatty foods. Patient education about smaller and more frequent meals and blander foods, combined with not eating immediately before retiring, is helpful. Antacids may be helpful, used judiciously in pregnancy.

## Constipation

**Constipation** is physiologic in pregnancy, associated with increased transit time, increased water absorption, and often decreased bulk. Dietary modifications, including increased fluid intake and increased bulk with such foods as fruits and vegetables, are usually helpful. Other useful interventions may include use of surface-active bowel softeners such as **docusate,** supplemental dietary fibers such as **psyllium hydrophilic mucilloid,** and lubricants.

## Fatigue

In early pregnancy, patients often complain of extreme **fatigue** that is unrelieved by rest. There is no specific treatment, other than adjustment of the woman's schedule to the extent possible to accommodate this temporary lack of energy. Patients can be reassured that the symptoms disappear in the second trimester.

## Leg Cramps

**Leg cramps,** usually affecting the calves, are common during pregnancy. A variety of treatments, including oral calcium supplement, potassium supplement, or tonic water have been proposed over the years, none of which are universally successful. Massage and rest are often advised.

## Back Pain

Lower back pain is common, especially in late pregnancy. The altered center of gravity caused by the growing fetus places unusual stress on the lower spine and associated muscles and ligaments. Treatment focuses on heat, massage, and limited use of analgesia. A specially fitted maternal girdle may also help, as will not wearing shoes with high heels.

## Round Ligament Pain

Sharp groin pain, especially as pregnancy advances, is common, often quite uncomfortable, and disturbing to patients. This pain is often more pronounced on the right side because of the usual dextrorotation of the gravid uterus. The woman should be reassured that the pain represents stretching and spasm of the round ligaments. Modification of activity, especially more gradual movement, is often helpful; analgesics are rarely indicated.

## Varicose Veins and Hemorrhoids

Varicose veins are not caused by pregnancy, but often first appear during the course of gestation. Besides the disturbing appearance to many patients, varicose veins can cause an aching sensation, especially when patients stand for long periods of time. A support hose can help diminish the discomfort, although it has no effect on the appearance of the varicose veins. Popular brands of support hose do not provide the relief that prescription elastic hose can. **Hemorrhoids** are varicosities of the hemorrhoidal veins. Treatment consists of sitz baths and local preparations. Varicose veins and hemorrhoids regress postpartum, although neither condition may abate completely. Surgical correction of varicose veins or hemorrhoids should not be undertaken for approximately the first 6 months postpartum to allow for the natural involution to occur.

## Vaginal Discharge

The hormonal milieu of pregnancy often causes an increase in normal vaginal secretions. These normal secretions must be distinguished from infections such as vaginitis, which has symptoms of itching and malodor, and bacterial vaginosis, which has been linked to preterm labor. Spontaneous rupture of membranes, which is characterized by leakage of thin, clear fluid, is another possible cause that must be considered.

## SUGGESTED READINGS

American College of Obstetricians and Gynecologists. Exercise during pregnancy and the postpartum period. ACOG Committee Opinion No. 267. *Obstet Gynecol.* 2002;99(1):171–173.

American College of Obstetricians and Gynecologists. Guidelines for diagnostic imaging during pregnancy. ACOG Committee Opinion No. 299. *Obstet Gynecol.* 2004;104(3):647–651.

American College of Obstetricians and Gynecologists. Immunization during pregnancy. ACOG Committee Opinion No. 282. *Obstet Gynecol.* 2003;101(1):207–212.

American College of Obstetricians and Gynecologists. Management of postterm pregnancy. ACOG Practice Bulletin No. 55. *Obstet Gynecol.* 2004;104(3):639–646.

American College of Obstetricians and Gynecologists. Nausea and vomiting of pregnancy. ACOG Practice Bulletin No. 52. *Obstet Gynecol.* 2004;103(4):803–815.

American College of Obstetricians and Gynecologists. Obesity in pregnancy. ACOG Committee Opinion No. 315. *Obstet Gynecol.* 2005;106(3):671–675.

American College of Obstetricians and Gynecologists. Prenatal and perinatal human immunodeficiency virus testing: expanded recommendations. ACOG Committee Opinion No. 304. *Obstet Gynecol.* 2004;104(5):1119–1124.

American College of Obstetricians and Gynecologists. Psychosocial risk factors: perinatal screening and intervention. ACOG Committee Opinion No. 343. *Obstet Gynecol.* 2006;108(2): 469–477.

American College of Obstetricians and Gynecologists. Rubella vaccination. ACOG Committee Opinion No. 281. *Obstet Gynecol.* 2002;100(6):1417.

American College of Obstetricians and Gynecologists Screening for fetal chromosomal abnormalities. ACOG Practice Bulletin No. 77. *Obstet Gynecol.* 2007;109(1):217–227.

American College of Obstetricians and Gynecologists. Smoking cessation during pregnancy. ACOG Committee Opinion No. 316. *Obstet Gynecol.* 2005;106(4):883–888.

American College of Obstetricians and Gynecologists. The importance of preconception care in the continuum of women's health care. ACOG Committee Opinion No. 313. *Obstet Gynecol.* 2005; 106(3):665–666.

*Antepartum Fetal Surveillance.* ACOG Practice Bulletin No. 9. Washington, DC: American College of Obstetricians and Gynecologists; 1999.

*Assessment of Fetal Lung Maturity.* ACOG Educational Bulletin No. 230. Washington, DC: American College of Obstetricians and Gynecologists; 1996.

*Fetal Macrosomia.* ACOG Practice Bulletin No. 22. American College of Obstetricians and Gynecologists; 2000.

# Assessment of Genetic Disorders in Obstetrics and Gynecology

By acquiring a basic knowledge of reproductive genetics, the learner will be able to better understand patterns of inheritance, learn the principles of prenatal testing and its application to the diagnosis of fetal anomalies.

Recent discoveries in the field of genetics have led to the increased use of genetic principles and techniques in all areas of medicine, including obstetrics and gynecology. In obstetrics, prenatal screening is routinely performed to detect genetic disorders such as Down syndrome and cystic fibrosis. In gynecology, clinicians can offer appropriate genetic testing for women deemed at high risk for genes that increase the risk of breast, bowel, and ovarian cancers. In the future, genetic evaluation may lead to earlier and more accurate diagnosis of conditions such as diabetes. Gene-based therapies may also be used to treat diseases with greater specificity and fewer side effects than conventional treatments.

## BASIC CONCEPTS IN GENETICS

Knowledge of the basic principles of genetics and an understanding of their application are essential in current medical practice. These principles form the basis for screening, diagnosis, and management of genetic disorders.

### Genes: Definition and Function

**Genes,** the basic units of heredity, are segments of deoxyribonucleic acid (**DNA**) that reside on **chromosomes** located in cell nuclei. DNA is a double-stranded helical molecule. Each strand is a polymer of nucleotides made up of three components: (1) a "base," which is either a purine (adenine [A] or guanine [G]) or a pyrimidine (cytosine [C] or thymine [T]); (2) a 5-carbon sugar; and (3) a phosphodiester bond. The strands of the DNA helix run in an antiparallel fashion, adenine binding to thymine and cytosine binding to guanine. These base pairs, in their nearly limitless combinations, constitute the **genetic code.**

The information in the DNA must be processed before it can be used by cells. **Transcription** is the process by which DNA is converted to a messenger molecule called ribonucleic acid (**RNA**). During transcription, the DNA molecule is "read" from one end (called the 5-prime [5′] end) to other end (called the 3-prime [3′] end). A **messenger RNA (mRNA)** molecule is formed that is exported from the cell nucleus into the cytoplasm. This mRNA contains a translation of the genetic code into "**codons.**" Transcription is regulated by promoter and enhancer sequences. **Promotor** sequences guide the direction of translation, from 5′ to 3′, and are located on the 5′ end. **Enhancer** sequences have the same function, but are found further down the 5′ end of the DNA molecule.

After transcription is complete, mRNA is used as a template to construct the amino acids that are the building blocks of proteins. In this process, called **translation,** each codon is matched to its corresponding amino acid. The amino acid strand grows until a "stop" codon is encountered. At this point, the now completed protein undergoes further processing and is then either used inside the cell or is exported outside the cell for use in other cells, tissues, and organs. Errors in the DNA replication process can occur in a variety of ways and lead to a **mutation,** a change in the normal gene sequence. Most DNA replication errors are rapidly repaired by enzymes that proofread and repair mistakes.

Replication errors are of four basic kinds: (1) **missense** mutations, in which one amino acid is substituted for another; (2) **nonsense** mutations, in which premature stop codons are inserted in a sequence; (3) **deletions;** and (4) **insertions.** An example of a replication error causing a recognized disease is Huntington disease, in which an abnormal number of CAG repeats occurs in the Huntington gene. DNA can also be damaged by environmental factors, such as ultraviolet light, ionizing radiation, or chemicals.

### Chromosomes

The genetic information in the human genome is packaged as **chromatin,** within which DNA binds with several chromosomal proteins to make **chromosomes.** A **karyotype** reveals the morphology and number of chromosomes. **Somatic cells** are all the cells in the human body that are not gametes (eggs or sperm). **Germ cells,** or gametes, contain a *single set* of chromosomes (*n* = 23) and are described as **haploid** in number. Somatic cells contain *two sets of chromosomes,* for a total of 46 chromosomes. These cells are **diploid,** signifying that they have a 2n chromosome complement (2n = 46). These chromosome pairs consist of 22 pairs of **autosomes,** which are similar in males and females. Each somatic cell also contains a pair of sex chromosomes. Females have two X sex chromosomes; males have an X and a Y chromosome.

### CHROMOSOME REPLICATION AND CELL DIVISION

Chromosomes undergo two types of **replication,** meiosis and mitosis, which are significantly different and produce cell types with crucially different capabilities. **Mitosis** is the replication of chromosomes in somatic cells. It is followed by **cytokinesis,** or cell division, that results in two daughter cells containing the same genetic information as the parent cell. **Meiosis** only occurs in germ cells. It is also followed by cytokinesis; but, in this case, cytokinesis results in four daughter cells with a haploid count.

   Somatic cells undergo cell division based on the cell cycle. There are four stages of the cell cycle: G1, S, G2, and M. G1, or gap 1, occurs immediately after mitosis and is a period of inactivity with no DNA replication. During **G1** all the DNA of each chromosome is present in the 2n form. The next phase is **S,** or synthesis, where the chromosomes double to become two identical sister chromatids with a 4n chromosome complement. During **G2,** or gap 2, the cells prepare for mitosis. G1, S, and G2 are also called **interphase,** which is the period between mitoses.

### *Mitosis*

The goal of mitosis is to form two daughter cells that have a complete set of genetic information. Mitosis is divided into five stages: prophase, prometaphase, metaphase, anaphase, and telophase. During **prophase** the chromatin swells, or condenses, and the two sister chromatids are in close approximation. The nucleolus disappears, and the mitotic spindle develops. Spindle fibers start to form centrosomes, microtubule-organizing centers that migrate to the poles of the cell. In **prometaphase** the nuclear membrane vanishes and the chromosomes begin to disperse. They will eventually attach to the microtubules that form the mitotic spindle. **Metaphase** is the stage of maximal condensation. The chromosomes are in a linear formation in the center of the cell, between the two spindle poles. It is during metaphase where cells can most easily be analyzed to obtain a karyotype from an amniocentesis or chorionic villus sampling (CVS). **Anaphase** is initiated when the two chromatids separate. They form daughter chromosomes that are drawn to opposite poles of the cell by the spindle fibers. Finally, **telophase** is when the nuclear membrane starts to reform around the independent daughter cells, which then go into interphase (Fig. 7.1).

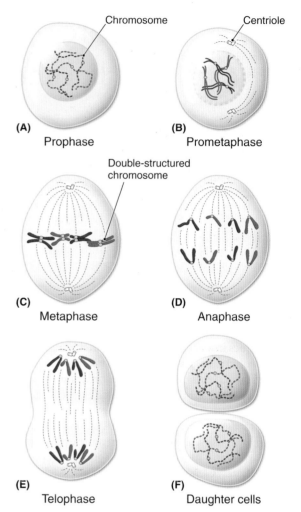

FIGURE 7.1. Stages of mitosis. (Modified from Sadler TW. *Langman's Medical Embryology.* 10th ed. Baltimore, MD: Lippincott Williams & Wilkins; 2006:12.)

### *Meiosis*

**Meiosis** differs from mitosis in that a haploid number of cells are initially produced in two successive divisions. ***The first division (meiosis I)*** *is termed a reduction division, because of the resulting decrease in chromosome number from diploid to haploid.* Meiosis I is also divided into four stages: prophase I, metaphase I, anaphase I, and telophase I. **Prophase I** is further divided into five substages: leptotene, zygotene, pachytene, diplotene, and diakinesis. In prophase I the chromosomes condense and become shorter and thicker. It is during the pachytene substage that **crossing over** takes place, resulting in four distinct gametes. However, it is during anaphase where most of the genetic variation occurs. In **anaphase I** the chromosomes go to opposite poles of the cell by **independent assortment,** signifying that there are $2^{23}$, or >8 million, possible variations. *Anaphase I is also the most error-prone step in meiosis.* The process of **disjunction,** where the chromosomes go to opposite poles of the cell, can result in nondisjunction, where both chromosomes go instead to the same pole. *Nondisjunction is a common cause of chromosomally abnormal fetuses.*

The **second meiotic division (meiosis II)** *is similar to mitosis, except that the process occurs within a cell with a haploid number of chromosomes.* Meiosis II is also divided into four stages: prophase II, metaphase II, anaphase II, and telophase II. The result of meiosis II is four haploid daughter cells. After anaphase II, the possibilities for genetic variation are further increased by $2^{23} \times 2^{23}$, ensuring genetic variation (Fig. 7.2).

## ABNORMALITIES IN CHROMOSOME NUMBER

*Any alteration in the chromosome number is called **heteroploidy**.* Heteroploidy can occur in two forms: euploidy and aneuploidy. In **euploidy,** the haploid number of 23 chromosomes is altered. An example of euploidy is triploidy, in which the haploid number has been multiplied by 3. The karyotype is 69,XXX or 69,XXY. Triploidy results from double fertilization of a normal haploid egg or from fertilization by a diploid sperm. Such abnormalities usually result in conceptions of partial hydatidiform moles and end spontaneously in the first trimester.

In **aneuploidy,** the diploid number of 46 chromosomes is altered. The **trisomies** are aneuploidies in which there are three copies of an autosome instead of two. Examples include **trisomy 21 (Down syndrome) trisomy 18 (Edward syndrome) trisomy 13 (Patau syndrome),** and **trisomy 16.** Most trisomies result from maternal meiotic nondisjunction, a phenomenon that occurs more frequently as a woman ages (Fig. 7.3 and Table 7.1).

Sex chromosome abnormalities occur in 1 of every 1000 births. The most common are 45,X; 47,XXY; 47,XXX; 47,XYY; and mosaicism (the presence of 2 or more cell populations with different karyotypes). Numeric sex chromosome abnormalities can result from either maternal or paternal nondisjunction.

## ABNORMALITIES IN CHROMOSOME STRUCTURE

Structural alterations in chromosomes are less common than numerical alterations. Structural abnormalities that

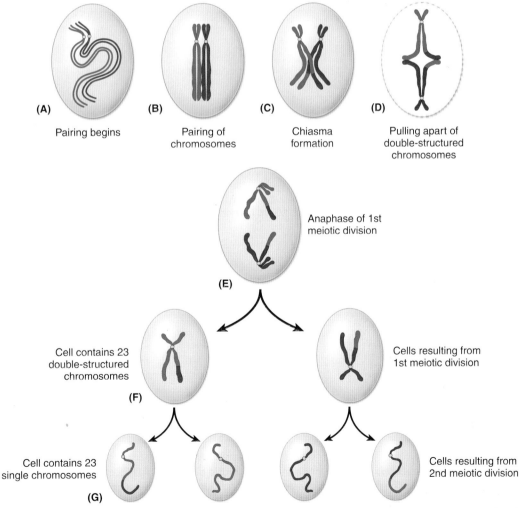

FIGURE 7.2. Stages of meiosis. (Modified from Sadler TW. *Langman's Medical Embryology.* 10th ed. Baltimore, MD: Lippincott Williams & Wilkins; 2006:13.)

| TABLE 7.1 | Commonly Diagnosed Chromosomal Abnormalities | |
| --- | --- | --- |
| **Chromosome Abnormality** | **Live Birth Incidence** | **Characteristics** |
| Trisomy 21 (Down syndrome) | 1:800 | Moderate to severe mental retardation; characteristic facies; cardiac abnormalities; increased incidence of respiratory infections and leukemia; only 2% live beyond 50 years |
| Trisomy 18 (Edwards syndrome) | 1:8000 | Severe mental retardation; multiple organic abnormalities; less than 10% survive 1 year |
| Trisomy 13 (Patau syndrome) | 1:20,000 | Severe mental retardation; neurologic, ophthalmologic, and organic abnormalities; 5% survive 3 years |
| Trisomy 16 | 0 | Lethal anomaly occurs frequently in first-trimester spontaneous abortions; no infants are known to have trisomy 16 |
| 45,X | 1:10,000 | Occurs frequently in first-trimester (Turner syndrome) sponta-neous abortions; associated primarily with unique somatic features; patients are not mentally retarded, although IQs of affected individuals are lower than those of siblings |
| 47,XXX; 47,XYY; 47,XXY (Klinefelter syndrome) | Each approximately 1:900 | Minimal somatic abnormalities; individuals with Klinefelter syndrome are characterized by a tall, eunuchoid habitus and small testes; 47,XXX and 47,XYY individuals do not usually exhibit somatic abnormalities, but 47,XYY individuals may be tall |
| del(5p) | 1:20,000 | Severe mental retardation, microcephaly, distinctive facial features, characteristic "cat's cry" sound (cri du chat syndrome) |

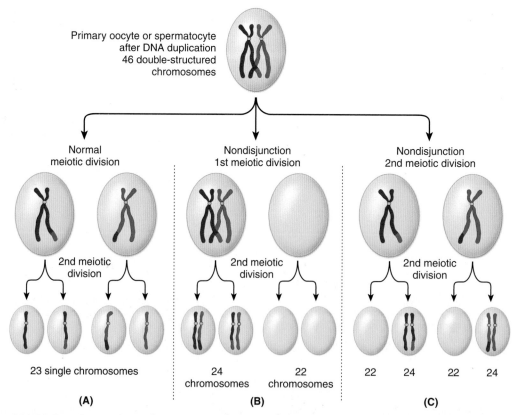

FIGURE 7.3. Comparison of normal and abnormal meiotic divisions. (A) Normal meiotic division. (B) Nondisjunction in the first meiotic division. (C) Nondisjunction in the second meiotic division. (Modified from Sadler TW. *Langman's Medical Embryology*. 10th ed. Baltimore, MD: Lippincott Williams & Wilkins; 2006:15.)

| TABLE 7.2 | Abnormalities in Chromosome Structure | |
|---|---|---|

| Abnormality in Chromosome Structure | Definition | Clinical Example |
|---|---|---|
| Deletion | Loss of a chromosome segment resulting in imbalance | Duchenne muscular dystrophy |
| Insertion | A segment removed from one chromosome is inserted into another | Hemophilia A |
| Inversion | A single chromosome has two breaks with reattachment in an inverted fashion | Inv(9); most common; no clinical sequelae |
| Robertsonian translocation | Loss of the short arm of two acrocentric chromosomes; the acrocentric chromosomes are 13, 14, 15, 21, and 22 | t(14q21q); one of the possible causes of Down syndrome |
| Reciprocal translocation | Breakage of nonhomologous chromosomes with a reciprocal exchange | Common (1 in 600 newborns); usually harmless |

affect reproduction occur in 0.2% of the population. A **deletion** occurs when a portion of a chromosome segment is lost (Table 7.2). In a **terminal deletion,** the missing portion of the chromosome is appended to the end of the long or short arm. If the missing portion of the chromosome is appended to both the long and short arms of the same chromosome, a **ring chromosome** can result. An **interstitial deletion** occurs when the deleted portion lacks a centromere, or in cases involving chromosomal breakage. **Insertions** occur when the portion of an interstitially deleted segment is inserted into a nonhomologous chromosome.

An **inversion** is the result of faulty repair of a chromosomal breakage. The broken portion is inserted into the chromosome in an inverted fashion. A **paracentric inversion** occurs when both breaks occur on one arm of a chromosome. These types of inversions do not include the **centromere,** the region where the chromosome pairs are joined. Paracentric inversions cannot be identified by a traditional karyotype because the arms appear to be of normal length. Fluorescence in situ hybridization (FISH) [see p. X] with locus-specific probes is used to detect this type of abnormality. A **pericentric inversion** involves a break in each arm. The centromere is included and a notable gain or loss of genetic material can be identified on a karyotype. For a parent with an inversion, the risk of having an abnormal child depends on the method of detection, the chromosome involved, and the size of the inversion. The observed risk is approximately 5% to 10% if the inversion is identified after the birth of an abnormal child, and 1% to 3% if identified at some other time. An exception is pericentric inversion of chromosome 9, which is not associated with genetic defects in offspring.

A **translocation** involves the transfer of two chromosome segments, usually between nonhomologous (non-paired) chromosomes. They are the most common form of structural rearrangements in humans. A translocation is described as **balanced** when equal amounts of genetic material are exchanged between chromosomes, and **unbalanced** when the chromosomes receive unequal amounts of genetic material. Two types of translocations are possible. A **Robertsonian translocation** only occurs in acrocentric chromosomes—those in which the centromere is located very near one end (chromosomes 13, 14, 15, 21, and 22). A person with a Robertsonian translocation is phenotypically normal, but the gametes they produce may be unbalanced. Whether the unbalanced gametes will result in abnormal offspring depends on the type of translocation, the chromosomes involved, and the sex of the carrier parent. The most clinically important Robertsonian translocations are those involving chromosome 21 and another acrocentric chromosome, most commonly chromosome 14. Carriers of these translocations are at increased risk of having a child with trisomy 21. The risk of trisomy 21 is 15% if the translocation is maternal and 2% or less if it is paternal.

**Balanced reciprocal translocations** may involve any chromosome and are the result of a reciprocal exchange of chromosome material between two or more chromosomes. Like those with Robertsonian translocations, individuals with a balanced reciprocal translocation are also phenotypically normal but may produce gametes with unbalanced chromosomes. The observed risk for a chromosomal abnormality in an offspring is less than the theoretical risk, because some of these gametes result in nonviable conceptions. In general, carriers of chromosome translocations identified after the birth of an abnormal child have a 5% to 30% risk of having unbalanced offspring. Children with an unbalanced chromosome translocation are at increased risk for mental retardation, neurodevelopmental delay, and other congenital abnormalities.

## Patterns of Inheritance

**Single-gene (Mendelian) disorders** display predictable patterns of inheritance related to the location of the gene (autosomal or X-linked) and the expression of the phenotype (dominant or recessive). Although Mendelian disorders were the first type of genetic disorders described, it is now known that there are many genetic and environmental factors that modify these genes, making true single-gene disorders relatively rare. Health care providers should be aware that many single-gene disorders are discovered each year and may be tracked using Internet databases, such as *Online Mendelian Inheritance in Man* (http://www.nslij-genetics.org/search_omim.html).

### AUTOSOMAL DOMINANT

Each gene occupies a specific position, or **locus,** on a chromosome. At each locus, there are two possible variations of the genes, or two **alleles.** If the phenotype of a disease is based on one allele in a gene pair, the gene is **dominant.** If the gene is located on an autosomal cell, its pattern of inheritance is described as **autosomal dominant.** Individuals with one dominant allele for a disorder (described as being **heterozygous** for the gene) will express disease and transmit the gene to 50% of their offspring (Box 7.1). Examples

---

### BOX 7.1
### Patterns of Inheritance

#### Characteristics of Autosomal Dominant Disorders
- Gene expression rarely skips a generation.
- An affected individual will transmit the gene to progeny 50% of the time.
- There should be equal sex distribution among affected relatives; males should be able to transmit to males and females to females.
- An unaffected first-degree relative will not transmit the gene to his or her progeny.

#### Characteristics of Autosomal Recessive Disorders
- Gene expression may appear to skip generations.
- Both males and females are affected.
- Neither parent is usually affected; affected individuals usually do not have affected children.
- If one parent is a carrier, half of the offspring will be carriers of the gene. If both parents are carriers, the risk of transmission of the disorder is 25%.
- If the suspected disorder is noted to be rare, consanguinity should be suspected.

---

of genetic disorders with autosomal dominant inheritance include Marfan syndrome, achondroplasia, and Huntington disease.

Phenotypic expression of autosomal dominant genes is not always straightforward and may vary depending on specific characteristics of the gene. **Variable expressivity** is the varying expression of a disease in an affected person. For example, some individuals with **neurofibromatosis** have only a few café au lait spots, whereas others have large tumors. Neurofibromatosis, however, demonstrates 100% penetrance. **Penetrance** describes the likelihood that a person carrying the gene will be affected. Retinoblastoma is an example of incomplete penetrance; not all affected individuals will express any obvious form of disease. **Anticipation** refers to an increase in severity and earlier expression of disease with each subsequent generation. An example of a genetic mutation that shows anticipation is Huntington disease, where an expansion of the trinucleotide repeat, CAG, leads to earlier expression of the disease in affected offspring.

### AUTOSOMAL RECESSIVE

An **autosomal recessive** *disease is only expressed when the affected individual carries two copies of the gene (described as being* **homozygous** *for the gene) (see Box 7.1). Individuals who are* **heterozygous** *for the gene express a normal phenotype.* During pregnancy, unless a woman has been screened for a particular disease based on her risk factors (e.g., sickle cell disease or cystic fibrosis), carriers of a recessive gene will not know they are carriers until they have affected offspring. Other examples of autosomal recessive disorders include Tay-Sachs disease and phenylketonuria.

### X-LINKED INHERITANCE

In **X-linked diseases,** the affected gene is located on the X chromosome. Because males only have one X chromosome, they will manifest disease if their X chromosome carries the affected gene. The male carrier status is considered **hemizygous,** while the female is almost always heterozygous.

X-linked recessive diseases are much more common than X-linked dominant diseases (Box 7.2). Some examples of X-linked recessive diseases are hemophilia and color blindness. Hypophosphatemia is an example of an X-linked dominant disease.

**Fragile X syndrome** is an X-linked disorder that causes mental retardation. It is caused by a repeat in the cytosine-guanine-guanine sequence in a specific gene located on the X chromosome. Transmission of the disease-producing genetic mutation to a fetus depends on the sex of the parent and the number of repeats in the parental gene. If the number of repeats is between 61 and 200, the individual is said to have a "premutation." These individuals are phenotypically normal, although women carrying the premutation are at increased risk for premature ovarian failure. A full mutation is characterized by more than 200 repeats. These individuals display the signs and symptoms of the disorder.

A male may transmit the unexpanded premutation gene to his offspring, but expansion to the full mutation is rare in a male with the premutation gene. A female with a premutation gene may also transmit the gene to her offspring; however, the premutation gene may expand during meiosis and result in a full mutation. Women with a family history of boys with developmental delay, extreme hyperactivity, and speech and language problems should be offered fragile X carrier testing. Women with ovarian failure or an elevated follicle-stimulating hormone level before 40 years of age without a known cause should be screened to determine whether they have the fragile X premutation.

### MITOCHONDRIAL INHERITANCE

**Mitochondrial inheritance** is different from other patterns of inheritance. Mitochondria contain unique DNA (called mitochondrial DNA) that differs from the DNA carried in the cell nucleus. Any mutations in this DNA are only transmitted from the mother to all of her offspring and, if a male fetus is affected, he will not pass it on to any of his offspring.

### MULTIFACTORIAL INHERITANCE

**Multifactorial disorders** are caused by a combination of factors, some genetic and some nongenetic (i.e., environ-mental). Multifactorial disorders recur in families, but are not transmitted in any distinctive pattern. Many congenital, single-organ system structural abnormalities are multifactorial, having an incidence in the general population of approximately 1 per 1000. Examples of multifactorial traits are cleft lip, with or without cleft palate; congenital cardiac defects; neural tube defects; and hydrocephalus.

### RISK FACTORS FOR GENETIC DISORDERS

Several factors have been identified that increase the risk of having a child with a chromosomal abnormality, including maternal or paternal age and exposure to certain drugs. Other factors, such as ethnicity or a family history of a disease, may indicate that an individual carries a gene for a Mendelian disorder. The first step in assessing risk is to document information about the patient's family and personal history (see Appendix 1, Antepartum Record). This record is an effective method for obtaining information concerning personal and family medical history, parental exposure to potentially harmful substances, or other issues that may have an impact on risk assessment and management. This information can be collected prior to conception during a preconception office visit, or during the first prenatal visit in the first trimester.

Some infectious diseases, including cytomegalovirus, rubella, and sexually transmitted diseases (see Chapter 15, Infectious Diseases in Pregnancy), as well as certain drugs (see Chapter 6, Preconception and Antepartum Care) have been linked to an increased risk of birth defects. Preexisting diabetes mellitus may also predispose a fetus to a congenital anomaly. Because these defects are not gene-based, family history and genetic testing procedures, such as amniocentesis or CVS, cannot be used to detect these abnormalities. Ultrasonography is the mainstay of surveillance for infectious and teratogen-induced congenital abnormalities.

### Advanced Maternal Age

The incidence of trisomy 21 (Down syndrome) among newborns of 35-year-old women is 1:385. Although the risk increases with age, the majority of cases of Down syndrome occur in women younger than 35 years of age (Fig. 7.4). In addition to Down syndrome, other chromosomal abnormalities increase in frequency with advanced maternal age (see Table 7.1).

### Previous Pregnancy Affected by Chromosomal Abnormality

Women who have had a previous pregnancy complicated by trisomy 21, 18, or 13 or any other trisomy in which the fetus survived at least to the second trimester, are at risk of having another pregnancy complicated by the same or different trisomy. The risk of trisomy recurrence is 1.6 to

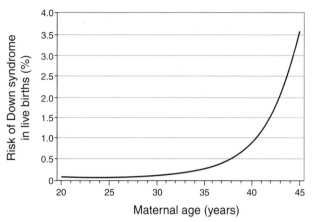

FIGURE 7.4. Estimated risk of Down syndrome according to maternal age. From Newberger DS. Down syndrome: prenatal risk assessment and diagnosis. *Am Fam Physician.* 2000;62(4):825. http://www.aafp.org/afp/20000815/825. html. Accessed October 20, 2008. Data from Cuckle HS, Wald NJ, Thompson SG. Estimating a woman's risk of having a pregnancy associated with Down's syndrome using her age and serum alpha-fetoprotein level. *Br J Obstet Gynaecol.* 1987;94(5):387–402.

8.2 times the maternal age risk, depending on several factors: the type of trisomy, whether the index pregnancy was a spontaneous abortion, maternal age at initial occurrence, and maternal age at subsequent prenatal diagnosis.

Some, but not all, sex-chromosome abnormalities carry an increased risk of recurrence. A pregnancy complicated by fetal XXX or XXY increases the recurrence risk by 1.6% to 2.5% the maternal age risk. Turner syndrome (monosomy X; XO) and XYY karyotypes impart a nominal risk of recurrence.

## History of Early Pregnancy Loss

At least half of all first-trimester pregnancy losses result from fetal chromosomal abnormalities. The most common are monosomy X; polyploidy (triploidy or tetraploidy); and trisomies 13, 16, 18, 21, and 22.

## Advanced Paternal Age

Increasing paternal age, particularly after age 50 years, predisposes the fetus to an increase in gene mutations that can affect X-linked recessive and autosomal dominant disorders, such as neurofibromatosis, achondroplasia, Apert syndrome, and Marfan syndrome.

## Ethnicity

Many Mendelian disorders occur more frequently in certain groups. African Americans are at increased risk of sickle

cell disease, the most common hemoglobinopathy in the United States. Approximately 8% of African Americans carry the sickle hemoglobin gene, which is also found with increased frequency in those of Mediterranean, Caribbean, Latin American, or Middle Eastern descent. Caucasians of Northern European descent are at increased risk of cystic fibrosis, with an estimated carrier percentage of 1 in 22. Tay-Sachs, Gaucher, and Niemann-Pick diseases occur with greater frequency in individuals of Ashkenazi Jewish descent. Other diseases associated with certain ethnic groups are β-thalassemia, found at increased frequency in individuals of Mediterranean origin and α-thalassemia in individuals of Asian origin.

## PRENATAL SCREENING

Obstetricians are responsible for determining if a woman is at increased risk for fetal abnormalities, and for describing and offering appropriate prenatal screening or diagnostic tests. *The purpose of prenatal genetic screening is to define the risk for a genetic disease in a low-risk population.* A **screening test** differs from a **diagnostic test** in that *screening tests only assess the risk that a child will have a genetic disease; they cannot confirm or rule out the presence of the disease. A diagnostic test is given if a screening test is positive, to assess whether the disease is present or absent in the developing fetus.* Genetic screening tests are routinely offered to all women to detect neural tube defects (NTDs), Down syndrome, and trisomy 18. In addition, individuals of certain ethnic groups can be tested to detect whether they carry a gene for a particular disorder.

## First-Trimester Screening

First-trimester screening tests are used to assess the risk of Down syndrome, trisomy 18, and trisomy 13 in a developing fetus. First-semester serum screening for Down syndrome consists of tests for levels of two biochemical markers: free or total **human chorionic gonadotropin (hCG)** and **pregnancy-associated plasma protein A (PAPP-A).** An elevated level of hCG (1.98 of the median observed in euploid pregnancies [MoM]) and a decreased level of PAPP-A (0.43 MoM) have been associated with Down syndrome. An ultrasonographic marker for Down syndrome is the size of the **nuchal transparency** (NT), a fluid collection at the back of the fetal neck that can be seen between 10 and 14 weeks of gestation (Fig. 7.5). An increase in the size of the NT between 10 4/7 and 13 6/7 weeks of gestation is recognized to be an early presenting feature of a variety of chromosomal, genetic, and structural abnormalities. When used alone, NT measurement has a detection rate for Down syndrome of 64% to 70%. Combining NT measurement with the other first-trimester biochemical markers yields an 82% to 87% detection rate of Down syndrome, with a 5% false-positive rate, which

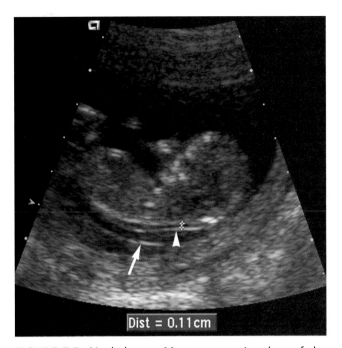

FIGURE 7.5. Nuchal area. Measurement is taken of the lucent area in the posterior neck (calipers), with the posterior caliper placed just inside the echogenic skin (arrowhead). The amnion (arrow) should not be mistaken for the skin. (From Doubilet PM, Benson CB. *Atlas of Ultrasound in Obstetrics and Gynecology.* Philadelphia, PA: Lippincott Williams & Wilkins; 2003:10f.)

is equal to or higher than second-trimester screening tests. Women found to have increased risk with first-trimester screening tests should be offered genetic counseling and the option of invasive fetal testing CVS in the first trimester or amniocentesis in the second trimester).

*An advantage of first-trimester screening is that the tests are performed early enough so that decisions can be made regarding continuing the pregnancy, if necessary* (Table 7.3). Disadvantages include the need for specialized training and appropriate ultrasound equipment to achieve optimal NT measurement and the availability of CVS. Detecting pregnancies at high risk for Down syndrome in the first trimester is of low utility if a diagnostic invasive test, i.e., CVS, cannot be performed to verify the findings.

Several other first-trimester ultrasonographic findings have been evaluated as potential markers for aneuploidy in the first trimester. Discovery of a structural malformation of a major fetal organ or structure (Table 7.4) or the finding of two or more minor malformations (e.g., choroid plexus cyst, extra digit, and single umbilical artery) increases the risk of aneuploidy sufficiently to warrant genetic testing of the fetus, regardless of maternal age or parental karyotype.

## Second-Trimester Screening

Second-trimester screening may be the only option if a woman is seen for the first time during the second trimester

| TABLE 7.3 | Down Syndrome Screening Tests and Detection Rates (5% Positive-Screen Rate) | |
| --- | --- |
| **Screening Test** | **Detection Rate (%)** |
| *First Trimester* | |
| NT measurement | 64–70* |
| NT measurement, PAPP-A, free or total β-hCG[†] | 82–87* |
| *Second Trimester* | |
| Triple screen (MSAFP, hCG, unconjugated estriol) | 69* |
| Quadruple screen (MSAFP, hCG, unconjugated estriol, inhibin A) | 81* |
| *First Plus Second Trimester* | |
| Integrated (NT, PAPP-A, quad screen) | 94–96* |
| Serum integrated (PAPP-A, quad screen) | 85–88* |
| Stepwise sequential | 95* |
| Contingent sequential | 88–94[‡] |

hCG = human chorionic gonadotropin; MSAFP = maternal serum alpha-fetoprotein; NT = nuchal translucency; PAPP-A = pregnancy-associated plasma protein A; quad = quadruple.
*From the FASTER trial (Malone F, Canick JA, Ball RH, Nyberg DA, Comstock CH, Buckowski R, et al; First- and Second-Trimester Evaluation of Risk (FASTER) Research Consortium. First-trimester or second-trimester screening, or both, for Down's syndrome. *N Engl J Med.* 2005;353(1):2001–2011. http://content.nejm.org/cgi/content/full/353/19/2001. Accessed October 20, 2008.)
[†]Also referred to as combined first-trimester screen
[‡]Modeled predicted detection rates (Cuckle H, Benn P, Wright D. Down syndrome screening in the first and/or second trimester: model predicted performance using meta-analysis parameters. *Semin Perinatol* 2005;29:252–257.)
From American College of Obstetricians and Gynecologists. Screening for fetal chromosomal abnormalities. ACOG Practice Bulletin 77. *Obstet Gynecol.* 2007;109(2):217–228.

**TABLE 7.4  Aneuploid Risk of Major Anomalies**

| Structural Defect | Population Incidence | Risk | Most Common Aneuploidy |
|---|---|---|---|
| Cystic hygroma | 1/120 EU–1/6000 B | 60–75% | 45X (80%) |
| Hydrops | 1/1500–1400 B | 30–80%* | 21, 18, 13, XXY |
| Hydrocephalus | 3–8/10,000 LB | 3–8% | 13, 21, 18, 45X |
| Hydranencephaly | 2/1000 IA | Minimal | 13, 18, triploidy |
| Holoprosencephaly | 1/16,000 LB | 40–60% | 13, 18, 18p- |
| Cardiac defects | 7–9/1000 LB | 5–30% | 21, 18, 13, 22, 8, 9 |
| Complete atrioventricular canal | | 40–70% | 21 |
| Diaphragmatic hernia | 1/3500–4000 LB | 20–25% | 13, 18, 21, 45X |
| Omphalocele | 1/5000 LB | 30–40% | 13, 18 |
| Gastroschisis | 1/10,000–15,000 LB | Minimal | |
| Duodenal atresia | 1/10,000 LB | 20–30% | 21 |
| Bladder outlet obstruction | 1–2/1000 LB | 20–25% | 13, 18 |
| Facial cleft | 1/700 | 1% | 13, 18, deletions |
| Limb reduction | 4–6/10,000 LB | 8% | 18 |
| Club foot | 1.2/1000 LB | 6% | 18, 13, 4p-, 18p- |
| Single umbilical artery | 1% | Minimal | |

Abbreviations: B, birth; EU, early ultrasonography; LB, livebirth; IA, infant autopsy
*30% if diagnosed at 24 weeks of gestation or later, 80% if diagnosed at 17 weeks of gestation or earlier
Data from Shipp TD, Benacerraf BR. The significance of prenatally identified isolated clubfoot: is amniocentesis indicated? *Am J Obstet Gynecol.* 1998;178(3): 600–602; and Nyberg DA, Crane JP. Chromosome abnormalities. In: Nyberg DA, Mahony BS, Pretorius DH. *Diagnostic Ultrasound of Fetal Anomalies: Text and Atlas.* Chicago, IL: Year Book Medical; 1990: 676–724.
From American College of Obstetricians and Gynecologists. Invasive prenatal testing for aneuploidy. ACOG Practice Bulletin 88. *Obstet Gynecol.* 2007;110(6):1459–1467.

of her pregnancy. Women who have had first-trimester screening for aneuploidy should not undergo independent second-trimester serum screening in the same pregnancy. When these test results are interpreted independently, the false-positive rates are additive, leading to many more unnecessary invasive procedures (11% to 17%). After first-trimester screening, subsequent second-trimester Down syndrome screening is not indicated, unless it is being performed as a component of an integrated test (explained below), stepwise sequential, or contingent sequential test.

TRIPLE AND QUADRUPLE SCREENING TESTS

An association between low maternal serum **alpha-fetoprotein (AFP)** levels and Down syndrome was reported in 1984. In the 1990s, hCG and unconjugated estriol were used in combination with maternal serum AFP to improve the detection rates for Down syndrome and trisomy 18. The average maternal serum AFP level in Down syndrome pregnancies is reduced to 0.74 MoM. Intact hCG is increased in affected pregnancies, with an average level of 2.06 MoM, whereas unconjugated estriol is reduced to an average level of 0.75 MoM. *When the levels of all three markers (**triple screen**) are used to modify the maternal age-related Down syndrome risk, the detection rate for Down syndrome is approximately 70%; approximately 5% of all pregnancies will have a positive screen result.* Typically, the levels of all three markers are reduced when the fetus has trisomy 18. *Adding inhibin A to the triple screen (**quadruple screen**) improves the detection rate for Down syndrome to approximately 80%.* The median value of the maternal inhibin A level is increased at 1.77 MoM in Down syndrome pregnancies, but inhibin A is not used in the calculation of risk for trisomy 18. These biochemical screening tests are performed at 15 to 20 weeks of gestation.

## ULTRASOUND SCREENING

*In the second trimester, gross abnormalities, such as cardiac defects, as well as a group of subtle sonographic markers (soft markers) may be associated with an increased risk for Down syndrome in certain women* (Box 7.3). Although findings of soft markers do not significantly increase the risk of Down syndrome, they should be considered in the context of first-trimester screening results, patient's age, and history. The significance of ultrasonographic markers identified by a second-trimester ultrasound examination in a patient who has had a negative first-trimester screening test result is unknown. Studies indicate that the highest detection rate is achieved with systematic combination of ultrasonographic markers and gross anomalies, such as thick nuchal fold or cardiac defects. However, an abnormal second-trimester ultrasound finding identifying a major congenital anomaly significantly increases the risk of aneuploidy and warrants further counseling and the offer of a diagnostic procedure.

## SCREENING FOR NTDs

*Maternal serum AFP is also used to screen for NTDs, congenital structural abnormalities of the brain and vertebral column.* NTDs occur in approximately 1.4–2 per 1000 births in the United States and are the second most common major congenital abnormality worldwide (cardiac malformations are the most common). Maternal serum AFP evaluation is an effective screening test for NTDs and should be offered to all pregnant women, unless they plan to have amniotic AFP measurement as part of prenatal diagnosis for chromosomal abnormalities or other genetic diseases. *Most affected pregnancies can be identified by an elevated maternal serum AFP level, defined as 2.5 MoM for a singleton pregnancy.* Women with a positive screening test should receive an ultrasound examination to detect identifiable causes of false-positive results (e.g., fetal death, multiple gestation, underestimate of gestational age) and for targeted study of fetal anatomy for NTDs and other defects associated with elevated maternal serum AFP.

---

**BOX 7.3**

**Some Ultrasonographic "Soft Markers" for Down Syndrome**

Nuchal fold
Intracardiac echogenic focus
Mild ventriculomegaly
Echogenic bowel
Shortened femur or humerus
Absent nasal bone
Pyelectasis

---

Approximately 90% of newborns with NTDs are born to women not offered amniocentesis because they have no family or medication history that would indicate them to be at increased risk. **Folic acid** has been shown to prevent recurrence and occurrence of neural tube defects. *Because most individuals at increased risk do not know it until they have an affected child, all women should be advised to take a vitamin that contains at least 0.4 mg of folic acid prior to conception.* For women who previously have had a child with a neural tube defect, the recommended dose is 4 mg daily.

### Integrated Screening

The results of both first-trimester and second-trimester screening and ultrasound can be combined to increase their ability to detect Down syndrome. *This "integrated" approach to screening uses both the first-trimester and second-trimester markers to adjust a woman's age-related risk of having a child with Down syndrome.* The results are reported only after both first-trimester and second-trimester screening tests are completed. Integrated screening provides the highest sensitivity with the lowest false-positive rate. The lower false-positive rate results in fewer invasive tests and, thus, fewer procedure-related losses of normal pregnancies. Although some patients value early screening, others are willing to wait several weeks if doing so results in an improved detection rate and less chance that they will need an invasive diagnostic test. Concerns about integrated screening include possible patient anxiety generated by having to wait 3 to 4 weeks between initiation and completion of the screening and the loss of the opportunity to consider CVS if the first-trimester screening indicates a high risk of aneuploidy.

## PRENATAL DIAGNOSIS OF GENETIC DISORDERS

Prenatal genetic diagnosis should be offered in circumstances in which there is a definable increased risk for a fetal genetic disorder that may be diagnosed by one or more methods. Prenatal screening or diagnosis should be voluntary and informed. In most circumstances, test results are normal and provide patients with a high degree of reassurance that a particular disorder does not affect a fetus, although there is no guarantee that the fetus is normal and with no abnormalities. Early prenatal genetic diagnosis also affords patients the option to terminate affected pregnancies. Alternatively, a diagnosis of a genetic disorder may allow a patient to prepare for the birth of an affected child and, in some circumstances, may be important in establishing a plan for care during pregnancy, labor, delivery, and the immediate neonatal period.

### Carrier Testing

*Individuals who have a family history of a specific genetic disorder but who show no signs of the disorder themselves, may undergo carrier testing to determine the risk of passing the disorder on to their offspring. In addition, individuals with certain ethnic backgrounds predisposed to genetic disorders may undergo carrier testing.* For example, ACOG recommends that individuals of Ashkenazi Jewish descent should be tested prior to pregnancy or early in pregnancy for Tay-Sachs disease, Canavan disease cystic fibrosis, and familial dysautonomia. There are also recommendations for other ethnic groups.

Carrier testing involves testing of cells obtained from a saliva or blood sample. Genes responsible for many diseases have been located, and **direct testing** for the presence of a specific mutation can be performed. Examples of diseases for which direct tests exist are Tay-Sachs disease, hemophilia A, cystic fibrosis, sickle cell disease, Canavan disease, familial dysautonomia, and thalassemia. For disorders where disease-causing mutations have not been delineated, indirect testing is required. **Indirect testing** refers to the process of determining DNA sequences of specific length that are linked to a mutation. These sequences, called **restriction fragment-length polymorphisms** (RFLPs), can be tested for by the Southern blot technique. Indirect testing is not as accurate as direct testing.

One partner is usually tested first. If one partner is found to be a carrier of a particular disorder, the other partner is tested as well. If both partners are carriers, a genetic counselor can provide more information regarding the risk of transmitting the disorder.

## Fetal Diagnostic Procedures

Prenatal analysis of DNA requires fetal nucleated cells, currently obtained by amniocentesis, CVS, or percutaneous umbilical blood sampling (PUBS).

### AMNIOCENTESIS

**Amniocentesis** is the withdrawal of 20 to 40 mL of amniotic fluid transabdominally, under concurrent ultrasound guidance, with a 20-gauge to 22-gauge needle. Traditional genetic amniocentesis is usually performed between 15 and 20 weeks' gestation. Direct analysis of the amniotic fluid supernatant is possible for AFP and acetylcholinesterase assays; such analyses permit detection of fetal NTDs and other fetal structural defects (e.g., omphalocele, gastroschisis).

*Studies have confirmed the safety of amniocentesis as well as its cytogenic diagnostic accuracy (greater than 99%).* The risk of pregnancy loss is less than 1%. Complications, which occur infrequently, include transient vaginal spotting or amniotic fluid leakage in approximately 1% to 2% of all cases, and chorioamnionitis in less than 1 in 1000 cases. The perinatal survival rate in cases of amniotic fluid leakage following midtrimester amniocentesis is greater than 90%.

Early amniocentesis performed from 11 weeks to 13 weeks of gestation has significantly higher rates of pregnancy loss and complications than traditional amniocentesis. For these reasons, early amniocentesis before 14 weeks of gestation should not be performed.

### CHORIONIC VILLUS SAMPLING

**Chorionic villus sampling** was developed to provide prenatal diagnosis in the first trimester. CVS is performed after 10 weeks of gestation by transcervical or transabdominal aspiration of chorionic villi (immature placenta) under concurrent ultrasound guidance. Recent multicenter trials have demonstrated transabdominal CVS to have similar safety and accuracy rates to that of traditional (i.e., performed at or after 15 weeks' gestation) amniocentesis; transcervical CVS carries a higher risk of pregnancy loss. Disorders that require analysis of amniotic fluid, such as NTDs, cannot be diagnosed with CVS. There is also a significant learning curve associated with the safe performance of CVS.

*The rate of pregnancy loss associated with CVS appears to approach, and may be the same as, the loss associated with midtrimester amniocentesis.* The most common complication of CVS is vaginal spotting or bleeding, which occurs in up to 32.2% of patients after transcervical CVS is performed. The incidence after transabdominal CVS is less. There have been reports that CVS performed before 10 weeks of gestation is associated with limb reduction and oromandibular defects. Although these associations are controversial, they should be discussed with the patient during counseling. Until further information is available, CVS should not be performed before 10 weeks of gestation.

### PERCUTANEOUS UMBILICAL BLOOD SAMPLING

**Percutaneous umbilical blood sampling (PUBS),** also known as **cordocentesis,** is usually performed after 20 weeks' gestation and has traditionally been used to obtain fetal blood for blood component analyses (e.g., hematocrit, Rh status, platelets), as well as cytogenetic and DNA analyses. The indications for PUBS are declining. One major benefit of PUBS is the ability to obtain rapid (18 to 24 hours) fetal karyotypes. However, with the advent of fluorescence in situ hybridization (FISH), PUBS has obviated the need for a procedure with more potential for complications. The procedure-related pregnancy loss rate has been reported to be less than 2%. Cordocentesis is rarely needed, but may be useful to further evaluate chromosomal mosaicism discovered after CVS or amniocentesis is performed.

Other prenatal diagnostic procedures include **fetal skin sampling, fetal tissue** (muscle, liver) **biopsy,** and **fetoscopy.** These procedures are used only for the diagnosis of rare disorders not amenable to diagnosis by less invasive methods.

### TESTS

Once fetal cells are obtained, a variety of tests and analyses can be performed. A **karyotype** is a photomicrograph of the chromosomes taken during metaphase, when the chromosomes have condensed. A separate image is made of each individual chromosome from this micrograph. The chromosomes are then matched to their homologue, so that the karyotype shows the chromosome pairs. Because most fetal cells in amniotic fluid specimens obtained through amniocentesis are not in metaphase, these cells must first be cultured (grown) in order to perform a karyotype analysis. An advantage of CVS over amniocentesis is that CVS allows for rapid cytogenetic and DNA analyses, because cytotrophoblasts obtained from first-trimester placentas are more likely to be in metaphase than amniotic fluid cells.

**Fluorescence in situ hybridization (FISH)** is a technique that involves fluorescent labeling of genetic probes for specific chromosomes, most commonly 13, 18, 21, X, and Y. FISH can identify abnormalities in chromosome number, and results are usually available by 48 hours. Although FISH analysis has been shown to be accurate, false-positive and false-negative results have been reported. Therefore, clinical decision making should be based on information from FISH and either a traditional karyotype, ultrasound findings, or a positive screening test result. **Spectral karyotyping (SKY)** is similar to FISH, but can be done for all chromosomes. SKY is useful in detecting translocations.

**Comparative genomic hybridization (CGH)** is an evolving method that identifies submicroscopic chromosomal deletions and duplications. This approach has proved useful in identifying abnormalities in individuals with developmental delay and physical abnormalities, when results of traditional chromosomal analysis have been normal. At present, the use of CGH in prenatal diagnosis is limited because of the difficulty in interpreting which DNA alterations revealed through CGH may be normal population variants. Until more data are available, use of CGH for routine prenatal diagnosis is not recommended.

## Genetic Counseling

Many couples at increased risk for having children with genetic disorders can benefit from genetic counseling, in which the primary health care provider, a medical geneticist, or other trained professional provides information and options to individuals or families about genetic disorders and risks. Ideally, this counseling takes place before conception. *The key elements in genetic counseling are accurate diagnosis, communication, and nondirective presentation of options.* The counselor's function is not to dictate a particular course of action, but to provide information that will allow couples to make informative decisions. Counseling is directed at helping the patient or family in the following areas:

- Comprehending the medical facts, including the diagnosis, probable course of the disorder, and available management
- Appreciating the way in which heredity contributes to the disorder and the risk of occurrence or recurrence in specific relatives
- Understanding the options for dealing with the risk of recurrence, including prenatal genetic diagnosis

- Choosing the course of action that seems appropriate in view of the risk and the family's goals and act in accordance with that decision
- Making the best possible adjustment to the disorder in an affected family member and to the risk of recurrence in another family member

Genetic counseling may also involve alternative reproductive options (e.g., pregnancy termination, permanent sterilization, selective pregnancy reduction, or donor insemination). Patients should also understand that outside parties, such as insurance companies, may be able to obtain the results of genetic testing.

## GENETICS IN GYNECOLOGY: CANCER SCREENING

*It is now known that certain breast and ovarian cancers have a genetic predisposition. Genetic tests have been developed for the detection of some of these genes.* Gynecologists play a key role in identifying individuals with a genetic disposition for cancer and ensuring that they receive the appropriate screening tests. The most important initial step in identifying women at high risk for hereditary cancers is a thorough family history. Clues to possible hereditary cancers include a history of cancers in first-degree relatives, cancers occurring at young ages, cancers in multiple generations, or many different cancers in one individual. Based on these findings, further testing and genetic counseling may be indicated.

The **BRCA1** and **BRCA2** genes have been identified as responsible for the hereditary forms of both breast and ovarian cancers. Clinically important *BRCA* mutations have been found in about 2% of Ashkenazi Jewish women, and are estimated to occur in about 1 in 300 to 500 women in the general non-Jewish US population. Criteria developed by the U.S. Preventative Services Task Force for *BRCA* testing referral are as follows:

- Two first-degree relatives with breast cancer, with at least one diagnosed at under age 50
- Three or more first-degree or second-degree relatives with breast cancer at any age
- A first-degree or second-degree relative with breast and ovarian cancer
- Two or more first-degree or second-degree relatives with ovarian cancer
- A male relative with breast cancer

Because the incidence of breast cancers linked to *BRCA* is higher in Ashkenazi Jewish women, the testing criteria for them are slightly different. Testing for BRCA in this population is indicated if the following are present:

- Any first-degree relative with breast or ovarian cancer
- Two second-degree relatives on the same side of the family with breast or ovarian cancer

In addition to breast cancer, other cancers have been found to have a hereditary component. A hereditary syndrome called hereditary nonpolyposis colorectal cancer type A **(HNPCC type A),** or **Lynch I syndrome,** increases the risk for developing colon cancer. A family history of colon, endometrial, ureteral, or renal cancers should alert the clinical to screen for the HNPCC-linked genes. **HNPCC type B,** or **Lynch II syndrome,** is an autosomal dominant inherited syndrome that increases the risk for all of the cancers in Lynch I syndrome, as well as for ovarian, gastric, and pancreatic cancers. Individuals or families who meet certain criteria, which include the presence of HNPCC in two successive generations and the diagnosis of HNPCC in at least three relatives, can undergo genetic testing to determine whether they have the defective gene.

## SUGGESTED READINGS

American College of Obstetricians and Gynecologists. Breast cancer screening. ACOG Practice Bulletin No. 42. *Obstet Gynecol.* 2003;101(4):821–832.

American College of Obstetricians and Gynecologists. Invasive prenatal testing for aneuploidy. ACOG Practice Bulletin No. 88. *Obstet Gynecol.* 2007;110(6):1459–1467.

American College of Obstetricians and Gynecologists. Neural tube defects. ACOG Practice Bulletin No. 44. *Obstet Gynecol.* 2003;102(1):203–213.

American College of Obstetricians and Gynecologists. Prenatal and preconceptional carrier screening for genetic diseases in individuals of Eastern European Jewish descent. ACOG Committee Opinion No. 298. *Obstet Gynecol.* 2004;104(2):425–428.

American College of Obstetricians and Gynecologists. *Screening for Birth Defects.* ACOG Patient Education Pamphlet No. 165. Washington, DC: American College of Obstetricians and Gynecologists; 2007.

American College of Obstetricians and Gynecologists. Screening for fetal chromosomal abnormalities. ACOG Practice Bulletin No. 77. *Obstet Gynecol.* 2007;109(1):217–227.

American College of Obstetricians and Gynecologists. Screening for fragile X syndrome. ACOG Committee Opinion No. 338. *Obstet Gynecol.* 2006;107(6):1483–1485.

American College of Obstetricians and Gynecologists. Update on carrier screening for cystic fibrosis. ACOG Committee Opinion No. 325. *Obstet Gynecol.* 2005;106(6):1465–1468.

*Guidelines for Perinatal Care.* 6th ed. Elk Grove Village, IL: American Academy of Pediatrics; Washington, DC: American College of Obstetricians and Gynecologists; 2007:105–111.

# 8 Intrapartum Care

**Topic 11:** Intrapartum Care

Students should understand and be able to describe the management of the normal events of labor and delivery, thus recognizing any abnormal events.

L abor is the progressive change in a woman's cervix in the setting of regular, rhythmic uterine contractions. This definition allows for a diagnosis of abnormal labor and, thus, for appropriate management, as discussed in the next chapter.

## MATERNAL CHANGES BEFORE THE ONSET OF LABOR

As patients approach term, they experience **uterine contractions** of increasing strength and frequency. Spontaneous uterine contractions, which are not felt by the patient, occur throughout pregnancy. Late in pregnancy they become stronger and more frequent, resulting in the patient's perception of discomfort. *These **Braxton Hicks contractions** (false labor) are not associated with dilation of the cervix, however, and do not fit the definition of labor.* It is frequently difficult for the patient to distinguish these often uncomfortable contractions from those of true labor. As a result, it is difficult for the physician to determine the true onset of labor by history alone. Braxton Hicks contractions are typically shorter in duration and less intense than true labor contractions, with the discomfort being characterized as over the lower abdomen and groin areas. It is not uncommon for these contractions to resolve with ambulation, hydration, or analgesia.

*True labor is associated with contractions that the patient feels over the uterine fundus, with radiation of discomfort to the low back and lower abdomen.*

These contractions become increasingly intense and frequent.

Another event of late pregnancy is termed **"lightening,"** in which the patient reports a change in the shape of her abdomen and the sensation that the baby is lighter, the result of the fetal head descending into the pelvis. The

patient may also report that the baby is "dropping." The patient often notices that her lower abdomen is more prominent, and she may feel a need to urinate more frequently as the bladder is compressed by the fetal head. The patient may also notice that she is breathing more easily, because there is less pressure on the diaphragm as the uterus becomes smaller.

Patients often report the passage of blood-tinged mucus late in pregnancy. This "bloody show" results as the cervix begins thinning (effacement) with the concomitant extrusion of mucus from the endocervical glands and a small amount of bleeding from small vessels in the area. Cervical effacement is common before the onset of true labor, when the internal os is slowly drawn into the lower uterine segment. The cervix is often significantly effaced before the onset of labor, particularly in the nulliparous patient. The mechanism of effacement and dilation and the vectors of the expulsive forces are demonstrated in Figure 8.1.

## EVALUATION FOR LABOR

Patients should be instructed to contact their health care provider for any of the following reasons: (1) if their contractions occur approximately every 5 minutes for at least 1 hour, (2) if there is a sudden gush of fluid or a constant leakage of vaginal fluid (suggesting rupture of membranes), (3) if there is any significant vaginal bleeding, or (4) if there is significant decrease in fetal movement.

### Initial Evaluation

At the time of initial evaluation, the prenatal records are reviewed to (1) identify complications of pregnancy up to that point, (2) confirm gestational age to differentiate preterm labor from labor in a term pregnancy, and (3) review pertinent laboratory information. A focused history helps in determining the nature and frequency of

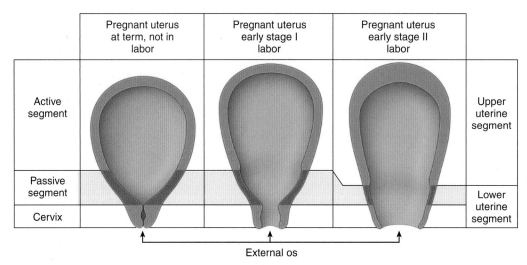

FIGURE 8.1. Mechanism of effacement, dilation, and labor. With continuing uterine contractions, the upper uterus (active segment) thickens, the lower uterine segment (passive segment) thins, and the cervix dilates. In this way, the fetus is moved downward, into and through the vaginal canal.

the patient's contractions, the possibility of spontaneous rupture of membranes or significant bleeding, or changes in maternal or fetal status. A focused review of systems should look for common complications of pregnancy resulting in altered labor management. A limited general physical examination is performed (with special attention to vital signs), along with the abdominal and pelvic examinations. If contractions occur during this physical examination, they may be palpated for intensity and duration by the examining physician. Auscultation of fetal heart tones is also of critical importance, particularly immediately following a contraction, to determine the possibility of any fetal heart rate deceleration. A limited transabdominal ultrasound may also be useful if there is a question of fetal lie, placental location, or decreased amniotic fluid volume or other abnormalities.

*The initial examination of the patient's abdomen may be accomplished using **Leopold maneuvers**, a series of four palpations of the fetus through the abdominal wall that helps accurately determine fetal lie, presentation, and position (see Figure 9.7).*

**Lie** is the relation of the long axis of the fetus with the maternal long axis. It is longitudinal in 99% of cases, occasionally transverse, and rarely oblique (when the axes cross at a 45-degree angle, usually converting to transverse or longitudinal lie during labor). **Presentation** is determined by the "presenting part," that is, that portion of the fetus lowest in the birth canal, palpated during the examination. For example, in a longitudinal lie, the presenting part is either breech or cephalic. The most common cephalic presentation is the one in which the head is sharply flexed onto the fetal chest such that the occiput or vertex pre-

sents. **Position** is the relation of the fetal presenting part to the right or left side of the maternal pelvis (Fig. 8.2).

The four Leopold maneuvers (see Fig. 9.7) include the following, facilitating several obstetric measurements:

1. Determining what occupies the fundus. In a longitudinal lie, the fetal head is differentiated from the fetal breech, the latter being larger and less clearly defined.
2. Determining location of small parts. Using one hand to steady the fetus, the fingers on the other hand are used to palpate either the firm, long fetal spine or the various shapes and movements indicating fetal hands and feet.
3. Identifying descent of the presenting part. Suprapubic palpation identifies the presenting part as the fetal head, which is relatively mobile, or a breech, which moves the entire body. The extent to which the presenting part is felt to extend below the symphysis suggests the station of the presenting part.
4. Identifying the cephalic prominence. As long as the cephalic prominence is easily palpable, the vertex is not likely to have descended to zero station.

Palpation of the uterus during a contraction may also be helpful in determining the intensity of that particular contraction. The uterine wall is not easily indented with firm palpation during a true contraction, but may be indented during a Braxton Hicks "contraction."

A digital vaginal examination allows the examiner to determine the consistency and degree of effacement and degree of dilation of the cervix. This examination should be avoided in women with premature rupture of membranes or vaginal bleeding. *Effacement is the shortening of the cervical canal from a length of about 2 cm to a mere circular orifice with almost paper-thin edges. Effacement is expressed as a percent of thinning from a perceived uneffaced state* (Fig. 8.3). A cervix that

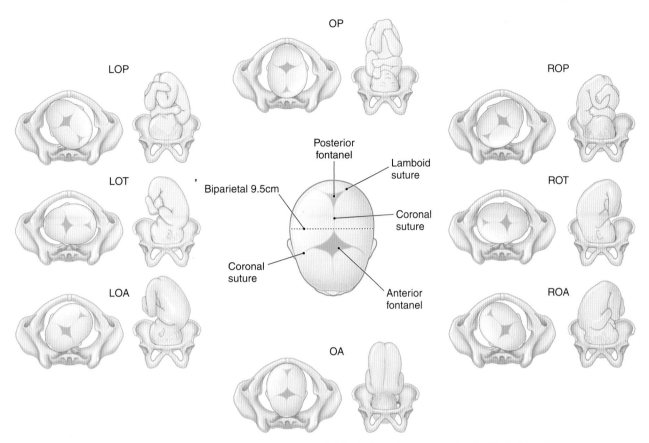

FIGURE 8.2. Various positions in vertex presentation. LOP = left occiput posterior; LOT = left occiput transverse; LOA = left occiput anterior; ROP = right occiput posterior; ROT = right occiput transverse; ROA = right occiput anterior.

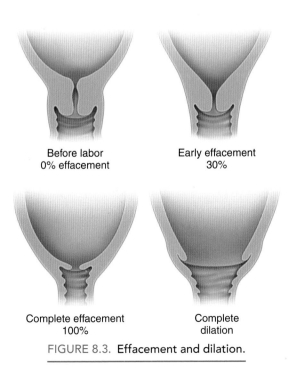

FIGURE 8.3. Effacement and dilation.

is not effaced, but is softened, is more likely to change with contractions than one that is firm, as it is earlier in pregnancy. If the cervix is not significantly effaced, it may also be evaluated for its relative position, that is, anterior, midposition, or posterior in the vagina. A cervix that is palpable anterior in the vagina is more likely to undergo change in labor sooner than one found in the posterior portion of the vagina. This suggests that the presenting part has descended into the pelvis, creating more pressure on the cervix, thereby rotating it anteriorly. With more effective force on the lower uterine segment, contractions would cause a greater change in dilation and effacement of the cervix.

## Fetal Station

Fetal station is determined by identifying the level of the fetal presenting part in the birth canal in relation to the ischial spines which are located approximately halfway between the **pelvic inlet** and the **pelvic outlet** (Fig. 8.4). *If the presenting part has reached the level of the ischial spines, it is termed zero station.* The distance between the ischial spines to the pelvic inlet above and the distance from the spines to the pelvic outlet below are divided into fifths, and

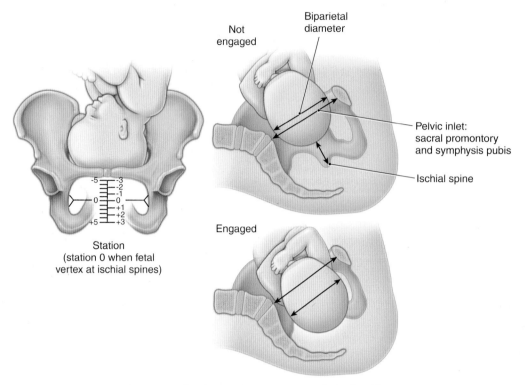

FIGURE 8.4. Station and engagement of the fetal head.

these measurements are used to further define station. These divisions represent centimeters above and below the ischial spines. Thus, as the presenting fetal part descends from the pelvic inlet toward the ischial spines, the designation is −5, −4, −3, −2, −1, then 0 station. Below the ischial spines, the presenting fetal part passes +1, +2, +3, +4, with +5 station corresponding to the fetal head being visible at the introitus. The clinical significance of the fetal head presenting at zero station is that the biparietal diameter of the fetal head, the greatest transverse diameter of the fetal skull, is assumed to have negotiated the pelvic inlet.

> *The fetal head is said to be engaged at zero station, a crucial functional "landmark" in the labor path.*

However, caput succedaneum, cephalohematoma, and molding of the fetal head may mislead the examiner to a greater station than has been obtained.

## STAGES OF LABOR

Although labor is a continuous process, it is divided into four functional stages because each has differing physiological activities and requires differing management.

- The **first stage of labor** is the interval between the onset of labor and full cervical dilation (10 cm). The first stage is further divided into two phases: (1) The **latent phase** of labor encompasses cervical effacement and early dilation, and (2) the **active phase** of labor, during which more rapid cervical dilation occurs, usually beginning at approximately 4 cm.
- The **second stage of labor** encompasses complete cervical dilation through the delivery of the infant.
- The **third stage of labor** begins immediately after delivery of the infant and ends with the delivery of the placenta.
- The **fourth stage of labor** is defined as the immediate postpartum period of approximately 2 hours after delivery of the placenta, during which time the patient undergoes significant physiologic adjustment.

Table 8.1 outlines the duration of various stages of labor, as first described in the research by Emmanuel Friedman, and Figure 8.5 represents this information graphically, known as the **Friedman curve.** New data, derived since the advent of epidural labor analgesia, suggest that the maximum slope of the normal labor curve during active phase may actually be slightly less steep.

## MECHANISM OF LABOR

The **mechanisms of labor** (also known as the **cardinal movements of labor** [Fig. 8.6]) refer to the changes of the position of the fetus as it passes through the birth canal. The fetus usually descends to where the occipital portion of the fetal head is the lowermost part in the pelvis, and it rotates toward the largest pelvic segment. *Because vertex presentation*

| | Latent Phase (hr) | Active Phase (hr) | Maximum Dilation (cm/hr) | Second Stage (hr) |
|---|---|---|---|---|
| **TABLE 8.1** Mean Duration of the Various Phases and Stages of Labor with Their Distribution Characteristics | | | | |
| Parity | | | | |
| Nulliparous | | | | |
| Mean | 6.5 | 4.5 | 3.0 | 1.0 |
| Upper limit* | 20.0 | 12.0 | 1.0 | 3.0 |
| Multiparous | | | | |
| Mean | 5.0 | 2.5 | 6.0 | 0.5 |
| Upper limit* | 13.5 | 5.0 | 1.5 | 1.0 |

*Fifth or 95th percentile.

*occurs in 95% of term labors, the cardinal movements of labor are defined relative to this presentation.* To accommodate to the maternal bony pelvis, the fetal head must undergo several movements as it passes through the birth canal. These movements are accomplished by means of the forceful contractions of the uterus. These cardinal movements of labor do not occur as a distinct series of movements, but rather as a group of movements that overlap as the fetus accommodates and moves progressively through the birth canal. These movements are

1. Engagement
2. Flexion
3. Descent
4. Internal rotation
5. Extension
6. External rotation or restitution
7. Expulsion

**Engagement** is defined as descent of the biparietal diameter of the head below the plane of the pelvic inlet, suggested clinically by palpation of the presenting part below the level of ischial spines (zero station). Engagement commonly occurs days to weeks prior to labor in women who have not delivered a child, whereas in women who have had children it more commonly happens at the onset of active labor. In any event, the importance of this event is that it suggests that the bony pelvis is adequate to allow significant descent of the fetal head, although the extension of this to the idea that delivery through the pelvis will happen in the labor does not follow. **Flexion** of the fetal head allows for the smaller diameters of the fetal head to present to the maternal pelvis. **Descent** of the presenting part is necessary for the successful completion of passage through the birth canal. *The greatest rate of descent occurs during the latter portions of the first stage of labor and during the second stage of labor.* **Internal rotation,** like flexion, facilitates presentation of the optimal diameters of the fetal head to the bony pelvis, most commonly from transverse to either anterior or posterior. **Extension** of the fetal head occurs as it reaches the introitus. To accommodate the upward curve of the birth canal, the flexed head now extends. **External rotation** occurs after delivery of the head as the head rotates to "face forward" relative to its shoulders. This is known as restitution, followed rapidly by delivery of the body, **expulsion.**

## NORMAL LABOR AND DELIVERY

Ideally, a pregnant woman has a principal, designated health care provider. Beginning with admission to the labor and delivery area, the obstetric team monitors the patient's progress. Once the patient is in active labor, her provider should be readily available.

### General Management

#### AMBULATION AND POSITION IN LABOR AND AT DELIVERY

Walking may be more comfortable than being supine during early labor. Women in early labor are confined to bed if they are too uncomfortable to move about safely or if care

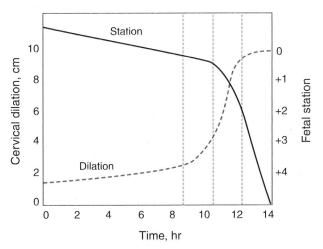

FIGURE 8.5. Graphic representation of cervical dilation and station during the first and second stages of labor.

FIGURE 8.6. Cardinal movements of labor: engagement (A), flexion (B), descent (C), internal rotation (D), extension (E), and external rotation (F).

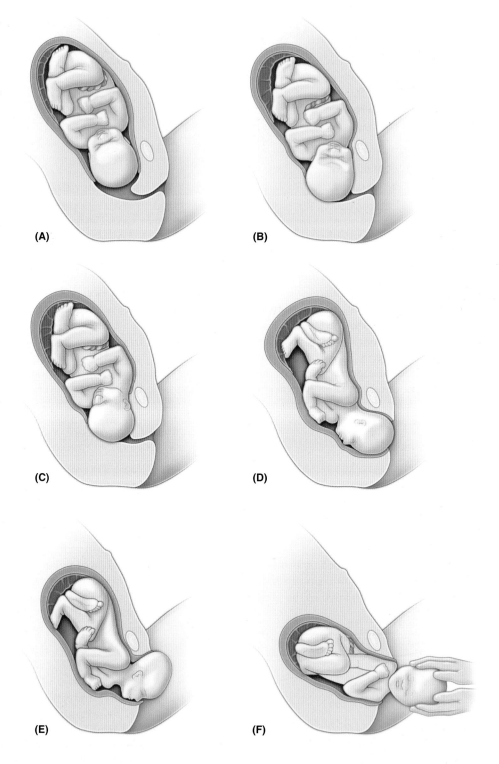

(A)

(B)

(C)

(D)

(E)

(F)

maneuvers require it. Supine labor is common in the United States. The left lateral position keeps the uterus off the inferior vena cava; this obstructs venous return, thence cardiac output, leading to hypotension (supine hypotensive syndrome). *The **dorsal lithotomy position** is most commonly used for spontaneous and operative vaginal delivery in the United States.* Elsewhere in the world, many other laboring positions are common, including sitting or crouching, in special "birthing chairs," on labor balls, or in variously configured tubs of warm water.

## FLUID MANAGEMENT AND ORAL INTAKE

Because labor is associated with decreased gastrointestinal peristalsis, there is concern about aspiration during the administration of anesthesia. Patients in active labor should avoid oral ingestion of anything except clear fluids (sips only), occasional ice chips, and preparations for moistening the mouth and lips.

When oral intake is not possible or is insufficient, intravenous therapy with ½ normal saline or D5 ½ normal saline is indicated. Normal saline can be used if increased oncotic pressure is desired, but lactated fluids are generally contraindicated because of the metabolic acid deficit incurred by the lactate administration.

## EVALUATION OF FETAL WELL-BEING

Measurement of the **fetal heart rate** and its changes during labor is the primary means of intrapartum assessment of fetal well-being. This may be done by intermittent auscultation with a stethoscope or hand-held Doppler, or by the use of electronic fetal monitoring. The method chosen may depend on risk assessment at admission, the preference of the patient and the obstetric staff, and department policy. Risk factors include vaginal bleeding, acute abdominal pain, temperature >100.4°F, preterm labor or rupture of membranes, hypertension, and nonreassuring fetal heart rate pattern.

In the absence of risk factors on admission, the standard approach to fetal monitoring is to determine, evaluate, and record the fetal heart rate every 30 minutes in the active phase in the first stage of labor, and at least every 15 minutes in the second stage. In the presence of risk factors, fetal surveillance should be performed using either intermittent auscultation or continuous fetal monitoring. During the active first stage of labor, auscultation should be performed every 15 minutes, preferably before, during, and after a contraction, and continuous monitoring should be evaluated at least every 15 minutes. During the second stage of labor, the fetal heart rate should be monitored every 5 minutes using either the intermittent or continuous procedure. If electronic fetal monitoring is used, an external tocodynamometer is initially used to assess uterine activity, providing information regarding the frequency and duration of contractions, but not their intensity. Electronic fetal monitoring is not necessary for a low-risk term pregnancy.

## Control of Pain

Management of discomfort and pain during labor is an essential part of good obstetric practice. Some patients tolerate pain by using techniques learned in childbirth preparation programs. It is important that bedside staff be knowledgeable about these pain management techniques and be supportive of the patient's decisions. Unless contraindicated, pharmacologic analgesics to ameliorate pain of contractions should be made available on request to women in labor.

During the first stage of labor, pain results from the contraction of the uterus and dilation of the cervix. This pain travels along the visceral afferents, which accompany

sympathetic nerves entering the spinal cord at T-10, T-11, T-12, and L-1. As the fetal head descends, there is also distension of the lower birth canal and perineum. This pain is transmitted along somatic afferents that comprise portions of the pudendal nerves that enter the spinal cord at S-2, S-3, and S-4. To provide relief from obstetric pain, the following methods of anesthesia and analgesia are used.

- **Epidural block:** infusion of local anesthetics or narcotics through a catheter into the epidural space. The most effective form of intrapartum pain relief in the United States, it can be used in either vaginal or abdominal deliveries and in postpartum procedures such as tubal ligation.
- **Spinal anesthesia:** a single injection of anesthetic
- **Combined spinal–epidural:** combination of the above two techniques
- **Local block:** local injection of anesthetic into the perineum or vagina. A **pudendal block** is a local block (Fig. 8.7).
- **General anesthesia:** inhaled or intravenous administration of anesthetic agents that results in a loss of maternal consciousness. This technique is reserved only for cesarean deliveries in selected cases.

To determine which method of obstetric pain control should be used, the positive and negative aspects of each should be considered. Of the regional modes of analgesia, epidural anesthesia is superior to spinal anesthesia in that it can be left as a continuous source of analgesia and anesthesia during both the labor and delivery process. The advantage of this technique is its ability to provide analgesia during labor as well as excellent anesthesia for delivery, yet maintain the patient's sense of touch, facilitating participation in the birth process. Spinal anesthesia provides good pain relief for procedures of limited duration, such as cesarean delivery or vaginal delivery when labor is rapidly progressing. Combined spinal–epidural anesthesia has advantages: the epidural catheter to titrate medications throughout labor and the rapid onset associated with spinal techniques. All of these types of regional anesthesia may be associated with a postdural puncture headache. However, combined spinal–epidural anesthesia avoids the risk of spinal headache in the mother and reduces the risk of sympathetic blockade, which could lead to hypotension. There is also less motor blockade than with spinal anesthesia. Local block may provide anesthesia for episiotomy and repair of vaginal and perineal lacerations; however, paracervical block may result in fetal bradycardia. General anesthesia is associated with complications such as maternal aspiration and neonatal depression. If properly administered, it is effective for most cesarean deliveries, but regional anesthesia is preferable.

## Management of Labor

### FIRST STAGE

Evaluation of the progress of labor is accomplished by means of a series of pelvic examinations. At the time of

FIGURE 8.7. Pudendal block. Local anesthesia can be administered easily at the time of delivery to provide perineal anesthesia for a vaginal delivery.

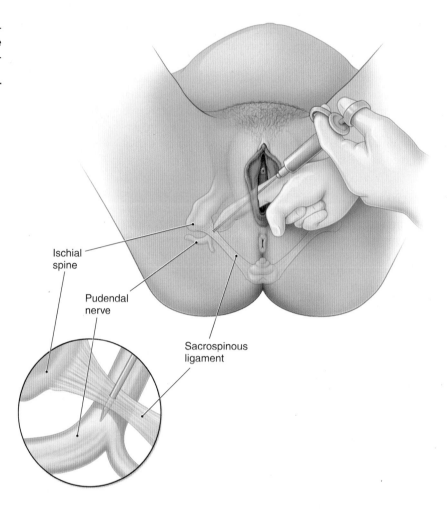

Ischial spine

Pudendal nerve

Sacrospinous ligament

each vaginal examination, a sterile lubricant is used. Each examination should identify cervical dilation, effacement, station, position of the presenting part, and the status of the membranes. These findings should be noted graphically on the hospital record, so that abnormalities of labor may be identified. *During the latter portions of the first stage of labor, patients may report the urge to push.* This may indicate significant descent of the fetal head with pressure on the perineum. More frequent vaginal examinations during this time may be necessary. Similarly, if there are significant fetal heart rate decelerations, more frequent examinations may be necessary to determine whether the umbilical cord is prolapsed or if delivery is imminent.

In addition to rupturing the membranes to insert an intrauterine pressure catheter or a fetal scalp monitor, if needed, artificial **rupture of membranes** many be beneficial in other ways. The **presence or absence of meconium** (fetal stool) can be identified. However, rupture of the membranes does carry some risk, because the incidence of infection may be increased if labor is prolonged, or umbilical cord prolapse may occur if rupture of the membranes is undertaken before engagement of the presenting fetal part. Spontaneous rupture of membranes has similar risks. The fluid should be observed for meconium and blood. Fetal heart tones should be assessed after membranes spontaneously rupture.

## SECOND STAGE

Once the **second stage** of labor has been reached (i.e., complete cervical dilation to 10 cm), voluntary maternal effort **(pushing)** can be added to the involuntary contractile forces of the uterus to facilitate delivery of the fetus. With the onset of each contraction, the mother is encouraged to inhale, hold her breath, and perform an extended Valsalva maneuver. This increase in intra-abdominal pressure aids in fetal descent through the birth canal.

It is during the second stage of labor that the fetal head may undergo further alterations. **Molding** is an alteration in the relation of the fetal cranial bones, even resulting in partial bone overlap (Fig. 8.8). Some minor degree of molding is common as the fetal head adjusts to the bony pelvis. The greater the disparity between the fetal head and the bony pelvis, the greater the amount of molding. **Caput succedaneum** is the edema of the fetal scalp caused by pressure on the fetal head by the cervix. *Molding and caput succedaneum are the two most common causes of overestimation of the amount of descent, that is, of station.* When there is a large amount of space "between the back of the fetal head and the curve of the sacrum," the physician is alerted to the possibility that the biparietal diameter of the fetal head is higher than might be thought based upon the physical level to which the presenting part's farthest dimension has reached. An

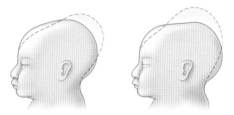

FIGURE 8.8. Molding of head.

extended second stage may last as long as 2 to 3 hours, and the prolonged resistance encountered by the fetal vertex may prevent appropriate identification of fontanels and sutures. Both caput and molding resolve in the first few days of life. If identified before the second stage of labor, these changes should be noted on the pelvic examination and may indicate a potential problem in negotiation of the birth canal.

An **episiotomy** facilitates delivery by enlarging the vaginal outlet and may be indicated in cases of instrumental delivery and/or protracted or arrested descent. With progressive labor and control of the fetal head and body at delivery, the risk of obstetric laceration with a normal-sized infant is low, so that the need for episiotomy is minimal. If an episiotomy is needed, it should be performed only after the perineum has been thinned considerably by the descending fetal head, and the incision should be somewhat longer on the mucosal as compared to the perineal surface of the incision (Fig. 8.9).

As the **fetal head crowns** (i.e., distends the vaginal opening), it is delivered by extension to allow the smallest diameter of the fetal head to pass over the perineum. This natural mechanism decreases the likelihood of laceration or extension of an episiotomy. To support the perineal

tissues and facilitate extension of the head, a **modified Ritgen maneuver** is performed (Fig. 8.10). This maneuver involves placing one hand over the vertex while the other hand exerts pressure through the perineum onto the fetal chin. A sterile towel is used to avoid contamination of this hand by contact with the anus. The chin can then be delivered slowly, with control applied by both hands.

After delivery of the head, the shoulders descend and rotate to a position in the anteroposterior diameter of the pelvis. The attendant's hands are placed on the chin and vertex, applying gentle downward pressure, thus delivering the anterior shoulder. To avoid injury to the brachial plexus, care is taken not to put excessive force on the neck. The posterior shoulder is then delivered by upward traction on the fetal head (Fig. 8.11). Delivery of the body now occurs easily in most cases. Immediately after delivery, the uterus significantly decreases in size.

## Third Stage

Delivery of the placenta is imminent when the uterus rises in the abdomen, becoming globular in configuration, indicating that the placenta has separated and has entered the lower uterine segment; a gush of blood and/or "lengthening" of the umbilical cord also occur. These are the three classic signs of placental separation. Pulling the placenta

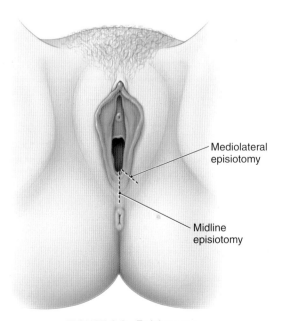

Mediolateral episiotomy

Midline episiotomy

FIGURE 8.9. Episiotomy.

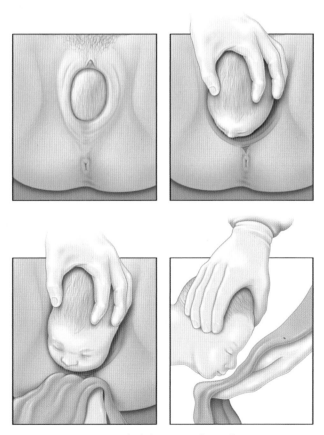

FIGURE 8.10. Vaginal delivery with midline episiotomy assisted by modified Ritgen maneuver.

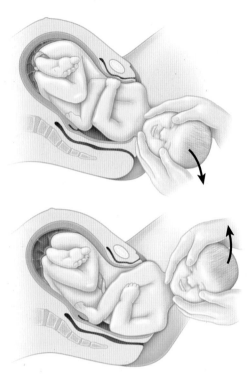

FIGURE 8.11. **Delivery of anterior and posterior shoulders.**

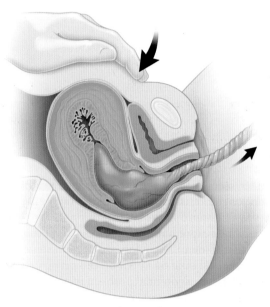

FIGURE 8.12. **Delivery of the placenta.**

from the uterus by excessive traction on the cord should be avoided. Inappropriate application of force may result in inversion of the uterus, an obstetric emergency associated with profound blood loss and shock. Instead, it is appropriate to wait for spontaneous extrusion of the placenta, sometimes up to 30 minutes. As the placenta passes into the lower uterine segment, gentle downward pressure is applied to the fundus of the uterus, and the placenta is guided by very gentle traction on the umbilical cord (Fig. 8.12). If necessary, the placenta may be removed manually. This is accomplished by passing a hand into the uterine cavity and using the side of the hand to develop a cleavage plane between the placenta and the uterine wall. Anesthesia may be required. The umbilical cord should be evaluated for the presence of the expected two umbilical arteries and one umbilical vein.

*After the placenta has been removed, the uterus should be palpated to ensure that it has reduced in size and become firmly contracted.* Excessive blood loss at this or any subsequent time should suggest the possibility of uterine atony. The use of uterine massage as well as oxytocic agents such as oxytocin, methylergonovine maleate (Methergine), or prostaglandins (carboprost or misoprostol) may be used routinely in the circumstance of excessive postpartum blood loss.

*Inspection of the birth canal should be performed in a systematic fashion.* The introitus, vagina, perineum, and the vulvar area, including the periurethral area, should be evaluated for lacerations. Ring forceps are commonly used to hold and evaluate the cervix. Lacerations, if present, are most commonly found at the 3 o'clock and

9 o'clock positions of the cervix. Repair is accomplished with an absorbable suture. Obstetric lacerations are classified in Table 8.2.

## Fourth Stage

*For the first hour after delivery, the likelihood of serious postpartum complications is at its greatest.* Postpartum uterine hemorrhage occurs in approximately 1% of patients. It is more likely to occur in cases of rapid labor, protracted labor, uterine enlargement (large fetus, polyhydramnios, multiple gestation), or intrapartum chorioamnionitis. Immediately after the delivery of the placenta, the uterus is palpated to determine that it is firm. Uterine palpation is done in this period to ascertain uterine tone. Perineal pads are applied and the amount of blood on these pads as well as pulse and blood

| TABLE 8.2 | Classification of Obstetric Lacerations |
|---|---|
| **Degree of Laceration** | **Description** |
| First degree | Involves the vaginal mucosa or perineal skin, but not the underlying tissue |
| Second degree | Involves the underlying subcutaneous tissue, but not the rectal sphincter or rectal mucosa |
| Third degree | Extends through the rectal sphincter, but not into the rectal mucosa |
| Fourth degree | Extends into the rectal mucosa |

pressure are monitored closely for the first several hours after delivery to identify excessive blood loss.

## LABOR INDUCTION

Labor can be induced when the benefits to either the woman or the fetus outweigh those of continuing the pregnancy. Labor induction can be achieved with intravenous oxytocin administration. The device used to administer oxytocin should permit precise control of the flow rate to ensure accurate, minute-to-minute control. Various regimens exist for stimulation of uterine contractions. These regimens vary in initial dose, amount of incremental dose increase, and interval between dose increases. Lower and less frequent dosage increases are associated with a lower incidence of uterine hyperstimulation. Higher and more frequent dosage increases may result in shorter time in labor and reduce the incidence of chorioamnionitis and the number of cesarean deliveries performed for dystocia (abnormal labor), but also in increased rates of uterine hyperstimulation.

**Cervical ripening** may be beneficial if the cervix is unfavorable for induction. Several techniques are available. Misoprostol, a prostaglandin E analog, is an effective agent for cervical ripening and induction of labor. It is administered vaginally. Prostaglandin E2 (PGE2) can also be administered vaginally or intracervically. Because of the increased risk of uterine hyperstimulation, both drugs are contraindicated in patients who have had a previous cesarean delivery or previous uterine surgery.

Cervical ripening also can be accomplished with mechanical dilation with laminaria. Laminaria are hygroscopic rods made from the stems of the seaweed *Laminaria japonica* that are inserted into the internal cervical os. As the rods absorb moisture and expand, the cervix is slowly dilated (Fig. 8.13). The risks associated with laminaria use include failure to dilate the cervix, cervical laceration, inadvertent rupture of the membranes, and infection. A synthetic form is also available. Placement of a 30 mL Foley catheter in the cervical canal is also used for cervical ripening.

Induction of labor by "stripping" or "sweeping" the amniotic membranes is a relatively common practice. Risks associated with this procedure include infection, bleeding from an undiagnosed placenta previa or low-lying placenta, and accidental rupture of membranes. Artificial rupture of membranes is another method of labor induction that may be used, particularly when the cervix is favorable. Routine early amniotomy results in a modest reduction in the direction of labor, but may result in an increased rate of intra-amniotic infection and cesarean delivery for fetal heart rate abnormalities. For these reasons, routine amniotomy is not recommended.

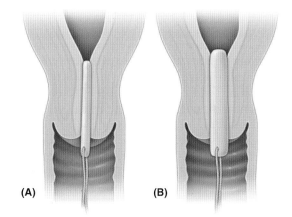

**(A)**            **(B)**

FIGURE 8.13. Use of laminaria. (A) Laminaria properly inserted just beyond the cervical os. (B) Properly placed laminaria that has expanded, causing cervical dilation.

## CESAREAN DELIVERY

**Cesarean delivery** is the most frequent major operation performed in the United States. Until 1965, the rate of cesarean delivery was stable at less than 5%, when it began to increase; it was more than 30% in 2005. Reasons for this increase include the ready availability of improved neonatal intensive care units in which infants with complications have a significantly greater survival rate, use in breech deliveries, and use in situations in which more sophisticated fetal monitoring is nonreassuring. However, no major improvements in newborn outcomes have occurred as a result.

The decision regarding mode of delivery should be made by the health care provider together with the patient. Advantages of a successful vaginal delivery include reduced risks of hemorrhage and infection; shorter postpartum hospital stay; and a less painful, more rapid recovery. However, cesarean delivery may be necessary. Examples of indications for cesarean delivery include hemorrhage from placenta previa, abruptio placentae, prolapse of the umbilical cord, and uterine rupture, as these conditions require prompt delivery. Planned vaginal delivery may be a reasonable approach for a fetus in breech presentation, but depends on the experience of the health care provider. In such circumstances, women should be informed that the risk of perinatal or neonatal mortality or short-term serious neonatal morbidity may be higher with a vaginal delivery than with a cesarean delivery, and the patient's informed consent should be documented.

An estimated 2.5% of all births in the United States are cesarean delivery on maternal request. This procedure should not be performed before 39 weeks of gestation, unless lung maturity can be documented. It is not recommended for women desiring several children, because the risks of placenta previa, placenta accreta, and gravid hysterectomy increase with each cesarean delivery.

Decisions regarding cesarean delivery have important ramifications, because the maternal mortality rate associated with cesarean delivery is two to four times that of a vaginal birth (i.e., 1 per 2500 to 1 per 5000 operations). Cesarean delivery can be performed through various incisions in the uterus. An incision through the thin, lower uterine segment allows for subsequent trials of vaginal birth after cesarean (VBAC) delivery if the patient has had one prior cesarean delivery. An incision through the thick, muscular upper portion of the uterus, a classical cesarean section, carries such a great risk of subsequent uterine rupture that repeat cesarean delivery for these patients is recommended.

## VAGINAL BIRTH AFTER CESAREAN DELIVERY (VBAC)

Cesarean deliveries may be performed as repeat procedures. Prior to the mid-1980s, it was believed that a previous cesarean delivery mandated that all subsequent deliveries be abdominal. Publication of data suggesting the safety of vaginal birth after cesarean (VBAC) led to a decade-long clinical trend away from the nearly 70-year-old adage: "Once a cesarean, always a cesarean." Success rates of VBAC were found to be 60% to 80%. More recently, the pendulum has again swung, resulting in an increasing trend for patients and their physicians to opt for scheduled elective repeat cesarean delivery.

The risks and benefits of a trial of labor versus repeat cesarean delivery should be discussed with the patient who has had a prior cesarean delivery. Although uterine rupture does occur more often with VBAC, the frequency is generally less than 1%.

The American College of Obstetricians and Gynecologists' guidelines for trial of VBAC include the availability of a 24-hour blood bank, continuous electronic fetal heart rate monitoring, a physician capable of performing a cesarean delivery, in-house anesthesia services, and ability to meet a 30-minute "decision-to-incision" time frame if cesarean delivery becomes necessary. Box 8.1 summarizes clinical considerations for VBAC.

---

> ## BOX 8.1
> ### Clinical Considerations in Vaginal Birth After Cesarean Delivery (VBAC)
>
> **Selection criteria useful in identifying candidates for VBAC:**
> - One previous low-transverse cesarean delivery
> - Clinically adequate pelvis
> - No other uterine scars or previous rupture
> - Physician immediately available throughout active labor who is capable of performing an emergency cesarean delivery
> - Availability of anesthesia, facility, and personnel for emergency cesarean delivery
>
> **Circumstances under which a trial of labor should not be attempted:***
> - Previous classical or T-shaped incision or extensive transfundal uterine surgery
> - Previous uterine rupture
> - Medical or obstetric complication that precludes vaginal delivery
> - Two prior uterine scars and no vaginal deliveries
> - Lack of anesthesia, facility, or personnel for an emergency cesarean delivery
>
> *Relative contraindications: two prior uterine surgeries with no previous vaginal delivery

American College of Obstetricians and Gynecologists. *Induction of Labor with Misoprostol.* ACOG Committee Opinion No. 228. Washington, DC: American College of Obstetricians and Gynecologists; 1999; reaffirmed 2008.

American College of Obstetricians and Gynecologists. Obstetric analgesia and anesthesia. ACOG Practice Bulletin No. 36. *Obstet Gynecol.* 2002;100(1):177–191.

American College of Obstetricians and Gynecologists. *Optimal Goals for Anesthesia Care in Obstetrics.* ACOG Committee Opinion No. 256. Washington, DC: American College of Obstetricians and Gynecologists; 2001; reaffirmed 2004.

American College of Obstetricians and Gynecologists. Vaginal birth after previous cesarean delivery. ACOG Practice Bulletin No. 54. *Obstet Gynecol.* 2004;104(1):203–212.

## SUGGESTED READINGS

American College of Obstetricians and Gynecologists. Cesarean delivery on maternal request. ACOG Committee Opinion no. 394. *Obstet Gynecol.* 2007;110(6):1501–1504.

## REFERENCE

1. *Guidelines for Perinatal Care.* 6th ed. Elk Grove Village, IL: American Academy of Pediatrics; Washington, DC: American College of Obstetricians and Gynecologists; 2007:139–162.

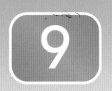
# Abnormal Labor and Intrapartum Fetal Surveillance

**Topic 22:** Abnormal Labor

**Topic 26:** Intrapartum Fetal Surveillance

Students should know how to differentiate between normal and abnormal labor and how to manage abnormal labor. They should know the basic physiology and pathophysiology of the fetal-uteroplacental unit leading to nonreassuring fetal status, the ways the fetal status may be monitored during labor, and the ways labor may be managed in the face of nonreassuring fetal status.

## ABNORMAL LABOR

**Abnormal labor,** or labor **dystocia** (literally, "difficult labor or childbirth") is characterized by the abnormal progression of labor. Dystocia is the leading indication for primary cesarean delivery in the United States. *Despite the high prevalence of labor disorders, considerable variability exists in the diagnosis, management, and criteria for dystocia that requires intervention.* Because dystocia can rarely be diagnosed with certainty, the relatively imprecise term "failure to progress" has been used, which includes lack of progressive cervical dilation or lack of descent of the fetal head or both.

### Factors That Contribute to Normal Labor— The Three Ps

**Labor** is the occurrence of uterine contractions of sufficient intensity, frequency, and duration to bring about demonstrable effacement and dilation of the cervix. Dystocia results from what have been categorized classically as abnormalities of the "power" (uterine contractions or maternal expulsive forces), "passenger" (position, size, or presentation of the fetus), or "passage" (pelvis or soft tissues).

#### UTERINE CONTRACTIONS ("POWER")

*Uterine activity can be monitored by palpation, external **tocodynamometry,** or by using **intrauterine pressure catheters (IUPCs)*** (Fig. 9.1). A tocodynamometer is an external strain

gauge that is placed on the maternal abdomen. It records the frequency of uterine contractions and relaxations, as well as the duration of each contraction. An IUPC, in addition to recording contraction frequency and duration, also directly measures the pressure generated by uterine contractions, via a catheter inserted into the uterine cavity. The catheter is attached to a gauge that measures intrauterine pressure in millimeters of mercury (mm Hg).

*Recent studies suggest that the use of an IUPC instead of external tocodynamometry does not affect the outcome in cases of abnormal labor.*

However, an IUPC may be useful in specific situations, such as maternal obesity or other factors that may prevent accurate clinical evaluation of uterine contractions.

For cervical dilation and fetal descent to occur, each uterine contraction must generate at least 25 mm Hg of peak pressure. Optimal intrauterine pressure is 50 to 60 mm Hg. The frequency of uterine contractions is also important in generating a normal labor pattern: the optimal frequency of uterine contractions is a minimum of three contractions in a 10-minute interval, often described as "adequate." Uterine contractions that are too frequent are not optimal, because they prevent intervals of uterine relaxation. During this "rest interval," the fetus receives unimpeded uteroplacental blood flow for oxygen and waste transport. Without these rest periods, fetal oxygenation may be compromised.

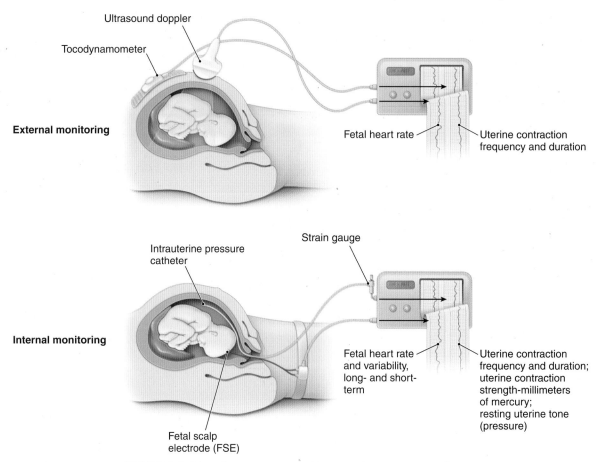

**External monitoring**

Ultrasound doppler

Tocodynamometer

Fetal heart rate

Uterine contraction
frequency and duration

**Internal monitoring**

Intrauterine pressure
catheter

Strain gauge

Fetal heart rate
and variability,
long- and short-
term

Uterine contraction
frequency and duration;
uterine contraction
strength-millimeters
of mercury;
resting uterine tone
(pressure)

Fetal scalp
electrode (FSE)

FIGURE 9.1. Tocodynamometer and intrauterine pressure catheter.

Another unit of measure commonly used to assess contractile strength is the **Montevideo unit (MVU).** This unit is the number of uterine contractions in 10 minutes times the average intensity (above the resting baseline intrauterine pressure). *Normal progress of labor is usually associated with 200 or more Montevideo units.*

## FETAL FACTORS ("PASSENGER")

Evaluation of the passenger includes clinical estimation of fetal weight and clinical evaluation of fetal lie, presentation, position, and attitude. *If a fetus has an estimated weight greater than 4000 to 4500 grams, the risk of dystocia, including shoulder dystocia and fetopelvic disproportion, is greater.* Because ultrasound estimation of fetal weight is often inaccurate by as much as 500 to 1000 grams when the fetus is near term (40 weeks' gestational age), this information must be used in conjunction with other parameters when making management decisions.

*Fetal attitude, presentation, and lie also play a role in the progress of labor* (Fig. 9.2). If the fetal head is asynclitic (turned to one side; **asynclitism**) or extended (**extension**), a larger

cephalic diameter is presented to the pelvis, thereby increasing the possibility of dystocia. A **brow presentation** (about 1 in 3000 deliveries) typically converts to either a vertex or face presentation, but, if persistent, may cause dystocia requiring cesarean delivery. Likewise, a **face presentation** (about 1 in 600 to 1000 deliveries) requires cesarean delivery in most cases. However, a **mentum anterior presentation** (chin toward mother's abdomen) may be delivered vaginally if the fetal head undergoes flexion, rather than the normal extension. *A persistent **occipitoposterior position** is also associated with longer labors (approximately 1 hour in multiparous patients and 2 hours in nulliparous patients).* In **compound presentations,** when one or more limbs prolapse alongside the presenting part (about 1 in 700 deliveries), the extremity usually retracts (either spontaneously or with manual assistance) as labor continues. When it does not, or in the 15% to 20% of compound presentations associated with umbilical cord prolapse, cesarean delivery is required.

Fetal anomalies, such as hydrocephaly and soft tissue tumors, may also cause dystocia. The routine use of prenatal ultrasound for other causes has allowed identification of these situations, significantly reducing the incidence of unexpected dystocia of this kind.

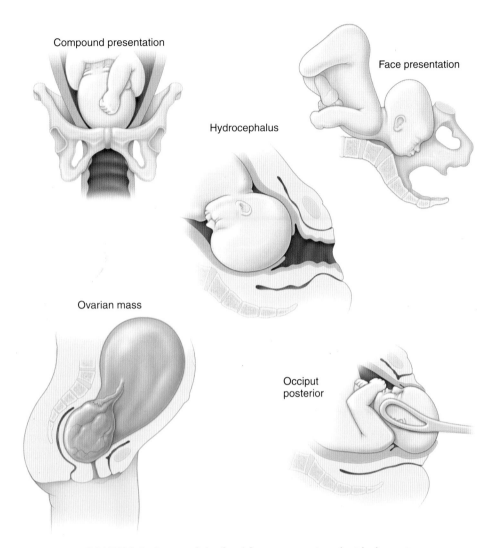

Compound presentation

Face presentation

Hydrocephalus

Ovarian mass

Occiput
posterior

FIGURE 9.2. Some of the fetal factors associated with dystocia.

## MATERNAL FACTORS ("PASSAGE")

A number of maternal factors are associated with dystocia. Dystocia can result from maternal skeletal or soft-tissue anomalies that obstruct the birth canal. **Cephalopelvic disproportion,** in which the size of the maternal pelvis is inadequate to the size of the presenting part of the fetus, may impede fetal descent into the birth canal.

*Clinical, radiographic, and CT measurements of the bony pelvis are poor predictors of successful vaginal delivery, due to the inaccuracy of these measurements as well as case-by-case differences in fetal accommodation and mechanisms of labor.*

**Clinical pelvimetry,** the manual evaluation of the diameters of the pelvis, is also a poor predictor of successful vaginal birth, except in rare circumstances when the pelvic

diameters are so small as to render the pelvis "completely contracted." Although radiographic and CT pelvimetry can be helpful in some cases, the progress of descent of the presenting part in labor is the best test of pelvic adequacy.

Soft-tissue causes of dystocia include abnormalities of the cervix, tumors or other lesions of the colon or adnexa, distended bladder, uterine fibroids, an accessory uterine horn, and morbid obesity. Epidural anesthesia may contribute to dystocia by decreasing the tone of the pelvic floor musculature.

## Risks

*Dystocia may be associated with serious complications for both the woman and the fetus.* Infection (chorioamnionitis) is a consequence of prolonged labor, especially in the setting of ruptured membranes. Fetal infection and bacteremia, including pneumonia caused by aspiration of infected amniotic fluid, is linked to prolonged labor. In addition, there are the attendant risks of cesarean or operative delivery, such as maternal soft tissue injury to the lower genital tract and fetal trauma.

## Diagnosis and Management of Abnormal Labor Patterns

Graphic documentation of progressive cervical dilation and effacement facilitates assessing a patient's progress in labor and identifying abnormal labor patterns. The Friedman Curve (see Chapter 8) is commonly used for this purpose. Labor abnormalities can be categorized into two general types: **protraction disorders,** in which labor is slow to progress, and **arrest disorders,** in which labor ceases to progress (Table 9.1). Protraction can occur during both the latent and active phases of labor, while arrest is recognized only in the active phase. Although the definition of the **latent phase** of labor is controversial, in general it can be defined as the phase in which the cervix effaces but undergoes minimal dilation (see Chapter 8).

Management of abnormal labor encompasses a wide range of options, from observation to operative or cesarean delivery. Management choice depends on several factors:

- Adequacy of uterine contractions
- Fetal malposition or cephalopelvic disproportion
- Other clinical conditions, such as nonreassuring fetal status or chorioamnionitis

Management decisions should be balanced between ensuring a positive outcome for mother and fetus and avoiding the concomitant risks of operative and cesarean delivery.

### FIRST-STAGE DISORDERS

*A **prolonged latent phase** is one that exceeds 20 hours in a nulliparous patient or 14 hours in a multiparous patient. A prolonged latent phase does not necessarily predict an abnormal active phase of labor.* Some patients who have initially been diagnosed as having a prolonged latent phase are subsequently found to have been in false labor. A prolonged latent phase does not in itself pose a danger to the mother or fetus. Options for management of women with a prolonged latent phase of labor include observation and sedation. With either of these options, the patient may stop having contractions, in which case she is not in labor; may go into active labor; or may continue experiencing prolonged labor into the active phase. In the latter case, other interventions as described below may be administered to augment uterine contractions.

*Once the patient is in active labor, the first stage is considered prolonged when the cervix dilates less than 1 cm per hour in nulliparous women, and less than 1.2 to 1.5 cm per hour in multiparous women.* Management options for a prolonged first stage include observation, augmentation by amniotomy or oxytocin, and continuous support. Cesarean delivery usually is warranted if maternal or fetal status becomes nonreassuring.

| TABLE 9.1 | Abnormal Labor Patterns | |
|---|---|---|
| | **Protraction Disorder** | **Arrest Disorder** |
| Latent phase | | — |
| Nulliparous | Duration of >20 hrs | |
| Multiparous | Duration of >14 hrs | |
| First stage | | No cervical dilation for more than 2 hours for both multiparous and nulliparous |
| Nulliparous | Cervical dilation rate of <1 cm per hr | |
| Multiparous | Cervical dilation rate of <1.2 to 1.5 per hr | |
| Second stage Nulliparous & multiparous | With regional anesthesia: Duration of >3 hrs<br><br>No regional anesthesia: Duration of >2 hrs or if fetus descends at a rate of less than 1 cm per hour | No descent after 1 hour of pushing |

From Shields SG, Ratcliffe SD, Fontain P, Leeman L. Dystocia in nulliparous women. *Am Fam Physician.* 2007;75:1671–1678.

*Augmentation* **Augmentation** refers to stimulation of uterine contractions when spontaneous contractions have failed to result in progressive cervical dilation or descent of the fetus. Augmentation can be achieved with **amniotomy** (artificial rupture of membranes) or oxytocin administration. *Augmentation should be considered if the frequency of contractions is less than 3 contractions per 10 minutes or the intensity of contractions is less than 25 mm Hg above the baseline or both.* Before augmentation, the maternal pelvis and cervix as well as fetal position, station, and well-being should be assessed. If there is no evidence of disproportion, oxytocin can be used if uterine contractions are judged to be inadequate. Contraindications to augmentation are similar to those for labor induction (see Chapter 8).

*If the membranes have not ruptured, amniotomy may enhance progress in the active phase and negate the need for oxytocin augmentation.* Amniotomy allows the fetal head, rather than the otherwise intact amniotic sac, to be the dilating force. It may also stimulate the release of prostaglandins, which could aid in augmenting the force of contractions.

Amniotomy is usually performed with a thin, plastic rod with a sharp hook on the end. The end is guided to the open cervical os with the examiner's fingers, and the hook is used to snag and disrupt the amniotic sac. Risks of amniotomy include fetal heart rate decelerations due to cord compression and an increased incidence of chorioamnionitis. For these reasons, amniotomy should not be routine and should be used for women with prolonged labor. The fetal heart rate (FHR) should be evaluated both before and immediately after rupture of the membranes.

*It has been shown that amniotomy combined with oxytocin administration early in the active stage reduces labor by up to 2 hours, although there is no change in the rate of cesarean delivery with this treatment protocol.*

The goal of oxytocin administration is to effect uterine activity sufficient to produce cervical change and fetal descent while avoiding uterine hyperstimulation and fetal compromise. Typically, a goal of a maximum of 5 contractions in a 10-minute period with resultant cervical dilation is considered adequate. Oxytocin may be administered in low-dose or high-dose regimens. Low-dose regimens are associated with a decreased incidence and severity of uterine hyperstimulation. High-dose regimens are associated with decreased labor times, incidence of chorioamnionitis, and cesarean delivery for dystocia.

*Continuous Labor Support* **Continuous** support during labor from caregivers (nurses, midwives, or lay individuals) may have a number of benefits for women and their newborns. Continuous care has been associated with reduced need for pain relief and oxytocin administration, lower rates of cesarean and operative deliveries, decreased incidence of 5-minute Apgar scores lower than 7, and increased patient satisfaction with the labor experience. However, there are insufficient data comparing differences in benefits on the basis of level of training of support personnel—that is, whether the caregivers were nurses, midwives, or doulas. There is no evidence of harmful effects from continuous support during labor.

### SECOND-STAGE DISORDERS

*A second-stage protraction disorder should be considered when the second stage exceeds 3 hours if regional anesthesia has been administered, or 2 hours if no regional anesthesia is used, or if the fetus descends at a rate of less than 1 cm per hour if no regional anesthesia is used. Second-stage arrest is diagnosed when there is no descent after 1 hour of pushing.* In the past, the fetus was thought to be at increased risk for morbidity and mortality when the second stage exceeded 2 hours. Currently, more intensive intrapartum surveillance provides the ability to identify the fetus that may not be tolerating labor well.

*Thus, the length of the second stage of labor is not in itself an absolute or even a strong indication for operative or cesarean delivery.*

As long as heart tones continue to be reassuring and cephalopelvic disproportion has been ruled out, it is considered safe to allow the second stage to continue. If uterine contractions are inadequate, oxytocin administration can be initiated or the dosage increased if already in place.

Bearing down efforts by the patient in conjunction with uterine contractions help bring about delivery. Labor positions other than the dorsal lithotomy position (e.g., knee-chest, sitting, squatting, or birth-chair) may bring about subtle changes in fetal presentation and facilitate vaginal delivery. Fetal accommodation may also be facilitated by allowing the effects of epidural analgesia to dissipate. The absence of epidural analgesia may increase the tone of the pelvic floor muscles, facilitating the cardinal movements of labor and restoring the urge to push. In some cases of fetal malpresentation, manual techniques can facilitate delivery. If the fetus is in the occipitoposterior position and does not spontaneously convert to the normal position, rotation can be performed to turn the fetus to the anterior position (Fig. 9.3).

The decision to perform an operative delivery in the second stage versus continued observation should be made on the basis of clinical assessment of the woman and the fetus and the skill and training of the obstetrician. Nonreassuring status of the fetus or mother is an indication for operative or cesarean delivery.

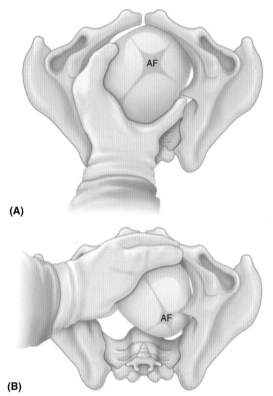

**(A)**

**(B)**

FIGURE 9.3. Manual rotation of a fetus in the occipitoposterior position to the occipitoanterior position. (A) The physician's hand is placed palm upward into the vagina. (B) The hand serves as a wedge to flex the fetal head while the fingers exert a rotating force to bring the occiput to anterior. (AF = anterior fontanel.) (Adapted from Shields SG, Ratcliffe SD, Fontain P, Leeman L. Dystocia in nulliparous women. *Am Fam Physician*. 2007;75(11):1675.)

## OPERATIVE DELIVERY

Operative vaginal deliveries are accomplished by applying direct traction on the fetal skull with forceps, or by applying traction to the fetal scalp by means of a vacuum extractor. The incidence of operative vaginal delivery in the United States is estimated to be 10% to 15%. *Although considered safe in appropriate circumstances, operative vaginal delivery has the potential for maternal and neonatal complications.* Operative vaginal delivery should be performed only by individuals with privileges for such procedures and in settings in which personnel are readily available to perform a cesarean delivery in the event the operative vaginal delivery is unsuccessful. However, the incidence of intracranial hemorrhage is highest among infants delivered by cesarean section following a failed vacuum or forceps delivery. The combination of vacuum and forceps has a similar risk for intracranial hemorrhage. Therefore, an operative vaginal delivery should not be attempted when the probability of success is very low.

## Classification

For both forceps and vacuum extraction deliveries, the type of delivery depends on the fetal station—the relationship between the leading portion of the fetal head and the level of the maternal ischial spines. **Outlet operative vaginal delivery** is the application of forceps or vacuum under the following conditions:

1. The scalp is visible at the introitus without separating labia.
2. The fetal skull has reached pelvic floor.
3. The sagittal suture is in anteroposterior diameter or right or left occiput anterior or posterior position.
4. The fetal head is at or on the perineum.
5. Rotation does not exceed 45°.

**Low operative vaginal delivery** is the application of forceps or vacuum when the leading point of the fetal skull is at station +2 or more and is not on the pelvic floor. This type of operative vaginal delivery has two subtypes:

1. Rotation 45° or less (left or right occiput anterior to occiput anterior, or left or right occiput posterior to occiput posterior)
2. Rotation greater than 45°

**Midpelvis operative vaginal delivery** is the application of forceps or vacuum when the fetal head is engaged but the leading point of the skull is above station +2. Under very unusual circumstances, such as the sudden onset of severe fetal or maternal compromise, application of forceps or vacuum above station +2 may be attempted while simultaneously initiating preparation for a cesarean delivery in the event that the operative vaginal delivery is unsuccessful.

## Indications and Contraindications

No indication for operative vaginal delivery is absolute. The following indications apply when the fetal head is engaged and the cervix is fully dilated:

• Prolonged or arrested second stage of labor
• Suspicion of immediate or potential fetal compromise
• Shortening of the second stage for maternal benefit

In certain situations, operative vaginal delivery should be avoided or, at the least, carefully considered in terms of relative maternal and fetal risks. Most authorities consider vacuum extraction inappropriate in pregnancies before 34 weeks of gestation because of the risk of fetal intraventricular hemorrhage. *Operative delivery also is contraindicated if a live fetus is known to have a bone demineralization condition (e.g., osteogenesis imperfecta) or has a bleeding disorder (e.g., alloimmune thrombocytopenia, hemophilia, or von Willebrand disease), and if the fetal head is unengaged or the position of the fetal head is unknown.*

## Forceps

**Forceps** are primarily used to apply traction to the fetal head to augment the expulsive forces, when the mother's voluntary efforts in conjunction with uterine contractions are insufficient to deliver the infant (Fig. 9.4). Occasionally, forceps are used to rotate the fetal head before applying traction to complete vaginal delivery. Forceps also may be used to control delivery of the fetal head, thereby avoiding precipitous delivery. Different types of forceps are available for the different degrees of molding of the fetal head.

Maternal complications of forceps delivery include perineal trauma, hematoma, and pelvic floor injury. Neonatal risks include injuries to the brain and spine, musculoskeletal injury, and corneal abrasion if the forceps are mistakenly applied over the neonate's eyes. The risk of **shoulder dystocia,** in which the fetus's anterior shoulder becomes lodged against the pubic symphysis, is increased in forceps deliveries of infants weighing over 4000 g.

## Vacuum Extraction

In **vacuum extraction,** a soft vacuum cup is applied to the fetal head and suction is exerted by means of a mechanical pump (Fig. 9.5). Vacuum extraction is associated with less maternal trauma than are forceps, but carries significant neonatal risks. Although the amount of traction applied to the fetal skull is less than that applied with forceps, it is still substantial and can cause serious fetal injury. Neonatal risks include intracranial hemorrhage, subgaleal hematomas, scalp lacerations (if torsion is excessive), hyperbilirubinemia, and retinal hemorrhage. In addition, separation of the scalp from the underlying structures can lead to cephalohematoma. *Overall, the incidence of serious complications with vacuum extraction is approximately 5%.* It is recommended that rocking movements or torque not be applied to the device and that only steady traction in the

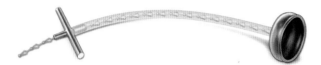

FIGURE 9.5. Vacuum extractor. Because the vacuum port can be bent at a 90-degree angle to the cup, it is useful in malpositions of the fetal head. (Adapted from Bofill JA. *Safe Vacuum Delivery* [Slide presentation]. Washington, DC: American College of Obstetricians and Gynecologists; 2001.)

line of the birth canal should be used. Clinicians caring for the neonate should also be alerted that an operative delivery has been used so that they can monitor the neonate for signs and symptoms of injury.

## BREECH PRESENTATION

**Breech presentation** occurs in about 2% of singleton deliveries at term and more frequently in the early third and second trimesters. In addition to prematurity, other conditions associated with breech presentation include multiple pregnancy, polyhydramnios, hydrocephaly, anencephaly, aneuploidy, uterine anomalies, and uterine tumors. The three kinds of breech presentation—frank, complete, and incomplete breech (Fig. 9.6)—are diagnosed by a combination of Leopold maneuvers, pelvic examination, ultrasonography, and other imaging techniques (Fig. 9.7). *The morbidity and mortality rates for mother and fetus, regardless of gestational age or mode of delivery, are higher in the breech than in the cephalic presentation.* This increased risk to the fetus comes from associated factors such as fetal anomalies, prematurity, and umbilical cord prolapse, as well as birth trauma.

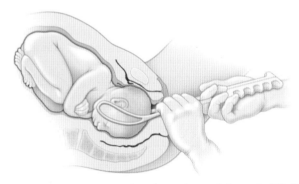

FIGURE 9.4. Forceps delivery. (Adapted from Bofill JA. *Forceps in Obstetrics* [Slide presentation]. Washington, DC: American College of Obstetricians and Gynecologists; 2001.)

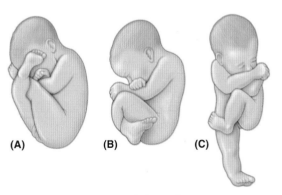

(A)          (B)          (C)

FIGURE 9.6. Types of breech presentations. (A) Frank breech, in which the feet are near the head; (B) complete breech, in which the legs are crossed; (C) footling breech, in which one or both feet are extended.

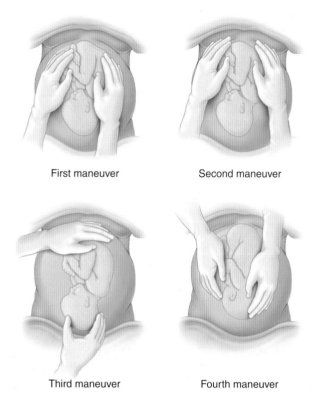

First maneuver

Second maneuver

Third maneuver

Fourth maneuver

FIGURE 9.7. Leopold maneuvers. The maneuvers are used to determine fetal position: 1) determination of what is in the fundus; 2) evaluation of the fetal back and extremities; 3) palpation of the presenting part above the symphysis; 4) determination of the direction and degree of flexion of the head.

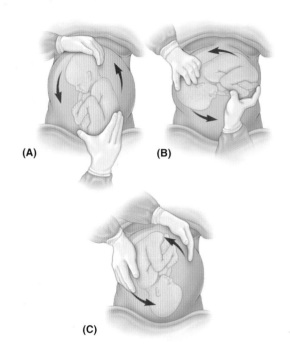

(A)    (B)

(C)

FIGURE 9.8. External cephalic version. In this maneuver, the fetus is converted from a breech to a vertex presentation.

*External cephalic version* (ECV) involves applying pressure to the mother's abdomen to turn the fetus in either a forward or backward somersault to achieve a vertex presentation prior to labor (Fig. 9.8). The goal of ECV is to increase the proportion of vertex presentations among fetuses that were formerly in the breech position near term. Once a vertex presentation is achieved, the chances for a vaginal delivery increase. *This maneuver is successful in approximately half of properly selected cases.* Patients who have completed 36 weeks of gestation are preferred candidates for ECV for several reasons. First, if spontaneous version is going to occur, it is likely to have taken place by 36 completed weeks of gestation. Second, risk of a spontaneous reversion is decreased after external cephalic version at term compared with earlier gestations. *Selection criteria include a normal fetus with reassuring fetal heart tracing, adequate amniotic fluid, presenting part not in the pelvis, and no uterine operative scars.* The risks include premature rupture of membranes, placental abruption, cord accident, and uterine rupture. External version is more often successful in parous women. *Existing evidence may support the use of a tocolytic agent (a drug that stops uterine contractions) during ECV attempts, particularly in nulliparous patients.*

Administration of anti-D immune globulin to Rh negative women is recommended.

In light of recent studies that further clarify the long-term risks of vaginal breech delivery, the decision regarding mode of delivery should depend on the experience of the healthcare provider. *Cesarean delivery will be the preferred mode for most physicians because of the diminishing expertise in vaginal breech delivery.* Planned vaginal delivery of a term singleton breech fetus may be reasonable under hospital-specific protocol guidelines for both eligibility and labor management. The following criteria have been suggested for vaginal breech delivery:

- Normal labor curve
- Gestational age greater than 37 weeks
- Frank or complete breech presentation. Because of the risk of umbilical cord prolapse, vaginal delivery of a fetus in the footling breech position is not recommended.
- Absence of fetal anomalies on ultrasound examination
- Adequate maternal pelvis
- Estimated fetal weight between 2500 g and 4000 g
- Documentation of fetal head flexion. Hyperextension of the fetal head occurs in about 5% of term breech fetuses, requiring cesarean delivery to avoid head entrapment.
- Adequate amniotic fluid volume (defined as a 3-cm vertical pocket)
- Availability of anesthesia and neonatal support

If a vaginal breech delivery is planned, the woman should be informed that the risk of perinatal or neonatal mortality or short-term serious neonatal morbidity may be higher in it than in a cesarean delivery, and the patient's informed consent should be documented.

## SHOULDER DYSTOCIA

Labor may sometimes arrest due to shoulder dystocia. Shoulder dystocia cannot be predicted or prevented, because accurate methods for identifying which fetuses will experience this complication do not exist. Antepartum conditions associated with shoulder dystocia include multiparity, postterm gestation, previous history of a macrosomic birth, and a previous history of shoulder dystocia. Although fetal macrosomia increases the risk of shoulder dystocia, elective induction of labor or elective cesarean delivery for all women suspected of carrying a fetus with macrosomia is not appropriate.

Diagnosis of shoulder dystocia has a subjective component, especially in less severe forms. The delivered fetal head may retract against the maternal perineum (turtle sign) and, if so, may assist in the diagnosis. Interventions that may be used to facilitate delivery include the McRoberts maneuver and the application of suprapubic pressure to assist in dislodging the impacted shoulder (Fig. 9.9). In contrast, fundal pressure may further worsen impaction of the shoulder and also may result in uterine rupture. Controversy exists as to whether episiotomy is necessary, because shoulder dystocia typically is not caused by obstructing soft tissue. Direct fetal manipulation with either rotational maneuvers or delivery of the posterior arm also may be used. In severe cases, more aggressive interventions, such as the Zavanelli maneuver (in which the fetal head is flexed and reinserted into the vagina to reestablish umbilical cord blood flow and delivery performed through cesarean section) or intentional

fracture of the fetal clavicle, may be performed. Regardless of the procedures used, brachial plexus injury is associated with shoulder dystocia; incidence ranges from 4% to 40%. However, most cases resolve without permanent disability; fewer than 10% of all cases of shoulder dystocia result in a persistent brachial plexus injury.

## INTRAPARTUM FETAL SURVEILLANCE

Evidence suggesting a **nonreassuring fetal status** during labor occurs in 5% to 10% of pregnancies. **Intrapartum fetal surveillance** is the indirect measurement of indicators of fetal status, such as fetal heart rate, blood gases, pulse rate, amniotic fluid volume, and fetal stimulation responses, during labor. *The goal of intrapartum fetal surveillance is to recognize changes in fetal oxygenation that could result in serious complications.* However, it is now recognized that many neurologic conditions previously attributed to **birth asphyxia** (defined as a situation of damaging acidemia, hypoxia, and metabolic acidosis) are in fact attributable to other causes not associated with labor, such as maternal infection, coagulation disorders, and autoimmune disorders; genetic causes; or low birth weight. Physicians should understand that intrapartum fetal surveillance is a tool for detection of events that occur during labor that could compromise fetal oxygenation and, in rare cases, lead to permanent neurologic disability.

### Pathophysiology

The **uteroplacental unit** provides oxygen and nutrients to the fetus while receiving carbon dioxide and wastes,

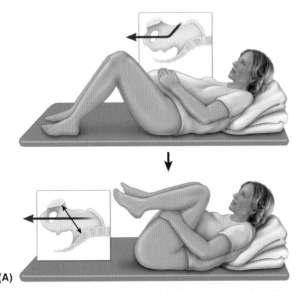

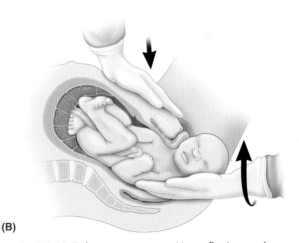

(A)          (B)

FIGURE 9.9. Procedures used to manage shoulder dystocia. (A) McRoberts maneuver. Hyperflexion and abduction of the hips cause cephalad rotation of the symphysis pubis and flattening of the lumbar lordosis that frees the impacted shoulder. (B) Suprapubic pressure plus cephalad rotation.

the products of the normal aerobic fetal metabolism. **Uteroplacental insufficiency** occurs when the uteroplacental unit is compromised. Initial fetal responses include fetal hypoxia (decreased blood oxygen levels); shunting of blood flow to the fetal brain, heart, and adrenal glands; and transient, repetitive, late decelerations of the FHR. If hypoxia continues, the fetus will eventually switch over to anaerobic glycolysis and develop metabolic acidosis. Lactic acid accumulates and progressive damage to vital organs occurs, especially the fetal brain and myocardium. If intervention is not timely, serious and possibly permanent damage and sometimes death can result.

**Neonatal encephalopathy** is a clinically defined syndrome of disturbed neurologic function in the earliest days of life in the term infant, manifested by difficulty with initiating and maintaining respiration, depression of tone and reflexes, subnormal level of consciousness, and sometimes seizures. Neonatal encephalopathy is not always associated with permanent neonatal neurologic impairment. **Hypoxic-ischemic encephalopathy (HIE)** is a subtype of neonatal encephalopathy for which the cause is considered to be limitation of oxygen and blood flow near the time of birth. Historically, it has been assumed that most cases of neonatal encephalopathy were hypoxic-ischemic encephalopathy, but epidemiologic studies have established that this assumption is incorrect.

> *Approximately 70% of cases of neonatal encephalopathy are caused by factors that were present before the onset of labor.*

It is estimated that the incidence of neonatal encephalopathy caused by intrapartum hypoxia is approximately 1.6/10,000, absent other coincident preconceptual or antepartum abnormalities. HIE is thus one item in the larger category of encephalopathies which may result from conditions such as prenatal stroke, prenatal infection, genetic abnormalities, and neonatal cerebral malformation. The criteria sufficient to suggest that an encephalopathy is associated with an acute intrapartum event are presented in Box 9.1.

**Cerebral palsy** is a chronic disability of the central nervous system (CNS) characterized by aberrant control of movement and posture appearing early in life and not as a result of progressive neurologic disease. Only one type of cerebral palsy, **spastic quadriplegia,** is associated with antepartum or intrapartum interruption of the fetal blood supply. Disorders not associated with intrapartum or peripartum asphyxia include dyskinetic or ataxic cerebral palsy (which commonly has a genetic origin) and epilepsy, mental retardation, or attention-deficit hyperactivity disorders.

## Intrapartum Fetal Heart Rate Monitoring

**Fetal heart rate (FHR) monitoring** is a modality intended to determine if a fetus is well-oxygenated. The majority of neonates (approximately 85%) born in the United States are assessed with **electronic fetal monitoring (EFM),** making it the most common obstetric procedure. **Intermittent auscultation** of the FHR after a contraction also is used to assess intrapartum fetal well-being. Beginning

---

**BOX 9.1**

**Criteria to Define an Acute Intrapartum Hypoxic Event as Sufficient to Cause Cerebral Palsy**

I. Essential criteria (must meet all four)
   a. Fetal metabolic acidosis demonstrated from umbilical cord arterial blood gas measurement (pH <7 and base deficit ≥12 mmol/L)
   b. Early-onset severe or moderate neonatal encephalopathy in newborn of ≥34 weeks gestational age
   c. Spastic or, less commonly, dyskinetic cerebral palsy
   d. Exclusion of other identifiable causes (trauma, coagulopathy, infection, or genetic anomaly)
II. Criteria non-specific to asphyxial insult, but suggestive of intrapartum timing (close proximity to labor and delivery, within 48 hours)

   a. Sentinel hypoxic event immediately before or during labor
   b. Sudden nonreassuring fetal heart rate pattern (e.g., sudden, sustained fetal bradycardia or absent variability in the presence of persistent late or variable decelerations)
   c. Apgar scores of 0–3 beyond 5 minutes
   d. Onset of multisystem illness (e.g., acute bowel injury, renal failure, hepatic failure, cardiac damage, hematologic abnormalities) within 72 hours of birth.
   e. Early cerebral imaging with evidence of acute nonfocal cerebral abnormality.

From ACOG Task Force on Neonatal Encephalopathy and Cerebral Palsy. *Neonatal Encephalopathy and Cerebral Palsy: Defining the Pathogenesis and Pathophysiology.* Washington, DC: American College of Obstetricians and Gynecologists; 2003:74.

in the 1980s, EFM became more common; rates of its use have doubled over the past 35 years.

EFM may be performed externally or internally. Most external monitors use a Doppler device with computerized logic to interpret and count the Doppler signals. Internal FHR monitoring is accomplished with a fetal electrode, which is a spiral wire placed directly on the fetal scalp or other presenting part.

Fetal heart rates by EFM are described in terms of baseline rate, variability, presence of accelerations, periodic or episodic decelerations, and the changes in these characteristics over time (Table 9.2) and classified by a three-tier fetal

| TABLE 9.2 | Definitions of Fetal Heart Rate Patterns |
|---|---|
| **Pattern** | **Definition** |
| Baseline | • The mean FHR rounded to increments of 5 beats per min during a 10 min segment, excluding:<br>  • Periodic or episodic changes<br>  • Periods of marked FHR variability<br>  • Segments of baseline that differ by more than 25 beats per min<br>• The baseline must be for a minimum of 2 min in any 10-min segment |
| Baseline variability | • Determined in a 10-minute window, excluding accelerations and decelerations.<br>• Variability is visually quantitated as the amplitude of peak-to-trough in beats per min<br>  • Absent—amplitude range undetectable<br>  • Minimal—amplitude range detectable but 5 beats per min or fewer<br>  • Moderate (normal)—amplitude range 6–25 beats per min<br>  • Marked—amplitude range greater than 25 beats per min |
| Acceleration | • A visually apparent increase (onset to peak in less than 30 sec) in the FHR from the most recently calculated baseline<br>• The duration of an acceleration is defined as the time from the initial change in FHR from the baseline to the return of the FHR to the baseline<br>• At 32 weeks of gestation and beyond, an acceleration has an acme of 15 beats per min or more above baseline, with a duration of 15 sec or more but less than 2 min<br>• Before 32 weeks of gestation, an acceleration has an acme of 10 beats per min or more above baseline, with a duration of 10 sec or more but less than 2 min<br>• Prolonged acceleration lasts 2 min or more, but less than 10 min<br>• If an acceleration lasts 10 min or longer, it is a baseline change |
| Bradycardia | Baseline FHR less than 110 beats per min |
| Decelerations | • Recurrent: occur with more than 50% of contractions during any 20-minute period<br>• Intermittent: occur with less than 50% of contractions during any 20-minute period |
| Early deceleration | • In association with a uterine contraction, a visually apparent, gradual (onset to nadir 30 sec or more) decrease in FHR with return to baseline<br>• Nadir of the deceleration occurs at the same time as the peak of the contraction |
| Late deceleration | • In association with a uterine contraction, a visually apparent, gradual (onset to nadir 30 sec or more) decrease in FHR with return to baseline<br>• Onset, nadir, and recovery of the deceleration occur after the beginning, peak, and end of the contraction, respectively |
| Tachycardia | Baseline FHR greater than 160 beats per min |
| Variable deceleration | • An abrupt (onset to nadir less than 30 sec), visually apparent decrease in the FHR below the baseline<br>• The decrease in FHR is 15 beats per min or more, with a duration of 15 sec or more, but less than 2 min<br>• When variable decelerations are associated with uterine contractions, their onset, depth, and duration commonly vary with successive uterine contractions. |
| Prolonged deceleration | • Visually apparent decrease in the FHR below the baseline<br>• Deceleration is 15 beats per min or more, lasting 2 min or more, but less than 10 min from onset to return to baseline |

Abbreviation: FHR, fetal heart rate.
Reprinted from National Institute of Child Health and Human Development Research Planning Workshop. Electronic fetal heart rate monitoring: research guidelines for interpretation. Am J Obstet Gynecol. 1997;177(6):1385–1390; with permission from Elsevier.

heart rate interpretation system (Box 9.2). *The goal of FHR monitoring is to detect signs of fetal jeopardy in time to intervene before irreversible damage occurs.* Despite the liberal use of continuous EFM in both high-risk and low-risk patients, there has been no consistent decrease in the frequency of cerebral palsy in the last two decades. Fetuses who are severely asphyxiated during the intrapartum period will have abnormal heart rate patterns.

*However, most patients with nonreassuring FHR patterns give birth to healthy infants. In addition, the false-positive rate of EFM for predicting adverse outcomes is high.*

Guidelines for intrapartum FHR monitoring are given in Table 9.3.

---

**BOX 9.2**
## Three-Tier Fetal Heart Rate Interpretation System

### Category I
*Category I fetal heart rate (FHR) tracings include <u>all</u> of the following:*
- Baseline rate: 110–160 beats per minute (bpm)
- Baseline FHR variability: moderate
- Late or variable decelerations: absent
- Early decelerations: present or absent
- Accelerations: present or absent

### Category II
*Category II FHR tracings include all FHR tracings not categorized as Category I or Category III. Category II tracings may represent an appreciable fraction of those encountered in clinical care. Examples of Category II FHR tracings include any of the following:*

**Baseline Rate**
- Bradycardia not accompanied by absent baseline variability
- Tachycardia

**Baseline FHR Variability**
- Minimal baseline variability
- Absent baseline variability not accompanied by recurrent decelerations
- Marked baseline variability

**Accelerations**
- Absence of induced accelerations after fetal stimulation

**Periodic or Episodic Decelerations**
- Recurrent variable decelerations accompanied by minimal or moderate baseline variability
- Prolonged deceleration ≥2 minutes but <10 minutes
- Recurrent late decelerations with moderate baseline variability
- Variable decelerations with other characteristics, such as slow return to baseline, "overshoots," or "shoulders"

### Category III
*Category III FHR tracings include either:*
- Absent baseline FHR variability and any of the following:
  – Recurrent late decelerations
  – Recurrent variable decelerations
  – Bradycardia
- Sinusoidal pattern

From Macones GA, Hankins GDV, Spong CY, Hauth J, Moore T. The 2008 National Institute of Child Health and Human Development Workshop Report on Electronic Fetal Monitoring: Update on Definitions, Interpretation and Research Guidelines. *Obstetrics & Gynecology.* 112(3):661–666, September 2008.

| TABLE 9.3 | Guidelines for Intrapartum Fetal Monitoring | | | |
|---|---|---|---|---|
| | **Auscultation** | | **Continuous Electronic Monitoring** | |
| | Low Risk | High Risk | Low Risk | High Risk |
| Active phase of first stage | Evaluate and record FHR every 30 min after a contraction | Evaluate and record FHR every 15 min, preferably after a contraction | Evaluate tracing at least every 30 min | Evaluate tracing at least every 15 min |
| Second stage | Evaluate and record FHR every 15 min | Evaluate and record FHR at least every 5 min | Evaluate tracing at least every 15 min | Evaluate tracing at least every 5 min |

Abbreviation: FHR, fetal heart rate.
American College of Obstetricians and Gynecologists. Fetal heart rate patterns: monitoring, interpretation, and management. ACOG Technical Bulletin 207. Washington DC: American College of Obstetricians and Gynecologists; 1995.

## FETAL HEART RATE PATTERNS

The normal baseline FHR is 120–160 beats per minute (bpm). An FHR less than 120 beats per minute is considered **bradycardia.** Fetal bradycardia between 100 and 120 beats per minute usually can be tolerated for long periods when it is accompanied by normal FHR variability. An FHR between 80–100 bpm is nonreassuring. An FHR that persists below 80 is an ominous sign and may presage fetal death.

An FHR above 160 beats per minute is considered **tachycardia.** The most common cause of fetal tachycardia is chorioamnionitis, but it also may be due to maternal fever, thyrotoxicosis, medication, and fetal cardiac arrhythmias. Fetal tachycardia between 160 and 200 beats per minute without any other abnormalities in FHR is usually well-tolerated.

## FETAL HEART RATE VARIABILITY

*Fetal heart rate variability* refers to the fluctuations in the FHR of two cycles or more, visually quantified as the amplitude of peak to trough in beats per minute. *FHR is graded according to amplitude range* (see Table 9.3; Fig 9.10).

*Moderate variability is an assuring sign that reflects adequate fetal oxygenation and normal brain function. In the presence of normal FHR variability, regardless of what other FHR patterns exist, the fetus is not experiencing cerebral tissue asphyxia.*

Decreased variability is associated with fetal hypoxia, acidemia, drugs that may depress the fetal CNS (e.g., maternal narcotic analgesia), fetal tachycardia, fetal CNS and cardiac anomalies, prolonged uterine contractions (uterine hypertonus), prematurity, and fetal sleep.

## PERIODIC FHR CHANGES

The FHR may vary with uterine contractions by slowing or accelerating in periodic patterns. These **periodic FHR changes** are classified as accelerations or decelerations, based on whether they are increases or decreases in the FHR and on their magnitude (in beats per minute).

*Accelerations* **Accelerations** *of the FHR are visually apparent increases (onset to peak in less than 30 seconds) in the FHR from the most recently calculated baseline* Accelerations are generally associated with reassuring fetal status and an absence of hypoxia and acidemia. Stimulation of the fetal scalp by digital examination usually causes heart rate acceleration in the normal fetus with an arterial fetal pH of >7.20 if delivery were to occur at the time of measurement. For this reason, fetal scalp stimulation is sometime used as a test of fetal well-being. External vibration stimulation, also termed **vibroacoustic stimulation,** elicits the same response and is also used for this purpose (see "Ancillary Tests," below).

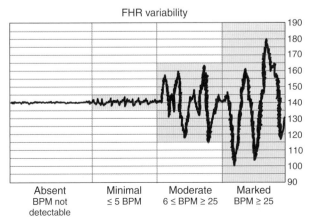

FIGURE 9.10. Fetal heart rate variability.

*Decelerations* Fetal heart rate **decelerations** *are visually apparent decreases in FHR from the baseline.* They can be either gradual (onset to nadir in 30 seconds or more) or abrupt (onset to nadir in less than 30 seconds). **Early decelerations** are associated with uterine contractions: the nadir of the deceleration occurs at the same time as the peak of the uterine contraction and, thus, is a "mirror image" of the contraction (Fig 9.11). Early decelerations are the result of pressure on the fetal head from the birth canal, digital examination, or forceps application that causes a reflex response through the vagus nerve with acetylcholine release at the fetal sinoatrial node. This response may be blocked with vagolytic drugs, such as atropine. Early FHR decelerations are considered physiologic, and are not a cause of concern.

**Late FHR decelerations** are visually apparent decreases in the fetal heart rate from the baseline fetal heart rate, associated with uterine contractions. The onset, nadir, and recovery of the deceleration occur, respectively, after the beginning, peak, and end of the contraction. *Late decelerations are considered significantly nonreassuring, especially when repetitive and associated with decreased variability.* Late decelerations are associated with uteroplacental insufficiency, as a result of either decreased uterine perfusion or decreased placental function, and thus with decreased intervillous exchange of oxygen and carbon dioxide and progressive fetal hypoxia and acidemia.

*Variable FHR decelerations* *are abrupt, visually apparent decreases in the fetal heart rate below the baseline fetal heart rate.* These variable decelerations may start before, during, or after uterine contraction starts, hence the term "variable." Variable decelerations are also mediated through the vagus nerve, with sudden and often erratic release of acetylcholine at the fetal sinoatrial node, resulting in their characteristic sharp deceleration slope. They are usually associated with umbilical cord compression, which may result from wrapping of the cord around parts of the fetus, fetal anomalies, or even knots in the umbilical cord. They are also commonly associated with oligohydramnios, in which the buffering space for the umbilical cord created by the amniotic fluid is lost. *Variable decelerations are the most common periodic FHR pattern.* They are often correctable by changes in the maternal position to relieve pressure on the umbilical cord. Infusion of fluid into the amniotic cavity (**amnioinfusion**) to relieve umbilical cord compression in cases of oligohydramnios or when rupture of membranes has occurred, has been shown to be effective in decreasing the rate of decelerations and cesarean delivery.

## Ancillary Tests

Because the rate of false-positive diagnosis of EFM is high, attempts have been made to find ancillary tests that help confirm a nonreassuring FHR tracing.

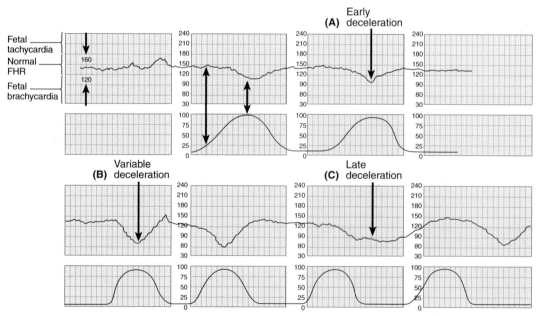

FIGURE 9.11. Fetal heart rate patterns. (A) Early deceleration. Notice how the nadir of the deceleration occurs at the same time as the peak of the uterine contraction; they are mirror images of each other. (B) Variable deceleration. These decelerations may start before, during, or after a uterine contraction starts (C) Late deceleration. The onset, nadir, and recovery of the deceleration occur, respectively, after the beginning, peak, and end of the contraction.

## FETAL STIMULATION

In the case of an EFM tracing with decreased or absent variability without spontaneous accelerations, an effort should be made to elicit one. Four techniques are available to stimulate the fetus: 1) fetal scalp sampling, 2) Allis clamp scalp stimulation, 3) vibro-acoustic stimulation, and 4) digital scalp stimulation. *Each of these techniques involves accessing the fetal scalp through the dilated cervix.* In vibroacoustic stimulation, the fetal scalp is stimulated with a vibratory device, and in digital scalp stimulation, the physician uses his or her finger to gently stroke the scalp.

Each of these tests is a reliable method to exclude acidosis if accelerations are noted after stimulation. Because vibroacoustic stimulation and scalp stimulation are less invasive than the other two methods, they are the preferred methods. When there is an acceleration following stimulation, acidosis is unlikely and labor can continue.

## DETERMINATION OF FETAL BLOOD pH OR LACTATE

When a nonreassuring FHR tracing persists without spontaneous or stimulated accelerations, a scalp blood sample for the determination of pH or lactate can be considered (Fig. 9.12). However, the use of scalp pH has decreased, and it may not be available at some tertiary hospitals. Furthermore, the positive predictive value of a low scalp pH to identify a newborn with HIE is only 3%.

## PULSE OXIMETRY

The use of pulse oximetry has been suggested as a modality to reduce the false-positive diagnosis of a nonreassuring FHR. However, research has demonstrated that neither the overall rate of cesarean delivery nor the rate of umbilical arterial pH less than 7 decreased when pulse oximetry was used in association with EFM in cases of nonreassuring fetal status. Because of the uncertain benefit of pulse oximetry and concerns about falsely reassuring fetal oxygenation, use of the fetal pulse oximeter in clinical practice cannot be supported at this time. Additional studies to test the efficacy and safety of fetal pulse oximetry are underway.

## Diagnosis and Management of a Persistently Nonreassuring FHR Pattern

A reassuring FHR pattern (Category I) may include a normal baseline rate, moderate FHR variability, persistence of accelerations, and absence of decelerations. Patterns believed to be predictive of current or impending fetal asphyxia (Category III) include recurrent late decelerations, recurrent severe variable decelerations, or sustained bradycardia with absent FHR variability. A nonreassuring pattern (Category II) is one that falls between these two extremes.

In the presence of a nonreassuring FHR pattern, the etiology should be determined, if possible, and an attempt should be made to correct the pattern by addressing the primary problem. If the pattern persists, initial measures include changing the lateral position to the left lateral position, administering oxygen, correcting maternal hypotension, and discontinuing oxytocin, if appropriate. Where the pattern does not respond to change in position or oxygenation, the use of tocolytic agents has been suggested to abolish uterine contractions and prevent umbilical cord compression. Uterine hyperstimulation can be identified by evaluating uterine contraction frequency and duration and can be treated with beta-adrenergic drugs. Amnioinfusion may also be used to prevent umbilical cord compressions. *Awaiting vaginal delivery is appropriate if it has been determined that delivery is imminent. If it is not, and there is evidence of progressive fetal hypoxia and acidosis, cesarean delivery is warranted.*

## MECONIUM

**Meconium** is a thick, black, tarry substance that is present in the fetal intestinal tract. It is composed of amniotic fluid, **lanugo** (the fine hair that covers the fetus), bile, and fetal skin and intestinal cells. The neonate's first stool consists of meconium. However, the fetus may pass the meconium in utero, which is a sign of fetal stress. Meconium passage is detected during labor when the amniotic fluid is stained dark green or black.

*Meconium-stained amniotic fluid is present in about 10% to 20% of births, and most meconium-stained neonates do not develop problems.*

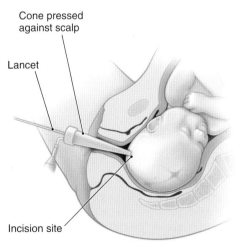

FIGURE 9.12. Fetal scalp sampling.

Cone pressed against scalp

Lancet

Incision site

**Meconium aspiration syndrome,** a condition caused by inhalation of meconium-stained amniotic fluid by the fetus, occurs in about 6% of births in which meconium is present. Severe cases of this syndrome may cause pneumonitis, pneumothorax, and pulmonary artery hypertension.

When there is thick meconium at delivery, interventions to prevent or decrease meconium aspiration syndrome should be considered. *Because meconium passage may predate labor, amnioinfusion should not be used as a preventive measure for meconium aspiration syndrome.* Suctioning of the upper airway should be performed after delivery of the head. If the infant is not vigorous and thick meconium is present, the fetus should be intubated and suctioning to remove material below the glottis should be performed before initiating positive-pressure ventilation. If the infant is active, suctioning and intubation are therapeutic options that are part of ongoing stabilization and care.

## SUGGESTED READINGS

ACOG Task Force on Neonatal Encephalopathy and Cerebral Palsy. *Neonatal Encephalopathy and Cerebral Palsy: Defining the Pathogenesis and Pathophysiology.* Washington, DC: American College of Obstetricians and Gynecologists; 2003.

American College of Obstetricians and Gynecologists. Amnioinfusion does not prevent meconium aspiration syndrome. ACOG Committee Opinion No. 346. *Obstet Gynecol.* 2006;108(4): 1053–1055.

American College of Obstetricians and Gynecologists. Analgesia and cesarean delivery rates. ACOG Committee Opinion No. 339. *Obstet Gynecol.* 2006;107(6):1487–1488.

American College of Obstetricians and Gynecologists. Dystocia and augmentation of labor. ACOG Practice Bulletin No. 49. *Obstet Gynecol.* 2003;102(6):1445–1454.

American College of Obstetricians and Gynecologists. External cephalic version. ACOG Practice Bulletin No. 13. Washington, DC: American College of Obstetricians and Gynecologists; 2000.

American College of Obstetricians and Gynecologists. Inappropriate use of the terms fetal distress and birth asphyxia. ACOG Committee Opinion No. 326. *Obstet Gynecol.* 2005;106(6):1469–1470.

American College of Obstetricians and Gynecologists. Intrapartum fetal heart rate monitoring. ACOG Practice Bulletin No. 70. *Obstet Gynecol.* 2005;106(6):1453–1461.

American College of Obstetricians and Gynecologists. Mode of term singleton breech delivery. ACOG Committee Opinion No. 340. *Obstet Gynecol.* 2006;108(1):235–237.

American College of Obstetricians and Gynecologists. Operative vaginal delivery. ACOG Practice Bulletin No. 17. Washington, DC: American College of Obstetricians and Gynecologists; 2000.

American College of Obstetricians and Gynecologists. Shoulder dystocia. ACOG Practice Bulletin No. 40. *Obstet Gynecol.* 2002; 100(5pt1):1045–1450.

American College of Obstetricians and Gynecologists. Vaginal birth after previous cesarean delivery. ACOG Practice Bulletin No. 54. *Obstet Gynecol.* 2004;104(1):203–212.

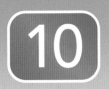

# Immediate Care of the Newborn

## INITIAL CARE OF THE WELL NEWBORN

### Delivery Room Assessment

In accordance with the American Heart Association (AHA) and the American Academy of Pediatrics (AAP), at least one person skilled in neonatal assessment and resuscitation should be available at every delivery to care for the newborn.

*Every delivering physician should be familiar with the initial assessment, resuscitation, and care of a newborn infant.*

The preterm newborn has special needs; these complications are discussed in the chapter on preterm birth (Chapter 20).

Immediately following delivery, the newborn infant should first be assessed to decide whether resuscitation is necessary. Four characteristics define a newborn who requires no additional resuscitation:

1. A full-term infant
2. Clear amniotic fluid with no evidence of meconium and infection
3. Spontaneous breathing and crying
4. Good muscle tone

In an effort to predict which newborns will require more intensive resuscitation, the gestational age should be estimated as accurately as possible prior to delivery. This allows the appropriate neonatal team to be present and prepared for resuscitation. It is also possible to assess the infant after delivery using the **Ballard scoring system,** which evaluates neuromuscular and physical maturity (Fig. 10.1).

The **Apgar Scoring system** is commonly used as an objective means to assess the newborn's condition (Table 10.1). Five signs are given scores of 0, 1, or 2, for a total of up to 10. Scores are assigned at 1 and 5 minutes, and at every 5 minutes until 20 minutes thereafter, if the 5-minute Apgar score is less than 7. Although these continued assess-ments are not part of the original Apgar scoring system, many clinicians find them to be of value in evaluating how an infant is responding to resuscitation. An Apgar score of 7 to 10 is indicative of an infant who requires no active resuscitative intervention; a score of 4 to 7 is considered indicative of a mildly to moderately depressed infant; and a score of less than 4 is suggestive of a severely depressed infant who requires immediate resuscitative efforts.

*The Apgar score should not be used to define birth asphyxia, because it is not designed to do so and, indeed, does not provide such information.*

Likewise, the Apgar score cannot be used to identify the causes of the newborn illness. In general, a low 1-minute Apgar score identifies the newborn who requires particular attention. The 5-minute Apgar score can be used to evaluate the effectiveness of any resuscitative efforts that have been undertaken, or to identify an infant who needs more evaluation and management. It should not be used to predict neurologic outcome in term infants.

### Routine Care

Basic routine care is necessary for all newborn infants, regardless of the need for resuscitative efforts. For infants who do not require resuscitation at birth, routine care is performed immediately following delivery.

First, the newborn infant is thoroughly dried to maintain appropriate body temperature. Warm blankets, skin-to-skin contact with the mother, or a radiant warmer can all accomplish this task.

*For healthy, vigorous, term neonates, skin-to-skin contact promotes maternal–infant bonding and initiation of breast-feeding in the first hour or life.*

**Neuromuscular maturity**

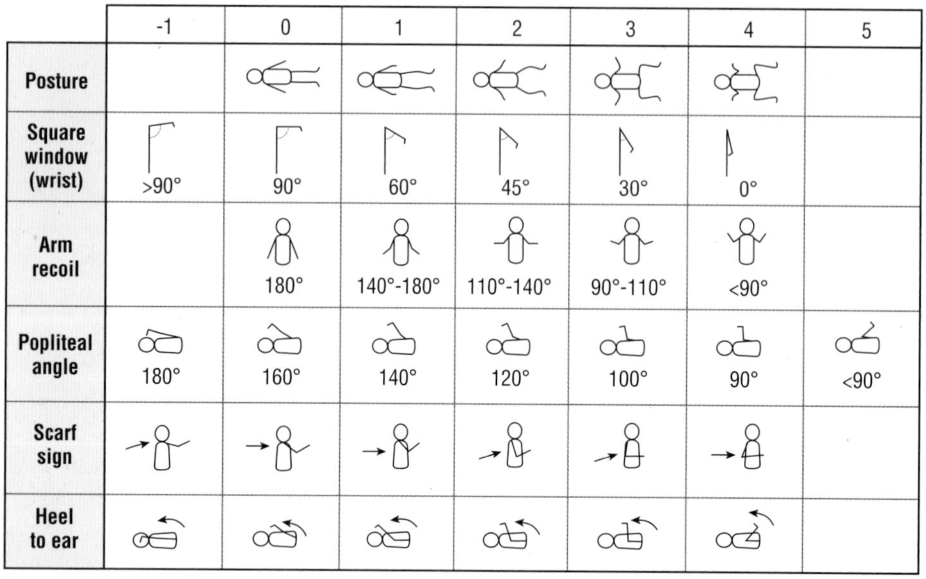

| | -1 | 0 | 1 | 2 | 3 | 4 | 5 |
|---|---|---|---|---|---|---|---|
| **Posture** | | | | | | | |
| **Square window (wrist)** | >90° | 90° | 60° | 45° | 30° | 0° | |
| **Arm recoil** | | 180° | 140°-180° | 110°-140° | 90°-110° | <90° | |
| **Popliteal angle** | 180° | 160° | 140° | 120° | 100° | 90° | <90° |
| **Scarf sign** | | | | | | | |
| **Heel to ear** | | | | | | | |

**Maturity rating**

| Score | Weeks |
|---|---|
| -10 | 20 |
| -5 | 22 |
| 0 | 24 |
| 5 | 26 |
| 10 | 28 |
| 15 | 30 |
| 20 | 32 |
| 25 | 34 |
| 30 | 36 |
| 35 | 38 |
| 40 | 40 |
| 45 | 42 |
| 50 | 44 |

**(B)**

**Physical maturity**

| | | | | | | | |
|---|---|---|---|---|---|---|---|
| **Skin** | Sticky friable, transparent | Gelatinous red, translucent | Smooth pink, visible veins | Superficial peeling or rash or both, few veins | Cracking pale areas, rare veins | Parchment deep cracking, no vessels | Leathery, cracked, wrinkled |
| **Lanugo** | None | Sparse | Abundant | Thinning | Bald areas | Mostly bald | |
| **Plantar surface** | Heel-toe 40-50 mm:-1 <40 mm:-2 | <50 mm, no crease | Faint red marks | Anterior transverse crease only | Creases on anterior 2/3 | Creases over entire sole | |
| **Breast** | Imperceptible | Barely perceptible | Flat areola- no bud | Stripped areola, 1-2 mm bud | Raised areola, 3-4 mm bud | Full areola, 5-10 mm bud | |
| **Eye/ear** | Lids fused loosely (-1) tightly (-2) | Lids open, pinna flat, stays folded | Slightly curved pinna, soft, slow recoil | Well curved pinna, soft but ready recoil | Formed and firm, instant recoil | Thick cartilage, ear stiff | |
| **Genitals male** | Scrotum flat, smooth | Scrotum empty, faint rugae | Testes in upper canal rare rugae | Testes descending, few rugae | Testes down, good rugae | Testes pendulous deep rugae | |
| **Genitals female** | Clitoris prominent, labia flat | Prominent clitoris, small labia minora | Prominent clitoris, enlarged minora | Majora & minora equally prominent | Majora large, minora small | Majora cover clitoris & minora | |

**(A)**

FIGURE 10.1. The Ballard score. The Ballard Scoring System uses points assigned to observations about neuromuscular maturity and physical maturity. (B) The points are summed yielding a score used to arrive at an estimated age in weeks. (*Guidelines for Perinatal Care.* 6th ed. Washington, DC: American College of Obstetricians and Gynecologists; 2007:216–217. Original source: Ballard JL, Khoury JC, Wedig K, Wang L, Eilers-Walsman BL, Lipp R. New Ballard Score expanded to include extremely premature infants. *J Pediatr.* 1991;119(3):417–423.)

| TABLE 10.1 | Apgar Scoring System | | |
|---|---|---|---|
| Sign | 0 | 1 | 2 |
| Color | Blue or pale | Acrocyanotic | Completely pink |
| Heart rate | Absent | <100 bpm | >100 bpm |
| Reflex activity response to stimulation | No response | Grimace | Cry or active withdrawal |
| Muscle tone | Limp | Some flexion | Active motion |
| Respirations | Absent | Weak cry; hypoventilation | Good, crying |

Bpm = beats per minute.

Premature infants have more difficulty maintaining their body temperature and are more susceptible to cold stress. These infants require warming pads, heated towels, and a preheated radiant warmer to stay warm.

Second, after the **umbilical cord** is clamped and cut, it is left exposed to air to facilitate drying and separation. Local application of antimicrobial agents (e.g., triple-dye, iodophor ointment, hexachlorophene powder) is common. The umbilical cord loses its bluish-white appearance within the first 24 hours after delivery. After a few days, the blackened, dried stump sloughs, leaving a granulating wound. If cord blood banking has been requested, the sample should be obtained and stored at this time.

Another essential component of routine care is the assessment of vital signs. An infant's temperature, heart and respiratory rate, core and peripheral color, level of alertness, tone, and activity should be monitored at delivery and every 30 minutes thereafter until these measures are stable for at least 2 hours.

If the mother plans to breastfeed, the newborn should be placed at the breast in the delivery room within the first hour after delivery. In general, healthy neonates should remain with their mothers.

## TRANSITIONAL CARE

Following the initial assessment and routine care of a healthy neonate, continued close observation is necessary for the subsequent stabilization-transition period (the first 6 to 12 hours after birth) to identify any problems that may arise. *The following findings should raise concern and result in closer observation: temperature instability; change in activity, including refusal of feeding; unusual skin coloration; abnormal cardiac or respiratory activity; abdominal distention; bilious vomiting; excessive lethargy or sleeping; delayed or abnormal stools; and delayed voiding.*

Following delivery, all newborns should receive prophylactic application of antibiotic ointment (containing erythromycin [0.5%] or tetracycline [1%]) to both eyes to prevent the development of **gonococcal ophthalmia neonatorum.** This is recommended regardless of the mode of delivery. This prophylactic measure can be delayed up to 1 hour to allow for breastfeeding.

Every newborn should also receive a parenteral dose of natural **vitamin K1** oxide (phytonadione, 0.5 to 1 mg) following delivery to prevent vitamin K-dependent hemorrhagic disease of the newborn. This form of administration is efficacious, and no commercial oral vitamin K preparation is approved for use in the United States at this time. This measure also can be delayed for up to 1 hour to allow breastfeeding in the first hour of life.

A newborn infant's voiding pattern and bowel movements should be closely observed within the first 24 hours following birth. Concern about an obstruction or congenital defect of the urinary tract is appropriate if voiding has not occurred within the first day of life. Ninety percent of newborns pass stool within the first 24 hours. A congenital abnormality such as **imperforate anus** should be considered if this does not occur. For the first 2 or 3 days of life, the stool is greenish-brown and tar-like in consistency. With the ingestion of milk, the stool becomes yellow in color and semisolid.

## Circumcision

**Circumcision** is the surgical removal of a distal portion of the foreskin. It is usually performed within the first 2 days of life on healthy term infants. *Circumcision is an elective procedure; therefore, parents should be given accurate and impartial information to allow them to make an informed decision.* Circumcision should always involve the administration of an anesthetic; both ring blocks and dorsal penile blocks have proved effective. Complications from circumcision are rare and include local infection and bleeding.

## Jaundice

Jaundice, which occurs in most newborns, is usually benign, but because of the potential toxicity of bilirubin, all newborns should be assessed prior to hospital discharge to identify those at high risk for severe **hyperbilirubinemia.** Two methods of assessment can be used: (1) predischarge measurement of total serum bilirubin or transcutaneous bilirubin levels in infants who are jaundiced in the first 24 hours, and (2) application of clinical risk factors for predicting severe hyperbilirubinemia. Late preterm (35 to 37 weeks gestation) infants are at higher risk for hyperbilirubinemia than are term infants. Acute bilirubin encephalopathy or kernicterus is associated with total serum bilirubin levels greater than 30 mg/dL.

If possible, the cause of the hyperbilirubinemia should be determined. Breastfeeding has a significant effect on unconjugated hyperbilirubinemia (breast milk jaundice and "breast-non-feeding jaundice"). Jaundice that persists for 2 weeks requires further investigation, including measurement of both total and direct serum bilirubin concentrations. Elevation of the direct serum bilirubin concentration always requires further investigation and possible intervention, which include phototherapy or exchange transfusion.

## INITIAL CARE OF THE ILL NEWBORN

Although most deliveries are uncomplicated, requiring only basic neonatal care, **resuscitation** may be necessary in up to 10% of all deliveries; 1% of these require major resuscitative efforts. The need for these efforts increases in circumstances such as premature birth, low–birth-weight infants, prolonged labor, and non-reassuring measures of fetal well-being. Not all deliveries occur in a setting with intensive pediatric care immediately available. In the absence of such staff and facilities, maternal transport to a facility with a greater capacity to provide appropriate care should be attempted before delivery. Alternatively, the transport of a neonatal team from a tertiary care center to the primary care site is an option.

## Neonatal Resuscitation

The normal newborn breathes within seconds of delivery and usually has established regular respirations within 1 minute of delivery. If the neonate is having difficulty breathing, ventilation, chest compression, and epinephrine should be instituted, as shown in the protocol in Figure 10-2. If an infant does not respond to epinephrine, hypovolemic shock should be considered, especially if there is evidence of blood loss. In this case, intravenous **normal saline** at 10 mL/kg should be given.

*The same principles of adult resuscitation (airway, breathing, and circulation) apply to neonatal resuscitation* (Figure 10.3). First, the newborn is transported to a radiant warming unit to be thoroughly dried. When drying the infant, it is important to remove wet towels to minimize the effect of evaporation that would otherwise lead to a rapid drop in core body temperature. The nose and oropharynx are suctioned to ensure an open airway as the infant is placed in the

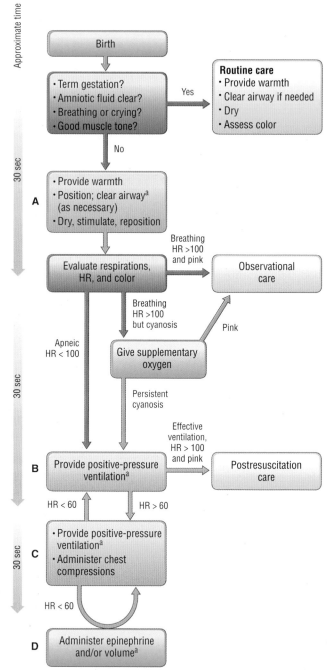

FIGURE 10.2. Algorithm for neonatal resuscitation. (Source: 2005 American Heart Association Guidelines for Cardiopulmonary Resuscitation and Emergency Cardiovascular Care, © 2005, American Heart Association.)

supine position. The head should be positioned with the neck slightly extended—the "sniffing position"—to allow for maximal air entry. Drying and suctioning, along with providing mild stimulation by rubbing the back or soles of the feet—or flicking the soles of the feet—help to stimulate the infant to breathe and cry.

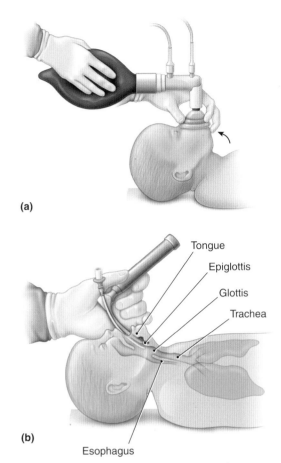

(a)

Tongue
Epiglottis
Glottis
Trachea

(b)
Esophagus

FIGURE 10.3. Airway management in newborn resuscitation. (A) Management with mask and Ambu bag. Most newborns can be safely and effectively managed with a face mask, elevating the chin [1] so that the airway is pulled up and opened [2] into the "sniffing position." (B) Management with endotracheal intubation. Intubation should only be performed by trained personnel to avoid iatrogenic injury.

Respiratory distress may occur as a consequence of maternal narcotic administration during labor. A **narcotic antagonist** can be considered only if severe respiratory pressure ventilation has improved the heart rate and color, and the mother received narcotics within 4 hours of delivery.

*In infants born to a narcotic-addicted mother, **naloxone is contraindicated** because the immediate withdrawal symptom that ensues can be life-threatening.*

## Umbilical Cord Blood Gases

During the resuscitation process, the metabolic well-being of an ill newborn is most accurately assessed using **umbilical cord blood gases.** Cord blood gases should be obtained in cases of cesarean delivery for fetal compromise, a low 5-minute Apgar score, severe growth restriction, abnormal fetal heart rate tracing, maternal thyroid disease, intra-

partum fever, and multifetal gestations. A segment of umbilical cord is double-clamped and cut and placed on the delivery table pending assessment of the 5-minute Apgar score, so that it may be taken for assessment of pH, $P_{O_2}$, $P_{CO_2}$, $HCO_3$, and base deficit. It should be remembered that, in the fetus, freshly oxygenated blood from the placenta travels to the fetus through the umbilical vein, and blood metabolized by the fetus travels back to the placenta through two umbilical arteries. *The most meaningful assessment of metabolic status of the infant at the time of delivery is through analysis of umbilical artery blood gases.* Analysis of paired arterial and venous specimens should prevent debate over whether a true arterial specimen was obtained. Therefore, where possible, obtaining both venous and arterial samples (paired specimen) is recommended. Normal values for umbilical arterial and venous samples are given in Table 10.2.

**Acidemia** is generally accepted as an increase in hydrogen ion concentration in an umbilical arterial sample resulting in a pH of <7.20. **Fetal asphyxia** is defined as a condition of impaired blood gas exchange leading to progressive hypoxemia and hypercapnia with a significant metabolic acidosis (base deficit ≥12 mmol/L).

*The base deficit can be used to predict metabolic acidosis significant enough to cause newborn complications.*

Ten percent of newborns with a base deficit of 12 to 16 mmol/L and 40% of newborns with a base deficit of >16 mmol/L will have moderate to severe complications, such as newborn encephalopathy and cardiovascular and respiratory complications. *The terms acidemia, acidosis, and asphyxia should be used carefully when applied to the newborn condition, because each term defines a series of changes that may or may not represent true metabolic compromise.*

## Umbilical Cord Blood Banking

Umbilical cord blood is now known to contain potentially life-saving hematopoietic stem cells for possible adult transplant for the correction of inborn errors of metabolism, hematopoietic malignancies, and genetic disorders of the blood and immune system. If a patient requests information

| TABLE 10.2 | Normal Umbilical Cord Blood Gas Values | |
|---|---|---|
| | Arterial | Venous |
| pH | 7.25–7.30 | 7.30–7.40 |
| $P_{CO_2}$ (mm Hg) | 50 | 40 |
| $P_{O_2}$ (mm Hg) | 20 | 30 |
| $HCO_3$ (mEq/hr) | 25 | 20 |

on umbilical cord banking, balanced and accurate information regarding the advantages and disadvantages of public or private banking should be provided. *The remote chance of an autologous unit of umbilical cord blood being used for a child or a family member (approximately 1 in 2700 individuals) should also be disclosed.*

## NEWBORN SCREENING

Newborn screening programs, which should be available to all newborns, include tests designed to detect infants with specific conditions who may benefit from early diagnosis and treatment. These conditions include disorders of metabolism, endocrinopathies, hemoglobinopathies, hearing loss, and cystic fibrosis. The tests may also identify parents who are carriers of inherited conditions.

To obtain a sample for testing, heel stick-derived blood is collected and placed onto filter paper. If the initial sample is collected before 12 to 24 hours after delivery, a second sample should be collected at 1 to 2 weeks of age to decrease the probability that phenylketonuria and other disorders with metabolite accumulation are missed as a result of early testing. Premature infants, neonates receiving parenteral feeding, or those treated for illness should have a newborn screening test performed at or near 7 days of age, regardless of feeding status.

Each state must have a system in place for notification, timely follow-up, and evaluation of any infant with a positive screening result. Positive results are usually reported to the newborn's primary care provider and the parents.

## SUGGESTED READINGS

American College of Obstetricians and Gynecologists. The Apgar score. ACOG Committee Opinion No. 333. *Obstet Gynecol.* 2005; 106(5):1141–1142.

American College of Obstetricians and Gynecologists. Circumcision. ACOG Committee Opinion No. 260. Obstet Gynecol 2001;98(4): 707–708.

American College of Obstetricians and Gynecologists. Newborn screening. ACOG Committee Opinion no. 393. *Obstet Gynecol.* 2007;110(6):1497–500.

American College of Obstetricians and Gynecologists. Umbilical cord blood banking. ACOG Committee Opinion No. 399. *Obstet Gynecol.* 2008;111(2):475–477.

*Guidelines for Perinatal Care.* 6th ed. Elk Grove Village, IL: American Academy of Pediatrics; Washington, DC: American College of Obstetricians and Gynecologists; 2007:205–302.

# 11 Postpartum Care

Topic 13: Postpartum Care

Topic 14: Lactation

Topic 29: Anxiety and Depression

The student should be familiar with normal postpartum events to provide optimal clinical care as well as be able to identify abnormal events.

*The **puerperium** is the 6- to 8-week-period following birth during which the reproductive tract, as well as the rest of the body, returns to the nonpregnant state.* Some of the physiologic changes of pregnancy have returned to normal within 1 to 2 weeks postpartum. The initial postpartum examination should be scheduled at 4–6 weeks after delivery.

## PHYSIOLOGY OF THE PUERPERIUM

### Involution of the Uterus

The uterus weighs approximately 1000 g and has a volume of 5000 mL immediately after delivery, compared with its nonpregnant weight of approximately 70 g and capacity of 5 mL. Immediately after delivery, the fundus of the uterus is easily palpable halfway between the pubic symphysis and the umbilicus. The immediate reduction in uterine size is a result of delivery of the fetus, placenta, and amniotic fluid, as well as the loss of hormonal stimulation. Further uterine involution is caused by autolysis of intracellular myometrial protein, resulting in a decrease in cell size but not in cell number. *As a result of these changes, the uterus returns to the pelvis by 2 weeks postpartum and is at its normal size by 6 weeks postpartum.* Immediately after birth, uterine hemostasis is maintained by contraction of the smooth muscle of the arterial walls and compression of the vasculature by the uterine musculature.

### Lochia

As the myometrial fibers contract, the blood clots from the uterus are expelled and the thrombi in the large vessels of the placental bed undergo organization. Within the first 3 days, the remaining decidua differentiates into a super-ficial layer, which becomes necrotic and sloughs, and a basal layer adjacent to the myometrium, which had contained the fundi of the endometrial glands. This basal layer is the source of the new endometrium.

*The subsequent discharge, called **lochia**, is fairly heavy at first and rapidly decreases in amount over the first 2 to 3 days postpartum, although it may last for several weeks.* Lochia is classically described as: (1) **lochia rubra**, menses-like bleeding in the first several days, consisting mainly of blood and necrotic decidual tissue; (2) **lochia serosa**, a lighter discharge with considerably less blood in the next few days; and (3) **lochia alba**, a whitish discharge which may persist for several weeks and which may be misunderstood as illness by some women, requiring explanation and reassurance. In women who breastfeed, the lochia seems to resolve more rapidly, possibly because of a more rapid involution of the uterus caused by uterine contractions associated with breastfeeding. In some patients, there is an increased amount of lochia 1 to 2 weeks after delivery, because the eschar that developed over the site of placental attachment has been sloughed. By the end of the third week postpartum, the endometrium is reestablished in most patients.

### Cervix and Vagina

Within several hours of delivery, the cervix has reformed, and by 1 week, it usually admits only one finger (i.e., it is approximately 1 cm in diameter). The round shape of the nulliparous cervix is usually permanently replaced by a transverse, fish–mouth-shaped external os, the result of laceration during delivery. *Vulvar and vaginal tissues return to normal over the first several days, although the vaginal mucosa reflects a hypoestrogenic state if the woman breastfeeds, because ovarian function is suppressed during breastfeeding.* The muscles of the pelvic floor gradually regain their tone.

*Vaginal muscle tone may be strengthened by the use of Kegel exercises, consisting of repetitive contractions of these muscles.*

## Return of Ovarian Function

The average time to ovulation is 45 days in nonlactating women and 189 days in lactating women. *Ovulation is suppressed in the lactating woman in association with elevated prolactin levels. In these women, prolactin remains elevated for 6 weeks, whereas in nonlactating women, prolactin levels return to normal by 3 weeks postpartum.* Estrogen levels fall immediately after delivery in all patients, but begin to rise approximately 2 weeks after delivery if breastfeeding is not initiated. *The likelihood of ovulation increases as the frequency and duration of breastfeeding decreases.*

## Abdominal Wall

Return of the elastic fibers of the skin and the stretched rectus muscles to normal configuration occurs slowly and is aided by exercise. The silvery **striae gravidarum** seen on the skin usually lighten in time. **Diastasis recti,** separation of the rectus muscles and fascia, also usually resolves over time.

## Cardiovascular System

Pregnancy-related cardiovascular changes return to normal 2 to 3 weeks after delivery. Immediately postpartum, plasma volume is reduced by approximately 1000 mL, caused primarily by blood loss at the time of delivery. During the immediate postpartum period, there is also a significant shift of extracellular fluid into the intravascular space. The increased cardiac output seen during pregnancy also persists into the first several hours of the postpartum period. The elevated pulse rate that occurs during pregnancy persists for approximately 1 hour after delivery, but then decreases.

*These cardiovascular events may contribute to the decompensation that sometimes occurs in the early postpartum period in patients with heart disease.*

Immediately after delivery, approximately 5 kg of weight is lost as a result of diuresis and the loss of extravascular fluid. Further weight loss varies in rate and amount from patient to patient.

## Hematopoietic System

*The **leukocytosis** seen during labor persists into the early puerperium for several days, thus minimizing the usefulness of identifying early postpartum infection by laboratory evidence of a mild-to-moderate elevation in the white cell count.*

There is some degree of autotransfusion of red cells to the intravascular space after delivery as the uterus contracts.

## Renal System

**Glomerular filtration rate** represents renal function and remains elevated in the first few weeks postpartum, then returns to normal. Therefore, drugs with renal excretion should be given in increased doses during this time. Ureter and renal pelvis dilation regress by 6 to 8 weeks. *There may be considerable edema around the urethra after vaginal delivery, resulting in transitory urinary retention.* About 7% of women experience urinary stress incontinence, which usually regresses by 3 months.

## MANAGEMENT OF THE IMMEDIATE POSTPARTUM PERIOD

### Hospital Stay

*In the absence of complications, the postpartum hospital stay ranges from 48 hours after a vaginal delivery to 96 hours after a cesarean delivery, excluding day of delivery.* Shortened hospital stays are appropriate when certain criteria are met to ensure the health of the mother and baby, such as the absence of fever in the mother; normal pulse and respiration rates and blood pressure level; lochia amount and color appropriate for the duration of recovery; absence of any abnormal physical, laboratory, or emotional findings; and ability of the mother to perform activities such as walking, eating, drinking, self-care, and care for the newborn. In addition, the mother should have adequate support in the first few days following discharge and should receive instructions about postpartum activity, exercise, and common postpartum discomforts and relief measures.

*During the hospital stay, the focus should be on preparation of the mother for newborn care, infant feeding including the special issues involved with breastfeeding, and required newborn laboratory testing.* When patients are discharged early, a home visit or follow-up telephone call by a healthcare provider within 48 hours of discharge is encouraged.

### Maternal–Infant Bonding

Shortly after delivery, the parents become totally engrossed in the events surrounding the newborn infant. The mother should have close contact with her infant. Obstetric units should be organized to facilitate these interactions by minimizing unnecessary medical interventions while increasing participation by the father and other family members. Nursing staff can observe the interactions between the infant and the new parents and intervene when necessary.

### Postpartum Complications

Infection occurs in approximately 5% of patients and significant immediate **postpartum hemorrhage** occurs in approximately 1% of patients (see Chapter 12, Postpartum

Hemorrhage). Immediately after the delivery of the placenta, the uterus is palpated bimanually to ascertain that it is firm. Uterine palpation through the abdominal wall is repeated at frequent intervals during the immediate postpartum period to prevent and/or identify uterine atony. Perineal pads are applied, and the amount of blood on these pads as well as the patient's pulse and pressure are monitored closely for the first several hours after delivery to detect excessive blood loss.

Some patients will experience an episode of increased vaginal bleeding between days 8 and 14 postpartum, most likely associated with the separation and passage of the placental eschar. This is self-limited and needs no therapy other than reassurance. Bleeding that persists or is excessive is called **delayed postpartum hemorrhage,** and it occurs in approximately 1% of cases. Treatment includes oxytocic therapy or suction evacuation of the uterus. Suction is successful in most cases, whether or not there is retained placental tissue, as is found in one-third of cases.

## Analgesia

After vaginal delivery, analgesic medication (including topical lidocaine cream) may be necessary to relieve perineal and episiotomy pain and facilitate maternal mobility. This is best addressed by administering the drug on an as-needed basis according to postpartum orders. Most mothers experience considerable pain in the first 24 hours after cesarean delivery. *Analgesic techniques include spinal or epidural opiates, patient-controlled epidural or intravenous analgesia, and potent oral analgesics.*

*Regardless of the route of administration, opioids can cause respiratory depression and decrease intestinal motility.*

Adequate supervision and monitoring should be ensured for all postpartum patients receiving these drugs.

## Ambulation

*Postpartum patients should be encouraged to begin ambulation as soon as possible after delivery.* They should be offered assistance initially, especially for patients who have delivered by cesarean section. Early ambulation helps avoid urinary retention and prevents puerperal venous thromboses and pulmonary emboli.

## Breast Care

**Breast engorgement** in women who are not breastfeeding occurs in the first few days postpartum and gradually abates over this period. If the breasts become painful, they should be supported with a well-fitting brassiere. Ice packs and analgesics may also help relieve discomfort. Women who do not wish to breastfeed should be encouraged to avoid nipple stimulation and should be cautioned against continued manual expression of milk.

A plugged duct (**galactocele**) and mastitis may also result in an enlarged, tender breast postpartum (Table 11.1). **Mastitis,** or infection of the breast tissue, most often occurs in lactating women and is characterized by sudden-onset fever and localized pain and swelling. Mastitis is associated with infection by *Staphylococcus aureus*, Group A or B streptococci, β *Haemophilus* species, and *Escherichia coli*. Treatment includes continuation of breastfeeding or emptying the breast with a breast pump and the use of appropriate antibiotics. Breast milk remains safe for the full-term, healthy infant.

Symptoms of a **breast abscess** are similar to those of mastitis, but a fluctuant mass is also present. Persistent fever after starting antibiotic therapy for mastitis may also suggest an abscess. Treatment requires surgical drainage of the abscess in addition to antibiotic therapy.

## Immunizations

Women who do not have antirubella antibody should be immunized for **rubella** during the immediate postpartum period. Breastfeeding is not a contraindication to this immunization. If a patient has not already received the **tetanus-diphtheria acellular pertussis vaccine,** and if it has been at least 2 years since her last tetanus-diphtheria booster, she should be given a dose before hospital discharge. If the woman is D-negative, is not isoimmunized,

| TABLE 11.1 | Differential Diagnosis of an Enlarged, Tender Breast Postpartum | | |
|---|---|---|---|
| **Finding** | **Engorgement** | **Mastitis** | **Plugged Duct** |
| Onset | Gradual | Sudden | Gradual |
| Location | Bilateral | Unilateral | Unilateral |
| Swelling | Generalized | Localized | Localized |
| Pain | Generalized | Intense, localized | Localized |
| Systemic symptoms | Feels well | Feels ill | Feels well |
| Fever | No | Yes | No |

and has given birth to a D-positive or weak-D-positive infant, 300 micrograms of **anti-D immune globulin** should be administered postpartum, ideally within 72 hours of giving birth.

*This dose may be inadequate in circumstances in which there is a potential for greater-than-average fetal-to-maternal hemorrhage, such as placental abruption, placenta previa, intrauterine manipulation, and manual removal of the placenta (see Chapter 19, Isoimmunization).*

Universal immunization with hepatitis B surface antigen (HbSAg1) is recommended for all newborns weighing 2000 g. In addition, all newborns receive a full range of screening tests.

## Bowel and Bladder Function

It is common for a patient not to have a bowel movement for the first 1 to 2 days after delivery, because patients have often not eaten for a long period. Stool softeners may be prescribed, especially if the patient has had a fourth-degree episiotomy repair or a laceration involving the rectal mucosa.

**Hemorrhoids** are varicosities of the hemorrhoidal veins. Surgical treatment should not be considered for at least 6 months postpartum to allow for natural involution. Sitz baths, stool softeners, and local preparations are useful, combined with reassurance that resolution is the most common outcome.

Periurethral edema after vaginal delivery may cause transitory urinary retention. *Patients' urinary output should be monitored for the first 24 hours after delivery.* If catheterization is required more than twice in the first 24 hours, placement of an indwelling catheter for 1 to 2 days is advisable.

## Care of the Perineum

During the first 24 hours, perineal pain can be minimized using oral analgesics and the application of an ice bag to minimize swelling. Local anesthetics, such as witch hazel pads or benzocaine spray, may be beneficial. Beginning 24 hours after delivery, moist heat in the form of a warm sitz bath may reduce local discomfort and promote healing.

*Severe perineal pain unresponsive to the usual analgesics may signify the development of a **hematoma,** which requires careful examination of the vulva, vagina, and rectum.*

Infection of the episiotomy is rare (<0.1%) and usually is limited to the skin and responsive to broad-spectrum antibiotics. **Dehiscence** (rupture of the incision) is uncommon,

with repair individualized on the basis of the nature and extent of the wound.

## Contraception

Postpartum care in the hospital should include discussion of **contraception.** *Approximately 15% of non-nursing women are fertile at 6 weeks postpartum.* Combined estrogen–progestin oral contraceptive preparations are not contraindicated by breastfeeding, although they may inhibit lactation slightly. Progestin preparations (oral norethindrone or depo-medroxyprogesterone acetate) have no effect or may slightly facilitate lactation. Women may consider initiating progesterone-only contraceptives at 6 weeks if breastfeeding exclusively or at 3 weeks if not exclusively. Once lactation is established, neither the volume nor the composition of breast milk are adversely affected by the administration of hormonal contraceptives, and there is no effect on the growth of breastfed infants. Insertion of intrauterine contraceptive 4 to 6 weeks postpartum is acceptable in the appropriately selected patient.

Postpartum sterilization is performed at the time of cesarean delivery or after a vaginal delivery and should not extend the patient's hospital stay. Ideally, postpartum minilaparotomy is performed before the onset of significant uterine involution but following a full assessment of maternal and neonatal well-being (see Chapter 25, Sterilization). Postpartum minilaparotomy may be performed using local anesthesia with sedation, regional anesthesia, or general anesthesia. Postpartum sterilization requires counseling and informed consent before labor and delivery. *Consent should be obtained during prenatal care, when the patient can make a considered decision, review the risks and benefits of the procedure, and consider alternative contraceptive methods.* In all cases of intrapartum or postpartum medical or obstetric complications, the physician should consider postponing sterilization to a later date. The federal and state regulations that address the timing of consent also are important to consider.

## Sexual Activity

Coitus may be resumed when the patient is comfortable; however, the *risks of hemorrhage and infection are minimal at approximately 2 weeks postpartum.* Women should be counseled, especially if breastfeeding, that coitus may initially be uncomfortable because of a lack of lubrication due to low estrogen levels, and that the use of exogenous, water-soluble lubrication is helpful. The lactating patient may also be counseled to apply topical estrogen or a lubricant to the vaginal mucosa to minimize the dyspareunia caused by coital trauma to the hypoestrogenic tissue. The female superior position may be recommended, as the woman is thereby able to control the depth of penile penetration.

## Patient Education

Patient education at the time of discharge should not be solely focused on postpartum and contraceptive issues. It is also a good opportunity to reinforce the value and need for healthcare of both mother and infant. Follow-up care that has been arranged for the newborn and frequency of healthcare for the new mother should be reviewed. High-risk behaviors such as alcohol, tobacco, and drug abuse should be discussed, along with appropriate interventions. Physicians should also assess the patient's mental state and her ease with care of the newborn. Infant safety concerns (e.g., automobile child restraints) are also appropriate topics of discussion. Postpartum follow-up of any preexisting medical conditions should also be reviewed and, when needed, the patient should be referred for care.

## Weight Loss

Maternal postpartum weight loss can occur at a rate of 2 lb per month without affecting lactation. On average, a woman will retain 2 lb more than her prepregnancy weight at 1 year postpartum. There is no relationship between body mass index or total weight gain and weight retention. Aging, rather than parity, is the major determinant of increases in a woman's weight over time.

Residual postpartum retention of weight gained during pregnancy that results in obesity is a concern. Special attention to lifestyle, including exercise and eating habits, will help these women return to a normal body mass index.

## Lactation and Breastfeeding

*Because breast milk is the ideal source of nutrition for the neonate, it is recommended that women breastfeed exclusively for the first 6 months and continue breastfeeding for as long as mutually desired.* Benefits of breastfeeding include decreased risks of otitis and respiratory infections, diarrheal illness, sudden infant death, allergic and atopic disease, juvenile-onset diabetes, and childhood cancers; fewer hospital admissions in the first year of life; and improved cognitive function. For premature infants, breast milk reduces the risk of necrotizing enterocolitis. Maternal benefits include improved maternal–child attachment, reduced fertility due to lactational amenorrhea, and reduced incidence of some hormonally sensitive cancers, including breast cancer.

There are few contraindications to breastfeeding. Women with HIV should not breastfeed due to the risk of vertical transmission. Women with active, untreated tuberculosis should not have close contact with their infants until they have been treated and are noninfectious; their breast milk may be expressed and given to the infant, except in the rare case of tuberculosis mastitis. Mothers undergoing chemotherapy, receiving antimetabolites, or who have received radioactive materials should not breastfeed until the breast milk has been cleared of these substances. Infants with galactosemia should not be breastfed due to their sensitivity to lactose. Mothers who use illegal drugs should not breastfeed their infants.

*Drugs in the breast milk are a common concern for the breastfeeding mother.* Less than 1% of the total dosage of any medication appears in breast milk. This should be considered when any medication is prescribed by a physician or when any over-the-counter medications are contemplated by the patient. Specific medications that would contraindicate breastfeeding include lithium carbonate, tetracycline, bromocriptine, methotrexate, and any radioactive substance. All substances of abuse are included as well, such as amphetamine, cocaine, heroin, marijuana, and phencyclidine (PCP).

At the time of delivery, the drop in estrogen levels and other placental hormones is a major factor in removing the inhibition of the action of prolactin. Also, suckling by the infant stimulates release of oxytocin from the neurohypophysis. The increased levels of oxytocin in the blood result in contraction of the myoepithelial cells and emptying of the alveolar lumen of the breast. The oxytocin also increases uterine contractions, thereby accelerating involution of the postpartum uterus. Prolactin release is also stimulated by suckling, with resultant secretion of fatty acids, lactose, and casein. **Colostrum** is produced in the first 5 days postpartum and is slowly replaced by maternal milk. Colostrum contains more minerals and protein but less fat and sugar than maternal milk, although it does contain large fat globules, the so-called colostrum corpuscles, which are probably epithelial cells that have undergone fatty degeneration. Colostrum also contains immunoglobulin A, which may offer the newborn some protection from enteric pathogens. Subsequently, on approximately the third to sixth day postpartum, milk is produced.

For milk to be produced on an ongoing basis, there must be adequate insulin, cortisol, and thyroid hormone, and adequate nutrients and fluids in the mother's diet. The minimal caloric requirement for adequate milk production in a woman of average size is 1800 kcal per day. In general, an additional 500 kcal of energy daily is recommended throughout lactation. All vitamins except K are found in human milk, but because they are present in varying amounts, maternal vitamin supplementation is recommended. Vitamin K may be administered to the infant to prevent hemorrhagic disease of the newborn. To maintain breastfeeding, the alveolar lumen must be emptied on a regular basis.

**Nipple care** is also important during breastfeeding. The nipples should be washed with water and exposed to the air for 15 to 20 minutes after each feeding. A water-based cream such as lanolin or A and D ointment may be applied if the nipples are tender. Fissuring of the nipple may make breastfeeding extremely difficult. Temporary cessation of breastfeeding, manual expression of milk, and use of a nipple shield will aid in recovery.

## ANXIETY, DEPRESSION, AND THE POSTPARTUM PERIOD

Although pregnancy and childbirth are usually joyous times, depression to some degree is actually common in the postpartum period. There is a wide spectrum of response to pregnancy and delivery, ranging from mild postpartum blues to postpartum depression (Table 11.2). Approximately 70% to 80% of women report feeling sad, anxious, or angry beginning 2–4 days after birth. These **postpartum blues** may come and go throughout the day, are usually mild, and abate within 1 to 2 weeks. Supportive care and reassurance are helpful in ensuring that symptoms are self-limited. Approximately 10% to 15% of new mothers experience **postpartum depression (PPD),** which is a more serious disorder and usually requires medication and counseling. *PPD differs from postpartum blues in the severity and duration of symptoms.* Women with PPD have pronounced feelings of sadness, anxiety, and despair that interfere with activities of daily living. These symptoms do not abate, but instead worsen over several weeks. **Postpartum psychosis** is the most severe form of mental derangement and is most common in women with preexisting disorders, such as manic–depressive illness or schizophrenia. This condition should be considered a medical emergency and the patient should be referred for immediate, often inpatient, treatment.

While the exact cause of PPD is unknown, several associated factors have been identified. The normal hormonal fluctuations that occur following birth may trigger depression in some women. Women who have a personal or family history of depression or anxiety may be more likely to develop PPD. Acute stressors, including those specific to motherhood (childcare), or other stressors (e.g., death of a family member) may contribute to the development of PPD. Having a child with a difficult temperament or health issues may lead the mother to doubt her ability to care for her newborn, which can lead to depression. The age of the mother may influence susceptibility to PPD, with younger women more likely to experience depression than older women. Toxins, poor diet, crowded living conditions, low socioeconomic status, and low social support may also play a role. *A strong predictor of PPD is depression during pregnancy.* It is estimated that half of all cases of PPD may begin during pregnancy. PPD may also be a continuation of a depressive disorder that existed prior to pregnancy, rather than a new disorder.

Treatment must be tailored to the patient's individual situation. Postpartum blues do not require treatment other than support and reassurance. Women with PPD should receive mental health counseling and medication, if warranted. Effective therapies for the treatment of PPD include cognitive-behavioral and interpersonal therapies.

## THE POSTPARTUM VISIT

At the time of the first postpartum visit, inquiries should be made into the following: status of breastfeeding, return of menstruation, resumption of coital activity, use of contraception, interaction of the newborn with the family, and resumption of other physical activities such as return to work. Observation about and appropriate questions concerning sadness and depression, anxiety, the parents' concerns about infant care, and the relationship of mother and her partner are also part of the first postpartum visit. Involutional changes will have occurred in most instances. Inflammatory changes because of the healing

| **TABLE 11.2** | Three Categories of Postpartum Mood Disorders | | |
|---|---|---|---|
| | **Postpartum Blues** | **Postpartum Depression** | **Postpartum Psychosis** |
| Incidence (%) | 70–80 | ≥10 | 0.1–0.2 |
| Average time | 2–4 days PP | 2 weeks to 12 months PP | 2–3 days PP |
| Average duration | 2–3 days, resolution within 10 days | 3–14 months | Variable |
| Symptoms | Mild insomnia, tearfulness, fatigue, irritability, poor concentration, depressed affect | Irritability, labile mood, difficulty falling asleep, phobias, anxiety; symptoms worsen in the evening | Similar to organic brain syndrome: confusion, attention deficit, distractibility, clouded sensorium |
| Treatment | None; self-limited | Antidepressant pharmacotherapy; psychotherapy | Antipsychotic pharmacotherapy; antidepressant pharmacotherapy (50% of patients also meet depression criteria) |

PP = postpartum.

of the cervix may result in minor atypia on a Pap smear performed at this time. Unless there is a history of significant cervical dysplasia, repeating the Pap smear in 3 months is appropriate.

## SUGGESTED READINGS

American College of Obstetricians and Gynecologists. *Use of Psychiatric Medications During Pregnancy and Lactation.* ACOG Practice Bulletin No. 92. Washington, DC: American College of Obstetricians and Gynecologists (ACOG); 2008.

American College of Obstetricians and Gynecologists. Depression during pregnancy and the postpartum period. In: American College of Obstetricians and Gynecologists. *Precis, Obstetrics: An Update in Obstetrics and Gynecology.* 3rd ed. Washington, DC: American College of Obstetricians and Gynecologists; 2006:180–187.

American College of Obstetricians and Gynecologists. The puerperium. In: American College of Obstetricians and Gynecologists. *Precis, Obstetrics: An Update in Obstetrics and Gynecology.* 3rd ed. Washington, DC: American College of Obstetricians and Gynecologists; 2006:188–195.

American College of Obstetricians and Gynecologists. *Guidelines for Perinatal Care.* 6th ed. Washington, DC: American College of Obstetricians and Gynecologists; 2007.

# Postpartum Hemorrhage

The prevention or management of postpartum hemorrhage is important, as it remains a major cause of maternal morbidity and mortality. Students should be able to explain the risk factors, differential diagnosis, and management of postpartum hemorrhage.

I t is estimated that, worldwide, 140,000 women die of **postpartum hemorrhage (PPH)** each year— 1 every 4 minutes. More than half of all maternal deaths occur within 24 hours of delivery, most commonly from excessive bleeding. *In addition to death, serious morbidity may follow postpartum hemorrhage. Sequelae include adult respiratory distress syndrome, coagulopathy, shock, loss of fertility, and pituitary necrosis (Sheehan syndrome).*

Hemorrhage can be sudden and profuse, or blood loss can occur more insidiously. PPH has been traditionally defined as a delivery-associated blood loss in excess of 500 mL for vaginal delivery and 1000 mL for cesarean birth; however, these estimates actually represent the average blood loss for each mode of delivery, respectively. The estimation of blood loss is subjective, introducing wide variance and inaccuracy.

Additionally, the same absolute volume loss for a patient weighing 50 kg may have vastly different effects than it would for someone weighing 75 kg, or for a patient with triplets versus a singleton. Thus, it is likely more appropriate and meaningful to use physiologic and objective criteria in defining clinical hemorrhage. Criteria in use include a 10% drop in hematocrit, need for transfusion, and signs and symptoms along the spectrum of physiologic effects of blood loss, described below.

## RECOGNITION AND EARLY DETECTION

*PPH is not a diagnosis, but a critically important sign that often occurs without warning and in the absence of risk factors.*

When present, however, these factors warrant heightened awareness about the risk of PPH (Box 12.1). Maternal hemodynamic responses to blood loss should also be monitored, as these responses are indicators of well-being, volume deficit, and prognosis. The loss of 10% to 15%

(500 mL for an average patient with singleton pregnancy) of blood volume may be tolerated with no signs or symptoms. As blood loss approaches 20%, the first signs of intravascular depletion become manifest, including **tachycardia, tachypnea,** and **delayed capillary refill,** followed by **orthostatic changes** and **narrowed pulse pressure** (due to elevated diastolic pressure secondary to vasoconstriction with maintenance of systolic pressure). Beyond approximately 30% volume loss, breathing and heart rate further increase, and overt hypotension develops. Finally, with profound blood loss above 40% to 50%, oliguria, shock, coma, and death may occur.

*The source and etiology of bleeding should be identified as soon as possible, and targeted interventions applied in order to minimize morbidity and prevent mortality.* The most common cause of PPH is uterine atony, representing about 80% of cases. Retained placenta, genital tract trauma (lacerations, rupture), and coagulation disorders are other causes. Hematomas can occur anywhere in the lower genital tract. Ruptured uterus and inverted uterus are rare but serious causes of PPH.

## GENERAL MANAGEMENT OF PATIENTS WITH POSTPARTUM HEMORRHAGE

*Postpartum hemorrhage is an unequivocal emergency; all available resources should be mobilized immediately upon its recognition.*

A general approach to management is outlined in Box 12.2. Because most cases of PPH are caused by **uterine atony,** the uterus should be palpated abdominally, seeking the soft, "boggy" consistency of the relaxed uterus. If this finding is confirmed, oxytocin infusion should be increased and either methylergonovine maleate or prostaglandins administered if excessive bleeding continues.

Other questions that may help direct assessment include:

- Was expulsion of the placenta spontaneous and apparently complete?
- Were forceps or other instrumentation used in delivery?
- Was the baby large or the delivery difficult or precipitous?
- Were the cervix and vagina inspected for lacerations?
- Is the blood clotting?

While the cause of the hemorrhage is being identified, general supportive measures should be initiated (see Box 12.2). Such measures include large-bore intravenous access; rapid crystalloid infusions; type, cross match, and administration of blood or blood components as needed; periodic assessment of hematocrit and coagulation profile; and monitoring of urinary output. The judicious use of blood component therapy is key to management. The mainstay of blood replacement therapy is packed red blood cells, with other components used as indicated for various disorders of the clotting cascade. See Table 12.1 for an outline of blood products and their effects.

*The management of PPH is greatly facilitated if patients at high risk are identified and preliminary preparations are made before the bleeding episode.* Box 12.3 reviews such preliminary, precautionary measures.

## MAJOR CAUSES OF POSTPARTUM HEMORRHAGE AND THEIR MANAGEMENT

### Uterine Atony

Ordinarily, the uterine corpus contracts promptly after delivery of the placenta, constricting the spiral arteries in the newly created placental bed, and preventing excessive

bleeding. This muscular contraction, rather than coagulation, prevents excessive bleeding from the placental implantation site. When contraction does not occur as expected, the resulting **uterine atony** leads to PPH.

Conditions that predispose to uterine atony include those in which there is extraordinary enlargement of the uterus (such as polyhydramnios or twins); abnormal labor (both precipitous and prolonged, or augmented by oxytocin); and conditions that interfere with contraction of the uterus (such as uterine leiomyomata or magnesium sulfate). The clinical diagnosis of atony is based largely on the tone of the uterine muscle on palpation. Instead of the normally firm, contracted uterine corpus, a softer, more pliable—often called "boggy"—uterus is found. The cervix is usually open. Frequently, the uterus contracts briefly when massaged, only to become relaxed again when the manipulation ceases.

*Because hemorrhage can occur in the absence of atony, other etiologies must be sought in the presence of a firm fundus.*

Management of uterine atony is both preventive and therapeutic. *Active management of the third stage of labor (the interval between the delivery of the fetus and delivery of the placenta), has been shown to reduce the incidence of PPH hemorrhage by as much as 70%.* The protocol for management of the third stage includes oxytocin infusion (usually 20 units in 1 liter of normal saline infused at 200–500 mL/hr) initiated immediately following delivery of the infant or its anterior shoulder, gentle cord traction, and uterine massage. Some physicians do not begin oxytocin infusion until after delivery of the placenta to avoid placental entrapment. However, there is no firm evidence that the rates of entrapment are higher with active management than with other strategies. Immediate breastfeeding may also enhance uterine contractility and, thus, reduce blood loss.

Once uterine atony is diagnosed, management can be categorized as medical, manipulative, or surgical. Management must be individualized in cases of severe uterine atony, taking into account the extent of hemorrhage, the overall status of the patient, and her future childbearing desires (see Box 12.2).

*Bimanual uterine massage alone is often successful in causing uterine contraction, and this should be done while preparations for other treatments are under way* (Fig. 12.1). **Uterotonic agents** include oxytocin, methylergonovine maleate, misoprostol (an analogue of prostaglandin $E_1$), dinoprostone (an analogue of prostaglandin $E_2$), and 15-methyl prostaglandin $F_{2\alpha}$, administered separately or in combination. **Methylergonovine maleate** is a potent uterotonic agent that can cause uterine contractions within several minutes. It is always given intramuscularly, because rapid intravenous administration can lead to dangerous hypertension, and its use is often avoided in those with hypertensive disorders. Though it should be avoided or used with extreme caution

## BOX 12.2
## Management of the Patient With Postpartum Hemorrhage

**General Measures:**
Evaluate excessive bleeding immediately
Assess overall patient status
Notify other members of obstetrics team
   (i.e., obtain help!)
Review clinical course for probable cause
- Any difficulty removing placenta?
- Were forceps used?
- Other predisposing factors?
Have operating room and personnel on standby
Monitor and maintain circulation
- Establish IV access: 2 large bore
- Type and cross-match blood
- Begin/increase crystalloid infusion
- Assess for clotting or check coagulation profile

**Evaluation: Perform in Rapid Succession**
Assess hemodynamic status
Bimanual examination: assess for atony
- May palpate for retained placental fragments
- May palpate uterine wall for rupture
Inspect perineum, vulva, vagina, and cervix
- Identify lacerations, hematomas, inversions
- Recruit assistance for exposure
- You or assistant may re-inspect placenta
Assess clotting

**Targeted Interventions**

**Atony**     (tone)
Immediate bimanual massage
Administer uterotonics (with requisite precautions)
- Oxytocin—IV: 10–40 units/1 L normal saline or
   lactated Ringer solution, continuous

- Methylergonovine—IM: 0.2 mg IM; may repeat
   in 2–4 hours
- 15-methyl PGF$_{2\alpha}$—IM 0.25 mg every 15 to
   90 minutes for up to 8 doses
- Dinoprostone—Suppository: vaginal or rectal;
   20 mg every 2 hours
- Misoprostol—800–1000 µg rectally; one dose
- Intrauterine tamponade—Bakri balloon, packing
Operative measures
Uterine compression sutures
Sequential arterial ligation or selective arterial
   embolization
Hysterectomy

**Retained placenta**     (tissue)
Manual removal; manage atony as above
Ultrasound assessment/guidance to assure
   complete removal
Suction curettage—ideally performed with ultra-
   sound guidance in operating room (OR)
Maintain suspicion for accreta—additional
   intervention required

**Genital tract lacerations and hematomas** (trauma)
Repair lacerations immediately
Exposure critical—get assistance, move to OR
No blindly placed sutures
Packing may be necessary
Observe stable, asymptomatic hematomas

**Coagulopathy**     (thrombin)
Appropriate factor replacement
Identify underlying cause
Hemorrhage, infection, amniotic fluid embolism,
   other

TABLE 12.1     Blood Component Therapy

| Product | Contents | Volume (mL) | Effect |
|---|---|---|---|
| Packed RBCs | RBCs, WBCs, plasma | 240 | Increase Hct 3%/unit, hemoglobin by 1 g/dL |
| Platelets | Platelets, RBCs, WBCs, plasma | 50 | Increase platelet count 5000–10,000/mm$^3$ per unit |
| FFP | Factors V and VIII, fibrinogen, antithrombin III | 250 | Increase fibrinogen by 10 mg/dL |
| Cryoprecipitate | Factors VIII and XIII, fibrinogen, vWF | 40 | Increase fibrinogen by 10 mg/dL |

FFP = fresh frozen plasma; Hct = hematocrit; RBC = red blood cell; vWF = von Willebrand factor;
WBC = white blood cell.

in those with cardiac, pulmonary, liver, or renal diseases, **15-methyl prostaglandin $F_{2\alpha}$** may be given intramuscularly or directly into the myometrium. **Dinoprostone** may be given by vaginal or rectal suppository. **Misoprostol** has recently been used for treatment and prevention of PPH. These prostaglandins result in strong uterine contractions. Typically, oxytocin is given prophylactically, as noted previously; if uterine atony occurs, the infusion rate is increased, and additional agents are given sequentially.

*Uterotonic agents are only effective for uterine atony. If the uterus is firm, the use of these agents is not necessary and other causes of bleeding should be explored.*

Occasionally, uterine massage and uterotonic agents are unsuccessful in bringing about adequate uterine contraction, and other measures must be used. Some practitioners use intrauterine compression with in utero packing or placement of a balloon compression device as a means of halting blood loss while preserving the uterus.

**Surgical management** of uterine atony may include uterine compression sutures (B-Lynch or multiple squares), sequential arterial ligation (ascending or descending branches of the uterine, utero-ovarian, then internal iliac arteries), selective arterial embolization, and hysterectomy (Fig. 12.2). *Very high success rates have been noted with surgical compression techniques, with consequent decreases in the use of hysterectomy and iliac artery ligations, both of which are associated with high rates of morbidity.* Additional advantages of compression techniques include rapid execution and preservation of fertility.

## Lacerations of the Lower Genital Tract

**Lacerations** of the lower genital tract are far less common than uterine atony as a cause of PPH, but they can be serious and require prompt surgical repair. *Predisposing factors include instrumented delivery, manipulative delivery such as a breech extraction, precipitous labor, presentations other than occiput anterior, and macrosomia.*

Although minor lacerations to the cervix are common in delivery, extensive lacerations and those that are actively bleeding usually require repair. To minimize blood loss caused by significant cervical and vaginal lacerations, all patients with any predisposing factors, or any patient in whom blood loss soon after delivery appears to be excessive despite a firm and contracted uterus, should have a careful repeat inspection of the lower genital tract. This vaginal examination may require assistance to allow adequate visualization. As a rule, repair of these lacerations is usually not difficult, if adequate exposure is provided.

Lacerations of the vagina and perineum (first-degree through fourth-degree vaginal and periurethral lacerations) are not common causes of substantial blood loss, although the steady loss of blood, which may come from

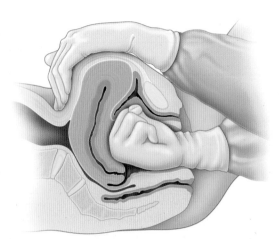

FIGURE 12.1. Management of uterine atony with manual massage. One hand gently compresses the uterus through the abdominal wall. The other is inserted so that pressure can be placed against the anterior lower uterine segment.

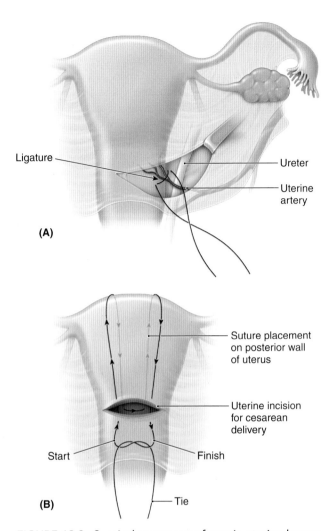

**(A)**

**(B)**

FIGURE 12.2. Surgical treatment of atonic uterine hemorrhage. (A) Ligation of the uterine artery. The artery crosses over the ureter and is ligated beyond this point at the uterine corpus. (B) "B-Lynch" suture.

deeper lacerations, may be so significant that their repair when bleeding is requisite. Periurethral lacerations may be associated with sufficient edema to occlude the urethra, causing urinary retention; a Foley catheter for 12 to 24 hours usually alleviates this problem.

## Retained Placenta

Normally, separation of the placenta from the uterus occurs because of cleavage between the **zona basalis** and the **zona spongiosa** facilitated by uterine contraction. Once separation occurs, expulsion is caused by strong uterine contractions. **Retained placenta** can occur when either the process of separation or the process of expulsion is incomplete. Predisposing factors to retained placenta include a previous cesarean delivery, uterine leiomyomata, prior uterine curettage, and succenturiate placental lobe.

Placental tissue remaining in the uterus can prevent adequate contractions, leading to atony and excessive bleeding.

> *After expulsion, every placenta should be inspected to detect missing placental cotyledons, which may remain in the uterus.*

Sheared or abruptly ending surface vessels may indicate an accessory, or **succenturiate,** placental lobe. If retained placenta is suspected—either because of apparently absent cotyledons or because of excessive bleeding—it can often be removed by inserting two fingers through the cervix into the uterine cavity, and manipulating the retained tissue downward into the vagina. If this is unsuccessful, or if there is uncertainty regarding the cause of hemorrhage, an ultrasound examination of the uterus can be helpful. Curettage with a suction apparatus and/or a large, sharp curette may be used to remove the retained tissue. Care must be exercised to avoid perforation through the uterine fundus.

Placental tissue may also remain in the uterus because separation of the placenta from the uterus may not occur normally. At times, placental villi penetrate the uterine wall to varying degrees. Specifically, abnormal adherence of the placenta to the superficial lining of the uterus is termed **placenta accreta;** penetration into the uterine muscle itself is called **placenta increta;** and complete invasion through the thickness of the uterine muscle is termed **placenta percreta.** If this abnormal attachment involves the entire placenta, no part of the placenta separates. Much more commonly, however, attachment is not complete and a portion of the placenta separates and the remainder remains attached. Major, life-threatening hemorrhage can ensue.

If a portion of the placenta separates and the remainder stays attached, hysterectomy is often required. However, an attempt to separate the placenta by curettage or other means of controlling the bleeding (such as surgical compression or sequential arterial ligation) is usually appropriate in trying to avoid a hysterectomy in a woman who desires more children.

## Other Causes of Postpartum Hemorrhage

### HEMATOMAS

**Hematomas** can occur anywhere from the vulva to the upper vagina as a result of delivery trauma. Hematomas may also develop at the site of episiotomy or perineal laceration. Hematomas may occur without disruption of the vaginal mucosa, when the fetus or forceps causes shearing of the submucosal tissues without mucosal tearing.

Vulvar or vaginal hematomas are characterized by exquisite pain with or without signs of shock. *Hematomas that are ≤5 cm in diameter and are not enlarging can usually be managed expectantly by frequent evaluation of the size of the hematoma and close monitoring of vital signs and urinary output.* Application of ice packs can also be helpful. Larger and enlarging hematomas must be managed surgically. If the hematoma is at the site of episiotomy, the sutures should be removed and a search made for the actual bleeding site, which is then ligated. If it is not at the episiotomy site, the hematoma should be opened at its most dependent portion and drained, the bleeding site identified, if possible, and the site closed with interlocking hemostatic sutures. Drains and vaginal packs are often used to prevent reaccumulation of blood. It should be noted that large amounts of blood can dissect and accumulate along tissue planes, especially into the ischiorectal fossa, precluding easy identification. This may be seen in those with trauma involving the vaginal side walls and sulci. Thus, careful monitoring of hemodynamic status is important in identifying those with occult bleeding.

## COAGULATION DEFECTS

Virtually any congenital or acquired abnormality in blood clotting can lead to PPH. Abruptio placentae, amniotic fluid embolism, sepsis, and severe preeclampsia are obstetric conditions associated with disseminated intravascular coagulopathy. The treatment of **coagulation disorders** involves correction of the coagulation defect with appropriate factor replacement.

> *When assessing a patient with PPH, a specimen of the blood that is passing from the genital tract should be obtained in a plain test tube to check whether the blood is clotting.*

It also should be recalled that profuse hemorrhage itself can lead to coagulopathy, thus creating a vicious cycle of bleeding.

## AMNIOTIC FLUID EMBOLISM

**Amniotic fluid embolism** is a rare, sudden, and often fatal obstetric complication thought to be caused primarily by entry of amniotic fluid into the maternal circulation. Significant biochemical, as well as physical, mediators are thought to be involved in the development of the clinical scenario, which unfolds as five findings that occur in sequence: (1) respiratory distress, (2) cyanosis, (3) cardiovascular collapse, (4) hemorrhage, and (5) coma. *The syndrome also often results in severe coagulopathy.* Treatment is directed toward total support of the cardiovascular and coagulation systems, although maternal mortality still approaches 30% to 50% in most series.

## UTERINE INVERSION

**Uterine inversion** is a rare condition in which the uterus literally turns inside out, with the top of the uterine fun-

dus extending through the cervix into the vagina and sometimes even past the introitus (Fig. 12.3). Hemorrhage with uterine inversion is characteristically severe and sudden. Treatment includes manual replacement, which frequently requires administration of an agent that causes uterine relaxation (such as terbutaline, magnesium sulfate, halogenated general anesthetics, and nitroglycerin). If manual replacement fails, surgery is required.

## UTERINE RUPTURE

Uterine rupture should be distinguished from dehiscence of a low transverse incision, as the clinical connotations are quite different. A **uterine rupture** is a frank opening between the uterine cavity and the abdominal cavity. A **uterine dehiscence** is a "window" covered by the visceral peritoneum. Significantly higher rates of maternal and fetal morbidity, and even maternal mortality, occur in cases of overt rupture.

Rupture can occur at the site of a previous cesarean delivery or other surgical procedure involving the uterine wall—from intrauterine manipulation or trauma, or from congenital malformation (small uterine horn), or spontaneously. Abnormal labor, operative delivery, and placenta accreta can lead to rupture. Surgical repair is required, with the specific approach tailored to reconstruct the uterus, if possible. Care depends on the extent and site of rupture, the patient's current clinical condition, and her desire for future childbearing. Rupture of a previous cesarean delivery scar often can be managed by revision of the edges of the prior incision, followed by primary closure. In addition to the myometrial disruption, consideration must be given to the

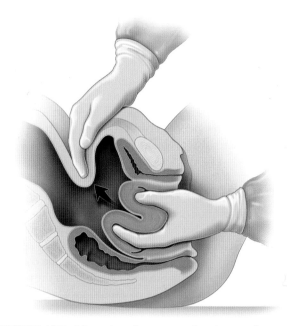

FIGURE 12.3. Manual replacement of an inverted uterus.

neighboring structures, such as the broad ligament, parametrial vessels, ureters, and bladder. Regardless of the patient's wishes for the avoidance of hysterectomy, this procedure may be necessary in a life-threatening situation. *Careful assessment in the face of maternal hemodynamic changes and monitoring other signs, such as acute abdominal pain, change in abdominal contour, non-reassuring fetal heart patterns, and loss of fetal station, are critical in early detection and intervention in such cases.*

## PREVENTION

Several preventive strategies can help curtail the incidence of delivery-associated hemorrhage, and many are quite effective. Active management of the third stage of labor, which involves immediate manual removal of the placenta and the administration of a uterotonic agent, has been shown to reduce the incidence of hemorrhage. In addition to preventing many cases of uterine atony, this approach will also reduce the incidence uterine inversion. The incidence of retained placenta is not increased with these techniques.

Finally, all obstetric units and practitioners must have the facilities, personnel, and equipment in place to manage PPH properly. Clinical drills to enhance the management of maternal hemorrhage are also recommended.

## SUGGESTED READING

American College of Obstetricians and Gynecologists. Postpartum hemorrhage. ACOG Practice Bulletin No. 76. *Obstet Gynecol.* 2006;108(4):1039–1047.

# 13 Ectopic Pregnancy and Abortion

The student should understand that ectopic pregnancy is a leading cause of maternal morbidity and mortality, and that early diagnosis and intervention can preserve fertility and save lives. Students should be able to define the types of spontaneous abortion (spontaneous, recurrent, incomplete, and septic) and explain their diagnosis and management, including the differential diagnosis of bleeding in the first trimester. Students should also be able to explain the indications, risks and benefits, and means for elective and therapeutic abortion. Students should be able to evaluate and manage fetal death in each trimester, including appropriate counseling for the parents.

## ECTOPIC PREGNANCY

An **ectopic** or **extrauterine pregnancy** is one in which the blastocyst implants anywhere other than the endometrial lining of the uterine cavity. As shown in Figure 13.1, 98% of ectopic pregnancies implant in the fallopian tube, with 80% occurring in the ampullary segment. Other locations include, but are not limited to, the ovary, cervix, and abdomen. In some form, they account for 1.3% to 2% of reported pregnancies in the United States.

In the past, ectopic pregnancy was life-threatening. Earlier diagnosis made possible by the new ability to detect the β-subunit of human chorionic gonadotropin (hCG), combined with high-resolution transvaginal sonography (TVS), has reduced this threat. Nevertheless, ectopic pregnancies remain an important cause of morbidity and mortality in the United States. The incidence of ectopic pregnancy has increased consistent with the rise in chlamydial infections.

### Tubal Ectopic Pregnancy

Without intervention, the natural course of a tubal pregnancy can lead to tubal abortion, tubal rupture, or spontaneous resolution. **Tubal abortion** is the expulsion of products of conception through the fimbriated end. This tissue can then either regress or reimplant in the abdominal cavity. **Tubal rupture** is associated with significant intra-abdominal hemorrhage, often necessitating surgical intervention.

### PATHOPHYSIOLOGY AND RISK FACTORS

An appreciation of risk factors for ectopic pregnancy leads to a timely diagnosis with improved maternal survival and future reproductive potential.

Inflammation has been implicated in the role of tubal damage that predisposes to ectopic pregnancies. Inflammatory processes, such as **salpingitis** and **salpingitis isthmica nodosa,** may also play a role. Acute pathology, such as **chlamydial infection,** causes intraluminal inflammation and subsequent fibrin deposition with tubal scarring. Despite negative cultures, persistent chlamydial antigens can trigger a delayed hypersensitivity reaction with continued scarring. Whereas endotoxin-producing *Neisseria gonorrhoeae* causes virulent pelvic inflammation with a rapid clinical onset, chlamydial inflammatory response is indolent and peaks at 7 to 14 days.

Although pregnancy after sterilization is rare, when it does occur, there is a substantial risk that the pregnancy will be ectopic. Most forms of **contraception** decrease the

FIGURE 13.1. Incidence of types of ectopic pregnancy by location. *ART* = assisted reproductive technologies

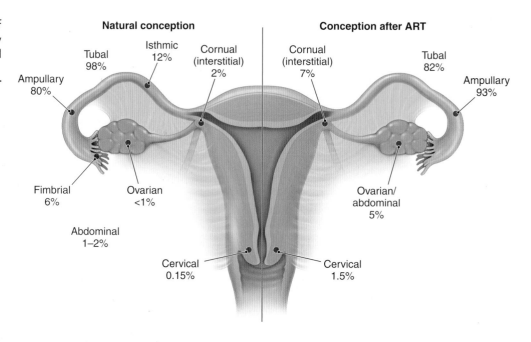

number of intrauterine pregnancies, thereby increasing the relative (but not absolute) incidence of ectopic pregnancy. Oral contraceptives prevent ovulation, significantly reducing pregnancies in all locations. Intrauterine devices do not increase the overall risk of ectopic pregnancy. Abortion does not predispose to ectopic pregnancy, although associated infection may do so.

A history of infertility, independent of tubal disease, and ovulation induction also appear to be risk factors in ectopic pregnancy. Additional risk factors include smoking, prior tubal surgery, diethylstilbestrol exposure, and advanced age.

## SYMPTOMS

With the availability of early pregnancy testing, the ability to diagnose ectopic pregnancy before rupture—even before the onset of symptoms—is not unusual. The classic symptoms associated with ectopic pregnancy are amenorrhea followed by vaginal bleeding and abdominal pain on the affected side. However, there is no constellation of symptoms that are diagnostic. Other pregnancy discomforts, such as breast tenderness, nausea, and urinary frequency, may accompany more ominous findings. These include shoulder pain worsened by inspiration, which is caused by phrenic nerve irritation from subdiaphragmatic blood, or vasomotor disturbances such as vertigo and syncope from hemorrhagic hypovolemia.

As long as placental hormones are produced, there is usually no vaginal bleeding. Irregular vaginal bleeding results from the sloughing of the decidua from the endometrial lining. Vaginal bleeding in patients with an ectopic gestation may range from little or none to heavy, menstrual-like flow. In some patients, the entire "decidual cast" is passed intact, simulating a spontaneous abortion. Histo-

logic evaluation of this tissue confirms whether placental villi are present. In any patient with a positive pregnancy test result, whenever evaluation of tissue passed spontaneously or obtained by curettage does not demonstrate villi, an ectopic implantation should be assumed to be present until proven otherwise.

Many women with a small unruptured ectopic pregnancy may have unremarkable clinical findings. Nevertheless, the diagnosis should be considered strongly when any of the above symptoms are reported by reproductive-age women, especially those with risk factors for an extrauterine pregnancy.

## CLINICAL FINDINGS

Abdominal and pelvic findings are notoriously scant in many women before tubal rupture. Prior to rupture, the diagnosis of an ectopic pregnancy is primarily based on laboratory and ultrasound findings. With rupture, however, nearly three-fourths of women will have marked tenderness on both abdominal and pelvic examination, and pain is aggravated with cervical manipulation. A pelvic mass, including fullness posterolateral to the uterus, can be palpated in about 20% of women. Initially, the ectopic pregnancy may feel soft and elastic, whereas extensive hemorrhage produces a firmer consistency. Many times, discomfort precludes palpation of the mass. Avoidance of pelvic examinations may actually help avert iatrogenic rupture.

Fever is not expected, although a mild elevation in temperature in response to intraperitoneal blood may occur. A temperature of 38°C may suggest an infectious cause to a patient's symptoms. Abdominal distension and tenderness, with or without rebound, rigidity, or decreased bowel sounds, may be seen in cases of intra-abdominal bleeding. Abdominal tenderness is variable; it is present in

50% to 90% of patients with ectopic pregnancies. Cervical motion tenderness caused by intraperitoneal irritation and adnexal tenderness are commonly found. An adnexal mass is present in roughly one-third of cases, but its absence does not rule out the possibility of an ectopic implantation. The uterus may enlarge and soften throughout the first trimester, thus simulating an intrauterine pregnancy. A slightly open cervix with blood or decidual tissue may be found and mistaken for a threatened and/or spontaneous abortion.

## DIFFERENTIAL DIAGNOSIS

Symptoms of ectopic pregnancy can mimic multiple entities. Early pregnancy complications (threatened, incomplete, or missed abortion), placental polyp, or hemorrhagic corpus luteal cyst are difficult to diagnose. Moreover, early bleeding occurs in about 20% of women with normal pregnancies. A number of nonpregnancy-related disorders, such as appendicitis and renal calculi, can mimic ectopic pregnancy.

*The rapid and accurate diagnosis of ectopic pregnancy is imperative to reduce the risk of serious complications or death.* Up to half of the women who have died as a result of ectopic pregnancy had a lag in treatment because of delayed or inaccurate diagnoses. Any sexually active woman in the reproductive age group who presents with pain, irregular bleeding, and/or amenorrhea should have ectopic pregnancy as a part of the initial differential diagnosis.

## DIAGNOSTIC PROCEDURES

TVS and serial serum β-hCG measurements are the most valuable diagnostic aids to confirm the clinical suspicion of an ectopic pregnancy.

The initial assessment in the otherwise hemodynamically stable patient must include a pregnancy test. A negative pregnancy test excludes the possibility of ectopic pregnancy. Urinary pregnancy tests, which detect hCG levels to 20 IU/L, are now commonly available. These tests detect hCG as early as 14 days after conception and are positive in more than 90% of cases of ectopic pregnancy. Serum assays can detect the presence of hCG as early as 5 days after conception, that is, before the missed menstrual cycle; however, because they require additional time and expertise to perform, they are often not used in a potentially emergent clinical setting.

If a positive pregnancy test is found when ectopic pregnancy is suspected, the remainder of the workup should focus on evaluating the viability and location of the pregnancy. In normal pregnancies, serum β-hCG levels rise in a log-linear fashion until 60 or 80 days after the last menses, at which time values plateau at about 100,000 IU/L. During this period a 66% or greater increase in serum β-hCG levels should be observed every 48 hours. Approximately 15% of normal intrauterine pregnancies are associated with less than a 66% increase in hCG, and 17% of ectopic

pregnancies have normal doubling times. Deviation from this pattern should raise suspicion for a pregnancy that is not proceeding normally, including ectopic pregnancy. *Although inappropriately rising serum β-hCG levels suggest (but do not diagnose) an abnormal pregnancy, they do not identify its location.*

A key adjunct to serial quantitative levels of hCG is pelvic ultrasonography (Fig. 13.2). High-resolution ultrasonography has revolutionized the clinical management of women with a suspected ectopic pregnancy. Using TVS, a gestational sac is usually visible between 4½ and 5 weeks from the last menstrual period, the yolk

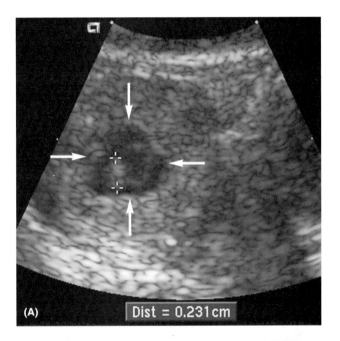

(A)    Dist = 0.231cm

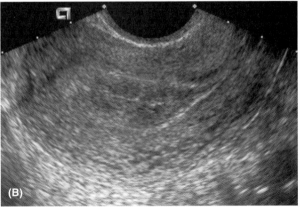

(B)

FIGURE 13.2. Ectopic pregnancy with an extrauterine gestational sac containing a live embryo. (A) Coronal transvaginal view of the right adnexa demonstrates an extrauterine sac (arrows) containing an embryo (calipers). (B) Sagittal transvaginal view of the uterus reveals no evidence of a gestational sac. (From Doubilet PM, Benson CB. *Atlas of Ultrasound in Obstetrics and Gynecology.* Philadelphia, PA: Lippincott Williams & Wilkins; 2003:319.)

sac appears between 5 and 6 weeks, and a fetal pole with cardiac activity is first detected at 5½ to 6 weeks. With transabdominal sonography these structures are visualized slightly later. Each institution must define a β-hCG **discriminatory value,** that is, the lower limit of hCG at which an examiner can reliably visualize pregnancy on ultrasound. The more sensitive transvaginal ultrasonography should show the pregnancy by the time the hCG level is 1000 to 2000 IU/L. Transabdominal ultrasonography should be able to identify an intrauterine gestation by the time the hCG level reaches 5000 to 6000 IU/L. Accurate diagnosis by sonography is three times more likely if the initial β-hCG level is above this value. The absence of uterine pregnancy with β-hCG levels above the discriminatory value signifies an abnormal pregnancy—ectopic, incomplete abortion, or resolving completed abortion. Care must be taken to differentiate between a uterine gestation and a **pseudogestational sac.** This one-layer sac is the result of an intracavitary fluid collection caused by sloughing of the decidua typically situated in the midline of the uterine cavity, whereas a normal gestational sac is eccentrically located (Fig. 13.3).

Serum progesterone concentration has also been used as a screening test for ectopic pregnancy. There is minimal variation in serum progesterone concentration between 5 and 10 weeks' gestation, thus a single value is sufficient. A serum progesterone level of <5 ng/mL has been used to identify a nonviable pregnancy with near-perfect specificity and with a sensitivity of 60%. Conversely, a serum progesterone of >20 ng/mL has a sensitivity of 95%, with a specificity of approximately 40% to identify a healthy pregnancy.

*Serum progesterone values cannot differentiate between an ectopic and intrauterine pregnancy.*

**Curettage** of the uterine cavity can also help rule out ectopic pregnancy but should only be undertaken after the possibility of interrupting an intact pregnancy has been considered. Although intrauterine and ectopic pregnancy can exist simultaneously in rare cases (heterotopic pregnancy), identification of chorionic villi in tissue samples identifies an intrauterine location of the pregnancy and essentially rules out ectopic pregnancy. The presumptive diagnosis of ectopic pregnancy is reportedly inaccurate in nearly 40% of cases without histologic exclusion of a spontaneous pregnancy loss. The **Arias-Stella reaction,** a hypersecretory endometrium of pregnancy seen on histologic examination, occurs with both ectopic and intrauterine pregnancies and, therefore, is not useful in identifying an ectopic pregnancy.

**Culdocentesis** can identify **hemoperitoneum** (blood in the peritoneal cavity), which may indicate a ruptured ectopic pregnancy, although it is also consistent with other causes, such as a ruptured corpus luteum cyst. An 18-gauge needle is inserted posterior to the cervix, between the uterosacral ligaments, and into the cul-de-sac of the peritoneal cavity (Fig. 13.4). Aspiration of clear peritoneal fluid (negative culdocentesis) indicates no hemorrhage into the abdominal cavity but does not rule out an unruptured ectopic pregnancy. Aspiration of blood that clots can indi-

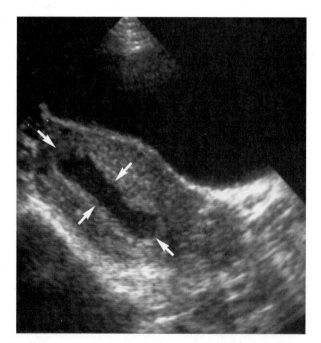

FIGURE 13.3. Pseudogestational sac. Sagittal transabdominal view of the uterus demonstrates a pseudogestational sac, a collection of fluid within the uterus. (From Doubilet PM, Benson CB. *Atlas of Ultrasound in Obstetrics and Gynecology.* Philadelphia, PA: Lippincott Williams & Wilkins; 2003:320.)

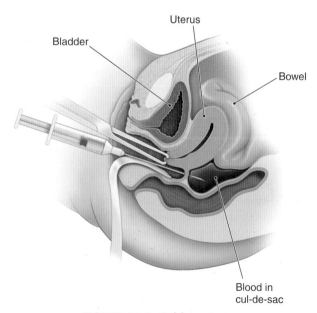

FIGURE 13.4. Culdocentesis.

cate either penetration of a vessel or such rapid blood loss into the peritoneal cavity that the blood clot has not had time to undergo fibrinolysis. Nonclotting blood is evidence of hemoperitoneum (positive culdocentesis), in which the blood clot has undergone fibrinolysis. If nothing is aspirated (equivocal or nondiagnostic culdocentesis), no information is obtained. Purulent fluid suggests a number of infection-related causes, such as salpingitis or appendicitis. Because no finding on culdocentesis can definitively confirm the presence or absence of ectopic pregnancy, its use in clinical practice has declined. When used, the primary utility of culdocentesis is that a positive culdocentesis identifies blood in the peritoneal cavity and confirms the need for further evaluation to identify the source of the bleeding.

The most accurate technique of identifying an ectopic pregnancy is by **direct visualization,** which is done most commonly via **laparoscopy.** Even laparoscopy, however, has a 2% to 5% misdiagnosis rate. For example, an extremely early tubal gestation may not be identified because it may not distend the fallopian tube sufficiently to be recognized as an abnormality (false-negative). Conversely, a false-positive diagnosis may result from a **hematosalpinx** (blood in the fallopian tube) being misinterpreted as an unruptured ectopic pregnancy or tubal abortion.

### MANAGEMENT

Management may be either surgical or medical, depending on a variety of factors. Surgery may be minimal or extensive, depending on the gestational age of the pregnancy and other factors. Due to the inherent risks of each, medical therapy is preferred over surgery in appropriate patients.

*Medical Management* **Methotrexate** is the medical treatment usually used as an alternative to surgical therapy. Methotrexate is a folic acid antagonist that competitively inhibits the binding of dihydrofolic acid to dihydrofolate reductase, which in turn reduces the amount of active intracellular metabolite, folinic acid.

The best candidate for medical therapy is the woman who is asymptomatic, motivated, and who has resources to be compliant with follow-up. Relative and absolute contraindications for medical management are listed in Box 13.1.

Factors that can be assessed in predicting the success of medical therapy include initial $\beta$-hCG level, size of ectopic pregnancy as determined by TVS, and presence or absence of fetal cardiac activity. The initial serum $\beta$-hCG level is the single best prognostic indicator of treatment success in women given single-dose methotrexate. An initial serum value <5000 IU/L is associated with a success rate of 92%, whereas an initial concentration >15,000 IU/L has a success rates of 68%. Although there are few data concerning the effect of ectopic pregnancy size on success

---

> ### BOX 13.1
> **Contraindications to Medical Therapy for Ectopic Pregnancy**
>
> **Absolute:**
> Breastfeeding
> Overt or laboratory evidence of immunodeficiency
> Alcoholism, alcoholic liver disease, or other chronic liver disease
> Preexisting blood dyscrasias, such as bone marrow hypoplasia, leukopenia, or thrombocytopenia, or significant anemia
> Known sensitivity to methotrexate
> Active pulmonary disease
> Peptic ulcer disease
> Hepatic, renal, or hematologic dysfunction
>
> **Relative:**
> Gestational sac greater than 3.5 cm
> Embryonic cardiac motion

rates with methotrexate, many early trials used "large size" as an exclusion criterion. Success rates with single-dose methotrexate were 93% in cases with ectopic masses <3.5 cm. Cardiac activity and size greater than 3.5 cm are considered relative contraindications to medical management because these findings are associated with a lower success rate.

The most common side effects of methotrexate include nausea, vomiting, diarrhea, gastric distress, dizziness, and stomatitis. Intramuscular methotrexate given as a single dose has been the most widely used medical treatment of ectopic pregnancy. Close monitoring is imperative. A serum $\beta$-hCG level is determined before administering methotrexate and is repeated on days 4 and 7 following injection. Levels may continue to rise until day 4. Comparison is then made between the day 4 and the day 7 serum values. If there is a decline by 15% or more, weekly serum $\beta$-hCG levels are measured until they are undetectable. If the $\beta$-hCG level does not decline, the patient may require either surgery or a second dose of methotrexate if no contraindications exist. If there is an adequate treatment response, hcG determinations are reduced to once a week. An additional dose of methotrexate may be given if $\beta$-hCG levels plateau or increase in 7 days. Surgical intervention may be required for patients who do not respond to medical therapy.

During the first few days following methotrexate administration, up to half of women experience abdominal pain that can be controlled with nonsteroidal anti-inflammatory drugs. This pain presumably results from tubal distention caused by tubal abortion or hematoma formation or both.

*Surgical Management* Women who are hemodynamically stable and in whom there is a small tubal diameter, no fetal cardiac activity, and serum β-hCG concentrations <5000 IU/L have similar outcomes with medical or surgical management. Conservative surgical techniques have been developed that maximize preservation of the fallopian tube. If removal is done through the laparoscope, definitive diagnosis and treatment can be accomplished at the same operation with minimal morbidity, cost, and hospitalization. In a **linear salpingostomy,** the surgeon makes an incision on the fallopian tube over the site of implantation, removes the pregnancy, and allows the incision to heal by secondary intention. A **segmental resection** is the removal of a portion of the affected tube (Fig. 13.5). **Salpingectomy** is removal of the entire tube, a procedure reserved for those cases in which little or no normal tube remains.

When conservative surgery or nonsurgical treatment is used, the patient must be followed posttherapy with serial quantitative β-hCG levels to monitor regression of the pregnancy. Subsequent surgery or methotrexate therapy is needed if trophoblastic function persists as evidenced by persistent or rising levels of hCG. Rh-negative mothers with ectopic pregnancy should receive **Rh immune globulin** to prevent Rh sensitization (see Chapter 19, Isoimmunization).

## Nonfallopian-Tube Ectopic Pregnancy

### OVARIAN PREGNANCY

Ectopic implantation of the fertilized egg in the ovary is rare. The recent increased incidence is likely due to improved imaging modalities. Risk factors are similar to those for tubal pregnancies. Diagnosis is based on the classical sonographic description of a cyst with a wide echogenic outer ring on or within the ovary.

### INTERSTITIAL PREGNANCY

Also termed **cornual pregnancy,** interstitial pregnancies implant in the proximal tubal segment that lies within the muscular uterine wall. Swelling lateral to the insertion of the round ligament is the characteristic anatomic finding. A pregnancy that implants in the cornual segment of the tube tends to present several weeks later in pregnancy, because the muscular cornu of the uterus is better able to expand and accommodate an enlarging pregnancy. As a result, rupture of a cornual (**isthmic**) pregnancy typically occurs between the eighth and sixteenth gestational weeks, and is often associated with massive hemorrhage, frequently requiring hysterectomy. Mortality rates are quoted as high as 2.5%.

### CERVICAL PREGNANCY

**Cervical pregnancy** occurs in 1 in 9000 to 12,000 pregnancies, when the ovum implants in the cervical mucosa below the level of the histologic cervical internal os. A risk factor unique to cervical pregnancy is a history of dilation and curettage, seen in nearly 70% of cases. Two diagnostic criteria are necessary for confirmation of cervical pregnancy: (1) the presence of cervical glands opposite the placental attachment site, and (2) a portion of or the entire placenta must be located below either the entrance of the uterine vessels or the peritoneal reflection on the anterior and posterior uterine surface. Medical management can be used if the previously described criteria are met.

FIGURE 13.5. Surgical management of ectopic pregnancy. (A) Site of linear incision for linear salpingostomy. (B) Linear incision. (C) Segmental resection. (D) Tubal reanastomosis.

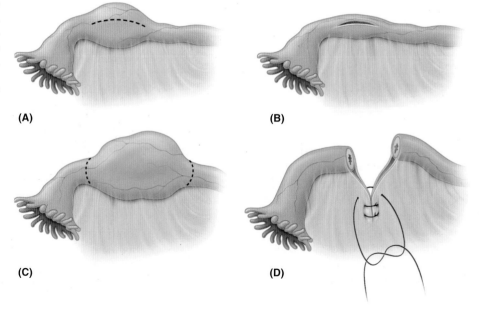

(A)

(B)

(C)

(D)

## HETEROTOPIC PREGNANCY

**Heterotopic pregnancy** (coincident or combined pregnancy) is the coexistence of an ectopic and intrauterine pregnancy. The incidence was previously estimated to be 1 in 30,000 pregnancies figuring incidences of dizygotic twinning and ectopic pregnancy of 1% each. As a result of assisted reproduction, however, the rate of heterotopic pregnancies has increased to 1 in 100 pregnancies. Mechanisms that have been proposed to explain this include: (1) hydrostatic forces delivering the embryo into the cornual or tubal area; (2) the tip of the catheter directing transfer towards the tubal ostia; or (3) reflux of uterine secretions leading to retrograde tubal implantation. In addition to the option of surgical management of the ectopic pregnancy while attempting to not disturb the intrauterine pregnancy, medical therapy in which potassium chloride can be injected into the pregnancy sac is a consideration.

*Methotrexate is contraindicated due to potential detrimental effects on the normal pregnancy.*

## ABDOMINAL PREGNANCY

The estimated incidence of **abdominal pregnancy** ranges from 1 in 10,000 to 1 in 25,000 live births. Abdominal pregnancies may result from primary implantation onto the peritoneal surface or secondary implantation via tubal rupture or tubal abortion. Physical findings and symptoms are widely variable, depending on gestational age and site of implantation. Diagnosis is confirmed primarily by ultrasonography.

Abdominal pregnancy is usually discovered long before fetal viability and removal of the pregnancy is the mainstay of therapy. Survival of the fetus occurs in only 10% to 20% of cases; up to one-half of those surviving have significant deformity. The patient is given the option of continuing the pregnancy to fetal viability with operative delivery, or operative termination of the pregnancy at the time of diagnosis. In either case, removal of the placenta is usually not attempted because of the risk of uncontrollable hemorrhage.

## SPONTANEOUS ABORTION

**Abortion** is the expulsion of the fetus prior to 20 weeks of gestation. **Spontaneous abortion** (miscarriage) occurs in the absence of intervention. An incidence of recognized spontaneous abortion of 15% to 25% is commonly cited, with approximately 80% occurring during the first 12 weeks of pregnancy. Approximately 50% of early spontaneous abortions are attributed to chromosomal abnormalities, most of which are trisomy.

Compared with first-trimester abortions, second-trimester abortions are less likely to be caused by chromosomal abnormalities and more likely to be caused by maternal systemic disease, abnormal placentation, or other anatomic considerations. This difference is clinically significant, because these conditions often can be treated and recurrent abortions can thereby potentially be prevented.

## Etiology

### INFECTIOUS FACTORS

Infections are an uncommon cause of early spontaneous abortion. *Chlamydia trachomatis* and *Listeria monocytogenes* have been associated with spontaneous abortion. Serological evidence supports a role for *Mycoplasma hominis* and *Ureaplasma urealyticum* in abortions. Finally, abortion is independently associated with serological evidence of syphilis, human immunodeficiency virus (HIV)-1 infection, and with vaginal colonization with group B streptococci.

### ENDOCRINE FACTORS

Thyroid autoantibodies are associated with an increased incidence of spontaneous abortion, even in the absence of clinical hypothyroidism. In women with type 1 diabetes, the degree of metabolic control in early pregnancy is associated with an increased risk of spontaneous abortion and major congenital malformation.

### ENVIRONMENTAL FACTORS

The abortion risk increases in a linear fashion with the number of cigarettes smoked per day. Both spontaneous abortion and fetal anomalies may result from frequent, high doses of alcohol use during the first 8 weeks of pregnancy. Radiation administered at therapeutic doses to treat cancer may be an abortifacient. It is important to note that exposure to less than 5 rads does not increase the risk for miscarriage.

### IMMUNOLOGIC FACTORS

There are a number of genetic disorders of blood coagulation that may increase the risk of both arterial and venous thrombosis. Some of the better studied thrombophilias are caused by mutations of the gene for factor V Leiden, prothrombin G20210A mutation, antithrombin III, proteins C and S, and methylene tetrahydrofolate reductase (hyperhomocysteinemia). These are most commonly associated with recurrent miscarriage.

### UTERINE FACTORS

Large and multiple **uterine leiomyomas** are common, and they may cause miscarriage. In most instances, their location is more important than their size, with submucous leiomyomata playing a more significant role than others, presumably because of their effect on implantation. In utero exposure to diethylstilbestrol (DES) has been associated with abnormally shaped uteri as well as cervical incompetence and spontaneous abortion. **Intrauterine synechiae** (Asherman syndrome), a condition that is caused by uterine curettage with subsequent destruction and scarring of the endometrium, may also be a cause of spontaneous abortion

## Classification and Differential Diagnosis of Spontaneous Abortions

Because the differential diagnosis of bleeding in the first trimester of pregnancy includes a wide range of possibilities, such as ectopic pregnancy, hydatidiform mole, cervical polyps, cervicitis, and neoplasm, the patient should be examined whenever there is bleeding in early pregnancy.

### TYPES OF SPONTANEOUS ABORTION

**Threatened abortion** is characterized by bleeding in the first trimester without loss of fluid or tissue. About half of women with a threatened abortion proceed to spontaneous abortion. Those who carry to viability a pregnancy complicated by threatened abortion are at greater risk for preterm delivery and an infant of low birth weight. There does not, however, appear to be a higher incidence of congenital malformations in these newborns. Some patients describe bleeding at the time of their expected menses, sometimes referred to as **implantation bleeding,** which may be related to implantation of the embryo in the endometrium.

In cases of miscarriage, bleeding usually begins first, and cramping abdominal pain follows a few hours to several days later. The pain may present as anterior and clearly rhythmic cramps; as a persistent low backache, associated with a feeling of pelvic pressure; or as a dull, midline, suprapubic discomfort. The combination of bleeding and pain usually indicates a poor prognosis for pregnancy continuation.

*Ectopic pregnancy should always be considered in the differential diagnosis of threatened abortion.*

An **inevitable abortion** is the gross rupture of the membranes in the presence of cervical dilation. Typically, uterine contractions begin promptly, resulting in expulsion of the products of conception. It is unusual for a pregnancy to successfully reach viability in this circumstance. Conservative management of these patients significantly increases the risk of maternal infection.

During an **incomplete abortion,** the internal cervical os opens and allows passage of blood. The products of conception may remain entirely in utero or may partially ex-

trude through the dilated os. Before 10 weeks, the fetus and placenta are commonly expelled together, but later they are delivered separately. In many cases, retained placental tissue remains in the cervical canal, allowing easy extraction from an exposed external os with ring forceps. If unsuccessful, a suction curettage effectively evacuates the uterus.

**Complete abortion** refers to a documented pregnancy that spontaneously passes all of the products of conception. Before 10 weeks, the fetus and placenta are often expelled in toto.

A **missed abortion** is the retention of a failed intrauterine pregnancy for an extended period, usually defined as more than two menstrual cycles. These patients have an absence of uterine growth and may have lost some of the early symptoms of pregnancy.

Many women have no symptoms during this period except persistent amenorrhea. If the missed abortion terminates spontaneously, and most do, the process of expulsion is the same as in any abortion.

### RECURRENT PREGNANCY LOSS

**Recurrent pregnancy loss** is a term used when a patient has had more than two consecutive pregnancy losses. The timing of the pregnancy losses may provide a clue to their cause. Genetic factors most frequently result in early embryonic losses, whereas autoimmune or anatomic abnormalities are more likely to result in second-trimester losses. Karyotyping is recommended for both parents when recurrent early abortion occurs, because there is a 3% chance that one parent is a symptomless carrier of a genetically balanced chromosomal translocation.

When recurrent pregnancy losses occur later than the first trimester of pregnancy, they can be caused by maternal medical conditions or anatomic anomalies, which may be treatable. Uterine anomalies, such as septate uteri, can be related to fetal wastage. In these cases, management including hysterography, operative hysteroscopy, or laparoscopy may be required to correct the problem. Intrauterine synechiae associated with Asherman syndrome may occur after a curettage procedure has denuded the endometrium past the layer of the basalis, so that webs of scar tissue develop across the uterine cavity (the synechiae). Asherman syndrome is associated with amenorrhea or irregular menses, infertility, and recurrent pregnancy loss. The diagnosis is confirmed by a hysterogram that shows the characteristic webbed pattern or by hysteroscopy. Treatment involves lysis of the synechiae and postoperative treatment with high doses of estrogen to facilitate endometrial proliferation, leading to the reestablishment of a normal endometrial layer.

Much attention has focused on the immune system and its role in recurrent pregnancy loss. **Antiphospholipid antibodies** are a family of autoantibodies that bind to negatively charged phospholipids. Lupus anticoagulant and anticardiolipin antibody have been linked with excessive pregnancy wastage. Treatment may include low-dose aspirin along with unfractionated heparin This therapy, begun when pregnancy is diagnosed, may be continued until delivery. Other immunologic defects associated with recurrent miscarriage are factor V Leiden defect and prothrombin gene mutation.

## Treatment

No intervention is necessary for patients with threatened abortion even if the bleeding is accompanied by low abdominal pain and cramping. If there is no evidence of significant abnormality on ultrasound evaluation, and if the pregnancy is found to be intact, the patient can be reassured and allowed to continue normal activities.

For an incomplete abortion, expectant, medical, and surgical management are all reasonable options, unless there is serious bleeding or infection. Surgical treatment is definitive and predictable but is invasive and not necessary for all women. Expectant and medical management may obviate curettage but are associated with unpredictable bleeding, and some women will need unscheduled surgery. In cases of significant pain, hemorrhage, or infection, prompt completion of abortion—either medically or surgically—is warranted.

Immediate considerations include control of bleeding, prevention of infection, pain relief, and emotional support. Bleeding is controlled by ensuring that the products of conception have been expelled or removed from the uterus. In cases of complete abortion, the uterus is small and firm, the cervix is closed, and ultrasound identifies an empty uterus. Curettage is a quick resolution that is almost 100% successful in completing early pregnancy losses. Hemostasis is enhanced through uterine contraction stimulated by oral methylergonovine. Removal of the products of conception and vaginal rest (no tampons, douches, or intercourse) decrease the risk of infection. A mild analgesic may be required and should be offered. Rh-negative mothers should receive Rh immune globulin (RhoGAM). Chromosomal evaluation of spontaneous abortions is not recommended, unless there is a history of recurrent abortion.

Emotional support is important for both the short- and long-term well-being of both the patient and her partner. No matter how well-prepared a couple is for the possibility of pregnancy loss, the event is a significant disappointment and cause of stress. When appropriate, the couple should be reassured that the loss was not precipitated by anything that they did or did not do, and that there was nothing that they could have done to prevent the loss.

A follow-up office visit is generally scheduled for 2 to 6 weeks after the loss of a pregnancy. This is an appropriate time to evaluate uterine involution, assess the return of menses, and discuss reproductive plans. The causes (or lack of causes) of the pregnancy loss should also be reiter-

ated. The impact of this loss on future childbearing should be discussed. A single pregnancy loss does not significantly increase the risk of future losses. Multiple pregnancy losses carry an increased risk for future pregnancies and warrant further evaluation for treatable etiologies.

## INDUCED ABORTION

Termination of an intact pregnancy before the time of viability can be done to safeguard the health of the mother, because of severe fetal abnormality, or on an elective, that is, voluntary basis. Elective abortion has been legal in the United States since the 1973 Supreme Court decision of *Roe v. Wade*. Since that time, various local and state laws have been proposed to significantly limit access to elective abortion. The health care provider should maintain a nonjudgmental position in treating women who may be considering elective termination of pregnancy.

**Induced abortion** is the medical or surgical termination of pregnancy before the time of fetal viability. In 2004, 839,226 legal induced abortions were reported to the CDC. Medical and/or surgical complications are associated with all choices, with the fewest complications related to elective abortion in the first trimester.

The most common form of suction curettage for first-trimester abortions, vacuum aspiration, requires a rigid cannula attached to an electric-powered vacuum source. Alternatively, manual vacuum aspiration uses a similar cannula that attaches to a handheld syringe for its vacuum source. Second-trimester abortions are most commonly performed through the cervix, using suction or extraction forceps, or by the use of prostaglandins, as in the form of intra-amniotic injections or vaginal suppositories.

Outpatient medical abortion is an acceptable alternative to surgical abortion in appropriately selected women with pregnancies less than 49 days of gestation (calculated from the first day of the last menstrual period). Beyond this point, surgical abortion is the preferred method of early abortion. Three medications for early **medical abortion** have been widely studied and used: the antiprogestin, **mifepristone (RU-486)**; the antimetabolite, **methotrexate**; and the prostaglandin, **misoprostol**. These agents cause abortion by increasing uterine contractility either by reversing the progesterone-induced inhibition of contractions—mifepristone and methotrexate, or by stimulating the myometrium directly—misoprostol. Abortion with this medical method is not always complete. As a result, the patient should be made aware that suction curettage may be required.

## Complications

The most common complications following an induced abortion include uterine perforation, cervical laceration, hemorrhage, incomplete removal of the fetus and placenta, and infection. In cases of postabortal infection, the patient usually presents with fever, pain, a tender uterus, and mild bleeding. Oral antibiotics and antipyretics are usually sufficient to manage these mild infections. If tissue remains in the uterus (incomplete abortion), a repeat suction curettage is necessary. The second most common complication following induced abortion is bleeding. Risk of death from abortion during the first 2 months of pregnancy is less than 1 per 100,000 procedures, with increasing rates as pregnancy progresses (versus 7.7 maternal deaths per 100,000 live births).

## Septic Abortion

An infected abortion, either complete or incomplete, is known as a **septic abortion.** Patients may present with sepsis, shock, hemorrhage, and possibly renal failure. It rarely occurs as a complication of a legal abortion, but is more commonly associated with criminal abortions, that is, those done illegally, under unsterile conditions, by persons who may have little or no knowledge of medicine or anatomy. *Broad-spectrum parenteral antibiotics, intravenous fluid therapy, and prompt evacuation of the uterus are indicated.* A careful evaluation for trauma, including perforation of the uterus, vagina, or intraabdominal structures, should also be carried out.

## Postabortal Syndrome

**Postabortal syndrome** develops when the uterus fails to remain contracted after spontaneous abortion (with or without suction curettage) or elective/therapeutic abortion. The patient presents with cramping pain and/or bleeding, and is found to have an open cervix, bleeding, and a large, "softer-than-expected" uterus, a result of the collection of blood in the uterus (hematometra). The clinical presentation is often indistinguishable from incomplete abortion. Suction curettage is the treatment for both conditions. Postevacuation treatment with an ergot derivative and an antibiotic reduces the risk of postabortal syndrome, further bleeding, and infection.

## SUGGESTED READINGS

American College of Obstetricians and Gynecologists. Management of recurrent early pregnancy loss. ACOG Practice Bulletin No. 24. *Obstet Gynecol.* 2001;97(2).

American College of Obstetricians and Gynecologists. Medical management of abortion. ACOG Practice Bulletin No. 67. *Obstet Gynecol.* 2005;106(4):871–882.

American College of Obstetricians and Gynecologists. Medical management of tubal pregnancy. ACOG Practice Bulletin No. 3. *Obstet Gynecol.* 1998;92(6):1–7.

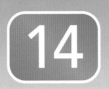

# Common Medical Problems in Pregnancy

**Topic 17:** Medical and Surgical Conditions in Pregnancy

For each of the following problems, students should be able to discuss the diagnosis during pregnancy, the impact of pregnancy on the condition and of the condition on the pregnancy (mother and fetus), and the initial management during pregnancy. The problems include hematologic diseases, diabetes mellitus, thyroid disease, urinary tract disorders, cardiac disease, asthma, surgical conditions, and trauma.

**M**aternal medical or surgical conditions can complicate the course of a pregnancy and/or can be affected by pregnancy. Physicians providing obstetric care must have a thorough understanding of the effect of pregnancy on the natural course of a disorder, the effect of the disorder on a pregnancy, and the change in management of the pregnancy and disorder caused by their coincidence.

## PRECONCEPTION CARE

*Preconception care includes the identification of those conditions that could affect a future pregnancy or fetus and that may be amenable to intervention.* Adverse effects on the fetus, including spontaneous abortion or congenital anomalies caused by medications or poorly controlled diabetes mellitus, can be reduced with proper care prior to pregnancy. Preconception care can be provided at any healthcare encounter during a woman's reproductive years. Complete information about preconception care and counseling can be found in Chapter 6, Preconception and Antepartum Care.

## HEMATOLOGIC DISEASE

### Anemia

The plasma and cellular composition of blood change significantly during pregnancy, with the expansion of plasma volume proportionally greater than that of the red blood cell mass. On average, there is a 1000-mL increase in plasma volume and a 300-mL increase in red-cell volume (a 3:1 ratio). Because the hematocrit (Hct) reflects the proportion of blood made up primarily of red blood cells, Hct demonstrates a "physiologic" decrease during pregnancy; therefore, this decrease is not actually an anemia.

*Anemia in pregnancy is generally defined as an Hct less than 30% or a hemoglobin of less than 10 g/dL.*

The direct fetal consequences of anemia are minimal, although infants born to mothers with iron deficiency may have diminished iron stores as neonates. The maternal consequences of anemia are those associated with any adult anemia. If anemia is corrected, the woman with an adequate red-cell mass enters labor and delivery better able to respond to acute peripartum blood loss and to avoid the risks of blood or blood product transfusion.

### IRON-DEFICIENCY ANEMIA

**Iron-deficiency anemia** is by far the most frequent type of anemia seen in pregnancy, accounting for more than 90% of cases. Because the iron content of the standard American diet and the endogenous iron stores of many American women are not sufficient to provide for the increased iron requirements of pregnancy, the National Academy of Sciences recommends 27 mg of iron supplementation (present in most prenatal vitamins) daily for pregnant women. Most prescription prenatal vitamin/mineral preparations contain 60 to 65 mg of elemental iron.

All pregnant women should be screened for iron-deficiency anemia. Severe iron-deficiency anemia is characterized by small, pale erythrocytes (Fig. 14.1) and red-cell indices that indicate a low mean corpuscular volume and low mean corpuscular hemoglobin concentration. Additional laboratory studies usually demonstrate decreased serum iron levels, an increased total iron-binding capacity, and a decrease in serum ferritin levels. A recent dietary history is obviously important, especially if pica (the consumption of non-nutrient substances such as starch, ice, or dirt) exists. Such dietary compulsions may contribute to iron deficiency by decreasing the amount of nutritious food and iron consumed.

Treatment of iron-deficiency anemia generally requires an additional 60 to 120 mg of elemental iron per day, in addition to the iron in the prenatal vitamin/mineral preparation. Iron absorption is facilitated by or with vitamin C supplementation or ingestion between meals or at bedtime on an empty stomach. The response to therapy is first seen as an increase in the reticulocyte count approximately 1 week after starting iron therapy. Because of the plasma expansion associated with pregnancy, the Hct may not increase significantly, but rather stabilizes or increases only slightly.

## FOLATE DEFICIENCY

*Adequate intake of folic acid (folate) has been found to reduce the risk of neural tube defects (NTDs) in the fetus.*

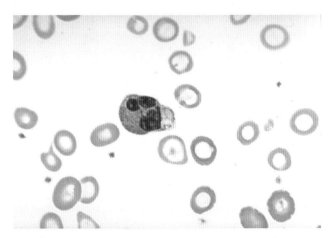

FIGURE 14.1. Peripheral blood smear of iron-deficiency anemia with microcytic, hypochromic erythrocytes. (From Rubin R, Strayer DS. *Rubin's Pathology: Clinicopathologic Foundations of Medicine.* 5th ed. Baltimore, MD: Lippincott Williams & Wilkins; 2007:20–22.)

The first occurrence of NTDs may be reduced by as much as 36% if women of reproductive age consume 0.4 mg of folate daily both before conception and during the first trimester of pregnancy. The Recommended Daily Dietary Allowance for folate for pregnant women is 0.6 mg. Folate deficiency is especially likely in multiple gestations or when patients are taking anticonvulsive medications. Women with a history of a prior NTD-affected pregnancy or who are being treated with anticonvulsive drugs may reduce the risk of NTDs by more than 80% with daily intake of 4 mg of folate in the months in which conception is attempted and for the first trimester of pregnancy.

Folate is found in green leafy vegetables and is now an added supplement in cereal, bread, and grain products. These supplements are designed to enable women to easily consume 0.4 mg to 1 mg of folate daily. Prescription prenatal vitamin/mineral preparations contain 1 mg of folic acid.

## OTHER ANEMIAS

The **hemoglobinopathies** are a heterogenous group of single-gene disorders that includes the structural hemoglobin variants and the thalassemias. **Hereditary hemolytic anemias** are also rare causes of anemia in pregnancy. Some examples are hereditary spherocytosis, an autosomal dominant defect of the erythrocyte membrane; glucose 6-phosphate dehydrogenase deficiency; and pyruvate kinase deficiency.

## The Hemoglobinopathies

More than 270 million people worldwide are heterozygous carriers of hereditary disorders of hemoglobin, and at least 300,000 affected homozygotes or compound homozygotes are born each year. The hemoglobinopathies include the thalassemias (α-thalassemia, β-thalassemia) and the sickle cell spectrum: sickle cell trait (Hb AS), sickle cell disease (Hb SS), and sickle cell disorders (Hb SC and sickle cell β-thalassemia) (Table 14.1).

Hemoglobin (Hb) consists of four interlocking polypeptide chains, each of which has an attached heme molecule. The polypeptide chains are called alpha, beta, gamma, delta, epsilon, and zeta. Adult hemoglobins consists of two alpha chains and either two beta chains (Hb A), two gamma chains (Hb F), or two delta chains (Hb $A_2$). The beta chains are the oxygen-carrying subunits of the hemoglobin molecule. Hb F is the primary hemoglobin of the fetus from 12 to 24 weeks of gestation. In the third trimester, production of Hb F decreases as production of beta-chains and Hb A begins.

**α-thalassemia** is generally caused by missing copies of the α-globin gene; however, occasionally point mutations can cause functional abnormalities in the protein. Humans normally have 4 copies of the α-globin gene. Those with 3 copies are asymptomatic, those with 2 copies

TABLE
**14.1**      The Hemoglobinopathies*

|  | Globin Abnormality | Genetics | Risk Groups |
|---|---|---|---|
| Sickle cell | **Hb S** (valine substituted for glutamic acid at the sixth position)—classic sickle cell<br>**Hb C** (lysine substituted for glutamic acid at the sixth position) | Autosomal recessive<br>**Sickle cell trait:** Hb AS heterozygous—one chain affected, <40% HbS<br>1/12 Black Americans<br>**Sickle cell disease:** Hb SS or Hb SC homozygous—both chains affected<br>1/600 Black Americans | African, Mediterranean, Turkish, Arabian, East Indian heritage |
| α-Thalassemia | Normal hemoglobin; production of α-globin chains is decreased | Autosomal recessive severity of disease depends on amount of globin produced<br>**Homozygous:** none = Hb Barts disease<br>**Heterozygous:** 25%–75% of normal amount | Asian, African, East Indian, Mediterranean heritage |
| β-Thalassemia | Normal hemoglobin; point mutations cause decreased production of β-globin chains | Autosomal recessive<br>**Homozygous:** β-thalassemia major (Cooleys anemia); no Hb A is produced = severe disease<br>**Heterozygous:** β-thalassemia minor; one normal and one abnormal β-globin allele = mild to moderate disease | Mediterranean, Middle Eastern, African, East Indian and Asian heritage |
| Sickle cell/β-thalassemia | One globin is Hb S and one globin codes for β-thalassemia | Autosomal recessive in 1/1700 pregnancies; severity of disease depends on the β-allele (no Hb A production = severe disease; moderate production = milder disease) | Same as for sickle cell and β-thalassemia |

*Hb A is normal adult hemoglobin.

have mild anemia, and those with 1 copy have hemolytic anemia. Individuals in whom the gene is absent have Hb Barts disease, which results in **hydrops fetalis** and intrauterine death.

Phenotypic expressions of **β-thalassemia** vary because of the many possible mutations in the β-globin gene. Some mutations cause an absence of the protein, while others result in a defective globin protein. β-thalassemia major occurs in homozygotes and is a severe disease, whereas a diagnosis of β-thalassemia minor (heterozygotes) may include asymptomatic to clinically anemic patients.

The **sickle cell disorders** are autosomal recessive disorders caused by point mutations that lead to functional abnormalities in the β-globin chains. Instead of normal Hb A, individuals with this disorder have abnormal Hb S. Hb S is unstable, especially under conditions of low oxygen tension. The unstable Hb S causes a structural change resulting in deformity of the normal spheroid shape of the red blood cell into the shape of a "sickle." These abnormally shaped cells lead to increased viscosity, hemolysis, and a further decrease in oxygenation. Sickling that occurs in small blood vessels can cause a **vaso-occlusive crisis,** in which the blood supply to vital organs is compromised.

Heterozygotic individuals (Hb AS) have **sickle cell trait** and are asymptomatic. The most severe form of the disease, which occurs in homozygotic individuals (Hb SS), is called **sickle cell anemia.** Sickle cell disorders are found not only in patients who have Hb SS, but also in those who have Hb S and one other abnormality of β-globin structure. The most common are Hb SC disease and Hb S/β-thalassemia.

*Women of Mediterranean, Southeast Asian, or African descent are at higher risk of being carriers for hemoglobinopathies and should be offered carrier screening.*

If both parents are deemed to be carriers of any hemoglobinopathy, genetic counseling is recommended. *For individuals of non African descent, initial testing should be done by complete blood count (CBC). Because individuals of African descent are at high risk for carrying a gene for sickle cell disease, these women should be offered hemoglobin electrophoresis in addition to a CBC.* Solubility testing, such as tests for the presence of Hb S (Sickledex), isoelectronic focusing, and high-performance liquid chromatography (HPLC) are inadequate for screening and fail to identify important transmissible hemoglobin gene abnormalities affecting fetal outcome.

Although the course of pregnancy can vary according to the type of hemoglobinopathy, there is also individual variation among patients with the same type of disorder. Besides the genetic implications, patients with the sickle cell trait (Hb AS) have an increased risk of urinary infections but experience no other pregnancy complications. Pregnancies in patients with HbS/β–thalassemia are generally unaffected. Patients who are Hb SS or Hb SC, in contrast, may suffer vaso-occlusive episodes. Infections are also more common due to functional asplenia caused by repetitive end-organ damage to the spleen. Infection should be ruled out before attributing any pain to a vaso-occlusive crisis.

Although prophylactic maternal red cell transfusions for women with hemoglobinopathies have been used in the past, *transfusions are, for the most part, reserved for complications of hemoglobinopathies such as congestive heart failure, sickle cell disease crises unresponsive to hydration and analgesics, and severely low levels of hemoglobin.* Because fetal outcomes such as preterm labor, intrauterine growth restriction, and low birth weight are more common in women with hemoglobinopathies, except those with sickle cell trait, antenatal assessment of fetal well-being and growth is an important part of managing patients with hemoglobinopathies.

## DIABETES MELLITUS

Approximately 2% of pregnancies are complicated by diabetes that either develops during pregnancy (gestational diabetes) or was antecedent to pregnancy (pregestational diabetes mellitus). *In either case, diabetes has significant implications for mother and fetus during pregnancy, and, conversely, pregnancy significantly affects diabetes.* Whether diabetes is newly diagnosed or long-standing, intense management may be stressful, and all those involved with obstetric care should be mindful of the extra emotional attention many of these patients need.

### Classification of Diabetes in Pregnancy

The American Diabetes Association (ADA) identifies three forms of glucose intolerance:

* **Type 1 diabetes mellitus** refers to diabetes diagnosed in childhood. It is thought to be caused by immunologic destruction of cells of the pancreas, resulting in necessary **insulin** replacement. **Diabetic ketoacidosis (DKA)** is more common in patients with this type of diabetes
* **Type 2 diabetes mellitus** is adult-onset glucose intolerance. Patients with type 2 diabetes mellitus are frequently overweight, and the disease can often be controlled with

weight control and a carefully followed diet. This type of diabetes is thought to result from insulin resistance and exhaustion of the cells, rather than their destruction.
* **Gestational diabetes mellitus (GDM)** refers to glucose intolerance identified during pregnancy. In most patients, it subsides postpartum, although glucose intolerance in subsequent years occurs more frequently in this group of patients.

### Physiology of Glucose Metabolism in Pregnancy

Dietary habits frequently change during pregnancy. Food intake may decrease early in pregnancy because of nausea and vomiting, and food preferences may change later in pregnancy. Several pregnancy-associated hormones also have a major effect on glucose metabolism. Most notable of these is **human placental lactogen (hPL),** which is produced in abundance by the enlarging placenta. HPL affects both fatty acid and glucose metabolism. It promotes lipolysis with increased levels of circulating free fatty acids and causes a decrease in glucose uptake. In this manner, hPL can be thought of as an anti-insulin. The increasing production of this hormone as pregnancy advances generally requires ongoing changes in insulin therapy to adjust for this effect.

Other hormones that have demonstrated lesser effects include **estrogen** and **progesterone,** which interfere with the insulin-glucose relation; and **insulinase,** which is produced by the placenta and degrades insulin to a limited extent. These effects of pregnancy on glucose metabolism make the management of pregnancy-associated diabetes difficult. DKA, for example, is more common in pregnant patients.

With increased renal blood flow, the simple diffusion of glucose in the glomerulus increases beyond the ability of tubular reabsorption, resulting in the **normal glucosuria of pregnancy,** commonly of approximately 300 mg/day. In patients with diabetes, this glucosuria may be much greater, but because of the poor correlation of pregnancy glucosuria values and simultaneous blood glucose concentrations, using urinary glucose levels is of little value in glucose management during pregnancy.

### Fetal Morbidity and Mortality in Pregestational and Gestational Diabetes

*Infants of mothers with diabetes are at a six-fold increased risk of congenital anomalies over the 1% to 2% baseline risk of all patients.* The most commonly encountered anomalies are cardiac and limb deformities. **Sacral agenesis** is a unique but rare anomaly for this group (Fig. 14.2).

The risk of **spontaneous abortion** is similar in patients with well-controlled diabetes and in patients without diabetes, but the risk is significantly increased for the patients

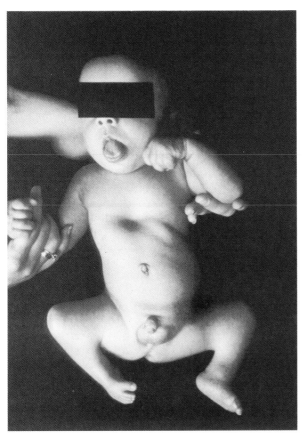

FIGURE 14.2. Infant born to a diabetic mother with poor glycemic control. Hypoplastic lower extremities and lack of lumbosacral spine are evident. (From Gabbe SG, Graves CR. Management of diabetes mellitus complicating pregnancy. *Obstet Gynecol*. 2003;102(4):857–868.)

with diabetes if glucose control is poor. *There is also an increased risk of intrauterine fetal demise and stillbirth, especially when diabetic control is inadequate.* Because of this potentially devastating outcome, beginning at approximately 30 to 32 weeks of gestation, various antepartum fetal tests may be initiated to monitor fetal health (see "Antepartum Fetal Monitoring" sections below).

Infections occur more frequently in mothers with diabetes. The glucose-rich urine is an excellent environment for bacterial growth; the risk of urinary tract infection (UTI) and pyelonephritis is approximately double that of nondiabetic pregnant patients. Patients should be told to promptly report any symptoms that suggest infection so that identification and treatment can be initiated.

*Excessive fetal growth, or* **macrosomia** *(usually defined as a fetal weight in excess of either 4000 or 4500 g), is more common in pregnant patients with diabetes because of the fetal metabolic effects of increased glucose transfer across the placenta.* However, intrauterine growth restriction can also occur due to uteroplacental insufficiency. For these reasons, serial ultrasonography is often performed to follow fetal growth. When the estimated fetal weight by ultrasound

late in pregnancy is greater than 4500 g, cesarean delivery is often recommended to avoid the risk of fetopelvic disproportion, shoulder dystocia, and other birth trauma associated with large infants.

*Another complication of pregnancy in patients with diabetes is an increase in amniotic fluid volume greater than 2000 mL, a condition known as hydramnios or* **polyhydramnios**. Encountered in approximately 10% of mothers with diabetes, the increases in amniotic fluid volume and uterine size are associated with an increased risk of placental abruption and preterm labor, as well as postpartum uterine atony. This condition is monitored while serial ultrasonography is performed for fetal growth, at which time the amount of amniotic fluid can be evaluated.

**Neonatal hypoglycemia** is often encountered in infants of women with diabetes. It results from the sudden change in the maternal-fetal glucose balance, in which an increased maternal glucose crossing the placenta is countered by an increase in fetal production of insulin. However, when the maternal supply of glucose is removed, this higher level of insulin can cause significant neonatal hypoglycemia. In addition, these newborns are subject to an increased incidence of neonatal hyperbilirubinemia, hypocalcemia, and polycythemia.

Infants of mothers with diabetes also tend to have an increased frequency of respiratory distress syndrome. The usual tests of lung maturity may be less predictive for these infants (see respiratory section below).

## Pregestational Diabetes

Approximately 1% of all pregnant patients are diabetic before pregnancy. Type 2 pregestational diabetes mellitus is most common. *Although 90% of diabetes cases encountered during pregnancy are GDM, more than one half of these eventually develop type 2 pregestational diabetes mellitus later in life.*

### Antepartum Fetal Monitoring

Women with pregestational diabetes should receive an ultrasound examination early in pregnancy to check for fetal viability and accurately date the gestational age. At 18 to 20 weeks of gestation, an ultrasound examination that focuses on identification of congenital anomalies, especially those of the heart and great vessels, is indicated. Echocardiography may also be done if there are suspected cardiac defects or when the fetal heart and great vessels could not be visualized by ultrasonography.

*Antepartum fetal monitoring, including fetal movement counting, the nonstress test, biophysical profile, and contraction stress test, performed at appropriate intervals, is a valuable approach and can be used to monitor women with pregestational diabetes.* This testing is usually initiated at 32 to 34 weeks of gestation, but can be undertaken earlier if other high-risk conditions exist.

## COMPLICATIONS

Pregnant patients with pregestational diabetes, especially type 1 diabetes, are at higher risk for diabetic ketoacidosis (DKA), the management of which is not altered in pregnancy. Fetal death can accompany DKA, so electronic fetal monitoring is essential until the maternal metabolic status is stabilized.

**Hypoglycemia** may also occur periodically, especially early in pregnancy, when nausea and vomiting interfere with caloric intake. Although hypoglycemia does not have adverse effects on the fetus, patients and family should be taught how to respond quickly and appropriately to hypoglycemia.

In addition to the added difficulties of glucose management and the increased risk of DKA during pregnancy, *mothers with pregestational diabetes have a two-fold increase in the incidence of pregnancy-induced hypertension, or* **preeclampsia,** *compared with patients without diabetes.* Because of this increased risk of preeclampsia, 24-hour urine collections to determine the level of proteinuria and creatinine clearance are often used in pregestational diabetics. Additionally, if patients have preexisting **diabetic nephropathy,** manifested by pre-pregnancy creatinine >1.5 or severe proteinuria, they are at an increased risk of progression to end-stage renal disease, and serial monitoring of renal function is warranted.

Diabetic **retinopathy** worsens in approximately 15% of pregnant patients with preexisting diabetes, some proceeding to proliferative retinopathy and loss of vision if the process remains untreated by laser coagulation. Therefore, women with pregestational type 1 or type 2 diabetes should have an ophthalmologic evaluation once in their first trimester if asymptomatic, and as needed if symptoms arise.

## MANAGEMENT

The patient with long-standing diabetes should realize that strict control of her glucose levels is advised during pregnancy, with greater attention to and more frequent monitoring of glucose values. *For these patients, management ideally begins before conception, with the goal of optimal glucose control before and during pregnancy.* Hemoglobin $A_{1c}$ levels can be measured to reflect average glucose values over the preceding 12 weeks. These levels can then be used to monitor glucose control both before and during pregnancy and to predict the likelihood of congenital anomalies in the fetus.

Excellent glucose control is achieved using a careful combination of diet, exercise, and insulin therapy. *Insulin requirements will increase throughout pregnancy, most markedly in the period between 28 to 32 weeks of gestation.*

The impact of pregnancy on diabetes, and vice versa, must also be emphasized to the pregnant patient with pregestational diabetes. Patients may need to be seen every 1 to 2 weeks during the first two trimesters and weekly after 28 to 30 weeks of gestation.

## Gestational Diabetes

The prevalence of GDM is estimated to be about 2%. GDM is usually identified by prenatal screening of pregnant patients. It may be suspected, however, in patients with known risk factors for GDM, which include age, ethnicity, past obstetric history (gestational diabetes in a previous pregnancy, a history of an infant weighing more than 4000 g at birth, repeated spontaneous abortions, or a history of unexplained stillbirth), a strong family history of diabetes, and obesity. However, 50% of patients identified as having gestational diabetes do not have such risk factors.

### LABORATORY SCREENING

*The most commonly used screening test for glucose intolerance during pregnancy is given at 24 to 28 weeks of gestation and consists of a 50-g, 1-hour oral glucose challenge.*

Patients whose glucose value exceeds 140 mg/dL (some use 130 or 135 mg/dL) require a standard 3-hour glucose tolerance test using 100 g of glucose. Two or more abnormal results of the 3-hour test establish the diagnosis of gestational diabetes.

In patients lacking any risk factors, the 1-hour glucose screening is usually performed between 24 and 28 weeks of gestation because glucose intolerance is generally evident by that time. Using this screening method, approximately 15% of patients have an abnormal screening test. Of those patients who then proceed to have the standard 3-hour oral glucose tolerance test, approximately 15% are diagnosed as having gestational diabetes. Although many practitioners choose to screen high-risk patients early in pregnancy, the benefit of early treatment of women with GDM identified early in pregnancy has not been demonstrated, but, rather, has been accepted on a theoretical basis.

### ANTEPARTUM FETAL MONITORING

*There is currently insufficient evidence to determine the optimal antepartum testing regimen for women with relatively normal glucose levels on diet therapy and no other risk factors.* Despite the lack of evidence, it is reasonable to conclude that women whose GDM is not well-controlled, who require insulin, or have other risk factors such as hypertension should receive the same antepartum testing regimen as women with pregestational diabetes. While ultrasonography can be used to assess congenital anomalies, the reliability of ultrasonography to estimate fetal weight and predict macrosomia prior to delivery has not been established.

## MANAGEMENT

*Often overlooked or underemphasized in the overall management of a patient whose pregnancy is complicated by diabetes mellitus is the importance of patient education.* The patient with newly diagnosed diabetes should receive general diabetic counseling, along with information about the unique features of the combination of diabetes and pregnancy. Home glucose monitoring is the norm, and instruction in technique should be provided.

The overall goal of managing GDM is to control glucose values within circumscribed limits: fasting glucose levels of less than 95 mg/dL or 1-hour postprandial levels of 130 to 140 mg/dL or 2-hour postprandial values less than 120 mg/dL. The mainstay of GDM management is diet. The recommended diet is about 30 Kcal/kg/day of ideal body weight, composed of approximately 45% complex carbohydrates, 35% fat, and 20% protein. *With careful attention to diet, many mothers with GDM do not require insulin.* Current available evidence does not support a recommendation for or against moderate caloric restriction in obese women with GDM. However, if caloric restriction is used, the diet should be restricted by no more than 33% of calories.

Patients are instructed to obtain a morning fasting glucose, along with pre- and postprandial glucose values throughout the day and evening. The precise goals for glucose control vary, but in general the fasting plasma glucose should be maintained in the 90 to 100 mg/100 mL range, and the postprandial values obtained throughout the day at <120 to 140 mg/100 mL. For those patients who are able to control their gestational diabetes with diet alone, the perinatal outcome is good. Pregnancy is allowed to continue to term, with delivery planned at that time.

*For patients with GDM whose glucose levels cannot be controlled with diet, exogenous insulin is needed.* Frequently, a combination of intermediate-acting NPH (neutral protamine Hagedorn) and fast-acting insulin (such as regular or lispro) is used together near breakfast and dinner in order to suppress gluconeogenesis in the liver as well as to counter the rises in glucose that occur with meals. This necessitates only twice-daily injections. However, some advocate splitting the evening insulin dose, giving the short-acting insulin at dinner, and then NPH at bedtime, in order to decrease the risk of nocturnal hypoglycemia. *Insulin does not cross the placenta and, therefore, does not directly affect the fetus.* However, glucose does cross the placenta (by facilitated diffusion); the higher the maternal glucose level, the higher the fetal glucose level. In response, the fetus produces more insulin. This increased insulin production converts glucose to fat, resulting in the heavier infants (macrosomia) often noted in patients with diabetes. Following delivery, the high

maternal glucose transfer ceases, but the continuing high fetal insulin concentration may lead to significant neonatal hypoglycemia temporarily.

Therapy with **oral hypoglycemic agents** is a newer aspect of diabetic therapy, and these agents are being used more commonly in pregnancy. Glyburide, which does not cross the placenta, has been shown to be comparable to insulin in both glucose control and adverse maternal and neonatal outcomes. Metformin has been used in many patients with polycystic ovary syndrome to achieve pregnancy, but is not used regularly after the first trimester for glucose control. As with pregestational diabetes, the use of these agents should be carefully considered and individualized.

*Patients with diabetes are monitored closely throughout pregnancy, usually at 1- to 2-week intervals.* Insulin adjustments are made on the basis of the glucose logs maintained by the patient. Also, as previously described, insulin requirements of a pregnant patient are expected to increase as pregnancy advances because of the rising production of hPL by the placenta, with its insulin-resistant effect.

## Labor and Delivery of the Patient with Diabetes

The goal is for the patient with diabetes to deliver a healthy child vaginally. The adequacy of glucose control, the well-being of the infant, estimated fetal weight by ultrasound, presence of hypertension or other complications of pregnancy, gestational age, presentation of the fetus, and status of the cervix are all factors involved in decisions regarding delivery. *In the well-controlled patient with diabetes who has no complications, induction at term (38 to 39 weeks) is often undertaken.* For women with GDM or pregestational diabetes and an estimated fetal weight of 4500 g or more, caesarean delivery may be considered. If an earlier delivery is deemed necessary for either fetal or maternal indications, fetal maturity studies may be performed on amniotic fluid obtained by amniocentesis. If antepartum steroids for fetal lung maturity become necessary (e.g., for patients with preterm labor), frequent glucose monitoring and, at times, increased doses of insulin are necessary to counter the hyperglycemic effects of corticosteroids.

*Whether the patient's labor begins spontaneously or is induced, the goal of intrapartum insulin therapy is strict glucose control.* Once active labor begins or glucose levels decrease to 70 mg/dL, a constant glucose infusion of a 5% dextrose solution delivered at a rate of 100 to 150 mL/hr is administered to maintain a glucose level of 100 mg/dL. The plasma glucose level should be assessed every 1 to 2 hours. Short-acting insulin may be administered, usually by constant intravenous infusion, if glucose levels exceed 100 mg/dL.

With delivery of the placenta, the source of the "anti-insulin" factors, most notably hPL, is removed. With its short half-life, the effect on plasma glucose is evident within hours. Many patients do not require any insulin for a few days postpartum. Routine management generally consists of frequent glucose assessments and a sliding scale approach with minimal insulin injections. The goals for optimal glucose values are less stringent in the puerperium than during pregnancy. For patients with gestational diabetes, no further insulin is required postpartum. In patients with pregestational diabetes, insulin is generally resumed at 50% of the pre-pregnant dose once a patient is consuming a normal diet. Thereafter, insulin can be adjusted over the ensuing weeks, with requirements usually reaching the pre-pregnancy level.

More than 95% of mothers with gestational diabetes return to a completely normal glucose status immediately postpartum; however, approximately 50% of these women go on to develop type 2 diabetes later in life and need to be educated about the importance of maintaining a healthy diet and regular exercise program. *Glucose tolerance screening is advocated 2 to 4 months postpartum to detect the 3% to 5% who remain diabetic and require treatment.* Typically, such screening involves a 75-g glucose load, followed by plasma glucose determination 2 hours later. A value above 140 mg/dL requires follow-up.

For contraception, barrier methods or intrauterine contraceptives are often chosen; patients who choose oral contraceptives should monitor their glucose values to identify an increase that is sometimes seen with this method (see Chapter 24, Contraception).

## THYROID DISEASE

As with diabetes mellitus, thyroid disease may predate pregnancy or may initially manifest during pregnancy. Obstetric conditions, such as gestational trophoblastic disease or hyperemesis gravidarum, may themselves affect thyroid function. All neonates of women with thyroid disease are at risk for neonatal thyroid dysfunction. For this reason, the neonate's pediatrician should be informed about the maternal diagnosis.

## Pathophysiology

**Thyrotoxicosis** is the condition that results from excess production of and exposure to thyroid hormone from any cause. **Hyperthyroidism** is thyrotoxicosis caused by hyperfunctioning of the thyroid gland. Graves disease is an autoimmune disease characterized by abnormal production of thyroid-specific immunoglobulins that either stimulate or inhibit thyroid function. Exacerbation of the signs and symptoms of hyperthyroidism is called a **thyroid storm**. **Hypothyroidism** is caused by inadequate thyroid hormone production. **Postpartum thyroiditis** is an autoimmune inflammation of the thyroid gland that presents as new-onset, painless hypothyroidism, transient thyrotoxicosis,

or thyrotoxicosis followed by hypothyroidism within 1 year postpartum.

Levels of thyroid-binding hormone (TBG) normally increase in pregnancy. Test results that change significantly in pregnancy are those influenced by TBG concentration, including total thyroxine (TT4), total triiodothyronine (TTd) and resin triiodothyronine uptake (TR3U). A transient increase may also occur in free thyroxine (FT4) and free thyroxine index (FTI) levels in the first trimester (Fig. 14.3).

Plasma iodide levels decrease during pregnancy, and this change may cause a noticeable increase in thyroid gland size (approximately 18% change) in 15% of women. However, in most women, the thyroid returns to normal size postpartum.

## Laboratory Screening

*There is insufficient evidence to warrant routine screening of asymptomatic pregnant women for hypothyroidism.*

Testing should be performed in women with a prior history of thyroid disease or symptoms of thyroid disease. Thyroid function is evaluated by measuring thyroid-stimulating hormone (TSH) levels. TSH does not cross the placenta, so this test is an accurate measure of hormone function during pregnancy. In pregnant women suspected of being hyperthyroid or hypothyroid, FT4 and FTI levels should be measured in addition to TSH.

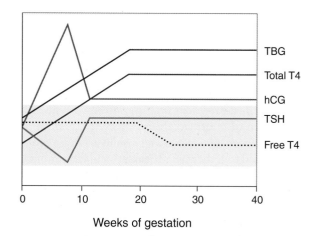

FIGURE 14.3. The pattern of changes in thyroid function and hCG concentration according to gestational age. The shaded area represents the normal range of thyroid-binding globulin, total thyroxine, thyroid-stimulating hormone, and free $T_4$ in the nonpregnant woman. TBG, thyroid-binding globulin; $T_4$, thyroxine; TSH, thyroid-stimulating hormone. (Modified from Brent GA. Maternal thyroid function: interpretation of thyroid function tests in pregnancy. *Clin Obstet Gynecol.* 1997;40(1):3–15.)

## Management of Existing Thyroid Disease in Pregnancy

Hyperthyroidism in pregnancy is treated with thioamides, specifically propylthiouracil (PTU) and methimazole. *The goal of treatment during pregnancy is to maintain the FT4 or FTI in the high normal range using the lowest possible dosage of thioamides to minimize fetal exposure.* Thioamide treatment for Graves disease in pregnancy may suppress fetal and neonatal thyroid function and has also been associated with fetal goiter. Neonatal hypothyroidism is usually transient and does not require treatment.

*Thyroid storm is a medical emergency characterized by an extreme hypermetabolic state. Although rare (it occurs in 1% of pregnancy patients with hyperthyroidism), it carries a high risk of maternal heart failure.* It is often precipitated by infection, surgery, labor, or delivery. Thyroid storm must be diagnosed and treated quickly in order to prevent shock, stupor, and coma (Box 14.1). Treatment of thyroid storm consists of a standard series of drugs, each of which plays a role in suppressing thyroid function. The underlying precipitating event should also be treated. The fetus should be appropriately evaluated with ultrasonography, biophysical profile, or nonstress test, depending on the gestational age.

*Treatment of hypothyroidism in pregnant women is the same as for nonpregnant women and involves administration of levothyroxine at sufficient dosages to normalize TSH levels.* Maternal thyroxine requirements increase in women with hypothyroidism diagnosed before pregnancy. Levothyroxine levels should be adjusted at 4-week intervals until TSH levels are stable. Thereafter, levels should be checked once per trimester.

## Management of Thyroid Disease Diagnosed During and After Pregnancy

Severe nausea and vomiting of pregnancy (**hyperemesis gravidarum**) may cause biochemical hyperthyroidism, in which levels of TSH are undetectable, or FTI levels are elevated, or both. This condition resolves spontaneously by 18 weeks of gestation. Routine measurements of thyroid function are not recommended in patients with hyperemesis gravidarum unless other overt signs of hyperthyroidism are evident.

*Postpartum thyroiditis occurs in 5% of women who have no prior history of thyroid disease.* Postpartum thyroiditis also may occur after pregnancy loss and has a 70% risk of recurrence. Almost half of women with postpartum thyroiditis have hypothyroidism, while the remaining women are evenly split between thyrotoxicosis and thyrotoxicosis followed by hypothyroidism. Postpartum thyrotoxicosis usually resolves on its own without treatment. Of those with hypothyroidism, approximately 40% of women require treatment for extremely high TSH levels or an increasing goiter size. Only 11% of women diagnosed with postpartum hypothyroidism develop permanent hypothyroidism.

## URINARY TRACT DISORDERS

**Urinary tract infections (UTIs)** are common in pregnancy. Approximately 8% of all women (pregnant and nonpregnant) have $>10^5$ colonies of a single bacterial species on a midstream culture. Approximately 25% of the pregnant women in this group develop an acute, symptomatic UTI. Other urinary tract disorders that may complicate pregnancy include urinary calculi, nephrolithiasis, and preexisting renal disease.

## Asymptomatic Bacteriuria and Uncomplicated Urinary Tract Infection

*Compared with nonpregnant women with similar colony counts on urine culture, asymptomatic bacteriuria in pregnancy is more likely to lead to* **cystitis** *and* **pyelonephritis**. The increased incidence of symptomatic infection during pregnancy is thought to be caused by pregnancy-associated urinary stasis and glucosuria. This relative urinary stasis in pregnancy is a result of progesterone-induced decreased ureteral tone and motility, mechanical compression of the ureters at the pelvic brim, and compression of the bladder and ureteral orifices. In addition, the pH of the urine is increased because of increased bicarbonate excretion, which also enhances bacterial growth.

*A urine culture is obtained at the onset of prenatal care and patients with asymptomatic bacteriuria are treated with ampicillin, cephalexin or nitrofurantoin.*

The most common organism identified is *Escherichia coli.* Approximately 25% to 30% of patients not treated for asymptomatic bacteriuria proceed to symptomatic UTI; hence, this treatment should prevent a significant number of symptomatic UTIs in pregnancy. However, 1.5% of patients with initial negative cultures also develop

---

**BOX 14.1**
## Symptoms of Thyroid Storm

Fever
Tachycardia out of proportion to the fever
Altered mental status, including restlessness, nervousness, confusion, and seizures
Vomiting
Diarrhea
Cardiac arrhythmia

symptomatic UTIs during pregnancy. Suppressive antimicrobial therapy is indicated if there are repetitive UTIs during pregnancy or following pyelonephritis during pregnancy. Consideration should be given to postpartum radiographic evaluation of these patients to identify renal parenchymal and urinary-collecting duct abnormalities.

**Acute cystitis** occurs in approximately 1% of pregnancies, and can manifest with dysuria, urinary frequency, and/or urgency. The treatment is the same as for asymptomatic bacteriuria.

## Pyelonephritis

Patients with **pyelonephritis** (inflammation of the renal parenchyma, calices, and pelvis) are acutely ill, with fever, costovertebral tenderness, general malaise, and often dehydration. Approximately 20% of these ill patients demonstrate increased uterine activity and preterm labor, and approximately 10% have positive blood cultures if they are obtained in the acute febrile phase of the disease. *Pyelonephritis occurs in 2% of all pregnant patients and is one of the most common medical complications of pregnancy requiring hospitalization, especially in its context as a major cause of maternal mortality (septic shock).*

After urinalysis and urine culture are obtained, patients are treated with intravenous hydration and antibiotics, commonly a cephalosporin or ampicillin and gentamicin. Uterine contractions may accompany these symptoms, and specific tocolytic therapy may be required if preterm labor ensues. It is known that *E. coli* can produce phospholipase A, which in turn can promote prostaglandin synthesis, resulting in an increase in uterine activity. Fever is also known to induce contractions, so antipyretics are required for a temperature >100.4°F. *Attention must be paid to the patient's response to therapy and her general condition; sepsis occurs in 2% to 3% of patients with pyelonephritis, and adult respiratory distress syndrome can occur.* If improvement does not occur within 48 to 72 hours, urinary tract obstruction or urinary calculus should be considered, along with a reevaluation of antibiotic coverage. Ultrasonography or other imaging study such as computed tomography will sometimes identify a calculus or abscess. The organisms most commonly cultured from the urine of symptomatic pregnant patients are *E. coli* and other gram-negative aerobes. Follow-up can be with either frequent urine cultures and/or empiric antibiotic suppression with an agent such as nitrofurantoin.

Recurrent symptoms or failure to respond to usual therapy suggests another cause for the findings. In these patients, a complete urologic evaluation 6 weeks after pregnancy may be warranted.

## Nephrolithiasis and Urinary Calculi

**Urinary calculi** are identified in approximately 1 in 1500 patients during pregnancy, although pregnancy per se does not promote stone development. Symptoms similar to those of pyelonephritis but without fever suggest urinary calculi. **Microhematuria** is more common with this condition than in uncomplicated UTI. *Renal colic (pain) is a typical symptom in nonpregnant women, but is seen less frequently in pregnant women because of the hormone-induced relaxation of ureteral tone.* Usually, hydration and expectant management, along with straining of urine in search of stones, suffice as management. Occasionally, however, the presence of a stone can lead to infection or complete obstruction, which may require urology consultation and drainage by either ureteral stent or percutaneous nephrostomy.

## Preexisting Renal Disease

During preconception counseling, patients who have preexisting renal disease (chronic renal failure or transplant) should be advised of the significant risks involved in a pregnancy. *Pregnancy outcome is related to the degree of serum creatinine elevation and the presence of hypertension.*

*Overall, pregnancy does not seem to have a negative impact on mild chronic renal diseases.* In general, patients with mild renal impairment (serum creatinine <1.5 mg/dL) have relatively uneventful pregnancies, provided other complications are absent. Patients with moderate renal impairment (serum creatinine 1.5 to 3.0 mg/dL) have a more guarded prognosis with an increased incidence of deterioration of renal function. Patients with severe renal impairment have the worst outcome. In approximately 50% of patients with renal disease, proteinuria is noted. An increase in proteinuria during pregnancy is not, by itself, a serious consequence. Many patients with renal disease also have preexisting or concurrent hypertension. These women are at increased risk for hypertensive complications of pregnancy.

*In addition to hypertension, there is an increased incidence of intrauterine growth restriction in patients with chronic renal disease.* Serial assessments of fetal well-being and growth are frequently performed. Pregnancy following renal transplantation is generally associated with a good prognosis if at least 2 years have elapsed since the transplant was performed, and thorough renal assessment reveals no evidence of active disease or rejection. Drug therapy should be minimal.

## CARDIAC DISEASE

With earlier diagnoses and more effective treatments, more women with congenital and acquired heart disease reach adulthood and may become pregnant. Patients with rheumatic heart disease (caused by untreated or delayed treatment of group A–hemolytic streptococcal [GAS] tonsillopharyngitis) and acquired infectious valvular heart disease (often associated with drug use) comprise only 50%

of pregnant cardiac patients. The remainder consists of other cardiac conditions that traditionally have been less commonly seen in pregnancy. *Because pregnancy is itself associated with an increase in cardiac output of 40%, the risks to mother and fetus are often profound for women with pre-existing cardiac disease.* Ideally, cardiac patients should have preconceptional care directed at maximizing cardiac function. They should also be counseled about the risks their particular heart disease poses in pregnancy.

## Classification of Heart Diseases in Pregnancy

The classification of heart disease by the New York Heart Association is useful to evaluate all types of cardiac patients with respect to pregnancy (Table 14.2). It is a functional classification and is independent of the type of heart disease. Patients with septal defects, patent ductus arteriosus, and mild mitral and aortic valvular disorders often are in classes I or II and tend to do well throughout pregnancy. *Primary pulmonary hypertension, uncorrected tetralogy of Fallot, Eisenmenger syndrome, Marfan syndrome with significant aortic root dilation, and certain other conditions are associated with a much worse prognosis (frequently death) through the course of pregnancy. For this reason, patients with such disorders are strongly advised not to become pregnant.*

## Management

General management of the pregnant cardiac patient consists of avoiding conditions that add additional stress to the workload of the heart beyond that already imposed by pregnancy, including prevention and/or correction of anemia, prompt recognition and treatment of any infections, a decrease in physical activity and strenuous work, and proper weight gain. Adequate rest is essential. For patients with class I or II heart disease, increased rest at home is advised; and in cases of higher class levels, hospitalization and treatment of cardiac failure may be required. Coordinated management between obstetrician, cardiologist, and anesthesiologist is especially important for patients with significant cardiac dysfunction.

The fetuses of patients with functionally significant cardiac disease are at increased risk for low birth weight and prematurity. *A patient with congenital heart disease is 1% to 5% more likely to have a fetus with congenital heart disease than is someone without this condition; antepartum fetal cardiac assessment using ultrasound is recommended.*

The antepartum management of pregnant cardiac patients includes serial evaluation of maternal cardiac status as well as fetal well-being and growth. Anticoagulation, antibiotic prophylaxis for subacute bacterial endocarditis, invasive cardiac monitoring, and even surgical correction of certain cardiac lesions during pregnancy can all be accomplished if necessary. The intrapartum and postpartum management of pregnant cardiac patients includes consideration of the increased stress of delivery and postpartum physiologic adjustment. Labor in the lateral position to facilitate cardiac function is often desirable. Every attempt is made to facilitate vaginal delivery because of the increased cardiac stress of cesarean section. Because cardiac output increases by 40% to 50% during the second stage of labor, shortening this stage by the use of forceps or vacuum extractor is often advisable. Epidural anesthesia to reduce the stress of labor is also recommended. Even with patients who are stable at the time of delivery, cardiac output increases in the postpartum period because of the additional 500 mL added to the maternal blood volume as the uterus contracts. Indeed, most obstetric patients who die with cardiac disease do so following delivery.

**Rheumatic heart disease** remains a common cardiac disease in pregnancy. *As the severity of the associated valvular lesion increases, the risk for thromboembolic disease, subacute bacterial endocarditis, cardiac failure, and pulmonary edema increases. A high rate of fetal loss also occurs in women with rheumatic heart disease.* Approximately 90% of these patients have mitral stenosis, whose associated mechanical obstruction worsens as cardiac output increases during pregnancy. Women with mitral stenosis associated with atrial fibrillation have an especially high risk of developing congestive heart failure.

**Maternal cardiac arrhythmias** are occasionally encountered during pregnancy. *Paroxysmal atrial tachycardia*

| TABLE 14.2 | New York Heart Association Functional Classification of Heart Disease |
|---|---|
| **Class** | **Description** |
| I | No cardiac decompensation |
| II | No symptoms of cardiac decompensation at rest; minor limitations of physical activity |
| III | No symptoms of cardiac decompensation at rest; marked limitations of physical activity |
| IV | Symptoms of cardiac decompensation at rest; increased discomfort with any physical activity |

is the most commonly encountered maternal arrhythmia and is usually associated with overly strenuous exercise. Underlying cardiac disease such as mitral stenosis should be suspected when atrial fibrillation and flutter are encountered.

**Peripartum cardiomyopathy** is an unusual but especially severe cardiac condition identified in the last month of pregnancy or the first 6 months following delivery. It is difficult to distinguish from other cardiomyopathies (e.g., myocarditis) except for its association with pregnancy. In many cases, no apparent cause can be determined. *Treatment is generally unchanged from cardiac failure unassociated with pregnancy, except that the use of angiotensin-converting enzyme inhibitors is avoided if the patient is pregnant.* Management includes bed rest, digoxin, diuretics, and, in some cases, anticoagulation. The mortality rate is high and is related to cardiac size 6 to 12 months later. If cardiac size returns to normal, prognosis is improved, although it remains guarded. Sterilization counseling is warranted for patients with cardiomyopathy.

## ASTHMA

**Asthma** is a restrictive-airways disease that is encountered in approximately 4% to 8% of pregnant patients. *The effects of pregnancy on asthma are variable—in general, about one third of patients worsen, one third improve, and the remaining one third are unchanged.* Women with mild or moderate asthma usually have excellent maternal and fetal outcomes (Table 14.3). However, suboptimal control of asthma during pregnancy may be associated with increased maternal or fetal risk. Decreased $FEV_1$ (forced expiratory volume in the first second of expiration) is associated with increased risk of low birth weight and prematurity.

> *Pregnant patients with asthma, even those with mild or well-controlled disease, should be monitored with PEFR or $FEV_1$ testing as well as by close symptom observation.*

Routine evaluation of pulmonary function in pregnant women with persistent asthma is recommended. Serial ultrasound examinations and antenatal fetal testing should be considered for women who have moderate or severe asthma during pregnancy beginning at 32 weeks of gestation or for women recovering from a severe asthma exacerbation

*The ultimate goal of asthma therapy in pregnancy is maintaining adequate oxygenation of the fetus by preventing hypoxic episodes in the mother.* Inhaled corticosteroid therapy, particularly budesonide, is the first-line controller treatment for persistent asthma during pregnancy. Inhaled albuterol is the recommended rescue therapy. *In the **step-care therapeutic approach**, the number and dosage of medications are increased with increasing asthma severity.* Once control of symptoms is achieved, a "step-down" approach is usually implemented in the nonpregnant patient. In pregnant patients, it may be prudent to postpone a reduction in a therapy that is effectively controlling a patient's asthma until after the birth. Patients should be instructed to identify and control or avoid factors, such as allergens and irritants, particular tobacco smoke.

Management of a severely asthmatic pregnant patient is similar to that of a nonpregnant patient. Evaluation consists of measurement of pulmonary function and arterial blood gases. Treatment may include administration of supplemental oxygen, treatment with nebulized β-agonists, corticosteroids (oral or intravenous), or intubation. *Women*

**TABLE 14.3    Classification of Asthma Severity and Control in Pregnant Patients**

| Asthma Severity* (Control†) | Symptom Frequency | Nighttime Awakening | Interference with Normal Activity | FEV₁ or Peak Flow (predicted percentage of personal best) |
|---|---|---|---|---|
| Intermittent (well controlled) | 2 days per week or less | Twice per month or less | None | More than 80% |
| Mild persistent (not well controlled) | More than 2 days per week, but not daily | More than twice per month | Minor limitation | More than 80% |
| Moderate persistent (not well controlled) | Daily symptoms | More than once per week | Some limitation | 60–80% |
| Severe persistent (very poorly controlled) | Throughout the day | Four times per week or more | Extremely limited | Less than 60% |

*Assess severity for patients who are not taking long-term-control medications.
†Assess control in patients taking long-term control medications to determine whether step-up therapy, step-down therapy, or no change in therapy is warranted.
American College of Obstetricians and Gynecologists. Asthma in pregnancy. ACOG Practice Bulletin No. 90. *Obstet Gynecol.* 2008;111(2):457–464.

*who are currently receiving or recently have taken systemic corticosteroids should receive intravenous administration of corticosteroids during labor and for 24 hours after delivery to prevent adrenal crisis.*

## SURGICAL CONDITIONS IN PREGNANCY

Patients who are pregnant can experience the same surgical conditions as those who are not pregnant, such as appendicitis, cholelithiasis, and bowel injury. In early gestation, ectopic pregnancy and torsion of the adnexa should be considered. Later in pregnancy, placental abruption and uterine rupture can cause acute abdominal signs and symptoms.

### Considerations for Pregnant Patients

*Surgical treatment of a pregnant woman should take into consideration both maternal and fetal health needs.* Radiographic or other studies should not be avoided just because the patient is pregnant, though precautions should be used. For procedures such as radiographs of the chest, an abdominal shield may be used to avoid unnecessary exposure to the fetus. Exposure to low doses of radiation is safe for the fetus when considered against failure to treat or to diagnose a condition requiring surgery.

*In the perioperative period, fetal heart tones should be monitored to the extent possible, consistent with the stage of gestation and need for intervention, usually by electronic fetal monitoring.*

The completely supine position should be avoided, if possible. Instead the patient should be placed in a decubitus lateral tilt to prevent the supine hypotensive syndrome, in which pressure on the vena cava reduces venous return to the heart, causing a drop in blood pressure and uterine blood flow. Oxygen administration may be helpful. In general, clinicians caring for these patients should be constantly aware of both maternal and fetal considerations. For example, the residual lung volume is diminished in pregnancy, which provides less reserve for respiratory function. Delayed gastric emptying makes aspiration of stomach contents during a surgical procedure more likely.

### Appendicitis in Pregnancy

**Appendicitis** is a common surgical problem in reproductive-aged women, and therefore a common surgical problem in pregnancy. Similar symptoms of the disease occur in pregnancy; of note, leukocytosis associated with appendicitis may be masked with the normal leukocytosis of pregnancy.

The appendix may be displaced upward as pregnancy advances, and can cause a shift in the location of abdominal pain associated with appendicitis, though pain is still most commonly located in the right lower quadrant. *When appendicitis is diagnosed and treated early (before appendiceal rupture and generalized peritonitis), fetal and maternal outcomes are good.* Surgical management has traditionally been with open appendectomy; however, laparoscopy is increasingly being utilized for management of appendicitis in pregnancy.

### Cholelithiasis in Pregnancy

Reproductive-aged women frequently have **gallstones.** *Cholelithiasis can be exacerbated during pregnancy due to hormonal effects that slow gallbladder emptying and cause an increase in residual gallbladder volume.* Asymptomatic cholelithiasis should be managed expectantly. If the patient develops biliary colic, attempts should be made to conservatively treat the patient with hydration, pain control, dietary restriction, and possible nasogastric tube. *However, if cholecystitis occurs with common bile duct obstruction, ascending cholangitis, pancreatitis, or acute abdomen, immediate surgical management is required.* Maternal and fetal outcomes tend to be excellent if surgical removal is undertaken before these serious consequences are allowed to worsen. As with appendicitis, traditional surgical management has been open cholecystectomy; however, in recent years, more evidence supports the safe use of laparoscopic cholecystectomy in pregnancy.

### Adnexal Masses in Pregnancy

Abnormal **ovarian** or **adnexal masses** can occur in pregnancy. Often, they are discovered during routine ultrasound examination of the fetus. Most of these masses are benign and spontaneously resolve during pregnancy. *For these reasons, expectant management is often advocated for adnexal masses in pregnancy.* Approximately 4% to 7% of persistent complex masses are malignant. With large masses, there is an increased risk of ovarian torsion or cyst rupture. In general, surgical management is best performed in the second trimester

## TRAUMA IN PREGNANCY

Maternal trauma is one of the leading causes of morbidity and mortality in pregnancy. *The most common cause of trauma in pregnancy is motor vehicle accidents. The second most common cause is physical violence against women, most frequently partner violence.* Traumatic injury can result in maternal injury and death, as well as placental abruption, uterine rupture, fetal–maternal hemorrhage, premature rupture of membranes, or preterm labor. In addition to the above conditions, which can compromise fetal well-being, direct fetal injury is also possible.

*The primary goal for evaluation of a pregnant trauma patient is maternal stabilization.* Management is essentially the same as for the nonpregnant patient. Vital signs should be assessed and the patient stabilized, followed by obstetric assessment. If the gestational age is 20 weeks or beyond, the patient should be placed in a decubitus lateral tilt position. If this is not feasible (for example due to cervical spine stabilization), manual displacement of the uterus off of midline will promote adequate maternal venous return. Fetal assessment includes verification of fetal heart tones with Doppler, followed by electronic fetal monitoring once the secondary survey is complete. Fetal ultrasound is also helpful for identifying location of placenta, fetal well-being, amniotic fluid volume, and estimated gestational age.

*After a minor trauma, electronic fetal monitoring (including tocometry) is recommended from 2 to 6 hours* (there are no large studies available to guide a consensus on the appropriate length of time for monitoring to occur). If, during that interval, there are any signs of uterine tenderness, irritability or contractions, vaginal bleeding, rupture of membranes, or non-reassuring fetal status, continued monitoring for at least 24 hours is advocated. Any moderate or major trauma necessitates at least 24 hours of continuous fetal monitoring.

**Feto-maternal hemorrhage** is another complication of maternal trauma, and determination of Rh status is an important part of the management. The extent of feto-maternal hemorrhage can be determined using one of several tests (e.g., the Kleihauer-Betke test). Most often a regular dose of Rh immunoglobulin is protective for all Rh-negative mothers.

If a pregnant woman undergoes cardiopulmonary arrest, attempts at resuscitation should begin immediately. *Emergent cesarean delivery should be considered after 4 minutes of failed resuscitation efforts if the patient is in the third trimester of pregnancy.* Maternal resuscitation is made easier once the fetus has been delivered. Fetal survival is not likely if maternal vital signs have been absent for more than 15 to 20 minutes.

## SUGGESTED READINGS

American College of Obstetricians and Gynecologists. Anemia in pregnancy. ACOG Practice Bulletin No. 95. *Obstet Gynecol.* 2008;112(1):201–207.

American College of Obstetricians and Gynecologists. Asthma in pregnancy. ACOG Practice Bulletin No. 90. *Obstet Gynecol.* 2008; 111(2):457–464.

American College of Obstetricians and Gynecologists. Gestational diabetes. ACOG Practice Bulletin No. 30. *Obstet Gynecol.* 2001; 98(2):525–538.

American College of Obstetricians and Gynecologists. Hemoglobinopathies in pregnancy. ACOG Practice Bulletin No. 78. *Obstet Gynecol.* 2007;109(1):229–237.

American College of Obstetricians and Gynecologists. Management of adnexal masses. ACOG Practice Bulletin No. 83. *Obstet Gynecol.* 2007;110(1):201–214.

American College of Obstetricians and Gynecologists. *Obstetric Aspects of Trauma Management.* Washington, DC: American College of Obstetricians and Gynecologists; 1998. ACOG Educational Bulletin No. 251.

American College of Obstetricians and Gynecologists. Pregestational diabetes mellitus. ACOG Practice Bulletin No. 60. *Obstet Gynecol.* 2005;105(3):675–685.

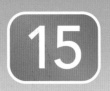
# Infectious Diseases in Pregnancy

Students should be able to recognize each of the following infectious diseases during pregnancy, discuss the impact of pregnancy on the condition and of the condition on the pregnancy (mother and fetus), and describe the initial management during pregnancy: group B streptococcus; herpes; rubella; hepatitis; human immunodeficiency virus, human papillomavirus, and other sexually transmitted infections; cytomegalovirus; toxoplasmosis; and varicella and parvovirus.

S creening for and preventing infectious disease is an integral part of routine prenatal care. Many of these agents can have devastating outcomes for mother, infant, or both. An understanding of the disease course in pregnancy, the maternal and fetal sequelae, and, most importantly, prevention and therapy are key to management of the pregnant patient and her fetus. Screening recommendations for common sexually transmitted diseases (STDs) in pregnancy are listed in Table 15.1. Infections involving specific organ systems and not associated with significant risk for fetal infection (i.e., urinary tract infections) are covered elsewhere (see Chapter 15, Medical and Surgical Complications in Pregnancy).

## GROUP B STREPTOCOCCUS

**Group B streptococcus (GBS)** (or *Streptococcus agalactiae*) is an important cause of perinatal infections. Asymptomatic lower genital tract colonization occurs in up to 30% of pregnant women, but cultures may be positive only intermittently, even in the same patient. Approximately 50% of infants exposed to the organism in the lower genital tract will become colonized. For most of these infants, such colonization is of no consequence, but without treatment, GBS sepsis occurs in approximately 0.2 infants per 1000 live births annually.

There are two manifestations of clinical infection of the newborn, termed early-onset and late-onset, occurring at roughly equal frequency. **Early-onset** infection manifests as septicemia and septic shock, pneumonia, or meningitis and occurs during the first week of life. Early-onset infection is much more common in preterm infants than in term infants. **Late-onset** infection occurs later, after delivery, and has been reported beyond 3 months (**late-late onset infection**) in very low–birth-weight preterm neonates. GBS disease in newborns may occur as a result of vertical transmission or nosocomial or community-acquired infection.

With prevention strategies, current rates of early-onset GBS disease of the newborn have decreased to approximately 0.3 per 1000 live births. Currently, the Centers for Disease Control and Prevention (CDC) and the American College of Obstetricians and Gynecologists (ACOG) recommend universal screening for GBS between 35 to 37 weeks of gestation.

*All women who are GBS positive by rectovaginal culture should receive antibiotic prophylaxis in labor or with rupture of membranes.*

If a patient's culture status is unknown, then prophylaxis should be given if any of the following conditions exists:

• Preterm labor (less than 37 weeks of gestation)
• Preterm premature rupture of membranes (PROM) (less than 37 weeks of gestation)

| TABLE 15.1 | Screening Recommendations for Sexually Transmitted Diseases in Pregnancy |
|---|---|
| **First prenatal visit** | |
| HIV | All women (CDC/ACOG) |
| Syphilis | All women (CDC/ACOG) |
| Hepatitis B | All women (CDC/ACOG) |
| Hepatitis C | High risk (CDC/ACOG) |
| HSV | Inquire about history, no routine screening (CDC/ACOG) |
| Chlamydia | All women (CDC/ACOG) |
| Gonorrhea | High risk (CDC/ACOG) |
| **Third trimester** | |
| HIV | High risk or if previously undocumented (CDC/ACOG) |
| Syphilis | High risk (CDC/ACOG) |
| Chlamydia | High risk (CDC/ACOG) |
| Gonorrhea | High risk (CDC/ACOG) |
| Group B Strep | All women at 35–37 weeks gestation (CDC/ACOG) |
| **Delivery/postpartum stay** | |
| HIV | High risk or if previously undocumented (CDC/ACOG) |
| Syphilis | High risk or if previously undocumented (CDC) All women (ACOG) |
| Hepatitis B | High risk or if previously undocumented (CDC/ACOG) |
| HSV | With prior history of genital HSV or new diagnosis in pregnancy, inquire about symptoms and perform careful inspection of lower genital tract and perineum before delivery (ACOG) |

Note: state or local laws may supersede these recommendations.
ACOG = American College of Obstetricians and Gynecologists; CDC = Centers for Disease Control and Prevention; HIV = human immunodeficiency virus; HSV = herpes simplex virus.

- Rupture of membranes 18 hours or longer
- Maternal fever during labor (at or above 38°C [100.4°F])

Women with GBS bacteriuria during their current pregnancy, or women who have previously given birth to an infant with early-onset GBS disease also are candidates for intrapartum antibiotic prophylaxis. When culture results are not available, intrapartum prophylaxis should be offered only on the basis of the presence of intrapartum risk factors for early-onset GMS disease. CDC Guidelines include recommended medication regimens.

In the mother, significant postpartum fever may indicate postpartum endometritis, sepsis, and, rarely, meningitis, which may be caused by infection with GBS. With endometritis, the onset is often sudden and within 24 hours of delivery. Significant fever and tachycardia are typically present; sepsis may follow.

## HERPES

**Herpes simplex virus (HSV)** is a double-stranded DNA virus that can be differentiated into HSV type 1 (HSV-1)

and HSV type 2 (HSV-2). Herpes simplex virus type 1 is the primary etiologic agent of herpes labialis, gingivostomatitis, and keratoconjunctivitis. Most genital infections with HSV are caused by HSV-2, but genital HSV-1 infections are becoming increasingly common, particularly among adolescent and young women. Up to 80% of new genital infections among women may be due to HSV-1, with the highest rates occurring in adolescents and young adults. Herpes infections are categorized as follows:

- **Primary** occurs in a woman with no evidence of prior HSV infection (seronegative to both HSV-1 and HSV-2).
- **Nonprimary first episode** occurs in a woman with a history of heterologous infection (first HSV-2 infection with a prior HSV-1 infection).
- **Recurrent** disease occurs in a woman with clinical or serologic evidence of prior genital herpes (of the same serotype).

The primary form poses the greatest risk to the fetus. The fetus/neonate is infected either from ascending infection following spontaneous rupture of membranes, or from passage through an infected lower genital tract at delivery. *With a primary infection at the time of delivery, the risk of neonatal infection approaches 50%; it is far lower (approximately 3%) with recurrent infection, as the size of the inoculum is much decreased.* In utero fetal infection can occur, although this is much less common. Most infants with localized herpes infection ultimately do well; as a rule, infants with disseminated infection do very poorly.

The diagnosis of HSV infection is suspected when clinical examination shows the characteristic tender vesicles with ulceration followed by crusting (Figure 15.1). Confirmation is by identification of the virus in cell culture, with most positive results reported within 72 hours. Polymerase chain reaction (PCR) testing is commercially available and is more sensitive than culture. Serologic testing for HSV-1 and HSV-2 immunoglobulin is also available and a helpful ancillary test because cultures of crusted or healing lesions can often be negative. Type-specific serologic testing that accurately distinguishes between anti-HSV-1 and -2 immunoglobulin is recommended.

All pregnant women should be asked about a history of HSV infection at their initial prenatal visit. *If infection with herpes virus is suspected during the course of pregnancy in a woman with undocumented history of HSV, a culture from a lesion should be obtained to confirm the diagnosis.* In such patients, or any patient with a history of herpes virus infection, careful inspection of the lower genital tract is important at the

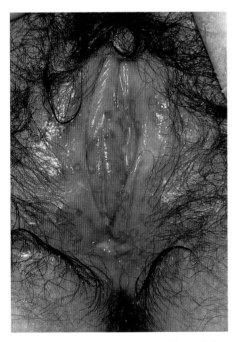

FIGURE 15.1. Herpes virus infection. Although herpes virus infection is primarily a blistering disease, on thin, moist skin, blisters quickly shear off to produce round, coalescing erosions. (Edwards L. *Genital Dermatology Atlas.* Philadelphia, PA: Lippincott Williams & Wilkins; 2004:90).

onset of labor or when rupture of membranes occurs. If no lesions are identified, vaginal delivery is deemed safe.

*Cesarean delivery is recommended if herpes lesions are identified on the cervix, in the vagina, or on the vulva at the time of labor or if spontaneous rupture of membranes occurs. This is true whether or not the lesions are associated with primary or recurrent infection due to the severity of neonatal disease.*

Acyclovir and related compounds are safe in pregnancy and can be used if symptoms are severe. Additionally, in patients with recurrent HSV, these medications should be offered for suppression of outbreaks starting at 36 weeks of gestation to reduce the risk of viral shedding and cesarean delivery due to active lesions. Routine antepartum genital HSV cultures in asymptomatic women are not recommended, as these tests do not predict viral shedding at delivery. *Routine type-specific serologic screening for HSV is not currently recommended.* However, serologic screening may be considered in certain populations to identify women who may benefit from suppressive therapy or preventive measures.

## RUBELLA

**Rubella** (German, or 3-day, measles) is an RNA virus with important perinatal impact if infection occurs during pregnancy. Widespread immunization programs in the last 30 years have prevented periodic epidemics of rubella, but some women of reproductive age lack immunity to this virus and are therefore susceptible to infection. Once infection occurs, immunity is life-long. A history of prior infection is an unreliable indicator of immunity.

If a woman develops rubella infection in the first trimester of pregnancy, there is an increased risk of both spontaneous abortion and congenital rubella syndrome. Although most infants with congenital rubella appear normal at birth, many subsequently develop signs of infection. Common defects associated with the syndrome include congenital heart disease (e.g., patent ductus arteriosus), mental retardation, deafness, and cataracts. The risk of congenital rubella is related to the gestational age at the time of infection; it is highest in the first month of pregnancy and decreases with increasing gestational age. Primary infection can be diagnosed by serologic testing for IgM and IgG antibodies during the acute and convalescent stages of infection.

*Because of the serious fetal implications, prenatal screening for IgG rubella antibody is routine. All pregnant women should be screened, unless they are known to be immune based on previous serologic testing.* Young women should be vaccinated when they are not pregnant, if they are susceptible. The vaccine uses a live attenuated rubella virus that induces antibodies in virtually all women who have been vaccinated.

Because of this, pregnant women should not be vaccinated. It is recommended that pregnancy be delayed 1 month following immunization, although congenital rubella syndrome following vaccination during an undiagnosed pregnancy has not been reported. In women whose prenatal screen identifies a lack of rubella antibody, vaccination postpartum at the time of hospital discharge is recommended. Such management poses no risk to the newborn or other children; breastfeeding is not contraindicated.

If rubella is diagnosed in a pregnant woman, the patient should be advised of the risk of fetal infection and counseled regarding options for continuing the pregnancy.

> *Because there is no effective treatment for a pregnant patient infected with rubella, patients who do not have immunity are advised to avoid potential exposure.*

Although immune globulin may be given to an infected woman, it does not prevent fetal infection. The absence of clinical signs in a woman who has received immune globulin does not guarantee that infection of the fetus has been prevented.

## HEPATITIS

Viral hepatitis is one of the most common and potentially serious infections that can occur in pregnant women. Six forms of viral hepatitis have now been identified, two of which, hepatitis A and hepatitis B, can be prevented effectively through vaccination.

### Hepatitis A

**Hepatitis A virus** (HAV) is transmitted from person to person primarily through fecal–oral contamination. Good hygiene and proper sanitation are important to prevent infection. However, vaccination is the most effective means of preventing transmission. The hepatitis A vaccine is available as both a single-antigen vaccine and as a combination vaccine (containing both HAV and HBV antigens). Prior to vaccine availability, HAV accounted for one-third of cases of acute hepatitis in the United States. HAV infection does not progress to chronic infection. Diagnosis is confirmed by demonstration of anti-HAV IgM antibodies. HAV infection has no specific effects on pregnancy or the fetus. *Vaccination safety during pregnancy has not been established, but the risk to the developing fetus is minimal because the vaccine contains inactivated purified viral proteins.* Vaccination is recommended for individuals who are intravenous (IV) drug users, who have certain medical disorders (chronic liver disease or receiving clotting factor concentrates), are employed in specific occupations (e.g., working in primate labs or research labs), and who travel to countries with endemic HAV infection. *HAV immune globulin is effective for both pre- and post-exposure prophylaxis and can be used during pregnancy.*

### Hepatitis B

**Hepatitis B virus** (HBV) infection is more serious than HAV infection regardless of pregnancy status. HBV is transmitted by the parenteral route and through sexual contact. Ten to fifteen percent of infected adults develop chronic infection and, of those, some will become carriers. *Testing for hepatitis B surface antigen (HBsAg) during pregnancy is routine, as about half of pregnant women infected lack traditional high-risk factors.* Vertical transmission of hepatitis occurs to a significant but variable extent and is related to the presence or absence of maternal HBeAg: if the patient is positive for the "e" antigen, indicating a high viral load and active viral replication, her fetus has 70% to 90% risk of becoming infected; and most of such infants will become chronic carriers. *The risk of fetal infection is higher if maternal infection occurs in the third trimester.* Neonatal infection can also occur via breast milk.

> *Women who are HBsAg negative with risk factors for HBV infection should be offered vaccination during pregnancy.*

Patients who have been exposed to HBV should be treated as soon as possible with hepatitis B immune globulin (HBIG) and begin the vaccination series. All infants now receive vaccination against hepatitis B, with the initial injection given between 2 days and 2 months of delivery. *Infants of mothers who are HBsAg positive should receive the vaccine and HBIG within 12 hours of birth.* Breastfeeding is not contraindicated in women who are chronic carriers if their infants have received both the vaccination and HBIG within 12 hours of delivery.

### Hepatitis C

**Hepatitis C virus** (HCV) infection is a growing problem in the United States and has obstetric implications. Similar to HBV in transmission (sexual, parenteral, vertical), HCV infection is often asymptomatic. Diagnosis is made by serologic evidence of anti-HCV IgG. However, antibodies may not be detectable until up to 10 weeks after onset of clinical illness. PCR identification of HCV RNA may be a useful adjunct to diagnosis in early and chronic infection. The presence of anti-HCV antibody does not confer immunity or prevent transmission of infection. Fifty percent of infected individuals go on to have chronic infection.

Screening for evidence of HCV infection is not routine. *However, the CDC recommends routine screening for certain groups* (Box 15.1). Vertical transmission occurs in 2% to 12% of cases, with the risk of fetal infection directly related to the quantity of hepatitis C RNA virus in maternal blood. Vertical transmission is rare with an undetectable hepatitis C RNA viral load. Maternal co-infection with **human immunodeficiency virus** (HIV) is also associated with a higher risk of vertical transmission of HCV. Other risk factors for fetal infection include prolonged rupture of membranes in labor and use of invasive fetal monitoring. *Currently, there are no preventive measures known to reduce the risk of mother-to-child transmission; cesarean delivery has not been consistently associated with a decreased rate of vertical transmission and should be performed for usual obstetric indications in HCV-infected women.* Breastfeeding is not contraindicated in women with HCV. Newer therapies for HCV infection that clear detectable virus in the blood and normalize transaminase levels are promising in nonpregnant adults. Immune globulin does not contain antibodies to HCV and has no role in postexposure prophylaxis.

## Hepatitis D and E

**Hepatitis D virus** (HDV) is an incomplete viral particle that can only cause infection in the presence of HBV. Transmission of HDV is through the parenteral route; chronic infection can occur, resulting in severe disease in 70% to 80% of chronically infected individuals and mortality rates as high as 25%. *Vertical transmission has been documented but is uncommon.* Diagnosis is made by identification of HDV antigen and anti-HDV IgM in acute disease; IgG antibodies develop, but are not protective. No vaccine is currently available. Measures to prevent HBV infection are effective in the prevention of HDV transmission.

**Hepatitis E virus** (HEV) infection is a waterborne disease and is uncommon in the United States. *The disease is typically self-limited, but has been associated with higher rates of fulminant hepatitis E and mortality in pregnant women, which can be as high as 20% after infection in the third trimester.* Co-infection with HIV results in severe disease and high mortality in pregnancy. Diagnosis is made by serologic testing for HEV-specific antibodies in women with travel exposure. The risk of vertical transmission is very low, but cases have been reported. No vaccine is currently available.

## HIV/AIDS SYNDROME

Worldwide, women account for nearly 50% of those infected with HIV. The CDC estimates that 27% of those living with acquired immune deficiency syndrome (AIDS) in the United States are women. Of these women, 71% were exposed through heterosexual contact and 27% through injection drug use. One percent of those living with AIDS are children under the age of 13, most of whom acquired the infection perinatally.

*The usual estimated latency period from untreated HIV to AIDS is about 11 years.* HIV infection becomes AIDS as the helper (CD4$^+$) lymphocyte count decreases and the host becomes more susceptible to other types of infections. With the availability of increasingly effective antiretroviral drugs, life span and quality of life have improved dramatically.

## Pathophysiology

HIV is a single-stranded, RNA, enveloped human retrovirus that has the ability to become incorporated into the cellular DNA of CD4$^+$ cells such as lymphocytes, monocytes, and some neural cells. Once infected, seroconversion usually occurs within 2 to 8 weeks, but it may take up to 3 months and in rare cases, 6 months. HIV infection appears to have no direct effect on pregnancy course or outcome. Likewise, pregnancy does not seem to affect the course of HIV. *Both HIV and pregnancy may affect the natural history, presentation, treatment, or significance of certain infections, and these, in turn, may be associated with pregnancy complications or perinatal infection.* These infections include vulvovaginal candidiasis, bacterial vaginosis, genital herpes simplex, human papillomavirus (HPV), syphilis, cytomegalovirus (CMV), toxoplasmosis, and hepatitis B and C. All women demonstrate a decline in absolute CD4$^+$ cell counts in pregnancy, which is thought to be secondary to hemodilution. On the other hand, the percentage of CD4$^+$ cells remains relatively stable. *Therefore, percentage, rather than absolute number, of CD4$^+$ cells may be a more accurate measure of immune function for HIV-infected women.*

The baseline rate of perinatal HIV transmission without prophylactic therapy is approximately 25%, and is generally related to higher viral loads and lower CD4$^+$ counts. *With zidovudine (ZDV) monotherapy, perinatal transmission is reduced to ~8%. Currently, with combination antiretroviral therapy and an undetectable viral load, perinatal transmission is reduced to 1% to 2%.* There is evidence that transmission can occur antepartum, intrapartum, or postpartum through breastfeeding; however, 66% to 75% of transmission appears to occur during or close to the intrapartum period, particularly in non-breastfeeding populations.

## Screening and Testing

Initial screening consists of **enzyme-linked immuno-sorbent assay (ELISA),** which is based on an antigen–antibody reaction. In 99% of cases, antibodies to HIV become detectable by 3 months after infection. If results of ELISA are positive, a **Western blot** test, which identifies antibodies to specific portions of the virus, is performed to confirm the diagnosis. A serologic test is reported as positive only if both the ELISA and the Western blot analyses are positive; this testing has a sensitivity and specificity of over 99%.

Universal, voluntary HIV screening for pregnant women is standard and should be part of the standard prenatal laboratory tests, unless a patient states that she does not want HIV testing. This "opt-out" approach is recommended by both ACOG and the CDC; however, state and local laws to the contrary may supersede these recommendations.

*Refusal of testing should be documented.*

Additionally, third-trimester repeat screening is recommended for at-risk populations (including women with an STD or women who use illicit drugs, exchange sex for money or drugs, have multiple sexual partners in pregnancy, or who have signs or symptoms suggesting acute HIV during pregnancy), as well as for women who declined testing in the first trimester or have undocumented HIV status at the time of labor and delivery.

**Rapid HIV testing** is a valuable alternative to the conventional testing previously discussed. Results can be available *within hours* after the blood sample is obtained, and thus is especially useful when a patient of unknown HIV status presents in labor.

*A positive rapid HIV test must be confirmed by Western blot analysis or immunofluorescence assay before the woman is deemed HIV positive; however, immediate antiretroviral treatment should be started as soon as a rapid HIV-positive result is noted in a laboring patient.*

## Management

Management involves antiretroviral therapy and taking precautions during delivery to avoid transmission.

*Antiretroviral therapy in pregnancy is a key component to reduction of perinatal transmission to as low as 1% to 2%.*

Effective combination antiretroviral therapy should be offered to all HIV-infected pregnant women, and is admin-

istered in the antepartum and intrapartum period as well as to the neonate. Other than maternal disease status and viral load, risks factors for increased vertical transmission of HIV include chorioamnionitis, prolonged rupture of membranes, invasive fetal monitoring, and mode of delivery.

Awareness of maternal HIV status can help guide management of labor and delivery to minimize risk of transmission to the fetus. The likelihood of transmission increases linearly with increasing duration of rupture of membranes. The use of fetal scalp electrodes or fetal scalp sampling increases exposure of the fetus to maternal blood and genital secretions, and may increase the risk of vertical transmission, depending on the serum and genital HIV viral load. These techniques should be avoided. Use of episiotomy or vacuum extraction or forceps may potentially increase risk of transmission by increasing exposure to maternal blood and genital secretions. However, these techniques may help shorten duration of labor or rupture of membranes with vaginal delivery and, thus, may decrease the likelihood of transmission. Finally, cesarean delivery performed before the onset of labor and rupture of membranes significantly reduces the risk of perinatal HIV transmission. Planned cesarean delivery at 38 weeks of gestation to prevent perinatal transmission of HIV is recommended for women who have a viral load >1000 copies/mL.

*Breastfeeding plays a significant role in perinatal HIV transmission;* it is estimated to have accounted for up to 50% of newly infected children globally. Breastfeeding in the setting of established maternal infection has a significant additional risk of transmission.

*When safe alternatives are available, breastfeeding should be avoided in HIV infection.*

The field of HIV care and management is rapidly advancing and care of HIV-infected pregnant women should be coordinated with a health care provider who regularly cares for HIV-infected women. Comprehensive information is also provided and regularly updated on the U.S. Department of Health and Human Resources Web site AIDS*info,* at www.aidsinfo.nih.gov, under "perinatal treatment guidelines."

## HUMAN PAPILLOMAVIRUS

More than one-third of sexually active women have been exposed to at least one type of the **human papillomavirus (HPV).** Genital wart lesions (**condyloma acuminata**) often increase in size and area during pregnancy due to relative immune suppression. If extensive, cesarean delivery may be necessary to avoid excessive trauma to the lower genital tract. In pregnancy, cryotherapy, laser therapy, and trichloroacetic acid may be used to treat genital HPV lesions. *Podophyllin, 5-fluorouracil, and interferon are not rec-*

*ommended, as they may be toxic to the fetus.* Because there are limited data regarding imiquimod use in pregnancy, it is generally avoided. Treatment of genital HPV lesions is often delayed until after pregnancy, as spontaneous resolution may occur. Transmission of HPV from mother to infant is very rare but manifests as laryngeal papillomatosis. Cesarean delivery does not prevent perinatal transmission of HPV.

Certain HPV types cause abnormal Pap test results and cervical dysplasia. *Management of abnormal Pap test results in pregnancy is similar to that in nonpregnant women; however, biopsies and other excisional procedures are often deferred until the postpartum period.* Close follow-up which may include a repeat Pap smear and/or colposcopy in pregnancy is often performed instead. HPV infection and abnormal Pap smears as well as recommendations regarding the **HPV vaccine** are discussed elsewhere in the text (see Chapters 27, Sexually Transmitted Diseases and 43, Cervical Neoplasia and Carcinoma).

## SYPHILIS

**Syphilis** is a systemic disease caused by the motile spirochete *Treponema pallidum.* The spirochete is transmitted by direct contact, invading intact mucous membranes or areas of abraded skin. A painless ulcer at the site of inoculation follows, usually within 6 weeks following exposure. The ulcer is firm, with elevated edges; it lasts for several weeks. One to 3 months later, a skin rash occurs, or, in some patients, raised lesions **(condyloma lata)** appear on the genitalia.

*T. pallidum* is generally considered to cross the placenta to the fetus after 16 weeks of gestation. Transmission can occur at any stage of maternal infection and has been documented at as early as 6 weeks of gestation.

Spontaneous abortion, stillbirth, and neonatal death are more frequent in any untreated patient, whereas neonatal infection is more likely in primary or secondary rather than latent syphilis. Newborns with congenital syphilis may be asymptomatic or have the classic signs of the syndrome, although most infants do not develop evidence of disease for 10 to 14 days after delivery. Early evidence of the disease includes a maculopapular rash, "snuffles," mucous patches on the oropharynx, hepatosplenomegaly, jaundice, lymphadenopathy, and chorioretinitis (Fig. 15.2). Later signs include Hutchinson teeth, mulberry molars, saddle nose, and saber shins.

**Congenital syphilis** is readily preventable with prompt and appropriate maternal treatment. Therefore, all pregnant women should be screened serologically as early as possible and again at delivery (and if exposed to an infected partner). Serologic testing is the mainstay of diagnosis. **Nontreponemal screening tests** (Venereal Disease Research Laboratory [VDRL], rapid plasma reagin [RPR]) are sometimes falsely positive; **treponemal-specific tests** (fluorescent treponemal antibody absorbed [FTA-ABS], *T. pallidum* particle agglutination [TP-PA]) are used to

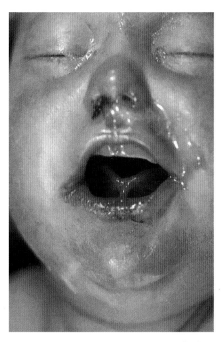

FIGURE 15.2. Congenital syphilis. Note the mucous patches on the oropharynx and the characteristic "snuffles." CDC/Dr. Norman Cole.

confirm infection and identify antibodies specific for *T. pallidum.* A positive treponemal-specific test result indicates either active disease or previous exposure; regardless of treatment, the test remains positive for life in most individuals.

Therapy differs by stage of disease and is generally the same as that recommended for nonpregnant adults. There are no proven alternative therapies to penicillin for treating syphilis in pregnancy. Therefore, patients with penicillin sensitivity require skin testing, followed by desensitization for those with a true penicillin allergy. The Jarisch-Herxheimer reaction occurs most often among patients with early syphilis and is an acute febrile reaction that typically occurs in the first 24 hours after treatment. *In pregnancy, this reaction may precipitate preterm labor or cause fetal distress and may warrant close observation of mothers after treatment.* Post-treatment titers (RPR or VDRL) should be followed serially for at least one year. A fourfold increase in serologic titer, or persistent or recurrent signs or symptoms, may indicate inadequate treatment or reinfection. Retreatment is indicated in either case. Response to therapy is again evaluated by following serologic titers.

## GONORRHEA

*Antepartum screening for* Neisseria gonorrhoeae *should be performed early in pregnancy for women with risk factors or symptoms and repeated in the third trimester for women at high risk* (see Table 16.1). Rates in pregnancy range from

1% to 7%, depending on the population. Diagnosis is made by PCR.

*All cases of gonorrhea must be reported to health care officials.*

Treatment is with an extended spectrum or 3rd-generation cephalosporin.

*Tetracyclines and fluoroquinolones are contraindicated in pregnancy.*

Infection above the cervix (i.e., of the uterus, including the fetus, and the fallopian tubes) is rare after the first weeks of pregnancy. At delivery, however, infected mothers may transmit the organism, causing gonococcal ophthalmia in the neonate. All neonates receive routine prophylactic treatment with sterile ophthalmic ointment containing erythromycin or tetracycline, which is generally effective in preventing neonatal gonorrhea.

## CHLAMYDIA

Antepartum screening for **Chlamydia trachomatis** should be performed early in pregnancy and repeated in the third trimester based on risk factors (see Table 16.1). It has been detected in 2% to 13% of pregnant women, depending on the population, and is generally found in 5% of all populations. In pregnant women, infection is often asymptomatic but may cause urethritis or mucopurulent cervicitis. Like gonorrhea, infection of the upper genital tract is uncommon during pregnancy, although chlamydia infection has been associated with postpartum endometritis and infertility. Diagnosis is made by culture, direct fluorescent antibody staining, enzyme immunoassay, DNA probe, or PCR.

Maternal chlamydia infection at the time of delivery results in colonization of the neonate in 50% of cases. Neonates colonized at birth may go on to develop purulent conjunctivitis soon after birth or pneumonia at 1 to 3 months of age. Routine prophylaxis against neonatal gonococcal ophthalmia is not generally effective against chlamydial conjunctivitis; systemic treatment of the infant is necessary. Fortunately, neonatal chlamydial ophthalmia and pneumonia are becoming less common with the institution of universal prenatal screening and treatment. Recommended treatment of genital infection with *C. trachomatis* in pregnancy includes azithromycin or amoxicillin.

*Doxycycline and ofloxacin are contraindicated during pregnancy.*

Repeat testing to confirm successful treatment, preferably by culture performed 3 to 4 weeks after completion of therapy, is recommended in pregnancy.

## CYTOMEGALOVIRUS

*Approximately 1% of all neonates are infected with CMV in utero and excrete CMV at birth. Although the majority of CMV infections are asymptomatic, 5% of infected neonates show symptoms at birth.* A DNA herpesvirus, CMV may be transmitted in saliva, semen, cervical secretions, breast milk, blood, or urine. CMV infection is often asymptomatic, although it can cause a short febrile illness. Similar to HSV, CMV may have dormant periods, only to reactivate at a later time. There are multiple serotypes and the presence of anti-CMV IgG does not confer immunity; recurrent infection may occur with a new strain of virus. The prevalence of antibodies to CMV is inversely proportional to age and socioeconomic status.

The risk of neonatal infection is significantly higher with primary maternal infection than with recurrent infection; with recurrent infection the risk of neonatal infection is much lower, at 2% or less. Intrauterine growth restriction is sometimes noted. Most infants are asymptomatic at birth; when signs occur, they include petechiae, hepatosplenomegaly, jaundice, thrombocytopenia, microcephaly, chorioretinitis, or nonimmune hydrops fetalis. Long-term sequelae include severe neurologic impairment and hearing loss.

There is no effective vaccine or treatment for maternal or fetal infection. Therefore, routine serologic screening for CMV in pregnancy is not recommended. Testing is generally limited to women in whom CMV infection is suspected and is done by culture or PCR. Antiviral agents have been used to treat neonate infection but remain experimental.

## TOXOPLASMOSIS

Infection with the intracellular parasite **Toxoplasma gondii** occurs primarily through ingestion of the infectious tissue cysts in raw or poorly cooked meat or through contact with feces from infected cats, which contain infectious sporulated oocytes. The latter may remain infectious in moist soil for more than 1 year. *Only cats that hunt and kill their prey are reservoirs for infection; those that eat prepared cat food are not.* In immunocompetent adult humans, infection is most commonly asymptomatic and disease is self-limited. Prior infection confers immunity, unless the individual is immunosuppressed. Approximately 15% of reproductive-age women have antibodies to toxoplasmosis.

Although congenital infection is more common following maternal infection in the third trimester, the sequelae following 1st-trimester fetal infection are more severe. Over half of infants whose mothers are infected during the last trimester of pregnancy have serologic evidence of infection, but three-fourths of these show no gross evidence of infection at birth. Signs of congenital infection include severe mental retardation, chorioretinitis, blindness, epilepsy, intracranial calcifications, and hydrocephalus.

In some regions with high prevalence of disease (France and Central America), screening is routine in pregnancy. In the United States, routine screening in pregnancy is not recommended except in the presence of maternal HIV infection. Because identification of the organism in tissue or blood is complex and infection is usually asymptomatic, diagnosis depends on demonstration of seroconversion. A positive IgG titer indicates infection at some time. A negative IgM effectively rules out recent infection; however, IgM may persist for long periods and a positive test is not reliable in assessing duration of disease. In addition, false-positive IgM results are common with commercially available assays. Confirmatory testing in pregnancy should be performed in a *Toxoplasma* reference laboratory prior to initiating any therapy.

Treatment of acutely infected pregnant women with spiramycin may reduce the risk of fetal transmission but does not prevent sequelae in the fetus if infection has occurred. This medication is only available through the FDA. If fetal infection has already been noted (through ultrasound findings or confirmed with testing of fetal blood or amniotic fluid), pyrimethamine and sulfadiazine therapy may decrease the risk of congenital infection and the severity of manifestations.

Prevention of infection should be an important part of prenatal care, including counseling regarding thoroughly cooking all meats, careful hand washing after handling raw meats, washing of fruits and raw vegetables before ingestion, wearing gloves when working with soil, and keeping cats indoors and feeding them only processed foods. If a cat is kept outside, someone other than a pregnant woman should feed and care for the cat and dispose of its wastes.

## VARICELLA

**Congenital varicella** (chicken pox) infection can be serious, but it is very uncommon due to high rates of immunity in women of reproductive age. Risk for congenital varicella syndrome (skin scarring, limb hypoplasia, chorioretinitis, microcephaly) is limited to maternal infection occurring in the first half of pregnancy. Most patients are immune, even if they or their families do not recall the patient having been infected. A pregnant patient exposed to varicella can have serologic testing (IgM and IgG), and can be given varicella zoster immune globulin within 72 hours of exposure to reduce the severity of maternal infection. *A pregnant patient who develops the characteristic varicella rash can be given oral acyclovir within 24 hours of the rash to decrease symptoms and duration of disease* (Figure 15.3). However, maternal acyclovir has not been shown to decrease the rate or severity of fetal infection.

If clinical infection occurs in a patient from 5 days prior to delivery to 2 days after delivery, neonatal infection can be severe, even deadly. Varicella zoster immune globulin is given to infants in such situations, though protection is not complete.

Severe complications of varicella including pneumonia and encephalitis are much more common in adults than in children. Varicella pneumonia seems to occur more fre-

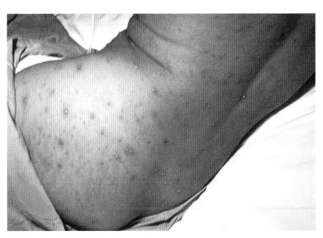

FIGURE 15.3. Varicella. Chickenpox lesions on day 6 of the illness. CDC/J. D. Millar.

quently with varicella infection during pregnancy and is associated with maternal mortality. Treatment is with intravenous acyclovir. Effective vaccination against varicella has been available since 1995 and should be offered to susceptible nonpregnant women.

*The vaccine is a live attenuated virus and should be avoided in pregnancy and within 1 month of conception; however, no adverse outcomes have been reported if given in pregnancy.*

Vaccination of susceptible household contacts of pregnant women is safe.

## PARVOVIRUS

Maternal **parvovirus B19** infection can cause devastating fetal outcomes such as spontaneous abortion, fetal nonimmune hydrops fetalis, and even death. Seroprevalence increases with age and is >60% in adolescents and adults. For susceptible pregnant women, the risk of seroconversion ranges from 20% to 50%, depending on closeness to the infectious contact (higher risk for closer contacts such as family members); however, the risk of transplacental infection is low. *Maternal immune status can be determined by serologic testing; IgM reflects recent infection and IgG indicates infection in the past and immunity.* Routine serologic screening in pregnancy is not recommended. Exposed pregnant women should be offered B19-specific IgM and IgG serologic testing. If IgM is positive or seroconversion is confirmed, ultrasound testing for 10 weeks to look for evidence of fetal hydrops (ascites, edema), placentomegaly, and growth disturbances is performed. Intrauterine transfusions may be necessary if hydrops develops. There is no specific treatment for parvovirus infection. If hydrops does not develop in the fetus, long-term outcomes are good with apparently normal development.

## SUGGESTED READINGS

American College of Obstetricians and Gynecologists. Human papillomavirus. ACOG Practice Bulletin No. 61. *Obstet Gynecol.* 2005;105(4):905–918.

American College of Obstetricians and Gynecologists. Immunization during pregnancy. ACOG Committee Opinion No. 282. *Obstet Gynecol.* 2003;101(1):207–212.

American College of Obstetricians and Gynecologists. Management of herpes in pregnancy. ACOG Practice Bulletin No. 82. *Obstet Gynecol.* 2007;109(6):1489–1498.

American College of Obstetricians and Gynecologists. Perinatal viral and parasitic infections. ACOG Practice Bulletin No. 20. *Obstet Gynecol.* 2000;96(3):1–13.

American College of Obstetricians and Gynecologists. Prenatal and perinatal human immunodeficiency virus testing: expanded recommendations. ACOG Committee Opinion No. 304. *Obstet Gynecol.* 2004;104(5):1119–1124.

American College of Obstetricians and Gynecologists. Prevention of early-onset group B streptococcal disease in newborns. ACOG Committee Opinion No. 279. *Obstet Gynecol.* 2002;100(6):1405–1412.

American College of Obstetricians and Gynecologists. Rubella vaccination. ACOG Committee Opinion No. 281. *Obstet Gynecol.* 2002;100(6):1417.

American College of Obstetricians and Gynecologists. Viral hepatitis in pregnancy. ACOG Practice Bulletin No. 86. *Obstet Gynecol.* 2007;110(4):941–956.

American College of Obstetricians and Gynecologists. Scheduled cesarean delivery and the prevention of vertical transmission of HIV infection. ACOG Committee Opinion No. 234. *Obstet Gynecol.* 2000;95(5) (Reaffirmed 2003).

American College of Obstetricians and Gynecologists. *Guidelines for Perinatal Care.* 6th ed. Elk Grove Village, IL: American Academy of Pediatrics; 2007.

Infection. In: American College of Obstetricians and Gynecologists. *Precis, Obstetrics: An Update in Obstetrics and Gynecology.* 3rd ed. Washington, D.C.: American College of Obstetricians and Gynecologists; 2006:121–136.

# 16 Hypertension in Pregnancy

Topic 18: Preeclampsia-Eclampsia Syndrome

Students should be able to define and classify hypertensive disease in pregnancy, including preeclampsia, eclampsia, and the HELLP syndrome; to discuss the pathophysiology of preeclampsia and its diagnosis, evaluation, and initial management, including labor management and the appropriate use of magnesium sulfate; and understand and be able to discuss the effects of preeclampsia on pregnancy (mother and fetus) and the converse.

H ypertensive disorders occur in approximately 12% to 22% of pregnancies and cause substantial perinatal morbidity and mortality for both mother and fetus. Hypertensive disease is directly responsible for approximately 20% of maternal deaths in the United States. The exact cause of hypertension in pregnancy remains unknown.

## CLASSIFICATION

Various classifications of hypertensive disorders in pregnancy have been proposed. Box 16.1 presents a commonly used classification. Because hypertensive disorders in pregnancy represent a spectrum of disease, classification systems should be used as a guide only.

### Chronic Hypertension

*Chronic hypertension is defined as hypertension present before the 20th week of pregnancy or hypertension present before pregnancy.* The categories of hypertension in pregnancy and the blood pressure (BP) criteria used to define each are as follows:

- Mild hypertension: Systolic pressure of ≥140–180 mm Hg or diastolic pressure of ≥90–100 mm Hg or both
- Severe hypertension: Systolic pressure of ≥180 mm Hg or diastolic pressure of ≥100 mm Hg

A major risk with chronic hypertension is the development of preeclampsia or eclampsia later in the pregnancy, which is relatively common and difficult to diagnose. The acute onset of proteinuria and worsening hypertension in women with chronic hypertension is suggestive of superimposed preeclampsia.

### Gestational Hypertension

*Hypertension that develops after 20 weeks of gestation in the absence of proteinuria and returns to normal postpartum is termed* **gestational hypertension.** Gestational hypertension develops in 5% to 10% of pregnancies that proceed beyond the first trimester, with a 30% incidence in multiple gestations, regardless of parity. Maternal morbidity is directly related to the severity and duration of hypertension.

*Approximately 25% of women with gestational hypertension develop superimposed preeclampsia or eclampsia.* It is often difficult to distinguish between preeclampsia and gestational hypertension when a patient is seen late in pregnancy with an elevated blood pressure level. In such cases, it is always wise to assume that the findings represent preeclampsia and treat accordingly.

### Preeclampsia

**Preeclampsia** *is the development of hypertension with proteinuria and edema after 20 weeks of gestation.* This condition can occur earlier in the presence of gestational trophoblastic disease (see Chapter 41, Gestational Trophoblastic Neoplasia). Risk factors for preeclampsia are in Box 16.2. The criteria for diagnosis of preeclampsia are:

- Blood pressure of ≥140 mm Hg systolic or ≥90 mm Hg diastolic that occurs after 20 weeks of gestation in a woman with previously normal blood pressure
- Proteinuria, defined as urinary excretion of 0.3 g protein or higher in a 24-hour urine specimen

**Severe preeclampsia** is characterized by one or more of the following:

- Blood pressure ≥160 mm Hg systolic or ≥110 mm Hg diastolic on two occasions at least 6 hours apart while the patient is on bed rest

**BOX 16.1**
**Hypertensive Disorders in Pregnancy**

Gestational hypertension
Preeclampsia
    Mild
    Severe
Eclampsia
Chronic hypertension preceding pregnancy (any cause)
Chronic hypertension (any cause) with superimposed gestational hypertension
    Superimposed preeclampsia
    Superimposed eclampsia

- Marked proteinuria (generally ≥5 g per 24-hour urine collection, or 3+ or more on two dipstick of random urine samples collected at least 4 hours apart)
- Oliguria <500 mL in 24 hours
- Cerebral or visual disturbances such as headache and scotomata ("spots" before the eyes)
- Pulmonary edema or cyanosis
- Epigastric or right-upper-quadrant pain (probably caused by subcapsular hepatic hemorrhage or stretching of Glisson capsule)
- Evidence of hepatic dysfunction
- Thrombocytopenia
- Intrauterine fetal growth restriction (IUGR)

These changes illustrate the multisystem involvement associated with preeclampsia. Severe preeclampsia is an indication for delivery, regardless of gestational age or maturity.

## Eclampsia

*Eclampsia is the additional presence of convulsions (**grand mal seizures**) in a woman with preeclampsia that is not explained*

**BOX 16.2**
**Risk Factors for Preeclampsia**

Nulliparity
Multifetal gestation
Maternal age over 35 years
Preeclampsia in a previous pregnancy
Chronic hypertension
Pregestational diabetes
Vascular and connective tissue disorders
Nephropathy
Antiphospholipid syndrome
Obesity
African-American race

*by a neurologic disorder.* Eclampsia occurs in 0.5% to 4% of patients with preeclampsia.

*Most cases of eclampsia occur within 24 hours of delivery, but approximately 3% of cases are diagnosed between 2 and 10 days postpartum.*

## HELLP Syndrome

**HELLP syndrome** *is the presence of **h**emolysis, **e**levated **l**iver enzymes, and **l**ow **p**latelet count.*

*HELLP syndrome, like severe preeclampsia, is an indication for delivery to avoid jeopardizing the health of the woman.*

This syndrome is now appreciated as a distinct clinical entity, occurring in 4% to 12% of patients with severe preeclampsia or eclampsia. Criteria for diagnosis are:

- Microangiopathic hemolysis
- Thrombocytopenia
- Hepatocellular dysfunction

## PATHOPHYSIOLOGY

Hypertension in pregnancy affects the mother and newborn to varying degrees. Given the characteristic multisystem effects, it is clear that several pathophysiologic mechanisms are involved (Fig. 16.1). *The predominant pathophysiologic finding in preeclampsia and gestational hypertension is **maternal vasospasm**.* Several potential causes for maternal vasospasm have been postulated:

1. **Vascular changes:** Instead of noting the physiologic trophoblast-mediated vascular changes in the uterine vessels (decreased musculature in the spiral arterioles leads to the development of a low-resistance, low-pressure, high-flow system), inadequate maternal vascular response is seen in cases of preeclampsia and/or intrauterine fetal growth restriction. Endothelial damage is also noted within the vessels.
2. **Hemostatic changes:** Increased platelet activation with increased consumption in the microvasculature is noted during the course of preeclampsia. Endothelial fibronectin levels are increased and antithrombin III and $\alpha_2$-antiplasmin levels are decreased, reflecting endothelial damage. Low antithrombin III levels are permissive for microthrombi development. Endothelial damage is then thought to promote further vasospasm.
3. **Changes in prostanoids:** Prostacyclin ($PGI_2$) and thromboxane ($TXA_2$) are increased during pregnancy, with the balance in favor of $PGI_2$. In patients who develop preeclampsia, the balance shifts to favor $TXA_2$. Again, $PGI_2$ functions to promote vasodilatation and

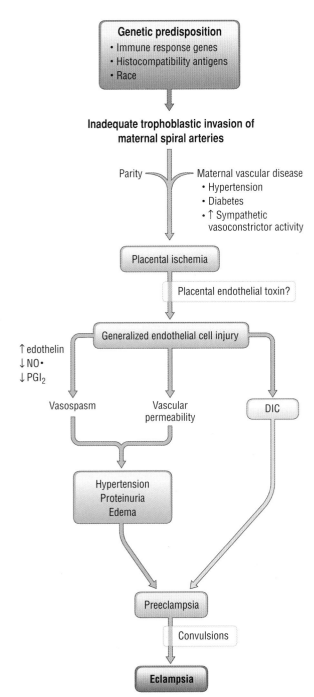

**FIGURE 16.1.** Proposed pathways and markers implicated in the development of preeclampsia and eclampsia. DIC = disseminated intravascular coagulation; NO· = nitric acid; PGI$_2$ = prostacyclin.

5. **Lipid peroxide, free radicals, and antioxidant release:** Lipid peroxides and free radicals have been implicated in vascular injury and are increased in pregnancies complicated by preeclampsia. Decreased antioxidant levels are also noted.

These five mechanisms, in any combination or permutation, are thought to contribute to the following common pathophysiologic changes seen in patients with preeclampsia:

1. **Cardiovascular effects:** Elevated blood pressure is seen as the result of potential vasoconstriction as well as an increase in cardiac output.
2. **Hematologic effects:** Plasma volume contraction may develop, with risk of rapid onset hypovolemic shock, if hemorrhage occurs. Plasma volume contraction is reflected in increased hematocrit values. Thrombocytopenia/disseminated intravascular coagulation may also develop from microangiopathic hemolytic anemia. Involvement of the liver may lead to hepatocellular dysfunction and further evolution of coagulopathy. Third spacing of fluid may be noted, because of increased blood pressure and decreased plasma oncotic pressure.
3. **Renal effects:** Decreased glomerular filtration rate (increasing serum creatinine) and proteinuria (urine protein levels greater than 300 mg per 24 hours) develop secondary to atherosclerotic-like changes in the renal vessels (glomerular endotheliosis). Uric acid filtration is decreased; therefore, elevated maternal serum uric acid levels may be an indication of evolving disease.
4. **Neurologic effects:** Hyperreflexia/hypersensitivity may develop. In severe cases, grand mal (eclamptic) seizures may develop.
5. **Pulmonary effects:** Pulmonary edema may occur and can be related to decreased colloid oncotic pressure, pulmonary capillary leak, left heart failure, iatrogenic fluid overload, or a combination of these factors.
6. **Fetal effects:** Decreased intermittent placental perfusion secondary to vasospasm is thought to be responsible for the increased incidence of intrauterine growth restriction (<10% estimated fetal weight for gestational age), oligohydramnios, and increased perinatal mortality of infants born to mothers with preeclampsia. An increased incidence of placental abruption is also seen. With the stress of uterine contractions during labor, the placenta may be unable to adequately oxygenate the fetus. This may result in signs of intrapartum uteroplacental insufficiency. Specifically, a nonreassuring fetal-heart-rate pattern may necessitate cesarean delivery.

*Presumably because of vasospastic changes, placental size and function are decreased.* The results are progressive fetal hypoxia and malnutrition, as well as an increase in the incidence of intrauterine growth restriction and oligohydramnios.

decrease platelet aggregation, and TXA$_2$ promotes vasoconstriction and platelet aggregation. Because of this imbalance, vessel constriction occurs.
4. **Changes in endothelium-derived factors:** Nitric oxide, a potent vasodilator, is decreased in patients with preeclampsia and may explain the evolution of vasoconstriction in these patients.

## EVALUATION

The history and physical examination are directed toward detection of pregnancy-associated hypertensive disease and its signs and symptoms. A review of current obstetric records, if available, is especially helpful to ascertain changes or progression in findings. *Visual disturbances, especially scotomata, or unusually severe or persistent headaches are indicative of vasospasm.* Right-upper-quadrant pain may indicate liver involvement, presumably involving distention of the liver capsule. Any history of loss of consciousness or seizures, even in the patient with a known seizure disorder, may be significant.

*The position of the patient influences blood pressure.* It is lowest with the patient lying in the lateral position, highest when the patient is standing, and at an intermediate level when she is sitting. The choice of the correct-size blood pressure cuff also influences blood pressure readings, with falsely high measurements noted when normal-sized cuffs are used on large patients. Also, during the course of pregnancy, blood pressure typically declines slightly in the second trimester, increasing to prepregnant levels as gestation nears term (Fig. 16.2). If a patient has not been seen previously, there is no baseline blood pressure against which to compare new blood pressure determinations, thereby making the diagnosis of pregnancy-related hypertension more difficult.

The patient's weight is compared with her pregravid weight and with previous weights during this pregnancy, with special attention to excessive or too-rapid weight gain.

Peripheral edema is common in pregnancy, especially in the lower extremities.

> *However, persistent edema unresponsive to resting in the supine position is not normal, especially when it also involves the upper extremities, sacral region, and face.*

Indeed, the puffy-faced, edematous, hypertensive pregnant woman is the classic picture of preeclampsia. Careful blood pressure determination in the sitting and supine positions is necessary. Funduscopic examination may detect vasoconstriction of retinal blood vessels indicative of similar vasoconstriction of other small vessels. Tenderness over the liver, attributed partly to hepatic capsule distension, may be associated with complaints of right-upper-quadrant pain. The patellar and Achilles' deep tendon reflexes should be carefully elicited, and hyperreflexia noted. The demonstration of clonus at the ankle is especially worrisome.

The maternal and fetal laboratory evaluations for pregnancy complicated by hypertension are presented in Table 16.1 and demonstrate, by the wide range of tests, the multisystem effects of hypertension in pregnancy. *Maternal liver dysfunction, renal insufficiency, and coagulopathy are significant concerns and require serial evaluation.* Evaluation of fetal well-being with ultrasonography, and a nonstress test and/or biophysical profile are important.

## MANAGEMENT

*The goal of management of hypertension in pregnancy is to balance the management of both fetus and mother and to optimize the outcome for each.* Maternal blood pressure should be monitored and the mother should be observed for the sequelae of the hypertensive disease. Intervention for maternal indications should occur when the risk of permanent disability or death for the mother without intervention outweighs the risks to the fetus caused by intervention. For the fetus, there should be regular evaluation of fetal well-being and fetal growth, with intervention becoming necessary if the intrauterine environment provides more risks to the fetus than delivery with subsequent care in the newborn nursery.

### Chronic Hypertension

*The management of patients with chronic hypertension in pregnancy involves closely monitoring maternal blood pressure and watching for the superimposition of preeclampsia or eclampsia, and following the fetus for appropriate growth and fetal well-being.* Medical treatment of essential hypertension has been disappointing, in that no significant improvement in pregnancy outcome has been demonstrated with treatment.

*Antihypertensive medication in women with chronic hypertension is generally not given unless the systolic blood pressure is 150 to 160 mm Hg or the diastolic blood pressure 100 to*

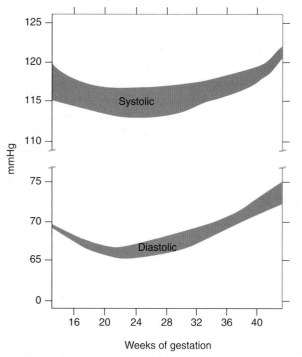

FIGURE 16.2. Range of blood pressures in normotensive pregnancy. Note the decrease in blood pressure in the second trimester.

| TABLE 16.1 | Laboratory Assessment of Pregnant Hypertensive Patients |
|---|---|

| Test or Procedure | Rationale |
|---|---|
| **Maternal studies** | |
| Complete blood count | Increasing hematocrit may signify worsening vaso-constriction and decreased intravascular volume |
| | Decreasing hematocrit may signify hemolysis |
| Platelet count | Thrombocytopenia is associated with worsening disease |
| Coagulation profile (PT, PTT) | Coagulopathy is associated with worsening disease |
| Liver function studies | Hepatocellular dysfunction is associated with worsening disease |
| Serum creatinine<br>Uric acid<br>24-hour urine<br>Creatinine clearance<br>Total urinary protein | Decreased renal function is associated with worsening disease |
| **Fetal studies** (To assess for pregnancy-associated hypertension effects on the fetus) | |
| Ultrasound examination<br>Fetal weight and growth<br>Amniotic fluid volume | IUGR<br>Oligohydramnios |
| NST and/or biophysical profile | Placental status (indirect assessment) |

IUGR = intrauterine growth restriction; NST = nonstress test; PT = prothrombin time; PTT = partial thromboplastin time.

*110 mm Hg.* The purpose of such medications is to reduce the likelihood of maternal stroke. Methyldopa is a commonly used antihypertensive medication for this purpose, although a combined alpha-and-beta-blocker (such as labetalol) and calcium-channel blockers (such as nifedipine) are also commonly used. It was formerly taught that diuretics were contraindicated during pregnancy, but diuretic therapy is no longer discontinued, and indeed is usually continued, in the patient who already has been on such therapy before becoming pregnant.

## Preeclampsia

The severity of the preeclampsia and the maturity of the fetus are the primary considerations in the management of preeclampsia. Care must be individualized, but there are well-accepted general guidelines.

*The mainstay of management for patients with mild preeclampsia is rest and frequent monitoring of mother and fetus. Testing for suspected fetal growth restriction or oligohydramnios and twice-weekly nonstress tests, biophysical profiles, or both, are commonly employed and should be repeated as indicated, according to maternal condition.* Testing is recommended twice weekly for suspected fetal growth restriction or oligohydramnios. Ultrasound examination for fetal growth and amniotic fluid assessment is recommended every 3 weeks. Daily fetal movement assessment also may prove useful.

Hospitalization is often initially recommended for women with new-onset preeclampsia. After maternal and fetal conditions are serially assessed, subsequent management may be continued in the hospital, at a day-care unit, or at home on the basis of the initial assessment.

*For the patient with worsening preeclampsia or the patient who has severe preeclampsia, management is often best accomplished in a tertiary-care setting.* Daily laboratory tests and fetal surveillance may be indicated. Stabilization with magnesium sulfate, antihypertensive therapy (as indicated), monitoring for maternal and fetal well-being, and delivery by either induction or cesarean delivery are required.

For almost a century, **magnesium sulfate** has been used to prevent and to treat eclamptic convulsions. Other anticonvulsants, such as diazepam and phenytoin, are rarely used because they are not as efficacious as magnesium and because they have potential adverse effects on the fetus. *Magnesium sulfate is administered by intramuscular or intravenous routes, although the latter is far more common.* In 98% of cases, convulsions will be prevented. *Therapeutic levels are 4 to 6 mg/dL with toxic concentrations having predictable consequences* (Table 16.2). Frequent evaluations of the patient's patellar reflex and respirations are necessary to monitor for manifestations of rising serum magnesium concentrations. In addition, because magnesium sulfate is excreted solely from the kidney, maintenance of urine output of at least 25 mL/hour will help avoid accumulation

| TABLE 16.2 | Magnesium Toxicity |
|---|---|
| **Serum Concentration (mg/dL)** | **Manifestation** |
| 1.5–3 | Normal concentration |
| 4–6 | Therapeutic levels |
| 5–10 | Electrocardiogram changes |
| 8–12 | Loss of patellar reflex |
| 9–12 | Feeling of warmth, flushing |
| 10–12 | Somnolence; slurred speech |
| 15–17 | Muscle paralysis; respiratory difficulty |
| 30 | Cardiac arrest |

of the drug. Reversal of the effects of excessive magnesium concentrations is accomplished by the slow intravenous administration of 10% calcium gluconate, along with oxygen supplementation and cardiorespiratory support, if needed.

Antihypertensive therapy is initiated if, on repeated measurements, the systolic blood pressure is >160 mm Hg or if diastolic blood pressure exceeds 105 to 110 mm Hg. Hydralazine is often the initial antihypertensive medication of choice, given in 5- to 10-mg increments intravenously until an acceptable blood pressure response is obtained. A 10- to 15-minute response time is usual. *The goal of such therapy is to reduce the diastolic pressure to the 90- to 100-mm Hg range.* Further reduction of the blood pressure may impair uterine blood flow to rates that are dangerous to the fetus. Labetalol is another agent used to manage severe hypertension (Table 16.3).

*Once anticonvulsant and antihypertensive therapies are established in patients with severe preeclampsia or eclampsia, attention is directed toward delivery.* Induction of labor is often attempted, although cesarean delivery may be needed either if induction is unsuccessful or not possible, or if the maternal or fetal status is worsening. At delivery, blood loss must be closely monitored, because patients with pre-eclampsia or eclampsia have significantly reduced blood volumes. After delivery, patients remain in the labor and delivery area for 24 hours (longer if the clinical situation warrants) for close observation of their clinical progress and further administration of magnesium sulfate to prevent postpartum eclamptic seizures. Approximately 25% of eclamptic seizures occur before labor, 50% occur during labor, and 25% occur in the first 24 hours after delivery. Usually, the vasospastic process begins to reverse itself in the first 24 to 48 hours after delivery, as manifested by a brisk diuresis.

## Eclampsia

The *eclamptic seizure* is life-threatening for mother and fetus. *Maternal risks include musculoskeletal injury (including biting the tongue), hypoxia, and aspiration.* Maternal therapy consists of inserting a padded tongue blade, restraining gently as needed, providing oxygen, assuring maintenance of an adequate airway, and gaining intravenous access. Eclamptic seizures are usually self-limited, so medical therapy should be directed to the initiation of magnesium therapy (4 to 6 g slowly, intravenously) to prevent further seizures. If a patient receiving magnesium sulfate experi-

| TABLE 16.3 | Antihypertensive Medications Used in Pregnancy | |
|---|---|---|
| **Medication** | **Mechanism of Action** | **Effects** |
| Thiazide | Decreased plasma volume and CO | CO decreased; RBF decreased; maternal depletion; neonatal thrombocytopenia |
| Methyldopa | False neurotransmission, CNS effect | CO unchanged; RBF unchanged; fever, maternal lethargy, hepatitis, and hemolytic anemia |
| Hydralazine | Direct peripheral vasodilation | CO increased; RBF unchanged or increased; maternal flushing, headache, tachycardia, lupus-like syndrome |
| Propranolol | β-adrenergic blocker | CO decreased; RBF decreased; maternal increased uterine tone with possible decrease in placental perfusion; neonatal depressed respirations |
| Labetalol | α- and β-adrenergic blocker | CO unchanged; RBF unchanged; maternal tremulousness, flushing, headache; neonatal depressed respirations; contraindicated in women with asthma and heart failure |
| Nifedipine | Calcium-channel blocker | CO unchanged; RBF unchanged; maternal orthostatic hypotension and headache (also a tocolytic); no neonatal effects known |

CNS = central nervous system; CO = cardiac output; RBF = renal blood flow.

ences a seizure, additional magnesium sulfate (usually 2 g slowly) can be given, and a blood level obtained. Other anticonvulsant therapy with diazepam or similar drugs is generally not warranted.

Transient uterine hyperactivity for up to 15 minutes is associated with fetal heart rate changes, including bradycardia or compensatory tachycardia, decreased variability, and late decelerations. These are self-limited and are not dangerous to the fetus unless they continue for 20 minutes or more. *Delivery during this time imposes unnecessary risk for mother and fetus and should be avoided.* Arterial blood gases are often obtained, any metabolic disturbance should be corrected, and a Foley catheter should be placed to monitor urinary output. If the maternal blood pressure is high, if maternal urinary output is low, or if there is evidence of cardiac disturbance, consideration of a central venous catheter and, perhaps, continuous electrocardiogram monitoring is appropriate.

## HELLP Syndrome

Patients with HELLP syndrome are often multiparous and have blood pressure recordings lower than those of many preeclamptic patients. The liver dysfunction may be manifest as right-upper-quadrant pain, and is all too commonly misdiagnosed as gallbladder disease or indigestion. Major morbidity and mortality with unrecognized HELLP make accurate diagnosis imperative. The first symptoms are often vague, including nausea and emesis and a nonspecific viral-like syndrome. *Treatment of these gravely ill patients is best done in a high-risk obstetric center and consists of cardiovascular stabilization, correction of coagulation abnormalities, and delivery.* Platelet transfusion before or after delivery is indicated if the platelet count is <20,000/mm$^3$, and it may be advisable to transfuse patients with a platelet count <50,000/mm$^3$ before proceeding with a cesarean birth. Management of cases of HELLP syndrome should be individualized based on gestational age at presentation, maternal symptoms, physical examination, laboratory findings, and fetal status.

## SUGGESTED READINGS

American College of Obstetricians and Gynecologists. Chronic hypertension in pregnancy. ACOG Practice Bulletin No. 29. *Obstet Gynecol.* 2001;98(1):177–185.
American College of Obstetricians and Gynecologists. Diagnosis and management of preeclampsia and eclampsia. ACOG Practice Bulletin No. 33. *Obstet Gynecol.* 2002;99(1):159–167.

This chapter deals primarily with APGO Educational Topic:

Topic 20:   Multifetal Gestation

Students should understand that multifetal gestations require modifications in antepartum, intrapartum, and postpartum care.

The overall incidence of multiple gestations in the United States is almost 3%, but these pregnancies account for a disproportionate share of perinatal morbidity and mortality. The natural rate of twinning is approximately 1 in 90, and is slightly higher in blacks than in whites. *The rate is rising as a result of an increase in maternal age and the more frequent use of assisted reproductive technologies (ART) and ovulation-induction agents.* Since 1980, there has been a 65% increase in the frequency of twins, and a 500% increase in triplet and high-order births. It is estimated that 43% of triplet and high-order gestations result from ART procedures and 38% from ovulation induction; spontaneous conception accounts for the remainder. Although the exact mechanism is not known, monozygotic twinning is also higher in pregnancies conceived using ART.

Twin gestations can be characterized as dizygotic (fraternal) or monozygotic (identical). **Dizygotic twins** occur when two separate ova are fertilized by two separate sperm. **Monozygotic twins** result from the division of the fertilized ovum after conception. There is a marked difference in the incidence of twinning in various populations, almost exclusively the result of the incidence of dizygotic twinning. The incidence of monozygotic twinning is fairly constant around the world, at approximately 1 in 250 pregnancies. *Increasing maternal age and increasing parity are independent risk factors for dizygotic twinning, and rates are higher among mothers of families with twins.*

## NATURAL HISTORY

The following describes the various developmental sequences possible when the monozygotic conceptus separates into twins (also called **chorionicity**) [Fig. 17.1]:

- **Diamnionic/Dichorionic:** If division of the conceptus occurs within 3 days of fertilization, each fetus will be surrounded by an amnion and chorion.

- **Diamnionic/Monochorionic:** If division occurs between the 4th and 8th day following fertilization, the chorion has already begun to develop, whereas the amnion has not. Therefore, each fetus will later be surrounded by an amnion, but a single chorion will surround both twins.

- **Monoamnionic/Monochorionic:** In 1% of monozygotic gestations, division occurs between days 9 and 12, after development of both the amnion and the chorion, and the twins will share a common sac. Division thereafter is incomplete, resulting in the development of **conjoined** twins. The fetuses may be fused in a number of ways, with the most common involving the chest and/or abdomen. This rare condition is seen in approximately 1 in 70,000 deliveries. This condition is associated with a mortality rate of up to 50%.

## RISKS OF MULTIFETAL GESTATION

Multifetal pregnancies are associated with increased perinatal morbidity, 3 to 4 times that of a comparable singleton pregnancy.

*The most significant cause of morbidity is preterm labor and delivery.*

Compared with singleton pregnancies, which are delivered at an average gestational age of 40 weeks, twins are delivered at an average of 37 weeks, triplets at 33 weeks, and quadruplets at an average of 29 weeks. Thus, with each additional fetus, the length of gestation is decreased by approximately 4 weeks. *Other associated morbidities include intrauterine growth restriction, hydramnios (in approximately 10% of multiple gestations, predominantly monochorionic gestations), preeclampsia (3 times more frequent in twin gestations), congenital anomalies, postpartum hemorrhage, placental abrup-*

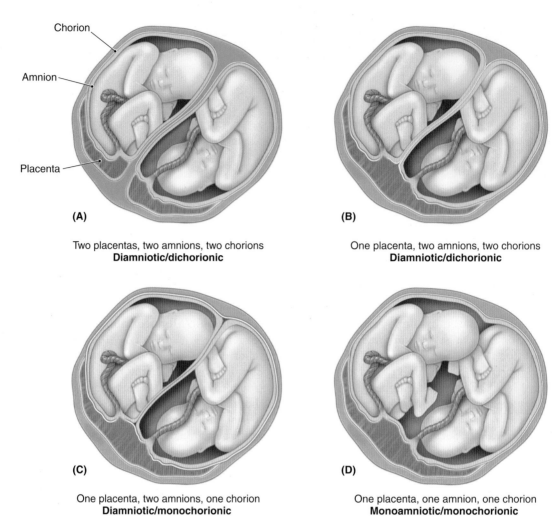

Chorion

Amnion

Placenta

**(A)**

Two placentas, two amnions, two chorions
**Diamniotic/dichorionic**

**(B)**

One placenta, two amnions, two chorions
**Diamniotic/dichorionic**

**(C)**

One placenta, two amnions, one chorion
**Diamniotic/monochorionic**

**(D)**

One placenta, one amnion, one chorion
**Monoamniotic/monochorionic**

FIGURE 17.1. Chorionicity in twin pregnancies. (A) Two placentas, two amnions, two chorions: diamniotic dichorionic. (B) One placenta, two amnions, two chorions: diamniotic/dichorionic. (C) One placenta, two amnions, one chorion: diamniotic/monochorionic. (D) One placenta, one amnion, one chorion: monoamniotic/monochorionic. (Based on American College of Obstetricians and Gynecologists. *Having Twins.* Patient Education Pamphlet AP092. Washington, DC: ACOG; 2004.)

*tion, and umbilical cord accidents.* Both spontaneous abortions and congenital anomalies are approximately twice as common in multiple gestations (Table 17.1).

## Twin–Twin Transfusion Syndrome

*As development of a monochorionic gestation progresses, various vascular anastomoses between the fetuses can develop that, in turn, can lead to a condition known as* **twin–twin transfusion syndrome.** In this circumstance, through arterial-venous anastomoses, there is net flow from one twin to another, often with untoward pregnancy outcomes. The so-called donor twin can have impaired growth, anemia, hypovolemia, and other problems. The recipient twin can develop hypervolemia, hypertension, polycythemia, and congestive heart failure as a result of this preferential transfusion. A sec-

ondary manifestation involves amniotic fluid dynamics. The hypervolemia in the recipient twin leads to an increase in urinary output and, in turn, to an increase in amniotic fluid volumes (hydramnios). The opposite effect may occur in the donor twin—hypovolemia leads to decreased urinary output and, possibly, a decrease in amniotic fluid volume (oligohydramnios). Hydramnios in the one twin compounds the risk of preterm labor already present for multifetal pregnancies. Traditionally, serial removal of amniotic fluid from the sac of the recipient twin has been the only treatment option with improved survival. However, intrauterine laser ablation of the vascular anastomoses has met with some success in treating this difficult problem, especially in the most severe cases. *Other vascular abnormalities include absence of an umbilical artery, which may be associated in 30% of cases with other congenital problems, especially renal agenesis. A single*

| TABLE 17.1 | Morbidity and Mortality in Multiple Gestation | | |
|---|---|---|---|
| **Characteristic** | **Twins** | **Triplets** | **Quadruplets** |
| Average birth weight[1] | 2347 g | 1687 g | 1309 g |
| Average gestational age at delivery[1] | 35.3 wk | 32.2 wk | 29.9 wk |
| Percentage with growth restriction[2] | 14–25 | 50–60 | 50–60 |
| Percentage requiring admission to neonatal intensive care unit[3] | 25 | 75 | 100 |
| Average length of stay in neonatal intensive care unit[3–9] | 18 days | 30 days | 58 days |
| Percentage with major handicap[9, 10] | — | 20 | 50 |
| Risk of cerebral palsy[9, 10] | 4 times more than singletons | 17 times more than singletons | — |
| Risk of death by age 1 year[11–13] | 7 times higher than singletons | 20 times higher than singletons | — |

[1]Martin JA, Hamilton BE, Sutton PD, Ventura SJ, Menacker F, Munson ML. Births: final data for 2002. *Natl Vital Stat Rep.* 2003;52(10):1–102.

[2]Mauldin JG, Newman RB. Neurologic morbidity associated with multiple gestation. *Female Pat.* 1998;23(4):27–28, 30, 35–36, passim.

[3]Ettner SL, Christiansen CL, Callahan TL, Hall JE. How low birthweight and gestational age contribute to increased inpatient costs for multiple births. *Inquiry.* 1997–98;34:325–339.

[4]McCormick MD, Brooks-Gunn J, Workman-Daniels K, Turner J, Peckham GJ. The health and developmental status of very low-birth-weight children at school age. *JAMA.* 1992;267:2204–2208.

[5]Luke B, Bigger HR, Leurgans S, Sietsema D. The cost of prematurity: a case-control study of twins vs singletons. *Am J Public Health.* 1996;86:809–814.

[6]Albrecht JL, Tomich PG. The maternal and neonatal outcome of triplet gestations. *Am J Obstet Gynecol.* 1996;174:1551–1556.

[7]Newman RB, Hamer C, Miller MC. Outpatient triplet management: a contemporary review. *Am J Obstet Gynecol.* 1989;161:547–553; discussion 553–555.

[8]Seoud MA, Toner JP, Kruithoff C, Muasher SJ. Outcome of twin, triplet, and quadruplet in vitro fertilization pregnancies: the Norfolk experience. *Fertil Steril.* 1992;57:825–834.

[9]Elliott JP, Radin TG. Quadruplet pregnancy: contemporary management and outcome. *Obstet Gynecol.* 1992;80(2):421–424.

[10]Grether JK, Nelson KB, Cummins SK. Twinning and cerebral palsy: experience in four northern California counties, births 1983 through 1985. *Pediatrics.* 1993;92:854–858.

[11]Luke B, Minogue J. The contribution of gestational age and birth weight to perinatal viability in singletons versus twins. *J Mat-Fetal Med.* 1994;3:263–274.

[12]Kiely JL, Kleinman JC, Kiely M. Triplets and higher order multiple births: time trends and infant mortality. *Am J Dis Child.* 1992;146:862–868.

[13]Luke B, Keith LG. The contribution of singletons, twins, and triplets to low birth weight, infant mortality, and handicap in the United States. *J Reprod Med.* 1992;37:661–666.

American College of Obstetricians and Gynecologists. Multiple gestation: complicated twin, triplet, and high-order multifetal pregnancy. ACOG Practice Bulletin No. 56. *Obstet Gynecol.* 2004;104(4):869–883.

*umbilical artery is seen in approximately 3% to 4% of twins, compared with 0.5% to 1% of singletons.*

## Death of One Fetus

*Multiple gestations, especially high-order gestations, are at increased risk of losing one or more fetuses remote from delivery.* No fetal monitoring protocol has been shown to predict most of these losses. In addition, authorities disagree about the preferred antepartum surveillance method and management once a demise has occurred. Some investigators advocate immediate delivery of the remaining fetuses. However, if the death is the result of an abnormality of the fetus itself rather than maternal or uteroplacental pathology, and the pregnancy is remote from term, expectant management may be appropriate. The most difficult cases are those in which the fetal demise occurs in one fetus of a monochorionic twin pair. Because virtually 100% of monochorionic placentas contain vascular anastomoses that link the circulations of the 2 fetuses, the surviving fetus is at significant risk of sustaining damage caused by the sudden, severe, and prolonged hypotension that occurs at the time of the demise or by embolic phenomena that occurs later. By the time the demise is discovered, the greatest harm has most likely already been done and there may not be any benefit in immediate delivery, especially if the surviving fetuses are very preterm and otherwise healthy. In such cases, allowing the pregnancy to continue may provide the most benefit.

## DIAGNOSIS AND ANTENATAL MANAGEMENT

Most multifetal pregnancies are diagnosed using ultrasound.

*On a clinical basis, twin pregnancy should be suspected when the uterine size is large for the calculated gestational age.*

A difference of 4 cm or more between the weeks of gestation and the measured fundal height should prompt evaluation with ultrasound to detect the cause (e.g., inaccurate gestational age, multiple gestation, hydramnios, gestational trophoblastic disease, or pelvic tumor).

Serial ultrasound assessments have shown that only 50% of twin pregnancies detected in the first trimester result in the delivery of viable twins. The other 50% of cases deliver a single fetus because of intrauterine demise and ultimate resorption of one embryo/fetus (vanishing twin syndrome). During the first ultrasonographic examination that confirms a twin gestation, chorionicity should be determined because the potential morbidity and mortality associated with a monochorionic gestation is different from that of a dichorionic gestation (described below). Chorionicity can be determined with almost 100% certainty as early as 9 to 10 weeks of gestational age.

Once the diagnosis of twin pregnancy has been made and chorionicity has been assigned, subsequent antenatal care addresses each of the potential concerns for mother and fetus, as listed in Table 17.2. Although the maternal blood volume is greater with a twin gestation than with a singleton pregnancy, the anticipated blood loss at delivery is also greater. Anemia is more common in these patients, and a balanced diet during pregnancy, which may include increased intake of iron, folate, and other micronutrients, is important. *Because of the increased risk for preterm labor in multiple gestations, careful attention to detection of uterine contractions is important, and the patient should be cautioned about signs and symptoms of preterm labor, such as low back pain, a thin or increase in vaginal discharge, and vaginal bleeding.* Cervical examinations to detect early effacement and dilation are often done every 1 to 2 weeks beginning in the midtrimester. When available, serial ultrasound assessments of endovaginal cervical length may be interspersed with the vaginal examinations.

Assessment of **fetal fibronectin** may aid in predicting preterm delivery in women, but it has limited predictive

| TABLE 17.2 | Antenatal Management of Twin Pregnancies |
|---|---|
| **Concern** | **Action** |
| Adequate nutrition | Balanced diet; additional 300 kcal in daily intake; multivitamin, and mineral supplements (e.g., folate) |
| Increased blood loss at delivery | Prevent anemia (iron) |
| Fetal growth | Increasing rest beginning at 24–26 weeks; the value of this is unclear, but also may decrease preterm labor |
| Preterm labor | Educate patient on signs of labor; increase bed rest; cervical examinations every 1–2 weeks alternating with cervical length ultrasounds; fetal fibronectin assessment |
| Pregnancy-induced hypertension | Frequent blood pressure determinations; frequent urinary protein assessment |
| Fetal growth, discordant growth | Periodic ultrasonographic examinations |

value in multifetal gestations. At each visit, blood pressure should be evaluated and, if elevated, urine protein should be assessed. Beginning at 30 to 32 weeks, daily fetal kick counts are usually begun to help assess fetal well-being.

*With multifetal gestations, periodic ultrasonographic examination should be performed approximately every 4 weeks, beginning at 16 to 18 weeks of gestation.* At each examination, growth of each fetus is assessed and an estimate of amniotic fluid volume is made. Discordant growth is defined as a 15% to 25% reduction in the estimated fetal weight of the smallest fetus compared with the largest. Ultrasonography should be performed more often in cases of discordant growth.

## INTRAPARTUM MANAGEMENT

*Intrapartum management is largely determined by the presentation of the twins.* In general, if the first (presenting) twin is in the cephalic (vertex) presentation, labor is allowed to progress to vaginal delivery, whereas if the presenting twin is in a position other than cephalic, cesarean delivery is often performed. During labor, the heart rate of both fetuses is monitored separately. *Approaches to the delivery of twins vary, depending on gestational age or estimated fetal weight, presentation of the twins, and the experience of the attending physicians.* Regardless of the delivery plan, access to full obstetric, anesthetic, and pediatric services is mandatory because cesarean delivery may be required on short notice. About 40% of all twin pairs enter labor with both in the cephalic (vertex) presentation. After delivery of the first twin, if the second fetus remains cephalic, vaginal delivery of the second twin generally proceeds smoothly. With proper monitoring of the second twin, there is no urgency in accomplishing the second delivery.

If the second twin is presenting in any way other than cephalic (40% of all twin deliveries), there are two primary manipulations that may affect vaginal delivery. The first is **external cephalic version.** Using ultrasonographic visualization, the fetus is gently guided into the cephalic presentation by abdominal massage and pressure (Figure 17.2A). The second maneuver is **breech extraction,** in which the physician reaches a hand into the uterine cavity, grasps the lower extremities of the fetus, and gently delivers the infant via breech delivery (Figure 17.2B). Delivering the second twin via cesarean delivery is another management option, but is usually reserved for inability to safely deliver vaginally.

The possibility of a prolapsed umbilical cord must always be borne in mind when delivery of twins is to be accomplished. Twin gestations in which the first twin is in the breech presentation (20% of all twin deliveries) are most often delivered via cesarean delivery. Some clinicians and their patients plan for cesarean delivery unless both fetuses are in a cephalic presentation.

Postpartum, the overdistended uterus may not contract normally, leading to uterine atony and postpartum hemorrhage (see Chapter 12, Postpartum Hemorrhage).

## SUGGESTED READING

American College of Obstetricians and Gynecologists. Multiple gestation: complicated twin, triplet, and high-order multifetal pregnancy. ACOG Practice Bulletin No. 56. *Obstet Gynecol.* 2004; 104(4):869–883.

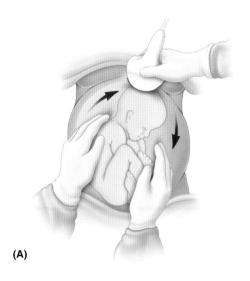

(A)

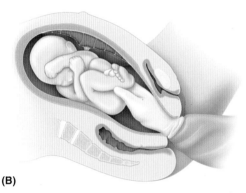

(B)

FIGURE 17.2. Twin delivery. (A) External cephalic version. (B) Breech extraction (internal podalic version).

# Fetal Growth Abnormalities: Intrauterine Growth Restriction and Macrosomia

Topic 31:  Fetal Growth Abnormalities

Fetal growth is multifactorial and can be altered by a variety of extrinsic and intrinsic factors. The maternal, placental, and fetal contributions to growth must all be considered. Students should be able to define the two major fetal growth abnormalities, macrosomia and fetal growth restriction, as well as discuss their evaluation and management. They should also be able to identify the major morbidities and causes of mortality for each condition.

## INTRAUTERINE GROWTH RESTRICTION

"Fetal growth restriction" describes infants whose weights are much lower than expected. Population-based norms are used to categorize abnormal growth. *A fetus or infant whose weight is less than the 10th percentile of a specific population at a given gestational age is designated as having* ***intrauterine growth restriction [IUGR]*** (Table 18.1). Therefore, careful assignment of gestational age is crucial to the diagnosis and management of patients with IUGR.

The term **"small for gestational age" (SGA)** is used to describe an infant with a birth weight at the lower extreme of the normal birth weight distribution. In the United States, the most commonly used definition of SGA is a birth weight below the 10th percentile for gestational age. The use of the terms "small for gestational age" (SGA) and "intrauterine growth restriction" has been confusing, and the terms often are used interchangeably. In this book, SGA will be used only in reference to the infant and IUGR to the fetus.

The use of gestational age percentiles remains limited for a number of reasons. First, by definition, the prevalence of IUGR will be 10%, but not all such neonates are pathologically small. Second, any percentile cut-off fails to take into account an individual's growth potential. Also, a simple percentile cannot take into account growth rate. The change in percentile over time or change in specific measurements may be more important. Finally, the time when the growth restriction is found may be a factor in morbidity and mortality: growth restriction at earlier gestational ages has greater effects on morbidity and mortality.

## Significance

*The goal of recognizing neonates with growth abnormalities is to identify infants at risk for increased short-term and long-term morbidity or mortality.*

In the short-term, the growth restricted fetus potentially lacks adequate reserves to continue intrauterine existence, to undergo the stress of labor, or to fully adapt to neonatal life. These conditions make the infant vulnerable to intrauterine fetal death, asphyxia, acidemia, and intolerance to labor. Neonatal complications, low Apgar scores, polycythemia, hyperbilirubinemia, hypoglycemia, hypothermia, apnea, respiratory distress, seizures, sepsis, meconium aspiration, and neonatal death.

Alterations in fetal growth may have lifelong implications. The antenatal response or fetal adaptation to the intrauterine nutritional and metabolic environment may predict or dictate the response to an extrauterine environment. Increasing evidence supports the concept of fetal origins for adult diseases and the association between birth size and long-term health. Associations have been reported between birth weight and adult obesity, cardiovascular disease (coronary heart disease, hypertension, and stroke), insulin resistance, and dyslipidemia. Therefore, intrauterine growth may reflect the foundation of many aspects of lifelong physiologic function.

*In general, the smaller the fetus with IUGR, the greater its risk for morbidity and mortality.* Perinatal morbidity and mortality is significantly increased in the presence of low birth weight for gestational age, especially with weights below the 3rd percentile for gestational age. One study found that 26% of all stillbirths were SGA. Thus, it is

| TABLE 18.1 | Definition of Commonly Used Fetal Growth Descriptors |
|---|---|
| **Growth Descriptor** | |
| Low birth weight | <2500 g |
| Intrauterine growth restriction | <10% |
| Macrosomia | >4000–4500 g |
| Large for gestational age | >90% |

important to identify such infants in utero so that management maximizes the quality of their intrauterine environment, permits planning and implementation of delivery using the safest means possible, and provides necessary care in the neonatal period.

## Pathophysiology

For a fetus to thrive in utero, an adequate number of fetal cells and cells that differentiate properly are both requisite. In addition, nutrients and oxygen must be available via an adequately functioning uteroplacental unit to allow an increase in the number of cells and in cell size. Early in pregnancy, fetal growth occurs primarily through **cellular hyperplasia,** or cell division, and early-onset IUGR may lead to an irreversible diminution of organ size and, perhaps, function. Early-onset IUGR is also more commonly associated with heritable factors, immunologic abnormalities, chronic maternal disease, fetal infection, and multiple pregnancies. Later in pregnancy, fetal growth depends increasingly on **cellular hypertrophy** rather than hyperplasia alone, so that delayed-onset IUGR may also result in decreased cell size, which may be more amenable to restoration of fetal size with adequate nutrition. The normal fetus grows throughout the pregnancy, but the rate of growth decreases after 37 weeks of gestational age as the fetus depletes fat for cellular growth.

The **placenta** grows early and rapidly compared with the fetus, reaching a maximum surface area of about 11 m² and weight of 500 g at approximately 37 weeks of gestational age. Thereafter, there is a slow but steady decline in placental surface area (and, hence, function), primarily because of microinfarctions of its vascular system. Late-onset growth restriction may therefore be primarily related to decreased function and nutrient transport of the uteroplacental unit, a condition termed **uteroplacental insufficiency.** In addition, because there is a close relationship between placental surface area and fetal weight, factors that act to decrease placental size are also associated with decreased (i.e., restricted) growth.

## Etiology

*IUGR is a descriptive term for a condition that has numerous potential causes.* Determining the specific diagnosis is impor-

tant for optimal management. Although a number of causes of IUGR have been recognized, a definite etiology of IUGR cannot be identified in approximately 50% of all cases. In addition, because the utilization of a percentile cut-off of 10% alone will result in a high proportion of false-positives, two-thirds or more of such fetuses categorized as IUGR will be simply constitutionally small and otherwise healthy.

Factors that affect fetal growth are extensive and include maternal, fetal, and placental causes; these are listed in Box 18.1.

### MATERNAL FACTORS

Maternal factors include viral infections, such as rubella, varicella, and cytomegalovirus, which are associated with high rates of growth restriction, particularly if infection occurs early in pregnancy. Although these infections may manifest only as mild "flu-like" illnesses, injury to the fetus during organogenesis can result in a decreased cell number, resulting in diminished growth with or without multiple congenital anomalies. Five percent or fewer of all cases of IUGR are related to early infection with these or other viral agents. Maternal substance abuse affects fetal growth and almost all infants with fetal alcohol syndrome will be growth-restricted. Women who smoke during pregnancy deliver babies 200 g smaller on average than do women who do not smoke; moreover, the rate of

---

**BOX 18.1**

**Risk Factors Associated With Intrauterine Growth Restriction**

- Maternal medical conditions
  - Hypertension
  - Renal disease
  - Restrictive lung disease
  - Diabetes (with microvascular disease)
  - Cyanotic heart disease
  - Antiphospholipid syndrome
  - Collagen-vascular disease
  - Hemoglobinopathies
- Smoking and substance use and abuse
- Severe malnutrition
- Primary placental disease
- Multiple gestation
- Infections (viral, protozoal)
- Genetic disorders
- Exposure to teratogens

American College of Obstetricians and Gynecologists. *Intrauterine Growth Restriction.* ACOG Practice Bulletin 12. Washington, DC: American College of Obstetricians and Gynecologists; 2000:2.

growth restriction is 3- to 4-fold greater among babies born to women who smoke during pregnancy. Women who use narcotics, heroin, methadone, or cocaine also have rates of growth-restricted babies ranging from as much as 30% to 50%. Medications known to be associated with IUGR include anticonvulsant medications, warfarin, and folic acid antagonists. Altitude may also affect fetal growth.

Other maternal factors that affect fetal growth and body composition include demographic factors and medical conditions. Extremes in maternal age (age younger than 16 years and older than 35 years) are associated with an increased risk of fetal growth restriction. Medical conditions that alter or affect placental function may also be causative factors.

Although one common pathway has not been clearly identified, many of these disorders occur together. Women with a history of prior obstetric complications have an increased risk of growth abnormalities. Maternal metabolism and body composition are two of the strongest regulators of fetal growth. Nutritional deficiencies and inadequate weight gain, particularly in teens or in underweight women, may result in IUGR.

## FETAL FACTORS

The inherent growth potential of the individual is determined genetically. Female fetuses are at greater risk for IUGR than males. In addition, up to 20% of growth-restricted fetuses have a chromosomal abnormality. In addition, single-gene mutations such as the glucokinase gene mutation, or genetic syndromes such as Beckwith-Wiedemann syndrome can also result in abnormalities of growth. Finally, multifetal pregnancies are at increased risk for growth restriction.

## PLACENTAL FACTORS

The placenta is critical for nutrient regulation and transportation from mother to fetus. Abnormalities in placentation or defective trophoblast invasion and remodeling may contribute to fetal growth restriction as well as other disorders of pregnancy. In addition, uterine anomalies (uterine septum or fibroids) may limit placental implantation and development and, consequently, nutrient transport, resulting in inadequate nutrition for the developing fetus. Finally, the genetic composition of the placenta is important and abnormalities such as confined placental mosaicism are associated with growth delay.

## Diagnosis

Assessment of gestational age is important in early pregnancy, because dating becomes increasingly imprecise at later gestational ages.

*Antenatal recognition of IUGR depends upon the recognition of risk factors and the clinical assessment of uterine size, followed by biometric measurements.*

Physical examination is limited in usefulness in recognizing IUGR or in making a specific diagnosis, but it is an important screening test for abnormal fetal growth. Maternal size and weight gain throughout pregnancy also have limited value, but access to such information is readily available; a low maternal weight or little or no weight gain during pregnancy may suggest IUGR. Serial measurements of **fundal height** are commonly used as a screening test for IUGR, but have high rates of false-negative and false-positive predictive values. Between 20 and 36 weeks of gestation, fundal height should increase approximately 1 cm per week, consistent with gestational age in weeks (Fig. 18.1). A discrepancy may be related to constitutional factors, but a significant discrepancy of more than 2 cm may indicate IUGR and the need for an ultrasound examination. Clinical estimations of fetal weight alone are not helpful in diagnosing IUGR, except when fetal size is grossly diminished.

*If IUGR is suspected based on risk factors and clinical assessment, ultrasonography should be performed to assess fetal size and growth.* Specific **fetal biometry measurements** are compared with standardized tables that reflect normal growth at a certain gestational age. The four standard fetal

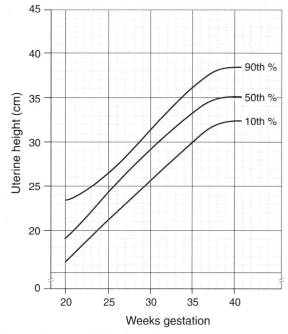

FIGURE 18.1. Fundal height evaluation as a screening test for intrauterine growth restriction. p = percentile. (Reprinted with permission from Scott JR, Di Saia PJ, Hammond CB, et al. *Danforth's Obstetrics and Gynecology.* 8th ed. Philadelphia, PA: Lippincott Williams & Wilkins; 1999.)

measurements include the (1) biparietal diameter, (2) head circumference (HC), (3) abdominal circumference (AC), and (4) femur length. Conversion of individual morphologic measurements to fetal weight using published equations or ratios of measurements can provide useful estimations of fetal size. An abdominal circumference within the normal range reliably excludes growth restriction, with a false-negative rate of less than 10%. A small abdominal circumference or fetal weight estimate below the 10th percentile suggests the possibility of growth restriction, with the likelihood increasing as the percentile rank decreases.

*When IUGR is suspected, serial measurements of fetal biometric parameters provide an estimated growth rate.* Such serial measurements are of considerable clinical value in confirming or excluding the diagnosis and assessing the progression and severity of growth restriction. Given the high incidence of genetic and structural defects associated with IUGR, a detailed ultrasound survey for the presence of fetal structural and functional defects may be indicated.

*Following recognition of altered fetal growth, a search for potential etiology should ensue.* Ultrasonography should include a detailed anatomic survey to evaluate for the presence of structural anomalies, given the high incidence of genetic and structural defects with IUGR. Ultrasound evaluation should also include an assessment of **amniotic fluid volume.** The combination of oligohydramnios (diminished amniotic fluid volume) and IUGR is associated with severe disease and increased morbidity. The mechanism of decreased amniotic fluid is thought to be decreased placental perfusion of oxygen and nutrients with a compensatory redistribution of fetal blood favoring the brain, adrenal gland, and heart. The consequent decrease in fetal blood to the kidneys leads to a reduction of urine output, which is the primary source of amniotic fluid in the second half of pregnancy.

Direct invasive studies of the fetus are useful in selected patients with IUGR. Amniocentesis for fetal lung maturity may assist delivery planning near term or when there is uncertainty regarding gestational age and concern for growth restriction. Fetal karyotyping and viral cultures and polymerase chain reactions can be performed on fluid obtained by amniocentesis. Rarely, **chorionic villus sampling** (biopsy of placenta) or direct blood sampling (**percutaneous umbilical blood sampling**) may be necessary for specific studies.

**Doppler velocimetry** of fetal vessels provides further insight into the fetal response to altered growth, and has become part of the standard assessment of the fetus once IUGR is diagnosed. Doppler velocimetry has been shown to both reduce interventions and improve fetal outcome in pregnancies at risk for IUGR. Fetal-placental circulation is evaluated in the umbilical artery and is measured by a systolic/diastolic (S/D) ratio. The S/D indirectly measures impedance or resistance downstream within the placental vessels. As placental resistance increases, diastolic flow decreases and the S/D ratio rises. *A normal S/D ratio at term is 1.8 to 2.0.* Fetuses with IUGR with absent or

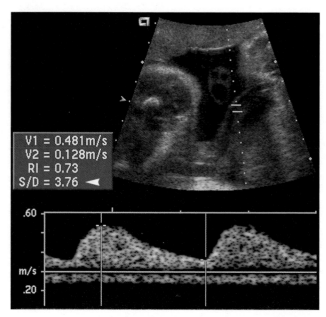

FIGURE 18.2. **Doppler volimetry.** Umbilical artery Doppler of a 35-week fetus demonstrates an elevated S/D ratio of 3.76 (arrowhead, calipers) due to diminished diastolic flow. (From Doubilet PM, Benson CB. *Atlas of Ultrasound in Obstetrics and Gynecology.* Philadelphia, PA: Lippincott Williams & Wilkins; 2003:227.)

reversed diastolic flow have progressively worse perinatal outcomes (Figure 18.2). The fetal middle cerebral artery is also evaluated and reflects fetal adaptation. The pathophysiologic response to reduced placental perfusion generally spares the fetal brain, resulting in an increase of diastolic and mean blood flow velocity in the middle cerebral artery. Ductus venosus may also be evaluated by Doppler ultrasound, and the fetus with abnormal ductus flow is at very high risk of adverse outcome.

## Management

*The goal of management of a growth-restricted fetus is to deliver the healthiest possible infant at the optimal time. Continued management of pregnancy with IUGR is based on the results of fetal testing.*

Serial evaluations of fetal biometry should be performed every 3 or 4 weeks to follow the extent of growth restriction. **Fetal monitoring** is important, and may include fetal movement counting, nonstress testing, biophysical profiles, and Doppler studies. There are no specific therapies that have proven beneficial for pregnancies complicated by IUGR.

*The fetus should be delivered if the risk of fetal death exceeds that of neonatal death, although in many cases these risks are difficult to assess.*

For example, a fetus with IUGR with normal anatomic survey, normal amniotic fluid volume, normal Doppler studies, and normal fetal testing may not benefit from early delivery. Conversely, the growth-restricted fetus with serial biometry measurements documenting decreasing growth rate and/or mildly abnormal Doppler studies may benefit from delivery, with or without fetal maturity documentation.

Neonatal management of IUGR infants may partially depend on gestational age, but includes preparation for neonatal respiratory compromise, hypoglycemia, hypothermia, and hyperviscosity syndrome. Growth-restricted fetuses have less fat deposition in late pregnancy, so newborn euglycemia cannot be maintained by the normal mechanism of mobilization of glucose by fat metabolism. **Hyperviscosity syndrome** results from the fetus's attempt to compensate for poor placental oxygen transfer by increasing the hematocrit to more than 65%. After birth, this marked polycythemia can cause multiorgan thrombosis, heart failure, and hyperbilirubinemia. Overall, growth-restricted infants who survive the neonatal period have a generally good prognosis.

## MACROSOMIA

Two terms have been used to define excessive fetal growth. **Fetal macrosomia** is based on weight alone and refers to a fetus with an estimated weight of 4000–4500 g or greater. **Large for gestational age (LGA)** generally implies a birth weight >90% for a given gestational age, and is dependent on both weight and gestational age with percentiles generated from population-specific norms (see Table 18.1). By definition, the prevalence of LGA is fixed, but not all neonates at the upper extreme of size are pathologically large. Growth potential, growth rate, and gestational age at onset may be important considerations.

### Etiology

Macrosomia, like fetal growth restriction, has multiple potential causes, categorized into fetal or maternal factors (Box 18.2). Similar to fetal growth restriction, fetal factors include the genetic composition or inherent growth potential of the individual, and genetic syndromes such as Beckwith-Wiedemann syndrome. Male fetuses are also more commonly affected than female fetuses.

Maternal factors include a history of macrosomia, maternal prepregnancy weight, weight gain during pregnancy, multiparity, male fetus, gestational age greater than 40 weeks, ethnicity, maternal birth weight, maternal height, maternal age younger than 17 years, and a positive 50-g glucose screen with a negative result on the 3-hour glucose tolerance test.

The magnitude of glucose intolerance during pregnancy and specific measures of control are correlated with fetal weight and fetal fat mass. Lipids are also associated with fetal size, with triglycerides and free fatty acids positively correlated to birth weight, and triglycerides inde-

---

**BOX 18.2**
**Risk Factors for Large for Gestational Age**

Fetal
    Genetic potential
    Specific gene disorders
    Male sex

Maternal
    History of previous macrosomic pregnancy
    Metabolism
    Body composition
    Pregnancy weight gain
    Parity

---

pendently associated with LGA infants. Maternal body composition and body mass index are major determinants of insulin sensitivity, independent of hypertension and pregestational or gestational diabetes. Also, maternal weight gain and pregravid weight contribute to the variance in fetal birth weight. Finally, increased parity is associated with larger babies.

### Significance

Macrosomia is associated with both increased maternal and fetal/neonatal risks. A patient with a macrosomic fetus has an increased risk of cesarean delivery, because of labor abnormalities. The risk of postpartum hemorrhage and vaginal lacerations are also elevated with macrosomia. Maternal infections associated with macrosomia include urinary tract infection in women undergoing elective caesarean section and puerperal fever in women undergoing a trial of labor. Risks to the fetus are shoulder dystocia and fracture of the clavicle, although brachial plexus nerve injury is rare. Macrosomic infants also have an increased risk for lower Apgar scores.

Other neonatal risks are partially dependent on the underlying etiology of macrosomia, such as maternal obesity or diabetes, and may include an increased risk of hypothermia, hyperbilirubinemia, hypoglycemia, prematurity, and stillbirth. The relationship between gestational age and fetal size is important. Macrosomic preterm infants remain at risk for complications of prematurity. Size and extent of maturity are independent. Long-term risks include overweight or obesity in later life, again illustrating that intrauterine growth may predict the foundation of many aspects of lifelong physiologic function.

### Diagnosis

Because the diagnosis of macrosomia is based on an estimated fetal weight above the 90th percentile and becomes increasingly imprecise at later gestational ages, careful dating of pregnancy is important. The two primary methods for clinical estimation of fetal weight are Leopold maneuvers (abdominal palpation; see Fig. 9.7) and measurement of the height of the uterine fundus above the maternal symphysis pubis.

*Measurement of the symphysis–fundal height alone is a poor predictor of fetal macrosomia and should be combined with clinical palpation of (Leopold maneuvers) to be useful.*

Clinical findings may be combined with ultrasound to diagnose macrosomia. Ultrasound-derived estimates of fetal weight are obtained by entering the measurements of various fetal body parts, usually including the abdominal circumference, into one of several popular regression equations. However, most of the regression formulas currently in use are associated with significant errors when the fetus is macrosomic. The superiority of ultrasound-derived estimates of fetal weight over clinical estimates has not been established.

*The true value of ultrasound in management of macrosomia is its ability to rule out the diagnosis.*

Differential diagnosis of an enlarged uterus includes a large fetus, more than one fetus (multiple gestation), extra amniotic fluid (polyhydramnios), large placenta (molar pregnancy), or large uterus (uterine leiomyomata, other gynecologic tumor, or uterine anomaly).

## Management

*For mothers without diabetes, no clinical interventions designed to treat or curb fetal growth when macrosomia is suspected have* *been reported.* Current evidence does not support early delivery for macrosomia alone, because induction of labor does not decrease maternal and neonatal morbidity; it does increase the rate of cesarean deliveries. In addition, the data do not support a specific estimated fetal weight at which women should undergo elective cesarean delivery.

*Given the limitations of ultrasound estimations and the association with increasing injury with increasing infant weight, the American College of Obstetricians and Gynecologists recommends that a cesarean delivery should be offered for estimated fetal weights greater than 5000 g in women without diabetes and greater than 4500 g in women with diabetes.*

Various techniques can be used to facilitate vaginal delivery in the case of shoulder dystocia, such as exaggerated flexion of the thighs (McRoberts maneuver), suprapubic pressure, various rotations, episiotomy, delivery of the posterior arm, and intentional clavicular fracture. The Zavanelli maneuver, cephalic replacement with subsequent cesarean delivery, has yielded mixed results. A prolonged second stage of labor or arrest of descent in the second stage is an indication for cesarean delivery. Postpartum or neonatal management depends on gestational age and underlying etiology.

## SUGGESTED READINGS

American College of Obstetricians and Gynecologists. *Fetal Macrosomia*. ACOG Practice Bulletin 22. Washington, DC: American College of Obstetricians and Gynecologists; 2000.

American College of Obstetricians and Gynecologists. *Intrauterine Growth Restriction*. ACOG Practice Bulletin 12. Washington, DC: American College of Obstetricians and Gynecologists; 2000.

American College of Obstetricians and Gynecologists. Shoulder dystocia. ACOG Practice Bulletin No. 40. *Obstet Gynecol.* 2002; 100(5 Pt 1): 1045–1050.

# 19 Isoimmunization

**Topic 19:** Isoimmunization

Incompatibility between circulating maternal antibodies and fetal red blood cell antigens may result in fetal hemolysis with a potential for severe fetal or newborn illness. Students should be able to describe the circumstances leading to isoimmunization (including specifically to the D antigen), its pathophysiology, techniques used to determine its presence and severity in the mother and fetus, and the appropriate indications for Rh D immunoglobulin prophylaxis.

When any fetal blood group factor inherited from the father is not possessed by the mother, antepartum or intrapartum fetal–maternal bleeding may stimulate an immune reaction in the mother. Maternal immune reactions also can occur from blood product transfusion. *The formation of maternal antibodies is called **isoimmunization**. It can lead to various degrees of transplacental passage of these antibodies into the fetal circulation, causing an **antibody response** sufficient to destroy fetal red cells.* Although early exposures to maternal antigens during pregnancy may occur in the same pregnancy, isoimmunization more commonly occurs in a subsequent pregnancy. The binding of maternal antibodies to fetal red blood cells leads to **hemolytic disease** in the fetus or newborn, characterized by **hemolysis, bilirubin release,** and **anemia.** The severity of the illness encountered by the fetus or newborn is determined by a number of factors, including the degree of immune response elicited (i.e., how much antibody is produced), how strongly the antibody binds the antigen, the gestational age at which the diagnosis is made, and the ability of the fetus to replenish the destroyed red cells to maintain a hematocrit sufficient for growth and development (Table 19.1).

## NATURAL HISTORY

Any of the many blood group antigen systems can lead to isoimmunization, but the number of antigens involved in fetal and neonatal hemolytic disease is limited. The most common antigen involved is part of the **Rh (CDE) system,** specifically the **D antigen.**

The Rh system is a complex of five antigens—including the **C, c, D, E,** and **e antigens**—each of which elicits a unique immune response. These antigens are inherited together in distinctive patterns reflecting the underlying genotypic makeup of the parents. C and c are alternate forms of the same antigen, as are E and e, but there is no

d antigen. The D antigen is either present or absent. *Patients with the D antigen are termed **Rh D-positive,** and those lacking this gene, and hence the antigen, are said to be **Rh D-negative.*** Approximately 15% of whites, 5% to 8% of African Americans, and only 1% to 2% of Asians and Native Americans are Rh D-negative.

*A variant of the D antigen called the **weak D antigen** (formerly Du) also exists. If not appropriately diagnosed, patients can be mistakenly classified as Rh D-negative. For this reason, patients should not be considered Rh D-negative unless efforts have been made to look for the weak D antigen. Patients who are Rh weak D-positive should be managed the same as those who are Rh D-positive.*

*Isoimmunization can occur when an Rh D-negative woman is pregnant with a fetus who has inherited the Rh D antigen from its father and is thus Rh D-positive. Any event associated with fetomaternal bleeding can potentially lead to maternal exposure to fetal red blood cells,* which can trigger a maternal immune response. These events include:

- Childbirth
- Delivery of the placenta
- Threatened, spontaneous, elective, or therapeutic abortion
- Ectopic pregnancy
- Bleeding associated with placenta previa or abruption
- Amniocentesis
- Abdominal trauma
- External cephalic version

The amount of Rh D-positive blood required to cause isoimmunization is small—less than 0.1 mL is sufficient.

## Effects of Antibody Development on the Fetus and Newborn

One study indicates that 17% of Rh D-negative women who do not receive anti-D immune globulin prophylaxis

| TABLE 19.1 | Atypical Antibodies and Their Relationship to Fetal Hemolytic Disease | | |
|---|---|---|---|
| | Antigens Related to Hemolytic Disease | Hemolytic Disease Severity | Proposed Management |
| Lewis | | Not associated | Routine care |
| I | | Not associated | Routine care |
| Kell | K | Mild to severe | Fetal assessment |
| | k | Mild | Routine care |
| Rh (non-D) | E | Mild to severe | Fetal assessment |
| | e | Mild to severe | Fetal assessment |
| | C | Mild to severe | Fetal assessment |
| | c | Mild to severe | Fetal assessment |
| Duffy | $Fy^a$ | Mild to severe | Fetal assessment |
| | $Fy^b$ | Not associated | Routine care |
| Kidd | $Jk^a$ | Mild to severe | Fetal assessment |
| | $Jk^b$ | Mild | Routine care |
| MNS | M | Mild to severe | Fetal assessment |
| | N | Mild | Routine care |
| | S | Mild to severe | Fetal assessment |
| Lutheran | $Lu^a$ | Mild | Routine care |
| | $Lu^b$ | Mild | Routine care |
| P | $PP^{1pk}$ | Mild to severe | Fetal assessment |

Adapted from Weinstein L. Irregular antibodies causing hemolytic disease of the newborn: a continuing problem. *Clin Obstet Gynecol.* 1982;25(2):321.

during pregnancy will become isoimmunized. As with other antibody-mediated immune responses, the first immunoglobulin (Ig) type produced is of the **IgM** isoform, which does not cross the placenta to any extent. The chance of significant fetal or newborn disease in a woman's first at-risk pregnancy is therefore low. It is, however, important to consider prior pregnancy losses or terminations as potential exposures, because they could influence the risk of fetal or newborn disease. In a subsequent pregnancy, passage of minute amounts of fetal blood across the placenta into the maternal circulation, a relatively common occurrence, can lead to an **anamnestic response** of maternal antibody production, which is more robust and rapid than the initial response.

In the case of some antigens, the mother continues to produce predominantly IgM antibodies that fail to cross the placenta. In other cases, the secondary antibody response is characterized by the production of **IgG** antibodies that freely cross the placenta, enter the fetal circulation, and bind to antigenic sites on fetal red cells. Red blood cells that are highly bound with antibody are hemolyzed in the fetal reticuloendothelial system and destroyed via complement-mediated pathways. Hemolysis releases bilirubin, and the fetus excretes the bilirubin and its break-

down products in urine. If the fetus is able to augment erythropoiesis to keep pace with the rate of hemolysis, serious anemia may not develop. However, if large amounts of antibody cross the placenta resulting in destruction of large numbers of fetal red cells, the fetus may be unable to sufficiently replenish the red cells and anemia may ensue.

Typically, the first affected pregnancy is characterized by mild anemia and elevated bilirubin at birth, often necessitating treatment for the newborn, such as ultraviolet light and exchange transfusion, as the newborn's liver may be unable to effectively metabolize and excrete the released bilirubin. Markedly elevated bilirubin levels can lead to **kernicterus** (bilirubin deposition in the basal ganglia) which can cause permanent neurologic symptoms or even death. This condition is rarely seen today in developed countries.

*In some first-affected pregnancies, and in many, but not all, subsequent pregnancies with an antigen-positive fetus, antibody production increases as a result of the anamnestic response, leading to more significant hemolysis and anemia.* Assessment of the amount of bilirubin excreted by these fetuses into the amniotic fluid is one method used to monitor fetal status (see below). When fetal anemia is significant, fetal hematopoiesis increases, including the recruitment of alternative sites for red cell production. The fetal liver is an important site of extramedullary hematopoiesis. When the liver produces red blood cells, the production of other proteins decreases, resulting in a lower oncotic pressure within the fetal vasculature. This consequence, in conjunction with the increase in intravascular resistance to flow caused by islands of hematopoietic cells in the liver, can lead to the development of ascites, subcutaneous edema, or pleural effusion.

Severe anemia affects fetal cardiac function in two ways. First, anemia can lead to a high-output cardiac failure. As the cardiac system attempts unsuccessfully to keep pace with the oxygen-delivery demands, the myocardium becomes dysfunctional, resulting in effusions, edema, and ascites due to hydrostatic pressure increases. Second, the anemia itself can cause myocardial ischemia, thereby directly damaging and compromising myocardial function. This combination of fluid accumulation in at least two extravascular compartments (pericardial effusion, pleural effusion, ascites, or subcutaneous edema) is referred to as **hydrops fetalis.**

*Isoimmunization usually progressively worsens in each subsequent pregnancy.* Fetal anemia may occur at the same gestational age or earlier than in the prior affected pregnancies.

## Significance of Paternal Antigen Status

*Determination of the father's antigen status is important in assessing whether the fetus is at risk for developing anemia.* Any individual can be either homozygous or heterozygous for a particular gene. If the father is heterozygous for the gene for the particular antigen of interest, there is a 50% chance that the fetus will not inherit the gene for that antigen. For many of the antigens, this information can be determined easily by looking at which antigens are expressed on the father's red blood cells. For example, C and c are coded by the same gene, but differ by a single base change. An individual can express C, c, or both. If he expresses both, he is heterozygous; if only one antigen is detected, then he must be homozygous. Unfortunately, the situation is not as straightforward with Rh D (because there is no **d** antigen). However, direct **genotype testing** can be performed to determine if the father is homozygous or heterozygous. In a pregnancy involving an isoimmunized patient, the first step in management is determination of the paternal erythrocyte antigen status. In pregnancies in which there is a heterozygous or unknown paternal genotype, the fetal antigen type should be assessed by genetic analysis of fetal cells obtained by **amniocentesis.**

*Regardless of the amount of maternal antibody present, if the subsequent fetus does not carry the antigen (because the father was a heterozygote or there is different paternity), then the fetus has a 98.5% probably of not being at risk.*

## DIAGNOSIS

*All pregnant women should be tested at the time of the first prenatal visit for ABO blood group and Rh-D type and screened for the presence of erythrocyte antibodies. These laboratory assessments should be repeated in each subsequent pregnancy.* Repeated antibody screening is also recommended before administration of anti-D immunoglobulin at 28 weeks of gestation, postpartum, and the time of any event in pregnancy. Patients who are weak-D positive are not at risk for isoimmunization and should not receive anti-D immunoprophylaxis.

Any antibodies potentially associated with fetal hemolysis found during this routine screening are further evaluated based on the strength of the antibody response, which is reported in titer format (1:4, 1:8, 1:16, etc.), with higher numbers indicative of a more significant antibody response. Although often encountered during the process of antibody screening, anti-Lewis and Anti-I antibodies are not associated with fetal hemolytic disease, and therefore are not evaluated further.

## ASSESSMENT

Although antibody titers reflect the strength and the amount of the maternal antibody response, their utility in pregnancy management is limited. *Titers provide no information about fetal status.* In an initial sensitized pregnancy, serial antibody titer values can assist in determining when the maternal antibody response is strong enough to represent a risk of fetal anemia. A **critical titer** is that titer associated with a significant risk for severe fetal hemolytic disease and hydrops fetalis. In most centers, this is between 1:8 and 1:32. If the initial antibody titer is 1:8 or less, the Rh D-negative patient can be monitored with titer assessment every 4 weeks. In a first-sensitized pregnancy, titers are generally performed every 4 weeks. With a history of an affected fetus or infant, titers are not helpful in predicting fetal hemolytic disease and further evaluation is warranted.

Evaluation for possible fetal anemia is usually undertaken in the second trimester, although management may be individualized depending on history and available expertise. Traditionally, amniotic fluid assessment of the level of bilirubin has been used as a measure of fetal status and an indirect means of estimating the potential for severe fetal anemia. In the second half of a normal pregnancy, the level of bilirubin in the amniotic fluid decreases progressively, whereas in an affected, isoimmunized patient, the amount of bilirubin detected can deviate significantly. The increase in the amniotic fluid bilirubin in affected pregnancies is a result of fetal urinary excretion of the increased amount of circulating bilirubin. Until recently, serial amniocenteses were performed to determine the level of bilirubin in the amniotic fluid, which in turn reflected the severity of fetal anemia.

*The current trend in management is the measurement of* **peak velocity** *of middle cerebral artery (MCA) flow using* **Doppler ultrasound.** The velocity of flow through the

MCA is related to the viscosity of the blood. In the setting of fetal anemia, the blood is less viscous due to fewer cells and, therefore, the velocity of flow increases. Gestational age-specific peak velocity normal curves have been derived and correlated with the fetal hematocrit. The degree of peak velocity elevation above the median for that gestational age can be used to estimate the fetal hematocrit and thus the risk of fetal anemia. Using the peak systolic velocity of the MCA, almost all fetuses with moderate to severe anemia can be identified (Figs. 19.1 and 19.2).

*Ultrasound assessment of the fetus is also helpful in detecting severe signs of hemolysis that have resulted in profound fetal anemia.* Occasionally, the first presenting signs of fetal hemolysis may be hydropic changes in the fetus including subcutaneous edema, pericardial and/or pleural effusions, and ascites. When these findings are identified and hydrops fetalis is diagnosed, the fetal hematocrit is typically <15%.

Regardless of the methods used to monitor pregnancies at risk for fetal anemia, all techniques are designed to determine the fetal hematocrit using indirect measures. *If the monitoring test indicates a risk for fetal anemia, or if hydrops is diagnosed, cordocentesis or **percutaneous umbilical blood sampling** (PUBS) is performed to directly measure the fetal hematocrit.* Under ultrasound guidance, a needle is advanced into the umbilical vein, a sample of fetal blood removed, and the hematocrit is measured. In general, the

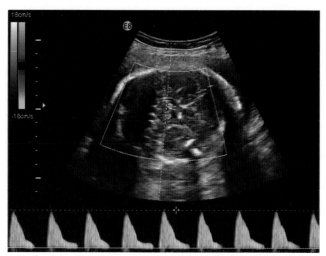

FIGURE 19.2. Image of fetal cerebral circulation demonstrating the middle cerebral artery and method of measuring peak flow. *PSV* = pressure supported ventilation.

average fetal hematocrit is 36% to 44% and, with severe anemia, it is less than 30% (Box 19.1). In addition to procedures to monitor the fetus for anemia, general tests for fetal well-being are indicated in all isoimmunized women with titers above the critical threshold, because the ability of an affected fetus, even if only mildly anemic, to withstand the stresses of pregnancy and labor may be compromised.

## MANAGEMENT

Previously, blood was transfused into the fetal abdominal cavity, where absorption of the red cells could take place over several days through the lymphatic channels.

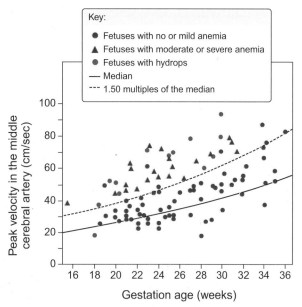

FIGURE 19.1. Peak velocity of systolic blood flow in the middle cerebral artery. Open circles indicate fetuses with no anemia or mild anemia; triangles indicate fetuses with moderate or severe anemia; and solid circles fetuses with hydrops. (From Mari G, Deter RL, Carpenter RL, et al. Noninvasive diagnosis by Doppler ultrasonography of fetal anemia due to maternal red-cell alloimmunization. Collaborative Group for Doppler Assessment of the Blood Velocity in Anemic Fetuses. *N Engl J Med.* 2000;342(1):9–14.)

---

> **BOX 19.1**
>
> **Evaluation of a Pregnancy With a Positive Maternal Antibody Screen**
>
> Maternal antibody identification and titer
> Careful obstetric history for prior affected fetus
>   Paternal antigen testing, possible fetal DNA testing
> Assessment of risk for fetal anemia if a critical titer is found or if there has been a prior affected child
>   Amniotic fluid bilirubin assessment
> Serial antibody titers, if first sensitized pregnancy
> Middle cerebral artery Doppler
> Ultrasound
> Cordocentesis/percutaneous umbilical blood sampling if monitoring test is abnormal

Currently, **transfusion** of antigen-negative red blood cells (depending on the blood group involved) to the fetus is indicated when PUBS determines that the fetus has moderate or severe anemia with a hematocrit less than 30%. *Direct transfusion under ultrasound guidance into the umbilical vein has become the preferred technique.* The procedure has a 1% to 3% risk of complications, including fetal death and preterm delivery, which must be weighed against the predicted course of the fetus if left untreated or delivered. The volume of red blood cells to be transfused can be calculated based on the gestational age, estimated fetal weight, the hematocrit of the unit of blood, and the difference between the current fetal hematocrit and the desired hematocrit. Because the transfused cells are antigen-negative, they are not subject to hemolysis by the maternal antibody and the predicted lifespan of the red cell is the only determinant of how long they persist in the fetal circulation. The timing and need for further transfusions can be based either on the predicted course given the severity of the disease, or on MCA Doppler assessments. After 2 to 3 transfusions, most of the circulating red cells in a fetus are transfused cells, as the hematopoietic system in the fetus has been suppressed.

## PREVENTION

Maternal exposure and subsequent sensitization to fetal blood usually occurs at delivery, but it can occur at any time during pregnancy. In the late 1960s, it was discovered that an antibody to the D antigen of the Rh system could be prepared from donors previously sensitized to the antigen. Administration of the **anti-D immune globulin** soon after delivery prevents an active antibody response to the D antigen by the mother in most cases.

> *Anti-D immune globulin is effective only for the D antigen of the Rh system. It is not effective in preventing sensitization to other Rh antigens or any other red cell antigens.*

It is now standard for Rh D-negative women who deliver Rh D-positive infants to receive a dose of 300 μg of anti-D immune globulin within 72 hours of delivery (Box 19.2). This practice reduces the risk of sensitization to the D antigen from around 16% to approximately 2%. The residual 2% risk is believed to result from sensitization occurring during the course of pregnancy, especially during the third trimester. *For this reason, it is standard practice to administer a 300-μg dose of anti-D immune globulin to all Rh D-negative women at about 28 weeks of gestation, unless it is certain that the father is Rh D-negative.* This prophylactic dose reduces the risk of sensitization from 2% to 0.2%. If there is any question regarding the need for prophylaxis, such as the certainty of paternity, anti-D immune globulin should be administered. Some authorities recommend that if

---

> **BOX 19.2**
> ### Indications for Anti-D Immune Globulin Administration in an Unsensitized Rh-Patient
>
> - At approximately 28 weeks of gestation
> - At time of procedures associated with possible fetal-to-maternal bleeding, such as amniocentesis or chorionic villus sampling
> - After ectopic pregnancy
> - After a threatened, spontaneous, or induced abortion
> - Within 72 hours of delivery of an Rh D-positive infant
> - Conditions associated with fetal-maternal hemorrhage (e.g., abdominal trauma, abruptio placentae)
> - Unexplained vaginal bleeding during pregnancy
>
> American College of Obstetricians and Gynecologists. *Guidelines for Perinatal Care.* 6th ed. Washington, DC: American College of Obstetricians and Gynecologists; 2007:104.

---

delivery has not occurred within 12 weeks of the injection at 28 weeks of gestation, a second 300 μg dose of anti-D immune globulin should be given.

*Because even a minute amount of fetal red cells can result in sensitization to the Rh D antigen, in any circumstance when a fetomaternal hemorrhage can occur, a prophylactic dose of 300 μg of anti-D immune globulin should be administered.* Each dose of anti-D immune globulin provides protection against sensitization for up to 30 mL of fetal blood or 15 mL of fetal red blood cells.

*In cases of trauma or bleeding during pregnancy in which there is a potential for more than a 30-mL fetomaternal transfusion, the extent of the fetomaternal hemorrhage can be assessed using the Kleihauer-Betke test.* This test identifies fetal erythrocytes in the maternal circulation. The number of fetal cells as a proportion of the total cells can be determined and the volume of fetomaternal hemorrhage can be estimated. Based on this estimation, the appropriate dose of Rh immune globulin can be determined. An indirect Coombs test can also be used to determine if the patient has received sufficient antibody. A positive test indicates that she has received an adequate dose.

## MANAGEMENT OF ISOIMMUNIZATION TO OTHER RED CELL ANTIGENS

Although the routine use of Rh immune globulin has decreased isoimmunization due to the D antigen, *iso-immunization due to other blood group antigens has proportionally increased.* The frequency of these antibodies varies depending on the frequency of the antigen in the general population and in various ethnic groups. In addition, the likelihood that these antibodies will result in significant fetal hemolytic disease depends on several factors, including the size of the sensitizing antigenic stimulus, the relative potency of the antigen, and the isoform (IgG or IgM) of antibody response.

Sensitization to any of these antigens can occur in any exposed women lacking the particular antigen, regardless of her ABO or Rh type. An antibody screen will detect the presence of these antibodies. *The most important cause of hemolytic disease of the fetus not associated with the D antigen is isoimmunization to the **Kell antigen*** (see Table 19.1). This sensitization commonly results from a prior blood transfusion. If a maternal antibody screen reveals the presence of an anti-Kell antibody, paternal blood typing for the Kell antigen should be performed. Because the direct phenotype of the erythrocyte for the Kell antigen and its complement—the Cellano antigen—can be performed, genotyping is not necessary. Ninety percent of individuals are Kell-negative, so if paternity is certain, no further evaluation is required. Even among those who carry the Kell antigen, 98% are heterozygous, so consideration should be given to fetal genotype determination.

Anemia resulting from Kell isoimmunization is unique in that the predominant effect of the antibody is destruction and suppression of hematopoietic precursor cells; hemolysis is only a minimal component of the fetal problem. For this reason, amniotic fluid surveillance of bilirubin may not be as useful in monitoring these pregnancies, and MCA Doppler is the preferred surveillance method. Most providers use a critical titer measurement of 1:8 to initiate further evaluation in Kell-sensitized pregnancies.

***ABO hemolytic disease,*** *due to maternal-fetal incompatibility for the major blood group antigens, can occur.* It is usually associated with mild fetal and newborn hyperbilirubinemia. Typically, it is not associated with severe fetal disease, because there are fewer A and B antigenic sites on fetal red blood cells than on adult blood cells. In addition, much of the anti-A and anti-B antibody produced is of the IgM isoform that does not cross the placenta to any extent.

## SUGGESTED READINGS

American College of Obstetricians and Gynecologists. Management of alloimmunization during pregnancy. ACOG Practice Bulletin No. 75. *Obstet Gynecol.* 2006;108(2):457–464.

American College of Obstetricians and Gynecologists. Prevention of Rh D Alloimmunization. ACOG Practice Bulletin 4. Washington, DC: American College of Obstetricians and Gynecologists; 1999.

# CHAPTER

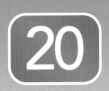

# Preterm Labor

**P**reterm birth is delivery that occurs prior to the completion of 37 weeks (259 days) of gestation. Because it is the most common cause of perinatal morbidity and mortality in the United States, prevention and treatment of preterm birth is a major focus of obstetric care. The consequences of preterm birth occur with increasing severity and frequency the earlier the gestational age of the newborn. In addition to perinatal death in the very young fetus, common complications of preterm birth include respiratory distress syndrome, intraventricular hemorrhage, necrotizing enterocolitis, sepsis, neurologic impairment, and seizures. Long-term morbidity associated with preterm delivery includes bronchopulmonary dysplasia and developmental abnormalities, including cerebral palsy. *The 11% to 12% of babies born prematurely account for 75% of all perinatal mortality and 50% of long-term neurologic impairment in children in the United States.*

Preterm births may be classified into two general presentations: **spontaneous** and **indicated.** Approximately 40% to 50% of preterm births result from spontaneous preterm labor with intact membranes; 25% to 40% result from preterm premature rupture of membranes (PROM) (see Chapter 22, Premature Rupture of Membranes). The remaining 20% to 30% occur following deliberate intervention for a variety of maternal or obstetric complications (e.g., eclampsia).

*Preterm labor is defined as the presence of regular uterine contractions that occur before 37 weeks of gestation and are associated with cervical changes.* It is often difficult to diagnose preterm labor because of the absence of definitive measurements. The lack of diagnostic criteria presents a problem, because treatment appears to be more effective when initiated early in the course of preterm labor.

## CAUSE, PREDICTION, AND PREVENTION OF PRETERM LABOR

### Causes

Preterm labor may represent a final common pathway for a number of pathogenic processes. The four main processes include: (1) activation of the maternal or fetal hypothalamic-pituitary-adrenal axis due to maternal or fetal stress, (2) decidual-chorioamniotic or systemic inflammation caused by infection, (3) decidual hemorrhage, or (4) pathologic uterine distention (Fig. 20.1). Numerous risk factors have been associated with preterm labor (Box 20.1). *The strongest risk factor is multifetal gestation.* With a prior preterm birth, the risk in a subsequent pregnancy increases and continues to increase with each subsequent pregnancy. African-American women have higher rates of preterm birth associated with preterm labor or preterm PROM, compared with other racial and ethnic groups. Subclinical intra-amniotic infection has also been associated with preterm labor and preterm PROM, especially when it occurs at earlier gestational ages. *In most cases, however, no cause or risk factor for preterm labor can be identified.*

Despite the lack of effective strategies to predict and prevent preterm labor, infant morbidity and mortality following preterm birth have decreased over the last several decades as the result of several factors. First, neonatal intensive care management of preterm infants has greatly improved outcomes. Therefore, maternal transport to a regional tertiary-care center is indicated for women in preterm labor presenting to hospitals without sophisticated neonatal intensive care. Second, the use of corticosteroids administered to a mother at immediate risk for preterm birth (such as a woman in preterm labor) has resulted in decreased incidence of respiratory distress

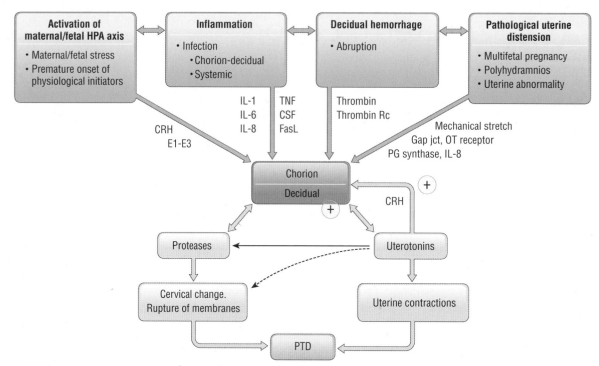

FIGURE 20.1. Preterm labor: Final common pathway. The four main processes include activation of the maternal or fetal hypothalamic-pituitary-adrenal axis (HPA), infection, decidual hemorrhage, and pathologic uterine distention. CRH = corticotropin-releasing hormone; CSF = colony-stimulating factor; E1= estrone, E3 = estriol; fasL = FAS ligand; IL = interleukin; jct = junction; OT = oxytocin receptor; PG = prostaglandin; PTD = preterm delivery; TNF = tumor necrosis factor.

### BOX 20.1
### Factors Associated With Preterm Labor

Prior history of preterm birth
Preterm uterine contractions
Premature rupture of membranes (PROM)
African-American race
Cervical insufficiency
- Primary
- Secondary to surgery (e.g., cone biopsy of cervix)
Infections
- Urinary
- Bacterial vaginosis
- Intra-amniotic
Excessive uterine enlargement
- Polyhydramnios
- Multiple gestation
Uterine distortion
- Leiomyomas
- Septate uterus, uterine didelphys, and other anomalies
Placental abnormalities
- Placental abruption
- Placenta previa
Maternal smoking (associated with PROM)
Iatrogenic: induction of labor

syndrome, intraventricular hemorrhage, and associated infant morbidity and mortality. A major goal of therapy to stop contractions in a woman in preterm labor (**tocolytic therapy**) is to prolong pregnancy for up to 48 hours in order to allow time to administer corticosteroids. Finally, prophylaxis against perinatal infection with group B streptococcus in women with preterm labor or preterm PROM has also decreased infant morbidity and mortality rates in the United States.

## Prediction of Preterm Labor

Patient and physician education has focused on recognition of the signs and symptoms that suggest preterm labor (Box 20.2). Patients with symptoms are counseled to seek prompt medical attention.

A number of factors are used to assess signs and symptoms and diagnose potential preterm labor. *An increase in the concentration of **fetal fibronectin** (fFN) in cervicovaginal secretions is found with preterm labor*. Fetal fibronectin is an extracellular glycoprotein normally found in the cervical mucus in early pregnancy and then again near term. A preterm rise in the concentration of fFN may be associated with an increased likelihood of birth between 22 and 34 weeks of gestation and birth within 7–14 days of the test. However, data combined from several studies reveal that the positive predictive value for delivery within a week is only 18%.

## BOX 20.2
### Symptoms and Signs of Preterm Labor

Menstrual-like cramps
Low, dull backache
Abdominal pressure
Pelvic pressure
Abdominal cramping (with or without diarrhea)
Increase or change in vaginal discharge (mucous, watery, light bloody discharge)
Uterine contractions, often painless

*The greatest benefit of fFN appears to be its negative predictive value: if fFN is absent (negative) in cervicovaginal secretions, the likelihood of delivery in the next 7 days is very low.*

Cervical length can also be used as a diagnostic factor. *As cervical length decreases in midpregnancy, the risk for preterm birth has been shown to increase in a continuous fashion.* **Transvaginal ultrasound** examination of the cervix is a reliable and reproducible method to assess cervical length. This test may be most helpful when evaluating women at high risk for recurrent preterm birth, those with uterine anomalies, and those who have had prior cervical cone biopsy or multiple dilation and curettage/evacuation procedures.

*Early asymptomatic dilation and effacement of the cervix* (**cervical insufficiency**) *may be associated with an increased likelihood of preterm labor and delivery.* Interventions such as prophylactic cervical cerclage (see Chapter 32, Gynecologic Procedures) on sonographic recognition of a shortened cervical length (often defined as less than 2.5 cm) has not improved outcomes.

**Bacterial vaginosis (BV)** is a common alteration of the vaginal flora that occurs in up to 40% of pregnant women and is associated with preterm labor and preterm PROM. *BV diagnosed in symptomatic pregnant patients should thus be treated.* Widespread screening and treatment for bacterial vaginosis in asymptomatic low-risk women and women with previous preterm birth has not been beneficial in decreasing the occurrence of preterm labor and is not recommended. *Treatment for BV may be considered for women at high risk for preterm labor.*

## Prevention

*There are currently no uniformly effective interventions to prevent preterm labor, regardless of risk factors.* Prophylactic therapy—including tocolytic drugs, bed rest, hydration, and sedation in asymptomatic women at high risk for preterm labor—has not been shown to be effective. However, in a select group of women at very high risk who have a documented history of preterm birth, the use of weekly intramuscular injections of progesterone (17-$\alpha$-hydroxyprogesterone caproate) starting at 16–20 weeks of gestation and continuing until 36 weeks appears to reduce spontaneous preterm birth. Vaginal progesterone supplementation in women with an ultrasonically determined shortened cervical length has also shown some benefit.

## EVALUATION OF A PATIENT IN SUSPECTED PRETERM LABOR

Prompt evaluation is critical in the patient who describes symptoms and signs suggestive of preterm labor. Use of an external electronic fetal monitor (**tocodynamometer**) may help to quantify the frequency and duration of contractions. The status of the cervix should be determined, either by visualization with a speculum or by gentle digital examination. Because digital examination may increase the risk of infection in the setting of PROM, speculum evaluation to assess cervical dilation and effacement should be performed first if there is suspicion of rupture of fetal membranes. Changes in cervical effacement and dilation on subsequent examinations are important in the evaluation of both the diagnosis of preterm labor, as well as the effectiveness of management. *Subtle changes are often of great clinical importance, so serial examinations by the same examiner are optimal, when this is possible.*

Because urinary infections can predispose a patient to uterine contractions, a urinalysis and urine culture should be obtained. A vaginal/rectal culture should be obtained for group B streptococcus (GBS). *Women with GBS bacteriuria are candidates for intrapartum antibiotic prophylaxis.* When indicated by history or physical examination findings, cultures for *Chlamydia* and *Neisseria gonorrhoeae* should be obtained.

Ultrasound examination is useful in assessing the gestational age of the fetus, estimation of the amniotic fluid volume (spontaneous rupture of membranes with fluid loss may precede preterm labor and may be unrecognized by the patient), fetal presentation, and placental location, as well as the existence of fetal congenital anomalies. *Patients should also be monitored for bleeding, as placental abruption and placenta previa may be associated with preterm labor* (see Chapter 21, Third-Trimester Bleeding).

Information concerning the length of the cervix can be obtained through ultrasound examination, although results are not particularly helpful unless the gestational age is less than 26 weeks. *Amniocentesis may be performed to assess for intra-amniotic infection.* Either clinical or subclinical infection of the amniotic cavity (chorioamnionitis) is thought to be associated with preterm labor. Amniotic fluid can be evaluated for the presence of bacteria, white blood cells, lactate dehydrogenase, and glucose. Evidence of white cells in the amniotic fluid, decreased glucose or elevated lactate dehydrogenase may indicate infection.

The presence of bacteria in amniotic fluid is correlated not only with preterm labor but also with the subsequent development of infection. A high suspicion of intrauterine infection should prompt delivery regardless of the gestational age. Tocolysis is not appropriate in the setting of intrauterine infection. At the time of amniocentesis, additional amniotic fluid may be obtained for fetal pulmonary maturity studies, which could influence subsequent management.

## MANAGEMENT OF PRETERM LABOR

*The purpose in treating preterm labor is to delay delivery, if possible, until fetal maturity is attained.*

Management involves two broad goals: (1) the detection and treatment of disorders associated with preterm labor, and (2) therapy for the preterm labor itself. *Fortunately, more than 50% of patients with preterm contractions have spontaneous resolution of abnormal uterine activity.* However, this complicates the evaluation of effectiveness of specific treatments, because it is unclear if the contractions would have resolved spontaneously or if their cessation was due to effective treatments.

Various tocolytic therapies have been used in the management of preterm labor (Table 20.1). Tocolytics have not been shown to prolong pregnancy beyond several days (only 2 to 7). Different treatment regimens address specific mechanisms involved in the maintenance of uterine contractions, and each, therefore, may be best suited for certain patients.

*Typically, patients with a diagnosis of preterm labor receive one form of tocolytic therapy, with the addition or substitution of other medications if the initial treatment is considered unsuccessful.*

Magnesium sulfate has been the most frequently used agent, but use of nifedipine is increasing. Evidence as to efficacy beyond several days is weak, but often management allows for administration of corticosteroid therapy. Adverse side effects, at times serious and even life-threatening to the mother, can occur. The gestational age of the fetus is always a consideration in deciding how vigorously to pursue therapy. For example, maternal risks may be more acceptable when treating a 26-week fetus as compared to a 32-week fetus.

Contraindications to tocolysis include conditions in which the adverse effects of tocolysis may be significant, such as advanced labor, a mature fetus, a severely anomalous fetus (from lethal congenital or chromosomal abnor-

### TABLE 20.1    Agents Used in Treating Preterm Labor

| Class (Example) | Action | Adverse Effects | Comments |
|---|---|---|---|
| Magnesium sulfate | Competes with calcium for entry into cells | May cause flushing or headaches; at high levels may cause respiratory or cardiac depression | High degree of safety; often used as first agent; contraindicated in patients with hypocalcemia or who have myasthenia gravis |
| Prostaglandin synthetase inhibitors (indomethacin) | Decreases PG production by blocking conversion of free arachidonic acid to PG | Premature constriction of ductus arteriosus possible especially after 34 weeks; reversible impaired fetal renal function and oligohydramnios with prolonged exposure (≥72 hours) | Second-line therapy |
| Calcium-channel blockers (nifedipine) | Prevents calcium entry into muscle cells | Hypotension and headache; possible decrease in uteroplacental blood flow, fetal hypoxia, and hypercarbia | May potentiate side effects of magnesium sulfate |
| β-adrenergic agents (ritodrine, terbutaline) | Increases cAMP concentration in cells, which decreases free calcium | Hypotension, tachycardia, anxiety, chest tightening or pain, ECG changes; increased pulmonary edema occurs very infrequently but is possible, especially with fluid overload; relatively contraindicated in patients with coronary artery disease and in those with renal failure | Less commonly used due to side effects |

cAMP, cyclic adenosine monophosphate; ECG, electrocardiogram; PG, prostaglandin.

malities), intrauterine infection, significant vaginal bleeding, and severe preeclampsia. In addition, a variety of obstetric complications, such as placental abruption, advanced cervical dilatation, or evidence of fetal compromise or placental insufficiency, may contraindicate delay in delivery.

From 24 to 32 to 34 weeks of gestation, management generally includes administration of **corticosteroids** (betamethasone or dexamethasone) to enhance fetal pulmonary maturity. *A single course of corticosteroids should be given to pregnant women between 24 and 32 weeks of gestation who are at risk of preterm delivery.* Both the incidence and severity of fetal respiratory distress syndrome are reduced with such therapy. Between 32 and 34 weeks of gestation,

the use of steroids to enhance fetal lung maturity is less certain. In addition, other sequelae of prematurity, such as interventricular hemorrhage and necrotizing enterocolitis, occur less frequently in infants whose mothers received corticosteroid therapy. Maximal benefit to the fetus occurs if the therapy is administered within 7 days of delivery; however, routine weekly courses are not recommended because of potential negative fetal effects.

## SUGGESTED READING

American College of Obstetricians and Gynecologists. Management of preterm labor. ACOG Practice Bulletin No. 43. *Obstet Gynecol.* 2003;101(5):1039–1047.

# 21 Third-Trimester Bleeding

---

**Topic 23:** Third-Trimester Bleeding

Students should be able to list the causes of bleeding in the third trimester, describe their evaluation and management, and discuss the maternal and fetal effects of such bleeding. They should also be able to describe the management of acute blood loss, including the proper use of blood and blood products.

---

Approximately 4% to 5% of pregnancies are complicated by vaginal bleeding in the third trimester. Bleeding ranges from spotting to life-threatening hemorrhage. Intercourse and recent pelvic examinations are common precipitants of spotting, as the cervix is more vascular and friable in pregnancy. Twenty percent of cardiac output is shunted to the pregnant uterus, so significant bleeding can be quickly catastrophic. Severe hemorrhage is much less common than spotting, but remains a leading cause of maternal and fetal morbidity and mortality. *The two most common causes of significant bleeding are placenta previa (in which the placenta is located close to or over the cervical os) and placental abruption (premature separation of the placenta).* Other important causes of bleeding are preterm cervical change, preterm labor, and uterine rupture (see Chapters 20, Preterm Labor, and 22, Premature Rupture of Membranes). In many cases, bleeding remains unexplained or is attributed to local lesions. Possible causes of third-trimester bleeding are listed in Box 21.1.

A focused but comprehensive history and physical exam are crucial in assessing obstetric bleeding once the patient is stable and a reassuring fetal heart rate pattern is confirmed. While diagnosis is rarely based solely on history, a differential diagnosis is usually possible after pertinent information has been gathered. It is always important to quantify bleeding and associated symptoms, such as abdominal pain. A personal or family history of bleeding with procedures may lead to a diagnosis of a bleeding disorder, whereas a history of cervical dysplasia and no recent pap tests would be worrisome for cervical cancer. It is also important to consider other origins of bleeding, such as hemorrhoids or bladder disorders.

A physical examination should always begin with vital signs. The fetal heart rate should be auscultated either by Doppler or electronic fetal monitor. A general review of respiratory and cardiovascular systems is warranted in all patients. Intravenous access should be established if the bleeding is heavy, estimated blood loss is significant, or the patient is unstable. A brief inspection for **petechiae** or **bruising** may be indicated if there is suspicion of a bleeding disorder. Particular attention should be paid to the abdomen and pelvis.

*Pelvic examination should not be undertaken until placental position is confirmed, as this could cause significant bleeding in a patient with placenta previa.*

Careful inspection of the vulva should be followed by a speculum examination of the vagina and cervix.

A common finding in pregnancy is a significant **ectropion** of the cervix, particularly among women with a history of using oral contraceptives. The ectropion is an area on the ectocervix where columnar epithelium has been exposed to vaginal acidity due to eversion of the endocervix. The ectropion may appear reddened and "raw looking." These findings may raise concerns about cancer, but they are actually benign.

Significant bleeding requires immediate management, including ongoing monitoring of vital signs and two large bore intravenous lines for administration of crystalloid fluid. Blood studies should include complete blood count, coagulation profile, and a type and cross match for 4 units. Regardless of the amount of bleeding, blood type and screen are necessary. *Patients who are Rh D-negative may require immunoglobulin to protect against the Rh D antigen and a **Kleihauer-Betke test** or other test to determine feto—maternal bleeding should be performed to determine the amount of immunoglobulin needed once the bleeding has been controlled* (see Chapter 20, Preterm Labor). Staff should be ready for delivery. Most likely, this will require an emergency caesarean delivery and, possibly, a general anesthetic. If the bleeding is not sufficient to warrant emergency delivery and/or the fetus is preterm, then blood studies should be continued and intervenous access maintained. An ultrasound examination should be performed to assess placental location and condition of the fetus. The patient should be admitted to the hospital to allow for close monitoring.

## PLACENTA PREVIA

*Placenta previa is a placental location close to or over the internal cervical os.* It can be classified as **complete,** in which the placenta completely covers the internal os, or **partial,** in which the placenta overlies part but not all of the internal os. A placenta that extends into the lower uterine segment but does not reach the internal os is called a **low-lying placenta.** (Fig. 21.1.)

> *Placenta previa classically presents with painless bleeding in the third trimester.*

In many cases there may be small amounts of bleeding prior to a more significant episode of bleeding. About 75% of women with placenta previa will have at least one episode of bleeding. On average this episode occurs at around 29 to 30 weeks of gestation. In general, placenta previa occurs in about 1 in 200 pregnancies. The incidence of placenta previa earlier in pregnancy (approximately 24 weeks) is 4% to 5% and decreases with increasing gestational age.

Complete placenta previa rarely resolves spontaneously, but partial and low-lying placenta previa will often resolve by 32 to 35 weeks of gestation. The mechanism does not involve an upward "migration" of the placenta, but rather a stretching and thinning of the lower uterine segment, which effectively moves the placenta away from the os.

**Transvaginal ultrasonography** is more accurate in diagnosing placenta previa than abdominal ultrasonography, which gives many false-positive results, particularly when the placenta is located posteriorly (Fig. 21.2). The etiology of placenta previa is not known; however, it may be associated with abnormal vascularization. **Risk factors** for placenta previa include placenta previa in a prior pregnancy (4% to 8% recurrence), prior cesarean delivery or other uterine surgery, multiparity, advanced maternal age, cocaine use, and smoking. Placenta previa has been associated with an increase in fetal anomalies, although the precise mechanism is unclear. These anomalies include severe cardiovascular, central nervous system, gastrointestinal, and respiratory abnormalities.

Bleeding usually ceases in 1 to 2 hours. Close observation, fluid administration, bed rest, and administration of steroids for fetal lung maturity may be appropriate if the fetus is premature and the bleeding is not heavy enough to warrant immediate delivery. The bleeding is usually painless, except when it is associated with labor or abruption (the premature separation of the placenta; see Table 21.1 for a comparison of placenta previa and placental abruption). *For patients in a stable condition, outpatient management may be considered if the patient is compliant, lives close to the hospital, and has someone with her at all times.* If the bleeding is severe or the fetus is at term, then delivery is appropriate.

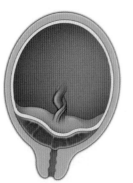 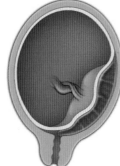 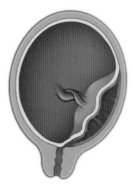 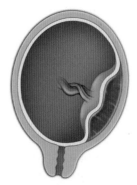

Complete       Partial       Marginal       Low lying

FIGURE 21.1.  Placenta previa. (Adapted from Oyelese Y, Smulian JC. Placenta previa, accreta, and vasa previa. *Obstet Gynecol.* 2006;10(4):927.)

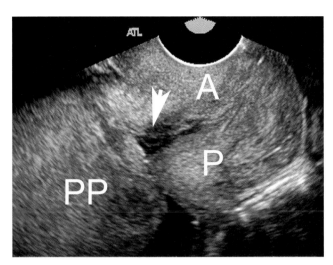

FIGURE 21.2. Transvaginal sonogram of a complete placenta previa *(PP)*. Note that both the placenta and the internal cervical os *(arrow)* are clearly depicted. *A,* anterior lip of cervix; *P,* posterior lip of cervix. The placenta just overlaps the internal os. (From Oyelese Y, Smulian JC. Placenta previa, accreta, and vasa previa. *Obstet Gynecol.* 2006;107(4):927.)

Placenta previa is associated with an increase in preterm birth and perinatal mortality and morbidity. Delivery is most often via caesarean birth. In a patient whose condition is stable, caesarean delivery can be undertaken at 36 to 37 weeks of gestation, following amniocentesis to confirm fetal lung maturity. If lung maturity is not demonstrated, the patient should be delivered at 37 to 38 weeks of gestation. Earlier caesarean delivery may be required if bleeding occurs or if the patient goes into labor. The number of bleeding episodes is unrelated to the degree of placenta previa or to fetal outcome.

Complications of placenta previa also include increased bleeding from the lower uterine segment where the placenta was attached at the time of cesarean delivery. The placenta may also be abnormally adherent to the uterine wall. This is termed **placenta accreta** if the placental tissue extends into the superficial layer of the myometrium, **placenta increta** if it extends further into the myometrium, or **placenta percreta** if it extends completely through the myometrium to the serosa, and sometimes into adjacent organs such as the bladder. The incidence of placenta accreta is about 1 in 2500 deliveries, but increases in patients with a history of cesarean delivery. The risk of requiring hysterectomy following a caesarean delivery for patients with placenta previa is increased, which in turn increases the risk of maternal and perinatal morbidity and mortality.

## PLACENTAL ABRUPTION

*Placental abruption refers to an abnormal premature separation of an otherwise normally implanted placenta.* There are various types of abruption, depending upon the extent and region of separation. A **complete abruption** occurs when the entire placenta separates. A **partial abruption** exists when part of the placenta separates from the uterine wall. A **marginal abruption** occurs when the separation is limited to the edge of the placenta (Fig. 21.3). A significant abruption requiring delivery occurs in 1% of births.

Abruption occurs when bleeding in the decidua basalis causes separation of the placenta and further bleeding. The classic presentation of abruption is vaginal bleeding with abdominal pain. Smaller or marginal abruptions may present with bleeding only. **Concealed hemorrhage** occurs when blood is trapped behind the placenta and is unable to exit. Painful uterine contractions, significant fetal heart rate abnormalities, and fetal demise may occur in severe cases.

Risk factors for placental abruption include chronic hypertension, preeclampsia, multiple gestation, advanced maternal age, multiparity, smoking, cocaine use, preeclampsia, and chorioamnionitis. Trauma is also a major risk factor.

| TABLE 21.1 | Characteristics of Placenta Previa and Placental Abruption | |
|---|---|---|
| **Characteristic** | **Placenta Previa** | **Placental Abruption** |
| Magnitude of blood loss | Variable | Variable |
| Duration | Often ceases within 1–2 hours | Usually continuous |
| Abdominal discomfort | None | Can be severe |
| Fetal heart rate pattern on electronic monitoring | Normal | Tachycardia, then bradycardia; loss of variability; decelerations frequently present; intrauterine demise not rare |
| Coagulation defects | Rare | Associated, but infrequent; DIC often severe when present |
| Associated history | None | Cocaine use; abdominal trauma; maternal hypertension; multiple gestation; polyhydramnios |

DIC = disseminated intravascular coagulation.

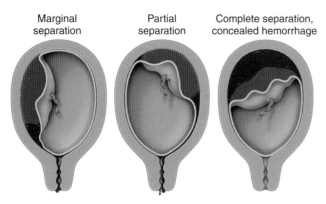

FIGURE 21.3. Types of placental abruption. Note that vaginal bleeding is absent when the hemorrhage is concealed.

Abruption in a prior pregnancy increases the risk of abruption in subsequent pregnancy by 15- to 20-fold.

*An elevated second-trimester maternal serum alpha-fetoprotein (AFP) level may be associated with up to a 10-fold increased risk of placental abruption due to possible entry of AFP into the maternal circulation through the placental uterine interface.*

Abruption is often diagnosed by clinical examination, although an ultrasound examination may be useful in less severe cases not requiring immediate delivery. Abruption may occur in the absence of ultrasound findings.

**Management** of patients with placental abruption includes monitoring of vital signs, fluid administration, and delivery for severe hemorrhage. Expectant management may be appropriate for preterm patients with less severe abruptions and minimal bleeding. Delivery is often by cesarean birth. Rarely, blood penetrates the uterus to such an extent that the serosa becomes blue or purple in color. This condition is called **Couvelaire uterus.** A Kleihauer-Betke or similar test is essential to determine the amount of fetal–maternal hemorrhage. Results guide decisions regarding administration of Rh D immunoglobulin in women who are Rh D-negative and determine the need for blood transfusion in the potentially anemic neonate. Coagulation abnormalities may also be associated with abruption (see Table 21.1). Abruption is the most common cause of coagulopathy in pregnancy. Platelet counts may be low and prothrombin time and partial thromboplastin time may be increased. Serum fibrinogen may also be depleted. Disseminated intravascular coagulation is a rare but extremely serious complication.

## VASA PREVIA

*Vasa previa describes the passage of fetal blood vessels over the internal os below the presenting part of the fetus.* It can occur with a **velamentous insertion,** in which the fetal blood vessels insert into the membranes between the amnion and chorion instead of into the placenta and are not protected by Wharton jelly (Fig. 21.4), or when there is a succenturiate lobe across the os from the main placenta. Vasa previa occurs in 1 in 2500 pregnancies. Rupture of a fetal vessel occurs rarely in pregnancy, but the risk is greatest with vasa previa. Rupture of a vessel can quickly lead to fetal death, as fetal blood volume is so small. Fetal mortality approaches 60% if rupture is not detected before delivery. When performing artificial rupture of membranes, it is important to ensure that no pulsating vessels are present which may represent a vasa previa.

*An **Apt test** can help distinguish fetal blood from maternal blood.*

This test mixes the blood specimen with water to achieve hemolysis. The centrifuged supernatant is mixed with sodium hydroxide (NaOH). Fetal blood remains pink and maternal blood turns yellow-brown.

## UTERINE RUPTURE

Most cases of uterine rupture occur in the site of a prior cesarean delivery. **Uteran rupture** describes a spontaneous

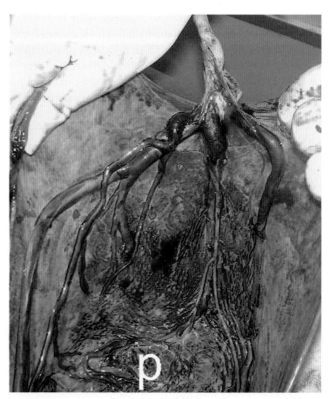

FIGURE 21.4. Vasa previa. Vessels are seen running unprotected through the membranes. *p*, placenta (From Oyelese Y, Smulian JC. Placenta previa, accreta, and vasa previa. *Obstet Gynecol.* 2006;107(4):927.)

complete transection of the uterus from endometrium to serosa. If the peritoneum remains intact, it is referred to as a **partial rupture** or **uterine dehiscence.** With complete rupture and fetal expulsion into the abdomen, mortality ranges from 50% to 75%. Fetal survival depends in large part on whether the placenta remains attached to the uterine wall. Cesarean delivery is imperative to ensure neonatal survival and decrease maternal morbidity.

## SUGGESTED READING

Oyelese Y, Smulian JC. Placenta previa, accreta, and vasa previa. *Obstet Gynecol.* 2006;10(4):927.

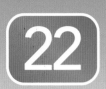

# Premature Rupture of Membranes

This chapter deals primarily with APGO Educational Topic:

**Topic 25:** Premature Rupture of Membranes

Students should be able to explain the risk factors associated with premature rupture of the membranes, its diagnosis by physical examination and laboratory study, and expectant versus immediate delivery managements. They should also be able to explain the risks and benefits for mother and infant from each kind of management and how to counsel patients about them.

A mniotic fluid is normally produced continuously, and after approximately 16 weeks' gestation is predominantly dependent on fetal urine production. However, passage of fluid across the fetal membranes, across the skin, and across the umbilical cord, as well as fetal saliva production and fetal pulmonary effluent, also contribute. Amniotic fluid protects against infection, fetal trauma, and umbilical cord compression. It also allows for fetal movement and fetal breathing, which, in turn, permits fetal lung, chest, and skeletal development. Decreased or absent amniotic fluid can lead to compression of the umbilical cord and decreased placental blood flow. Disruption (rupture) of the fetal membranes is associated with loss of protective effects and developmental roles of amniotic fluid.

*Premature rupture of membranes (PROM)* is the rupture of the chorioamnionic membrane before the onset of labor. PROM occurs in approximately 12% of all pregnancies. PROM is associated with about 8% of term pregnancies (37 weeks or more of gestational age) and is generally followed by the onset of labor. *Preterm PROM, defined as PROM that occurs before 37 weeks of gestation, is a leading cause of neonatal morbidity and mortality, and is associated with approximately 30% of preterm deliveries.* PROM leading to preterm delivery is associated with neonatal complications of prematurity such as respiratory distress syndrome, intraventricular hemorrhage, neonatal infection, necrotizing enterocolitis, neurologic and neuromuscular dysfunction, and sepsis. *The major complication of PROM is intrauterine infection.* The presence of lower genital tract infections with *Neisseria gonorrhoeae* and group B streptococcus as well as bacterial vaginosis increase the risk of intrauterine infection associated with PROM. Other complications include prolapsed umbilical cord and abruptio placentae.

Consequences of preterm PROM depend on the gestational age at the time of occurrence. Midtrimester preterm PROM (between 16 and 26 weeks of gestational age) complicates about 1% of all pregnancies. PROM that occurs early in pregnancy following midtrimester genetic amniocentesis is very likely to seal with reaccumulation of amniotic fluid. Persistent oligohydramnios at <22 weeks of gestation is associated with incomplete alveolar development and the development of pulmonary hypoplasia. *Survival is likely in the 24-week to 26-week group, although the morbidities of extreme prematurity in this group of neonates are more substantial.* Infants born with pulmonary hypoplasia cannot be adequately ventilated, regardless of the gestational age at birth, and soon succumb to hypoxia and barotrauma from high-pressure ventilation.

## ETIOLOGY

The cause of PROM is not clearly understood. Sexually transmitted diseases and other lower genital tract conditions, such as bacterial vaginosis, may play a role, as such infections are more commonly found in women with PROM than in those without sexually transmitted disease or bacterial vaginosis. However, intact fetal membranes and normal amniotic fluid do not fully protect the fetus from infection, because it appears that subclinical intraamniotic infection may contribute to PROM. Metabolites produced by bacteria and inflammatory mediators may either weaken the fetal membranes or initiate uterine contractions through stimulating prostaglandin synthesis. *The risk of PROM is at least doubled in women who smoke during pregnancy. Other risk factors for PROM include prior PROM (approximately twofold), short cervical length, prior preterm delivery, hydramnios, multiple gestations, and bleeding in early pregnancy (threatened abortion).* There is an inverse relationship between gestational age and latency (time from PROM until delivery). It also appears that the more severe the resilient oligohydramnios, the greater the risk of infection and, consequently, the shorter the latency.

**Chorioamnionitis,** infection of the fetal membranes and amniotic fluid, poses a major threat to the mother and fetus. Fetal sepsis is associated with an increased risk for morbidity, particularly neurologic abnormalities such as periventricular leukomalacia and cerebral palsy. This seems to be associated with inflammatory mediators in the fetal environment. Patients with intra-amniotic infection often experience significant fever (≥100.5°F), tachycardia (maternal and fetal), and uterine tenderness. Purulent cervical discharge is usually a very late finding. The maternal white blood cell (WBC) count is generally elevated, but this finding is nonspecific in pregnancy and may be the result of antenatal corticosteroids administration and may be misleading. Patients with chorioamnionitis frequently enter spontaneous and often dysfunctional labor. Once the diagnosis of chorioamnionitis is made, treatment consists of intravenous antibiotic therapy and prompt delivery, either by induction or augmentation of labor, if needed, or cesarean delivery, either for a primary indication or if vaginal delivery is expected to be substantially delayed.

## DIAGNOSIS

> *Fluid passing through the vagina must be presumed to be amniotic fluid until proved otherwise.*

At times, patients describe a "gush" of fluid, whereas at other times they note a history of steady leakage of small amounts of fluid. Intermittent urinary leakage is common during pregnancy, especially near term, and this can be confused with PROM. Likewise, the normally increased vaginal secretions in pregnancy as well as perineal moisture (especially in hot weather) may be mistaken for amniotic fluid.

The **nitrazine test** uses pH to distinguish amniotic fluid from urine and vaginal secretions. Amniotic fluid is alkaline, having a pH above 7.1; vaginal secretions have a pH of 4.5 to 6.0, and urine has a pH of ≤6.0. To perform the nitrazine test, a sample of fluid obtained from the vagina during a speculum examination is placed on a strip of nitrazine paper. If the pH is 7.1 to 7.3, reflecting that of amniotic fluid, the paper turns dark blue. Cervical mucus, blood, and semen are possible causes of false-positive results (Table 22.1).

The **fern test** is also used to distinguish amniotic fluid from other fluids. It is named for the pattern of arborization that occurs when amniotic fluid is placed on a slide and is allowed to dry in room air. The resultant pattern, which resembles the leaves of a fern plant, is caused by the sodium chloride content of the amniotic fluid. The ferning pattern from amniotic fluid is fine, with multiple branches, as shown in Figure 22.1; cervical mucus does not fern or, if it does, the pattern is thick with much less branching. This test is considered more indicative of rup-

| TABLE 22.1 | Causes of False–Positive and False–Negative Nitrazine Tests | |
|---|---|
| **False–Positive** | **False–Negative** |
| Basic urine | Remote PROM with no residual fluid |
| Semen | Minimal amniotic fluid leakage |
| Cervical mucus | |
| Blood contamination | |
| Some antiseptic solutions | |
| Vaginitis (especially trichomonas) | |

PROM, premature rupture of membrane.

tured membranes than the nitrazine test, but as with any test it is not 100% reliable.

Ultrasonography can be helpful in evaluating the possibility of rupture of membranes. If ample amniotic fluid around the fetus is visible on ultrasound examination, the diagnosis of PROM must be questioned. However, if the amount of amniotic fluid leakage is small, sufficient amniotic fluid will still be visible on scan. When there is less than the expected amount of fluid seen on ultrasound, the differential diagnosis of oligohydramnios, including PROM must be considered. *When the clinical history or physical examination is unclear, membrane rupture can be diagnosed unequivocally with ultrasonographically guided transabdominal instillation of indigo carmine dye, followed by observation for passage of blue fluid from the vagina.* This procedure is performed very infrequently, however.

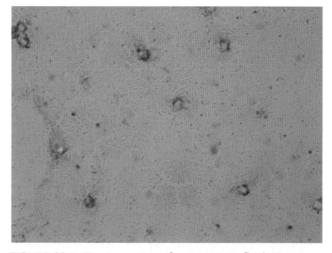

FIGURE 22.1. Ferning pattern from amniotic fluid. (Courtesy of Dr. Dwight Rouse. Scott JR, Gibbs RS, Karlan BY, Haney AH. *Danforth's Obstetrics and Gynecology.* 9th ed. Philadelphia, PA: Lippincott Williams & Wilkins; 2003:40.)

The **differential diagnoses** for PROM include urinary incontinence, increased vaginal secretions in pregnancy (physiologic), increased cervical discharge (pathologic, e.g., infection), exogenous fluids (such as semen or douche), and vesicovaginal fistula.

## EVALUATION AND MANAGEMENT

Factors to be considered in the management of the patient with PROM include the gestational age at the time of rupture, assessment of fetal well-being, the presence of uterine contractions, the likelihood of chorioamnionitis, the amount of amniotic fluid around the fetus, and the degree of fetal maturity. These management factors, together with the patient's history, must be carefully evaluated for information relevant to the diagnosis and approach. Abdominal examination includes palpation of the uterus for tenderness and fundal height measurement for evaluation of gestational age and fetal lie.

A sterile speculum examination is performed to assess the likelihood of vaginal infection and to obtain cervical or vaginal cultures for *N. gonorrhoeae*, β-hemolytic streptococcus, and *Chlamydia trachomatis*. The cervix is visualized for its degree of dilation as well as for the presence of free-flowing amniotic fluid. Fluid is obtained from the vaginal vault for nitrazine and/or fern testing. Because of the risk of infection, **digital examination** should be kept to a minimum and is best avoided until the patient is in active labor.

Ultrasound examination can be helpful in determining gestational age, verifying the fetal presentation, and assessing the amount of amniotic fluid remaining within the uterine cavity. It has been shown that labor and infection are less likely to occur when an adequate volume of amniotic fluid remains within the uterus.

## Term Premature Rupture of Membranes

If PROM occurs at term (≥37 weeks of gestation), spontaneous labor will ensue in 90% of women within about 24 hours.

*Awaiting the onset of spontaneous labor for 12 to 24 hours is reasonable, unless there are risk factors such as previous or concurrent vaginal infection (such as Group B streptococcus) or multiple digital pelvic examinations.*

However, with informed consent, induction of labor at any time after presentation of a PROM at term is also considered appropriate. Information that the physician should share with the patient as this decision is considered includes, in addition to the risk of infection, that oxytocin administration is associated with a decreased risk of chorioamnionitis and endometritis, and that there appears to be a decrease in the incidence of cesarean delivery in patients managed expectantly. Serial evaluation for the development of intrauterine infection (fever, uterine tenderness, and maternal and/or fetal tachycardia) and other complications of PROM is requisite with expectant management, which, in most cases, should not extend beyond 24 hours in term pregnancy. *When the decision to deliver is made, group B streptococcal prophylaxis should be given based on prior culture results or risk factors, if cultures have not been previously performed.*

## Preterm Premature Rupture of Membranes

The time from PROM to labor is called the **latency period** and is inversely related to gestational age. Between 28 weeks and term, about 50% of patients go into labor within 24 hours and 80% within 1 week. Only 50% of patients whose gestational age is 24 to 28 weeks go into labor within 1 week of PROM.

Amniocentesis can be helpful in assessing fetal lung maturity (FLM), but can be difficult in the setting of PROM and oligohydramnios. In addition to tests of FLM, evaluation for intra-amniotic infection (using the presence of bacteria on Gram stain, elevated WBC count, low glucose level, or a positive culture) can also be performed. If there is sufficient volume, FLM tests can also be performed on amniotic fluid obtained vaginally.

If there is strong clinical suspicion for the presence of uterine infection, delivery should be effected as soon as possible, regardless of gestational age.

*If the evaluation suggests intrauterine infection, intravenous antibiotic therapy and delivery are indicated, regardless of gestational age.*

The antibiotic prescribed should have a broad spectrum of coverage, because of the polymicrobial nature of the infection. The effect of tocolysis to permit antibiotic and antenatal corticosteroid administration in the patient with preterm PROM who is having contractions has yet to be conclusively evaluated; therefore, specific recommendations for or against tocolysis administration cannot be made.

*If the gestational age is thought to be in the transitional time of fetal maturity (i.e., from 34 to 36 weeks), the management is variable, depending on individual circumstances* (Table 22.2).

Because of the increased risk of chorioamnionitis and because steroids are not recommended after 34 weeks to increase fetal maturity, delivery is recommended when PROM occurs at or beyond 34 weeks of gestation. If PROM occurs at 32 to 33 completed weeks of gestation, the risk of severe complications of prematurity is low if FLM is evident by amniotic fluid samples collected vaginally or by amniocentesis. *The efficacy of corticosteroid use at 32 to 33 weeks of gestation has not been specifically addressed for women with PROM, but is recommended by some experts.*

| TABLE 22.2 | Management of Premature Rupture of Membranes Chronologically |
| --- | --- |

| Gestational Age | Management |
| --- | --- |
| Term (37 weeks or more) | Proceed to delivery, usually by induction of labor, if spontaneous labor does not occur soon after ROM |
| | Group B streptococcal prophylaxis recommended |
| Near term (34 weeks to 36 completed weeks) | Same as for term |
| Preterm (32 weeks to 33 completed weeks) | Expectant management, unless fetal pulmonary maturity is documented |
| | Group B streptococcal prophylaxis recommended |
| | Corticosteroid—no consensus, but some experts recommend |
| | Antibiotics recommended to prolong latency, if there are no contradictions |
| Preterm (24 weeks to 31 completed weeks) | Expectant management |
| | Group B streptococcal prophylaxis recommended |
| | Single-course corticosteroid use recommended |
| | Tocolytics—no consensus |
| | Antibiotics recommended to prolong latency, if there are no contradictions |
| Less than 24 weeks* | Patient counseling |
| | Expectant management or induction of labor |
| | Group B streptococcal prophylaxis is not recommended |
| | Antibiotics—data are incomplete on use in prolonging latency |

*The combination of birth weight, gestational age, and sex provide the best estimates of changes of survival and should be considered in individual cases.
From American College of Obstetricians and Gynecologists. Premature rupture of membranes. ACOG Practice Bulletin No. 80. *Obstet Gynecol.* 2007;109(4):1007–1019.

If PROM occurs at 24 to 31 completed weeks of gestation, patients should be cared for expectantly, if no maternal or fetal contraindications exist, until 33 completed weeks of gestation. Prophylaxis using antibiotics to prolong latency and a single course of antenatal corticosteroids can help reduce the risks of infection and gestational age-dependent neonatal morbidity. Patients are assessed carefully on a daily basis for uterine tenderness as well as maternal or fetal tachycardia. WBC counts may be obtained and compared with baseline, although the maternal WBC count is again nonspecific and can be affected by glucocorticoid administration. Intermittent ultrasound assessment helps to determine amniotic fluid volumes, because leaking of fluid from the vagina may cease and allow amniotic fluid to re-accumulate around the fetus. Daily fetal movement monitoring by the mother can also be helpful to assess fetal well-being. In the absence of sufficient amniotic fluid to buffer the umbilical cord from external pressure, compression of the cord can lead to fetal heart rate decelerations. If these are frequent and severe, there should be early and expeditious delivery to avoid fetal compromise or death. Unfortunately, such an umbilical cord accident often is unrecognized for a time, regardless of the monitoring regimen instituted. Electronic fetal monitoring is used frequently during the initial evaluation period to search for any fetal heart rate decelerations, although the fetal cardiac control mechanisms are often insufficiently developed in preterm fetuses to allow meaningful evaluation for fetal heart rate variability and reactivity.

PROM at very early gestational ages, such as before 20 to 22 weeks of gestation, presents additional problems.

Along with the risks of prematurity and infection already discussed, the very premature fetus faces the further hazards of pulmonary hypoplasia, skeletal malformations, and other consequences of prolonged oligohydramnios. The relation of PROM with both of these entities is both interesting and important. The inability of the fetus to move freely within the amniotic sac can lead to skeletal contractures, which can become permanent deformities. For normal fetal lung development to occur, fetal breathing must occur. During intrauterine life, the fetus normally inhales and exhales amniotic fluid, with the net movement out into the amniotic fluid space. This adds substances generated in the respiratory tree to the amniotic fluid pool, including the phospholipids that form the basis for many of the fetal maturity tests. If rupture of fetal membranes occurs before 22 weeks of gestation, the lack of amniotic fluid interferes with respiratory efforts and, thus, with sufficient pulmonary development. The result is a failure of normal growth and differentiation of the respiratory tree and fetal chest. If severe, pulmonary hypoplasia may occur, which leads to an inability to maintain ventilation.

Women presenting with PROM before potential viability should be counseled regarding the impact of immediate delivery and the potential risks and benefits of expectant management. Counseling should include a realistic appraisal of neonatal outcomes, including the availability of obstetric monitoring and neonatal intensive care facilities. Because of advances in perinatal care, morbidity and mortality rates continue to decline. An attempt should be made to provide parents with the most up-to-date information possible. Women with previable preterm PROM are usually managed expectantly, either at home or in the hospital. Once the pregnancy has reached viability, administration of antenatal corticosteroids for fetal maturation is appropriate, given that early delivery remains likely.

## SUGGESTED READING

American College of Obstetrics and Gynecology. Premature rupture of membranes. ACOG Practice Bulletin 80. *Obstet Gynecol.* 2007; 109(4):1007–1019.

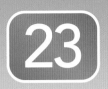

# 23

# Postterm Pregnancy

**Topic 30:** Postterm Pregnancy

Students should be able to identify the normal period of gestation, understand the evaluation and management of a pregnancy when gestation extends beyond the normal period, and discuss the maternal and fetal complications of postterm gestation.

Normal full-term pregnancy lasts from 38 to 42 weeks. The "due date" or "estimated date of delivery" (EDD) is calculated to be 40 weeks from the first day of the last menstrual period (LMP), presuming regular, 28-day cycles, and without recent, prior use of oral contraceptives. ***Postterm pregnancy*** *is a pregnancy that persists beyond 42 completed weeks of gestation.* This condition occurs in approximately 10% of pregnancies and carries with it an increased risk of adverse outcome. The increased morbidity and mortality in a small percentage of cases, however, warrants careful evaluation of all postterm pregnancies. In addition, postterm pregnancies can create significant stress for the patient, her family, and those caring for her. Therefore, the physician should understand the condition and the options for management.

*"Postdates" is a commonly used, but misleading synonym, and should be avoided.*

## CAUSE

*The most common "cause" of postterm pregnancy is inaccurate estimation of gestational age (dating.)* Inaccurate dating is more likely in women with irregular menses and, thus, inconsistent ovulation; women who seek prenatal care later in pregnancy; women with delayed ovulation (for example, women who have recently discontinued oral contraceptives); and women who inaccurately recall their LMP. Inaccurate dating that leads to the erroneous classification of a pregnancy as postterm has important sequelae. These pregnancies are labeled "high-risk." Costly increased evaluations are undertaken and the likelihood of intervention increases, specifically, delivery by induction of labor or by cesarean section, which are potentially associated with

increased maternal and fetal morbidity. Other less common causes of postterm pregnancy are listed in Table 23.1.

Whatever the cause, there is a tendency for recurrence of postterm pregnancy. *Approximately 50% of patients who have one postterm pregnancy will experience prolonged pregnancy with the next gestation.* Other important risk factors include maternal obesity, nulliparity, and postterm delivery of the mother. There also appears to be a genetic influence, based on twin studies.

## EFFECTS

*Compared with term pregnancies, the morbidity and mortality rates for both mother and fetus increase several-fold with postterm pregnancy.* Risks of maternal vaginal trauma, labor dysfunction, and cesarean delivery increase. Cesarean delivery carries increased risks of infection, bleeding, thromboembolic phenomenon, and visceral injury. Stillbirth and neonatal mortality rates increase steadily after 37 weeks, approaching 1 in 300 at 42 weeks, and increasing several-fold as the 44th week approaches. It is impossible to discuss postterm gestations without discussing macrosomia, shoulder dystocia, meconium aspiration syndrome (MAS), dysmaturity syndrome, and oligohydramnios, as these comorbidities are closely related.

***Macrosomia*** *is defined as an abnormally large infant size, specifically, an infant weighing 4000 g to 4500 g or greater.* It occurs in approximately 2.5% to 10% of postterm pregnancies. Maternal obesity, diabetes mellitus, or a previous macrosomic infant further raise the risk. Macrosomia is associated with an increased incidence of birth trauma, particularly if the infant is delivered vaginally. Such trauma includes shoulder dystocia; fracture of the clavicle; and associated brachial plexus injury, specifically Erb–Duchenne palsy.

**Shoulder dystocia** is an obstetrical emergency caused by impaction of the anterior fetal shoulder behind the

| TABLE 23.1 | Factors Associated With Postterm Pregnancy |
|---|---|
| **Factor** | **Discussion** |
| Inaccurate or unknown dates | Most common cause; high association with major risk factor of late or no prenatal care |
| Irregular ovulation; variation in length of follicular phase | Results in overestimation of gestational age |
| Anencephaly | Decreased production of 16α-hydroxydehydroepiandrosterone beta-sulfate, a precursor of estriol |
| Fetal adrenal hypoplasia | Decreased fetal production precursors of estriol |
| Placental sulfatase deficiency | X-linked disease prevents placenta conversion of sulfated estrogen precursors |
| Extrauterine pregnancy | Pregnancy not in uterus, no labor (see Chapter 13, Ectopic Pregnancy and Abortion) |

symphysis pubis during the process of vaginal delivery. A series of particular maneuvers can be accomplished to release this impaction. Brachial plexus injury is reported in approximately 0.85 to 1.89 per 1000 term deliveries, but increases 18- to 21-fold in macrosomic infants delivered vaginally; it can also occur during cesarean deliveries. In **Erb-Duchenne palsy,** paralysis, stretch, or tear injury to the upper roots of the brachial plexus, at C5 and C6, results in paralysis of the deltoid and infraspinatus muscles and flexor muscles of the forearm, causing the limb to hang limply close to the side, with the forearm extended and internally rotated; finger function is usually retained. Less frequently, damage is limited to the lower nerves of the brachial plexus, C8 and T1, causing **Klumpke paralysis,** or paralysis of the hand. Because most brachial injuries are mild, treatment is expectant, with splints and physical therapy in anticipation of complete or nearly complete recovery in 3 to 6 months. *Eighty to 90% of brachial plexus injuries completely resolve by 1 year of age.* Maternal risks with fetal macrosomia include a two-fold risk of cesarean delivery—with its associated operative risks and maternal trauma, particularly involving perineal lacerations if the fetus is delivered vaginally.

Another special concern in postterm pregnancies is **meconium passage** and **meconium aspiration syndrome.** MAS can lead to severe respiratory distress from mechanical obstruction of both small and large airways, as well as to meconium chemical pneumonitis. Meconium passage is not limited to postterm pregnancies, although prolonged pregnancy, particularly in the setting of oligohydramnios, is a substantial risk factor. Meconium passage occurs in 12% to 22% of women in labor, with aspiration occurring in up to 10% of these infants. The incidence of meconium passage increases as pregnancy becomes prolonged, as does the incidence of meconium aspiration syndrome.

**Dysmaturity syndrome,** which refers to infants with characteristics resembling chronic growth restriction, affects up to 20% of postterm pregnancies. These pregnancies are at increased risk of umbilical cord compression from oligohydramnios, meconium aspiration, and short-term neonatal complications (such as hypoglycemia, seizures, and respiratory insufficiency) and have an increased incidence of nonreassuring fetal testing, both antepartum and intrapartum.

**Oligohydramnios** is defined as decreased amniotic fluid for gestational age, and is generally quantified as an amniotic fluid index less than 5 cm. This is measured by dividing the gravid abdomen into quadrants and totaling the measurements of the largest vertical pockets of fluid in each of those quadrants. Amniotic fluid is a reflection of fetal swallowing, fetal breathing, fluid transfer across the amniotic sac, and, especially, fetal urination. The amniotic fluid reaches its maximum volume at approximately 34 to 36 weeks, and stays constant or slightly decreases from there for the remainder of the pregnancy. Any alterations in the above processes can cause changes in amniotic fluid volume. *Oligohydramnios is associated with poor outcomes secondary to umbilical cord compression, uteroplacental insufficiency, and meconium aspiration.* Because of these risks, after 40 weeks of gestation, close antepartum surveillance is warranted if pregnancy is allowed to continue. At term, oligohydramnios is an indication for delivery.

## DIAGNOSIS

*The diagnosis of postterm pregnancy rests on establishment of the correct gestational age.*

The first step in management of a patient with suspected postterm pregnancy is a careful review of the criteria used to establish the gestational age. The most common information used to determine gestational age include the patient's reported LMP and the first trimester ultrasound.

Ultrasound is most accurate for determining dating for gestational age when it is performed from 6 to 12 weeks of gestation. If the patient's LMP predicts an estimated date of delivery (EDD) that is within 10 days of an EDD determined by an ultrasound performed between 12 and 20 weeks of gestation, then the gestational age is considered fairly accurate. Once the EDD is determined, it should not be changed unless more accurate information is disclosed.

With improved access to prenatal care and greater importance placed on accurate gestational age assessment, the percentage of patients in whom postterm pregnancy is suspected has diminished. Nonetheless, a substantial number of patients do not seek prenatal care early in pregnancy or do not have an accurate gestational age determination. The prevalence of postterm pregnancy varies regionally, depending on the use of first-trimester ultrasound for gestational dating and routine labor induction.

## MANAGEMENT

Once the gestational age is believed to be firmly established and the patient approaches 41 weeks of gestation, management options include induction of labor or **antepartum fetal surveillance,** which continue either until spontaneous labor occurs or until approximately 42 weeks. In the United States, very few pregnancies are allowed to progress beyond 42 weeks and virtually none beyond 43 weeks. *Factors that influence management include the patient's concerns, the assessment of fetal well-being, and the status of the patient's cervix.* Induction of labor is appropriate if the cervix is favorable and if the patient prefers such management. The risk of failed induction is low with a favorable cervix, and most authorities believe it is low enough to recommend delivery in light of the risk of increased fetal morbidity in the postterm period.

The data on preventing postterm pregnancy are controversial. Some studies show that **sweeping the membranes** may decrease postterm pregnancy; other studies differ. Sweeping the membranes is a procedure by which the amniotic sac is gently detached from the uterine wall at the level of the cervix. This procedure is thought to release prostaglandins, thus increasing cervical dilatation, making the cervix more favorable and sometimes leading to the onset of labor. Sweeping the membranes should not be performed until gestational age can be verified and the maturity of the fetus ensured.

*If the gestational age is not well-established and the menstrual history and early ultrasound findings are not available, there is little additional information that can be used to determine the best estimate of gestational age.* Amniocentesis is not especially helpful, because fetal lung maturity is rarely a question in the postterm evaluation. Once the best date is selected, a management plan similar to that for a postterm pregnancy with well-established gestational age is used.

*If the cervix is not favorable, fetal well-being is monitored while awaiting spontaneous labor or ripening of the cervix, which makes induction appropriate.*

Fetal evaluation has not been shown to decrease mortality in postterm pregnancy; however, it is also not associated with any negative outcomes. A variety of management schemes have been devised to monitor fetal well-being, though none has been shown to be superior. Thus, it is common practice to assess fetal well-being using several methods. Weekly monitoring of **amniotic fluid volume** is commonly used, as oligohydramnios at term is a sufficient indication for delivery. **Nonstress tests** (fetal heart rate monitoring), **biophysical profiles** (ultrasound evaluation of fetal fluid, movement, tone, and breathing), or oxytocin challenge tests may be used once or twice a week. Another option is the combination of amniotic fluid assessment and nonstress test, known as the **modified biophysical profile.** Doppler flow studies of the umbilical artery are not considered useful. These studies are discussed in greater detail in Chapter 6, Preconception and Antepartum Care. **Daily fetal movement counting** is included in most management plans, with decreased perceived fetal movement being an indication for further, timely evaluation of fetal well-being. Results of these tests are most useful when considered within the context of other conditions affecting the mother and the fetus. If fetal test results are nonreassuring, delivery is indicated.

The patient with an unfavorable cervix should be counseled about risks of induction of labor and the risks of continuing pregnancy with fetal evaluation to help in clinical decision making. Both management plans—inducing labor and continued fetal surveillance—are associated with low rates of maternal and fetal morbidity in the low-risk patient. Although there is no absolute time by which labor must be induced, most physicians believe that delivery should occur between 41 and 42 completed weeks. *Compared with expectant management, several studies of routine induction at 41 weeks, using cervical ripening agents, have demonstrated lower cesarean delivery rates, lower perinatal mortality, decreased length of hospital stay, decreased hospital cost, and higher patient satisfaction.* Several different agents are now available for cervical ripening, including intracervical or intravaginal preparation of prostaglandin; Foley bulb placed through the cervix; and misoprostol. Oxytocin should ideally be initiated after the cervix is ripened.

*Induction at 41 weeks is quickly becoming the preferred management.*

Because of the risk of macrosomia-associated birth trauma, ultrasonographic estimation of fetal weight should be obtained before induction of labor in a postterm pregnancy when macrosomia is suspected. If the estimated fetal weight is more than 5000 g in a woman who does not have diabetes or 4500 g in a woman with diabetes, cesarean delivery should be considered. *There is no accurate way of estimating fetal weight at term;* ultrasonographic estimates have a calculation error up to 500 g late in pregnancy. Clinically determined estimated fetal weights by palpation of the patient's abdomen and Leopold maneuvers are similarly inaccurate.

For patients who are postterm, special precautions are taken at the time of delivery to provide prompt evaluation of the infant in the event of meconium passage. In a depressed infant, aggressive suctioning of the fetus with a laryngoscope decreases, but does not eliminate, the likelihood of meconium aspiration syndrome

*In a vigorous infant with meconium passage, laryngoscopy and aggressive suctioning have not been shown to decrease the risk of meconium aspiration syndrome, and are no longer recommended.*

Similarly, routine amnioinfusion during labor with meconium passage is not recommended.

## SUGGESTED READINGS

American College of Obstetricians and Gynecologists. Management of postterm pregnancy. ACOG Practice Bulletin No. 55. *Obstet Gynecol.* 2004;104(3):639–646.

*Guidelines for Perinatal Care.* 6th ed. Elk Grove Village, IL: American Academy of Pediatrics; Washington, DC: American College of Obstetricians and Gynecologists; 2007.

# 24 Contraception

**Topic 33:** Contraception and Sterilization

Students should be able to list the various methods of contraception by type and describe their mechanisms of action, effectiveness, risks, and benefits, as well as indications and contraindications.

In the past 15 years several new contraceptive options have been introduced in the United States, and several that were available have left the market for various reasons. Many methods are very reliable, although no method is effective if it is not used correctly. *The goal of all contraception is obviously to prevent the sperm and oocyte from uniting.* This goal is accomplished by several mechanisms of action: (1) inhibiting the development and release of the egg (via oral contraceptives, long-acting progesterone injection, or contraceptive patch and ring), or (2) imposing a mechanical, chemical, or temporal barrier between sperm and egg (via condom, diaphragm, spermicide, natural family planning, and intrauterine contraception). As a secondary mechanism, some methods also alter the ability of the fertilized egg to implant and grow (e.g., intrauterine contraception and postcoital oral contraceptives). Each approach may be used, individually or in combination, to prevent pregnancy, and each method has its own advantages and disadvantages, risks, and benefits.

Before advising a woman or couple on contraceptive options, the physician must understand the physiologic or pharmacologic mechanism of action, the effectiveness, the indications and contraindications, complications, and advantages and disadvantages of the contraceptive methods available, as well as the cultural context of the person or persons desiring contraception. When comparing methods, both the **method failure rate** (the failure rate inherent in the method if the patient uses it correctly 100% of the time) and the **typical failure rate** (the failure rate seen as the method is actually used by patients, that is, factoring in the mistakes in usage everyone will make from time to time, and even actual noncompliance) should be considered, as described in Table 24.1.

## FACTORS AFFECTING CHOICE OF CONTRACEPTIVE METHOD

Although efficacy is important in the choice of contraceptive methods, other factors to be considered include safety, availability, cost, and personal acceptability to patient and partner. Although we tend to think of safety in terms of significant health risks, for many patients this also includes the possibility of side effects. For a couple to use a method, it must be accessible and affordable for the patient. How and when the method is used also can determine acceptability. Options vary from methods that are coitus-dependent (barriers) to methods that are placed by a healthcare provider and last for up to 10 years (intrauterine contraception). Some women prefer methods they control. They can choose an oral daily preparation, while others consider the weekly transdermal (contraceptive patch) or the monthly transvaginal (contraceptive ring) forms easier to use successfully. Other women elect to use a method administered by their healthcare provider, such as injections, implants, or intrauterine contraception. Sterilization is discussed in Chapter 25.

The ability of a contraceptive method to provide some protection against sexually transmitted diseases (STDs) may also be relevant. Career or other life choices, as well as plans for future fertility, may influence the type and duration of the method chosen. Finally, the couple's feelings about which partner should take responsibility for contraception may be important. The clinician must be sensitive to all these factors that might influence the decision and provide factual information that fits the needs of the patient and her partner. A decision tree based on this concept is presented in Figure 24.1.

## HORMONAL CONTRACEPTIVES

For many women, "birth control" is synonymous with oral contraceptives (OCs) or hormonal contraception. Hormone-dependent choices now also include injectable hormonal preparations, an implantable hormonal rod, contraceptive patches, hormone-containing intrauterine systems, and contraceptive rings.

### Oral Contraceptives

About one-third of all sexually active women in the United States use oral contraceptives, with over one half of young women 20 to 24 years old using these contraceptives.

| TABLE 24.1 | Contraceptive Technique Pregnancy Rates in the First Year of Use in the United States | |

| Method | Percentage of Women Experiencing an Unintended Pregnancy Within the 1st Year of Use | |
| | Typical Use* | Perfect Use† |
| --- | --- | --- |
| No method of contraception | 85.0 | 85.0 |
| Hormonal contraceptives | | |
|   Combination pill | 8 | 0.3 |
|   Progestin-only pill | 8 | 0.3 |
|   Contraceptive patch | 8 | 0.3 |
|   Contraceptive ring | 8 | 0.3 |
|   DMPA | 3 | 0.3 |
|   Implantable contraceptive rods | 0.05 | 0.05 |
| Barrier contraceptives | | |
|   Spermicides | 29 | 18 |
|   Male condom (without spermicide) | 15 | 2 |
|   Female condom | 21 | 5 |
|   Diaphragm and spermicide | 16 | 6 |
| Intrauterine devices (IUDs) | | 3.0 |
|   Progesterone IUD | 0.2 | 0.2 |
|   Copper T-380A | 0.8 | 0.6 |
|   Withdrawal | 27 | 4 |
| Natural family planning | | |
|   Calendar | 5 | |
|   Ovulation method | 3 | |
|   Symptothermal | 2 | |
| Postcoital contraception/emergency | 25 | |
| Permanent—sterilization | | |
|   Male | 0.15 | 0.10 |
|   Female | 0.5 | 0.5 |

DMPA = Depo medroxyprogesterone acetate.
*Among typical couples who initiate use of a method (not necessarily for the first time), the percentage who experience an accidental pregnancy during the 1st year if they do not stop use for any other reason.
†Among couples who initiate use of a method (not necessarily for the first time) and who use it perfectly (both consistently and correctly), the percentage who experience an accidental pregnancy during the first year if they do not stop use for any other reason.
Adapted from American College of Obstetricians and Gynecologists. *Guidelines for Women's Health Care.* 3rd ed. Washington, DC. American College of Obstetricians and Gynecologists;2007:184–185.

Hormonal contraceptives have many health benefits, including decreasing a woman's risk of ovarian and uterine cancer. Although hormonal contraceptive methods are associated with risks, for most women the use of one of these agents is safer than pregnancy.

Hormone-based contraceptives provide the most effective reversible pregnancy prevention available. Method (theoretical) failure rates for oral, transdermal, and transvaginal contraceptives are in the range of ≤1%. Longer-acting hormonal methods (injections, implants, and intrauterine contraception) have effectiveness rates that equal or even surpass those of sterilization. Because OC failures are usually related to missed pills, injectable long-acting agents, patches, implants, intrauterine contraception, and rings share the additional advantage of lack of a need for daily compliance.

Hormonal contraceptives do not protect against STDs. Women who use these techniques should be counseled about high-risk behaviors and the need to use condoms for additional protection.

### MECHANISMS OF ACTION

Most of the oral contraceptives are combinations of an **estrogen** and a **progestin,** although there are also progestin-only products. Combination oral contracep-

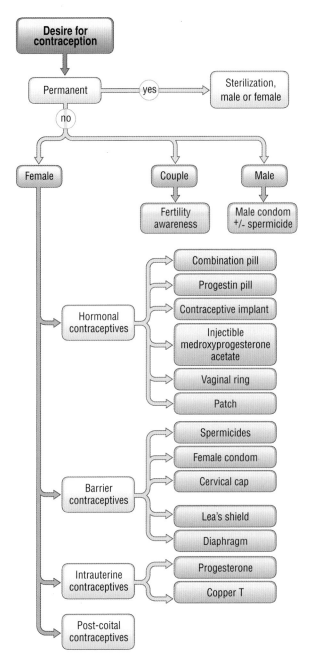

FIGURE 24.1. Decision tree for choosing a contraceptive method.

the progestational agent. The estrogen provides an additional modest contraceptive effect, thus increasing the efficacy of this method.

Common progestin compounds used in hormonal contraceptives include, in descending order of biologic progestin activity: norgestrel, ethynodiol diacetate, norethindrone acetate, norethynodrel, and norethindrone. Oral contraceptives using the less androgenic agents, desogestrel, norgestimate, and drospirenone, are also available if less androgenic activity is desired.

Many oral contraceptives contain a fixed ratio of estrogen and progestin, although **"phasic"** formulations have been introduced that vary this ratio during the course of the month. This leads to a slight decrease in the total dose of hormones used per month but is also associated with a slightly higher rate of **break-through bleeding** (bleeding not related to the menstrual period in a woman using oral contraceptives) between periods.

The classic regimen for hormonal contraception has been 21 days of active hormone (pill, patch, and ring) and 7 days of placebo or no hormones. Hormone regimens are also available that produce shorter or less frequent menstrual periods. These new regimens shorten the withdrawal bleed and decrease menstrual-related symptoms. Another formulation is a monophasic ethinyl estradiol/levonorgestrel preparation that extends the cycle to 3 months. Some women may prefer this usage pattern, although they should be aware that there is a higher incidence of break-through bleeding in the first 12-week cycle, compared with the 4-week cycle preparations. New preparations continue to be developed with the ultimate goal of maximizing benefits and minimizing side effects.

**Progestin-only contraceptives** (progestin-only "minipill") act primarily by making the cervical mucus thick and relatively impermeable. Ovulation continues normally in about 40% of patients using the progestin-only formulation. These oral contraceptives are of special usefulness in two clinical situations: lactating women and women over 40. In the former group, the progestin effect coincides with the prolactin-induced suppression of ovulation; in the latter group, the inherent reduced fecundity adds to the progestin effect. There is no effect on the quality or quantity of breast milk or any evidence of short- or long-term adverse effects on infants, and the progestin-only pill may be started immediately after delivery in the breast-feeding mother. *The progestin-only pill is also a good choice for women in whom estrogen-containing formulations are contraindicated.* Because of the low dosages of progestin, the minipill must be taken at the same time each day, starting on the first day of menses. If a woman is more than 3 hours late in taking the minipill, a back-up contraceptive method should be used for 48 hours.

## EFFECTS OF HORMONAL CONTRACEPTIVES

Hormonal contraception affects more than just the reproductive system. *Estrogens affect lipid metabolism, potentiate sodium and water retention, increase renin substrate, stimulate*

tive preparations contain **ethinyl estradiol** as the estrogen component and one of the 19-**nortestosterones** or a **spironolactone derivative (drospirenone)** as the progestin product. The progestational component provides the major contraceptive effect, acting primarily by suppressing secretion of luteinizing hormone, and, in turn, ovulation. The progestational agent also provides the secondary effect of thickening the cervical mucus and also alters fallopian tube peristalsis, inhibiting sperm movement and fertilization, if ovulation were to occur. The estrogenic component acts by suppressing secretion of follicle-stimulating hormone (FSH), preventing maturation of a follicle, as well as by potentiation of the action of *the cytochrome P-450 system, increase sex hormone-binding globulin, and can reduce antithrombin III.* Progestins increase sebum, stimulate the growth of facial and body hair, induce smooth muscle relaxation, and increase the risk of cholestatic jaundice. The newer progestational agents—desogestrel, norgestimate, and drospirenone—have less metabolic impact.

*Oral contraceptives have many beneficial effects.* Menstrual periods are predictable, shorter, and less painful and, as a result, the risk of iron-deficiency anemia is reduced. Oral contraceptive users have a lower incidence of endometrial and ovarian cancers, benign breast and ovarian disease, and pelvic infection. By decreasing conception, the risk of ectopic pregnancy is reduced, along with the complications of undesired intrauterine pregnancies.

Break-through bleeding occurs in 10% to 30% of women taking low-dose oral contraceptives during the first 3 months of use. Although it is an especially worrisome symptom, it is not associated with decreased efficacy as long as the pill-taking regimen is maintained. The abnormal bleeding pattern is the most common reason for discontinuation of contraception and women should be counseled to expect irregularities before hormones are initiated. If break-through bleeding does occur, it is best managed by encouragement and reassurance, because it usually resolves spontaneously. Break-through bleeding after approximately 3 months is associated with progestin-induced decidualization, with the shallow and fragile endometrium prone to asynchronous breakdown and bleeding. A short course of exogenous estrogen (1.25 mg conjugated estrogen for 7 days), given while the patient continues oral contraceptive use, usually stabilizes the endometrium and stops the bleeding. Taking two or three of the pills each day is not an effective therapy for break-through bleeding, because the progestin component will predominate, often worsening the problem by causing further decidualization of the endometrium.

**Amenorrhea** occurs in approximately 1% of users of low-dose oral contraceptives in the first year of use, reaching perhaps 5% of users after several years of use. Contraceptive efficacy is maintained if the pill regimen is followed. Changing to a higher estrogen-containing pill or use of exogenous estrogen may be employed to induce bleeding, if the patient wishes. A pregnancy test should precede therapy.

Serious complications (such as venous thrombosis, pulmonary embolism, cholestasis and gallbladder disease, stroke, and myocardial infarction) are more likely for women using high-dose formulations. However, these complications also can occur occasionally in patients taking low-dose formulations. Hepatic tumors have also been associated with the use of high-dose oral contraceptives. Although all of these complications are from 2 to 10 times more likely in pill-users, they are still uncommon.

Less serious but more common side effects also depend on the dosage and type of hormones used. Estrogens may cause a feeling of bloating and weight gain, breast tenderness, nausea, fatigue, or headache. Studies have demonstrated no overall weight gain in pill users despite the perception of weight gain. Altering the dose or composition of the progestational agent used may relieve some of these minor side effects.

The therapeutic principle of contraception is to select the method providing effective contraception with the greatest margin of safety, and then to use it as long as the patient wishes contraception or beneficial menstrual-related changes. If the patient experiences new signs or symptoms while using hormonal contraception, further evaluation or cessation of the chosen hormonal method may be required (Box 24.1).

## PATIENT EVALUATION FOR COMBINED HORMONAL CONTRACEPTIVE USE

Before considering estrogen- and progestin-containing contraceptives for a patient, a careful evaluation is required. Not only are hormones relatively or absolutely contraindicated in some patients, but also factors such as previous

---

**BOX 24.1**

**Management of New Symptoms in Patients Using Oral Contraceptives**

**Discontinue OCP; start nonhormonal methods, immediate evaluation**

| | |
|---|---|
| Loss of vision, diplopia | (Possible retinal artery thrombosis) |
| Unilateral numbness, weakness | (Possible stroke) |
| Severe chest/neck pain | (Possible myocardial infarction) |
| Slurring of speech | (Possible stroke) |
| Severe leg pain, tenderness | (Possible thrombophlebitis) |
| Hemoptysis, acute shortness of breath | (Possible pulmonary embolism) |
| Hepatic mass, tenderness | (Possible hepatic neoplasm, adenoma) |

**Continue OCP; immediate evaluation**

| | |
|---|---|
| Amenorrhea | (Possible pregnancy) |
| Breast mass | (Possible breast cancer) |
| Right-upper-quadrant pain | (Possible cholecystitis, cholelithiasis) |
| Severe headache | (Possible stroke, migraine headache) |
| Galactorrhea | (Possible pituitary adenoma) |

OCP = oral contraceptive pill.

menstrual history may have an impact on the choice of these agents. Combined oral conceptive use is contraindicated in women over age 35 years who smoke or who have had a thromboembolism, and in women with a history of coronary artery disease, congestive heart failure, or cerebral vascular disease (Box 24.2).

---

**BOX 24.2**

**Absolute and Relative Contraindications to the Use of Combination Oral Contraceptives***

**Absolute**
- Thrombophlebitis, thromboembolic disease
- Undiagnosed abnormal vaginal bleeding
- Cerebral vascular disease
- Known or suspected pregnancy
- Coronary occlusion
- Smokers >35 years old
- Impaired liver function
- Congenital hyperlipidemia
- Known or suspected breast cancer
- Hepatic neoplasm

**Relative**
- Severe vascular headache (classic migraine, cluster)
- Severe hypertension (if <35–40 years of age and in good medical control, can elect OCP)
- Diabetes mellitus (prevention of pregnancy outweighs the risk of complicating vascular disease in diabetics younger than 35–40 years)
- Gallbladder disease (may exacerbate emergence of symptoms when gallstones are present)
- Obstructive jaundice in pregnancy (some patients will develop jaundice)
- Epilepsy (do not exacerbate epilepsy, but antiepileptic drugs may decrease effectiveness of OCPs)
- Morbid obesity (must monitor glucose and lipoprotein profiles regularly)

**Conditions No Longer Considered Contraindications**
- Uterine leiomyoma (low-dose formulations not associated with growth; reduced bleeding may help in management)
- Sickle cell disease or sickle C disease
- Before elective surgery (theoretical association with thrombosis outweighed in most cases by avoiding pregnancy)

OCP = oral contraceptive pill.
*Risk primarily related to the estrogenic component.

---

Approximately 3% of patients may experience problems with resumption of their periods after prolonged contraceptive use (**postpill amenorrhea**). Younger women and those who had irregular periods before the use of oral contraceptives are more likely to experience this problem after discontinuing their use. These patients should be counseled about this potential complication.

*Hormonal contraceptives may interact with other medications that the patient is taking.* This interaction may reduce the efficacy of either the contraceptive or the other medications. Examples of drugs that decrease the effectiveness of contraceptives include barbiturates, benzodiazepines, phenytoin, carbamazepine, rifampin, and the sulfonamides. Drugs that may show retarded biotransformation when contraceptives are also used include anticoagulants, methyldopa, phenothiazines, reserpine, and tricyclic antidepressants. Antibiotics may alter the intestinal flora and are thought to interfere with hormone absorption, but efficacy is not reduced. *Before prescribing medications to women using contraceptives, the clinician should consider possible drug interactions.*

## Ring and Patch

The **transdermal contraceptive patch** contains synthetic estrogen and progestin and remains effective for an entire week (Fig. 24.2). The patient should start the patch on the first day of her menstrual period and replace it weekly for 3 weeks. The fourth week is patch-free to allow a with-

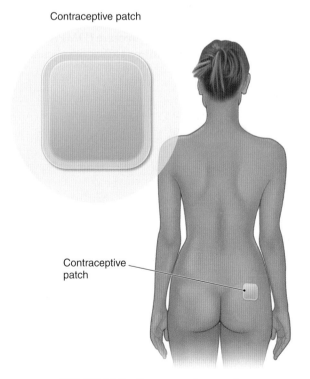

Contraceptive patch

Contraceptive patch

FIGURE 24.2. Contraceptive patch.

drawal bleed. Placement on clean, dry skin located on the buttocks, upper outer arm, or lower abdomen is recommended. Because of its ease of application and improved compliance, the "method failure" and "patient failure" of the patch are almost identical. Caution should be used when prescribing the patch for women weighing more than 90 kg (198 pounds) because of its decreased efficacy. Side effects and contraindications are similar to the OCs. A complaint specific to the patch, however, includes skin irritation from adhesive residue at the application site.

The **contraceptive vaginal ring** releases a sustained amount of synthetic estrogen and progestin daily (Fig. 24.3). Comparable with oral contraceptives in efficacy, the ring is associated with greater compliance because of its once-a-month usage. Placed into the vagina by the patient at the beginning of her menses, it is left in place for 3 weeks. Removal of the device results in a withdrawal bleed. The ring can be taken out of the vagina for up to 3 hours, if desired, without altering its efficacy. Because it is colorless and odorless, with a 2-inch diameter, most patients and their partners are unaware of the presence of the ring. An advantage of the ring over OCs is a decreased incidence of break-through bleeding.

Because the hormones in the vaginal ring and the transdermal patch do not get absorbed through the gastrointestinal tract, some of the medication interactions that occur with combined oral contraceptives may not apply. However, metabolism still occurs in the liver and, therefore, caution must be used.

## Injectable and Implantable Hormonal Contraceptives

**Depo medroxyprogesterone acetate** (DMPA) is an injectable progestin given in intramuscular or subcutaneous

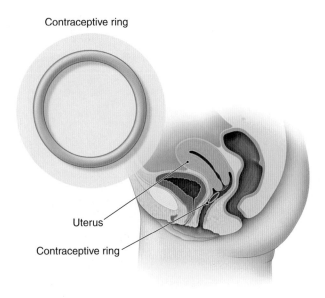

Contraceptive ring

Uterus

Contraceptive ring

FIGURE 24.3. **Contraceptive ring.**

injections every 3 months. It maintains a contraceptive level of progestin for at least 14 weeks, providing a useful "safety" margin in case an injection is not administered within precisely 3 months. The injection should be given within the first 5 days of the current menstrual period, and, if not, a back-up method of contraception is necessary for 2 weeks. DMPA is not a sustained-release preparation, relying instead on higher peaks and sustained levels of progestin. In addition to thickening of the cervical mucus and decidualization of the endometrium, DMPA also acts by maintaining a circulating level of progestin high enough to block the luteinizing hormone surge and, thus, ovulation. FSH suppression does not occur with DMPA as it does with combination oral contraceptives.

Recently, concerns have been raised about adverse effects of DMPA on bone mineral density resulting from alterations in bone metabolism associated with the reduced estrogen levels. Special concern has been raised about this effect during adolescence, a critical period of bone accretion, although the decrease in bone mineral density appears to be substantially reversible after discontinuation of this injectable contraceptive. Nonetheless, the U.S. Food and Drug Administration (FDA) has added a warning to this formulation, that use beyond 2 years should be carefully considered and alternate contraceptive methods be evaluated. In addition, women at special risk for osteoporosis should be especially careful when considering the use of DMPA. Concern about the use of DMPA in adolescents should be weighed against the advantages of compliance and effective contraception. In addition, noncontraceptive benefits of DMPA include decreased risk of endometrial carcinoma and iron-deficiency anemia. It may also improve management of pain associated with endometriosis, endometrial hyperplasia, and dysmenorrhea. As with all contraceptive options, the balance of overall risk to benefit for DMPA should be weighed on an individual, patient basis (Box 24.3).

The efficacy of DMPA is roughly equivalent to that of sterilization (see Table 24.1) and is not affected by weight or altered by patients taking medications that alter hepatic function. Contraindications of DMPA are similar to those of other hormonal contraceptives. DMPA injections may cause irregular bleeding, which decreases with each injection so that 80% of women are amenorrheic after 5 years. Because 25% of users discontinue DMPA within the first year of use owing to this problem, extensive pre-initiation counseling and, if needed, treatment with 7 days of conjugated estrogen (1.25 mg/day) may be useful. When DMPA is discontinued, about 50% of patients resume normal menses within 6 months. Twenty-five percent do not resume menses for more than 1 year. These patients should be evaluated to detect other possible causes.

The **implant contraceptive system** releases a daily dose of progestin and estrogen per day. This method is easier to insert and remove than previous implantable systems (Fig. 24.4). It works primarily by thickening the

---

**BOX 24.3**
**Indications and Contraindications for DMPA Contraception**

| Indications | Discussion |
|---|---|
| Desire for >1 year of contraception has been one of the indications until the recent concerns about effect on bone density. Now, use beyond 2 years should be individualized and considered carefully. | Short- or long-term use of DMPA should not be considered as an indication for dual-energy x-ray absorptiometry or other tests that assess bone mineral density. |
| Women for whom compliance with other methods has been problematic | One injection every 3 months, 2-week "safety" interval (i.e., can be delayed up to 2 weeks without loss of efficacy) |
| Breast feeding | No effect on quality of breast milk or on baby; increases quantity of breast milk; can be administered immediately postpartum |
| Women for whom estrogen-containing preparations are contraindicated | See below for absolute contraindications |
| Women with seizure disorders | Anti-seizure medications unaffected, and sedative effects of progestins may aid in seizure control |
| Sickle cell anemia | Probable in vivo inhibition of sickling |
| Anemia secondary to menorrhagia | Decreased menstrual flow |

**Contraindications**
- High risk for osteoporosis
- Known or suspected pregnancy
- Undiagnosed vaginal bleeding
- Known or suspected malignancy of the breast
- Active thrombophlebitis, or current or past history of thromboembolic disorders, or cerebral vascular disease
- Liver dysfunction or disease
- Known sensitivity to DMPA or any of its other ingredients

---

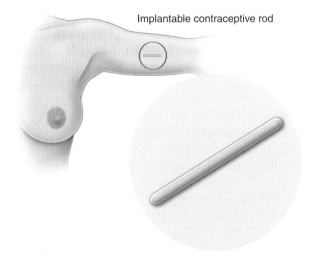

Implantable contraceptive rod

FIGURE 24.4.  Contraceptive implant.

cervical mucus and inhibiting ovulation. Unlike DMPA, it does not affect bone mineral density. The most common side effect is irregular, unpredictable vaginal bleeding that may continue even after several months of use.

## BARRIER CONTRACEPTIVES

Among the oldest and most widely used contraceptive methods are those that provide a barrier between sperm and egg. These barriers include condoms, diaphragms, and cervical caps. *Each of these methods depends on proper use before or at the time of intercourse and, as such, is subject to a higher failure rate than noncoitus-dependent methods.* This is the result of inconsistent or incorrect use as well as actual damage to the barrier material itself. For example, the latex in condoms, diaphragm, and cervical cap can be damaged by the application of oil-based lubricants. Despite this, these methods provide relatively good protection from unwanted pregnancy, are inexpensive, and most require little or no medical consultation. In addition, condoms and diaphragms provide some protection against the transmission of STDs, including gonorrhea, herpes, chlamydia, human immunodeficiency virus (HIV), and human papillomavirus infection.

## Condoms

**Condoms** are sheaths worn over the erect penis (male condom) or inside the vagina (female condom) to prevent sperm from reaching the cervix and upper genital tract. Although almost one half of all condoms are sold to women, the condom is the only reliable, nonpermanent method of contraception available to men. Condoms are widely available and inexpensive and may be made of latex, nonlatex or, less commonly, animal membrane (usually sheep cecum). A reservoir tip reduces the likelihood of breakage. Only latex condoms protect against HIV.

The condom is well-tolerated, with only rare reports of skin irritation or allergic reaction. Some men complain of reduced sensation with the use of condoms, but this may actually be an advantage for those with rapid or premature ejaculation. The slippage and breakage rate in normal use is estimated at 5% to 8%. In these cases, couples should be counseled to seek medical care within 72 hours so that emergency contraceptive methods may be used.

The **female condom** is a sheath, or vaginal liner, that fits into the vagina before intercourse (Fig. 24.5). All have slippage and breakage rates of about 3%, and, as in the case of diaphragms and cervical caps, it is recommended that they be left in place 6 to 8 hours after coitus.

## The Diaphragm, Cervical Cap, and Sponge

The **diaphragm** is a small, latex-covered, dome-shaped device. Proper use of a diaphragm includes applying a contraceptive jelly or cream containing spermicide into the center and along the rim of the device, which is then inserted into the vagina, over the cervix, and behind the pubic symphysis. In this position, the diaphragm covers the anterior vaginal wall and cervix.

The diaphragm can be inserted up to 6 hours before intercourse and must be left in place for 6 to 8 hours afterward, but not more than 24 hours. It may then be removed, washed, and stored. Users should be cautioned not to use talc to dry the diaphragm. If additional intercourse is desired during the 6- to 8-hour waiting time, additional spermicide should be applied without removing the diaphragm, and the waiting time should be restarted.

*There are several sizes of diaphragm available and one must be fitted to the individual patient.* Fit may change with significant weight change, vaginal birth, or pelvic surgery. The diaphragm should be the largest that can be comfortably inserted, worn, and removed. If the diaphragm is too small, it may slip out during coitus because of vaginal elongation; if it is too large, it may buckle, causing discomfort, irritation, and leakage. The patient must be initially instructed in the proper positioning of the diaphragm, with the correct position subsequently verified by the patient each time it is used. If the cervix can be felt through the dome of the diaphragm, the positioning is correct. If a diaphragm is fitted in the postpartum period, its sizing should be reevaluated in 2 to 3 months, because vaginal dimensions and support may change in the interval. Correct positioning of a diaphragm is shown in Figure 24.6.

Women who use diaphragms are approximately twice as likely to have urinary tract infections as women using hormonal contraception. The increased risk of UTI may be caused by a combination of pressure against the urethra, causing urinary stasis, and an effect of spermicides on the normal vaginal flora, increasing the risk of *Escherichia coli* bacteriuria and infection.

The **cervical cap** is a smaller version of the diaphragm that is applied to the cervix itself. This method is associated with a relatively high degree of displacement as well as with cervicitis and toxic shock syndrome. It also requires considerable effort to fit. The cervical cap should also be used in conjunction with spermicide. It must be left in place for 6 hours after intercourse, but not longer than 48 hours. Additional spermicide does not need to be applied with repeated acts of intercourse during that time. Correct positioning of the cervical cap is shown in Figure 24.7.

The **contraceptive sponge** is a small, pillow-shaped sponge containing spermicide. The sponge has a dimple that is designed to fit over the cervix and remain in place during intercourse. The opposite side has a loop to facilitate removal. The sponge is only available in one size, which may explain why it is more effective in a nulliparous woman than in one who has had children. The sponge is moistened prior to insertion and can be used for repeated acts of intercourse in a 24-hour period. The sponge should be left in place for at least 6 hours after intercourse, but

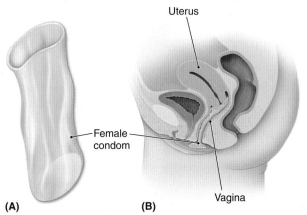

FIGURE 24.5. The female condom. (A) Preparation for insertion. (B) Condom in proper position.

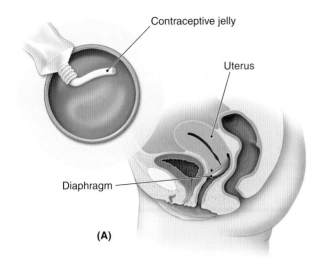

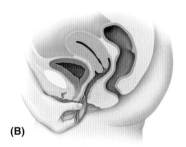

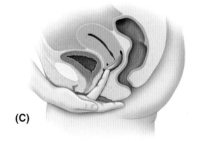

FIGURE 24.6. Diaphragm. (A) Diaphragm in place. (B) Insertion of the diaphragm. (C) Checking to ensure the diaphragm covers the cervix.

wearing it for more than 24 hours is not recommended because of the risk of toxic shock syndrome.

## Spermicides

**Spermicides** are preparations that contain an active chemical that kills sperm as well as some type of carrier or base (e.g., gel, foam, cream, film, suppository, or tablet). In the United States the active ingredient is nonoxynol-9 (N-9). Foams and tablets should be inserted high into the vagina against the cervix, from 10 to 30 minutes before each act of intercourse. The duration of maximal spermicidal effectiveness is usually no more than 1 hour. Douching should be avoided for at least 8 hours after use. There is

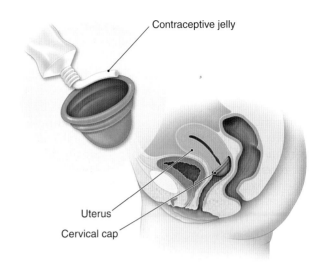

FIGURE 24.7. Cervical cap.

no known association between spermicide use and congenital malformation.

Spermicides are economical, well-tolerated, and effective in protection against pregnancy. *Spermicides used in combination with condoms have failure rates that approach those of hormonal methods.* Spermicides provide little, if any, protection against sexually transmitted infections when used alone.

## INTRAUTERINE CONTRACEPTION

**Intrauterine contraceptives,** also known as **intrauterine devices (IUDs),** are among the most commonly used and safe methods of interval contraception worldwide (Fig. 24.8). Two types of IUDs are available in the United

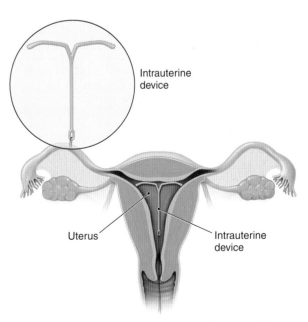

FIGURE 24.8. Intrauterine device.

States. Both are T-shaped. One releases a small amount of levonorgestrel into the uterus, and the other releases a small amount of copper into the uterus.

The Lippe loop is an unmedicated IUD available throughout the world except in the United States. The levonorgestrel-containing device primarily works by preventing the sperm and egg from meeting. It also thickens the cervical mucus and creates an unfavorable uterine environment. The copper in the copper-containing device can prevent the egg from being fertilized or from attaching to the wall of the uterus. It also prevents sperm from going into the uterus and the fallopian tube, reducing the sperm's ability to fertilize an egg. The copper-containing IUD is also used postcoitally as emergency contraception.

A clinically important side effect of the levonorgestrel-containing IUD is a decrease in menstrual blood loss (up to 50%) and severity of dysmenorrhea. Serum progesterone levels are not affected. IUD removal is followed by rapid reversal of these effects and return to a normal intrauterine environment and normal fertility. This system is used to relieve pain related to endometriosis and adenomyosis as well as for endometrial protection for women taking hormone replacement therapy who cannot take oral progestins (Box 24.4). Increased vaginal bleeding and menstrual pain are experienced by 5% to 10% of women and often result in their request to discontinue IUD use.

The progestin IUDs have a lesser incidence of this problem, because of the progestin effect on the endometrium.

Bacteria from the endogenous cervicovaginal flora can be introduced into the uterus during IUD insertion and may cause infection. Prophylactic antibiotics have not been shown to decrease the incidence of this type of infection. Sterile technique and a vaginal prep with Betadine should be used prior to insertion of an IUD. Pelvic infection occurring 3 or more months after IUD insertion may be presumed to be an acquired STD and treated accordingly. Women at high risk for STDs may benefit from screening prior to insertion. Asymptomatic IUD users with positive cervical cultures for gonorrhea or chlamydia, or with bacterial vaginosis, should be treated promptly. The IUD may remain in place unless there is evidence of spread of the infection to the endometrium or fallopian tubes and/or failure of treatment with appropriate antibiotics.

*The IUDs presently available in the United States are highly effective.* The copper-containing IUD has a recommended lifespan of 10 years and demonstrates a pregnancy rate of 0.5% to 0.8%. The levonorgestrel-releasing IUD lasts for up to 5 years and has a pregnancy rate of 0.2%. The overall expulsion rate for IUDs is 1% to 5%, with the greatest likelihood in the first few months of use. Expulsion is often preceded by cramping, vaginal discharge, or bleeding, although it may be asymptomatic, with the only evi-

---

## BOX 24.4
## Indications and Contraindications for Intrauterine Device Use

**Indications**
- Multiparous and nulliparous women at low risk for sexually transmitted diseases
- Women who desire long-term reversible contraception
- Women with the following medical conditions, for which an intrauterine device may be an optimal method:
  - Diabetes*
  - Thromboembolism†
  - Menorrhagia/dysmenorrhea‡
  - Breastfeeding§
  - Breast cancer ||
  - Liver disease¶

**Contraindications**
- Pregnancy
- Pelvic inflammatory disease (current or within the past 3 months)
- Sexually transmitted diseases (current)
- Puerperal or postabortion sepsis (current or within the past 3 months)
- Purulent cervicitis
- Undiagnosed abnormal vaginal bleeding
- Malignancy of the genital tract
- Known uterine anomalies or fibroids distorting the cavity in a way incompatible with intrauterine device (IUD) insertion
- Allergy to any component of the IUD or Wilson disease (for copper-containing IUDs)

§Copper only until 4–6 weeks postpartum.
||Copper only for current breast cancer.
¶The levonorgestrel intrauterine system is not recommended for current liver disease.
Data from The intra-uterine device: Canadian Consensus Conference on Contraception. *J SOGC.* 1998;20(7):769–773; IMAP statement on intrauterine devices. International Planned Parenthood Federation (IPPF). International Medical Advisory Panel (IMAP). *IPPF Med Bull.* 1995;29(6):1–4; and World Health Organization. Medical eligibility criteria for contraceptive use. 3rd ed. Geneva: WHO; 2004.
Adapted from American College of Obstetricians and Gynecologists. *Guidelines for Women's Health Care.* 3rd ed. Washington, DC. American College of Obstetricians and Gynecologists;2007:192–193.

dence being the observed lengthening of the IUD string or the partner feeling the device during intercourse. Patients should be counseled to see their clinician if expulsion is suspected.

The IUDs do not increase the overall risk of ectopic pregnancy. However, because the IUD offers greater protection against intrauterine than extrauterine pregnancy, the relative ratio of extrauterine pregnancy is greater in a woman who uses an IUD than in a woman not using contraception. Therefore, in the rare instance that a woman with an IUD in place becomes pregnant, that pregnancy would have a high risk of being extra-uterine.

About 40% to 50% of patients who become pregnant with an IUD in place will spontaneously abort in the first trimester. Because of this risk, patients should be offered IUD removal if the string is visible; this is associated with a decreased spontaneous abortion rate of about 30%. If the IUD string is not visible, instrumental removal may be performed, but the risk of pregnancy disruption is increased. If the IUD is left in place, pregnancy may proceed uneventfully. There is no evidence of an increased risk of congenital anomalies with either medicated or unmedicated devices. There is, however, an approximate twofold to fourfold increase in the incidence of preterm labor and delivery.

Patient selection and skillful insertion are crucial to the successful use of the IUD as a method of contraception. The risk of sexually transmitted infections is the most important factor in patient selection, not age and parity.

IUD insertion is best accomplished when the patient is menstruating. This timing is beneficial because it confirms the patient is not pregnant and her cervix is usually slightly open. If that timing cannot be achieved, it can be done at other times in the cycle as the patient is switching from another reliable method of contraception. The devices may also be inserted in breastfeeding women, who, in fact, demonstrate a lower incidence of postinsertional discomfort and bleeding. All IUD insertion techniques share the same basic rules: careful bimanual examination before insertion to determine the likely direction of insertion into the endometrial cavity, proper loading of the device into the inserter, careful placement to the fundal margin of the endometrial cavity, and proper inserter removal while leaving the IUD in place.

The IUD is removed by simply pulling on the string. If the string is not visible, rotating two cotton-tip applicators in the endocervical canal will often retrieve the strings. If this is not possible, a fine probe may be inserted, the IUD felt, and then removed with an "IUD hook" or small forceps. If needed, ultrasound guidance can assist in this process. Infrequently, IUDs become embedded in the uterine wall and require hysteroscopic removal. Even less frequently, an IUD perforates the uterus (at insertion, but is not always recognized) and requires laparoscopic removal.

## NATURAL FAMILY PLANNING

*"Natural family planning" refers to methods that seek to prevent pregnancy by either avoiding intercourse around the time of ovulation or using knowledge of the time of ovulation to augment other methods, such as barriers or spermicides.* These methods are safe, cost little, and may be more acceptable for couples who wish a natural method. However, the failure rate with typical use is high. For couples who are highly motivated and for women with a regular menstrual cycle, these methods may provide acceptable contraception.

Several methods are in use, and all are based on estimation of the woman's fertile period:

* Calendar method
* Basal body temperature method
* Cervical mucus method
* Symptothermal method

The calendar method is based on calculation of a woman's fertile period. For a woman with a regular 28-day cycle, the fertile period would last from days 10 through 17. Additional days are added to the fertile period based on the time of shortest and longest menstrual interval. Basal body temperatures and changes in cervical mucus are used to detect ovulation. A rise in basal body temperature of 0.5°F to 1°F, or the presence of thin, "stretchy," clear cervical mucus, indicates ovulation. The symptothermal method combines assessment of cervical mucus and basal body temperature methods.

Couples using these methods avoid intercourse until a suitable period after ovulation, that is, 2 to 3 days after temperature rise or from the first awareness of the clear, copious mucus associated with ovulation until 4 to 5 days thereafter, indicated by the appearance of the milky or opaque mucus seen in the postovulatory, or "safe," interval. These methods are especially difficult to use in the postpartum period, when menstrual regularity has not yet resumed and cervical secretions are varied in appearance. Ovulation can occur as early as the fifth week postpartum. Lactation may temporarily suppress ovulation for up to six months in women who are exclusively breastfeeding. Lactation as a method of contraception is unpredictable because a woman may begin ovulation before she resumes menstruation.

## POSTCOITAL/EMERGENCY CONTRACEPTION

**Postcoital or emergency contraception (ECP)** may be used for women who experience unprotected sexual intercourse. Making postcoital contraception widely and easily available is one of the most important steps that can be taken to reduce the high rates of unintended pregnancy and abortion. It is estimated that the regular use of postcoital contraception would prevent more than 1.5 million unintended pregnancies in the United States each year.

Combined oral conceptive regimens used for emergency contraception, known collectively as the Yuzpe method, were first reported by Albert Yuzpe in 1974. These regimens require taking 2 tablets within 72 hours of unprotected intercourse, followed by another two tablets in 12 hours. Subsequently, the use of a progestin-only regimen, known as **"Plan B,"** was approved for behind-the-counter dispensing to women over 18 years of age without a prescription. Plan B consists of two tablets of levonorgestrel taken 12 hours apart. This method is associated with a lower incidence of nausea and emesis than the Yuzpe method and with greater effectiveness. Both methods act by preventing ovulation and fertilization, and will not terminate an existing pregnancy. Emergency contraception can also be accomplished with a copper-containing IUD.

The failure rate for the Yuzpe regimen is estimated at 25%; for Plan B, 11%. Multiple unprotected coital events or an interval greater than 72 hours may be associated with an increasing failure rate, although some evidence of success is seen out to 120 hours after unprotected intercourse. If the woman is already pregnant, these medications have no ill effect on the fetus. The amount of hormone in these regimens is not associated with alterations in clotting factors or teratogenic risk.

The copper IUD is another recommended option for emergency contraception (except in patients with Wilson disease) and, in limited studies, has a failure rate of approximately 0.1%. An additional advantage of IUD insertion is the contraceptive effect that is provided for up to 10 years.

Before using this method, a pregnancy test is required because of the risk to an implanted pregnancy.

## INEFFECTIVE METHODS

The clinician must be prepared to counsel against routine use of less-than-effective, folklore-based techniques such as postcoital douching, withdrawal before ejaculation (coitus interruptus), makeshift barriers (such as food wrap), and various contraceptive coital positions. Contraceptive counseling should address effective methods compatible with the patient and her partner.

## SUGGESTED READINGS

American College of Obstetricians and Gynecologists. Emergency contraception. ACOG Practice Bulletin No. 69. *Obstet Gynecol.* 2005;106(6):1443–1452.

American College of Obstetricians and Gynecologists. *Guidelines for Women's Health Care.* 3rd ed. Washington, DC: American College of Obstetricians and Gynecologists; 2007.

American College of Obstetricians and Gynecologists. Intrauterine device. ACOG Practice Bulletin No. 59. *Obstet Gynecol.* 2005; 105(1):223–232.

American College of Obstetricians and Gynecologists. Noncontraceptive uses of the levonorgestrel intrauterine system. ACOG Committee Opinion No. 337. *Obstet Gynecol.* 2006; 107(6):1479–1482.

American College of Obstetricians and Gynecologists. Use of hormonal contraception in women with coexisting medical conditions. ACOG Practice Bulletin No. 73. *Obstet Gynecol.* 2006; 107(6):1453–72.

# 25 Sterilization

This chapter deals primarily with APGO Educational Topic:

Topic 33: Contraception and Sterilization

Students should be able to list the various methods of sterilization by type and describe their mechanisms of action, effectiveness, risks and benefits, and indications and contraindications.

Sterilization offers highly effective birth control without continuing expense, effort, or motivation. *It is the most frequently used method of controlling fertility in the United States.* Approximately one in three married couples have chosen surgical sterilization as their method of contraception. Sterilization is the leading contraceptive method for couples when the wife is older than 30 years and who have been married more than 10 years.

All available surgical methods of sterilization prevent the union of sperm and egg, either by preventing the passage of sperm into the ejaculate (vasectomy) or by permanently occluding the fallopian tube (tubal ligation and hysteroscopic sterilization).

*Although it is possible to reverse some forms of sterilization, the difficulty of doing so, combined with the generally poor rate of success and the financial expense, demands that patients consider the procedure permanent.*

The physician should counsel couples who are considering surgical sterilization and assist them in determining the best method.

Changes in operative techniques; anesthesia methods; and attitudes of the public, insurance providers, and physicians have contributed to the rapid increase in the number of sterilization procedures performed each year. Modern methods of surgical sterilization are less invasive, less expensive, safer, and as effective—if not more effective—than those used in the past (Table 25.1).

## STERILIZATION OF MEN

About one-third of all surgical sterilization procedures are performed on men. The technique for **vasectomy** varies and includes excision and ligation, electrocautery, and me-

chanical or chemical occlusion of the vas deferens. Because vasectomy is performed outside the abdominal cavity, the procedure is safer, more easily performed in most cases, less expensive, and generally more effective than procedures done on women. Vasectomy is also more easily reversed than most female sterilization procedures (Fig. 25.1). The main benefit of tubal ligation over vasectomy is immediate sterility.

*Minor postoperative complications occur in 5% to 10% of cases, and include bleeding, hematomas, acute and chronic pain, and local skin infections.* Some authors report a greater incidence of depression and change in body image after vasectomy than after female sterilization. This risk may be minimized with preoperative counseling and education. Concern has been raised about the formation of sperm antibodies in approximately 50% of patients, but no adverse long-term effects of vasectomy have been identified. Likewise, concerns about an increased risk of prostate cancer following vasectomy are not supported in literature; indeed, in countries with the highest rates of vasectomy, there is no increase in the incidence of prostate cancer.

*Pregnancy after vasectomy occurs in about 1% of cases.* Many of these pregnancies result from intercourse too soon after the procedure, rather than from recanalization. Vasectomy is not immediately effective. Multiple ejaculations are required before the proximal collecting system is emptied of sperm. Couples should use another method of contraception until male sterility is reasonably assured or postoperative azoospermia is confirmed by semen analysis (50% at 8 weeks, 100% at 10 weeks postprocedure).

## STERILIZATION OF WOMEN

Surgical sterilization techniques for women can be performed by laparoscopy, hysteroscopy, minilaparotomy, or transvaginally. *Sterilization can be performed as an interval procedure, after a spontaneous or elective abortion, or as a post-*

| TABLE 25.1 | Failure Rates (10-year) per 1000 procedures and Complications for Sterilization Methods | |
|---|---|---|
| **Tubal Ligation** | **10-Year Failure Rates per 1000 Procedures** | **Complications** |
| Bipolar coagulation | 24.8 | Injury to gastrointestinal and urinary systems, anesthesia-associated complications, hemorrhage, infection, ectopic pregnancy |
| Silicone band methods | 17.7 | |
| Spring clip | 36.5 | |
| Ligation methods -Postpartum -Interval | 7.5 20.1 | |
| Micro-insert (by hysteroscopy) | Not yet available | Uterine perforation, bleeding, and infection |
| **Vasectomy** | 10 | Infection, bleeding, hematoma formation, granuloma formation |

*partum procedure at the time of caesarean delivery or following vaginal delivery.* Some nonsurgical methods based on principles of immunization as well as sclerosing agents are under investigation, but remain experimental although promising. Regardless of the method chosen, patients should be counseled about the various components of the procedure, effectiveness rates, and possible complications. Failure rates of tubal sterilization are roughly comparable with those of the intrauterine contraceptive (IUC). Pregnancy should also be ruled out prior to performing any sterilization procedure.

## Laparoscopy

Performed as an outpatient interval procedure, laparoscopic techniques may be carried out under local, regional, or general anesthesia (see Chapter 32, Gynecologic Procedures). Small incisions, a relatively low rate of complications, and a degree of flexibility in the procedures have led to high physician and patient acceptability.

**Occlusion of the fallopian tubes** may be accomplished through the use of electrocautery (unipolar or bipo-lar) or the application of a plastic and spring clip (Filshie clip) or silastic band (Yoon or Falope ring). The choice among laparoscopic methods and cautery or occlusive device is often based more on operator experience, training, and personal preference than on outcome data.

**Electrocautery-based methods** are fast, but they carry a risk of inadvertent electrical damage to other structures, poorer reversibility, and greater incidence of ectopic pregnancies when failure does occur. Most operators coagulate at the isthmus, taking care that the coagulation forceps is placed over the entire fallopian tube and onto the mesosalpinx so that the entire tube and its lumen are coagulated >3 cm in length. Bipolar cautery is safer than unipolar; it has less risk of spark injury to adjacent tissue, because the current passes directly between the blades of the coagulation forceps (Fig. 25.2). *Unipolar cautery, however, has a lower failure rate than bipolar.* The surgeon, therefore, needs to carefully weigh the risk of the individual procedure with its respective effectiveness.

The **Hulka clip** is the most readily reversible method because of its minimal tissue damage, but it also carries the greatest failure rate (>1%) for the same reason. As in coagulation, care must be taken to place the jaws of the Hulka clip over the entire breadth of the fallopian tube at a 90-degree angle. This can be especially difficult when performed immediately postpartum, due to the natural edematous dilation of the tubes.

The **Falope ring** is intermediate for both reversibility and failure rates. Patients may, however, have a higher incidence of postoperative pain, requiring strong analgesics. Care must be taken to draw a sufficient "knuckle" of fallopian tube into the Falope ring applicator so that the band is placed below the outer and inner borders of the fallopian tube, thus occluding the lumen completely (Fig. 25.3A). Bleeding is a potential complication if too much pressure is placed on the mesosalpinx during the application of the ring.

The **Filshie clip** has a lower failure rate than the Hulka clip, because of its larger diameter, ease of application, and atraumatic locking device (Fig. 25.3B). To max-

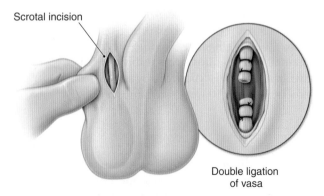

Scrotal incision

Double ligation of vasa

FIGURE 25.1. Vasectomy.

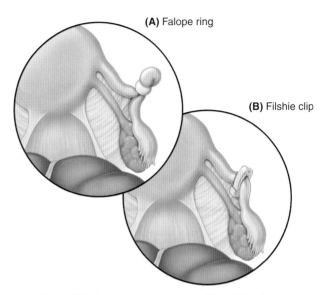

**(A)** Falope ring

**(B)** Filshie clip

FIGURE 25.3. (A) Falope ring. (B) Filshie clip.

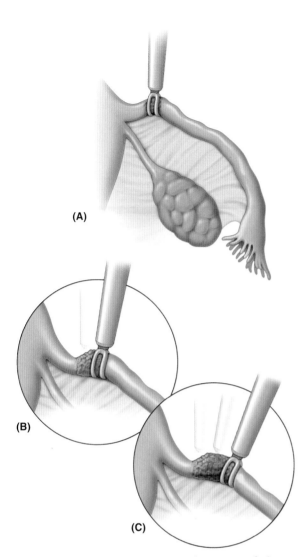

**(A)**

**(B)**

**(C)**

FIGURE 25.2. Electrocautery. (A) Placement of electro-cautery forceps. (B) Cauterization of the fallopian tube. (C) Tube coagulated to >3 cm in length.

imize effectiveness, this clip should be placed at the isthmic portion of the fallopian tube.

## Minilaparotomy

*Minilaparotomy is the most common surgical approach for tubal ligation throughout the world.* Minilaparotomy can be accomplished with a small infraumbilical incision made in the postpartum period or a small lower abdominal suprapubic incision used as an interval procedure, both of which provide ready access to the uterine tubes. Occlusion of the fallopian tubes may then be accomplished by excision of all or part of the fallopian tube or the use of clips, rings, or cautery.

*A common method of tubal interruption done in minila-parotomy is the Pomeroy tubal ligation* (Fig. 25.4). In this pro-cedure, a segment of tube from the midportion is elevated, and an absorbable ligature is placed across the base, forming a loop, or knuckle, of tube. This knuckle is then excised. Because of the similarity in appearance between the fallopian tube and the round ligament, this tissue is sent for histologic confirmation. When healing is complete, the ends of the tube will have sealed closed, with a 1- to 2-cm gap between the ends. Electrocoagulation or the application of clips or bands may also be accomplished through a minilaparotomy incision, although these are more widely used with laparoscopy.

## Transvaginal Approach

The thin wall of tissue between the vaginal canal and the posterior cul-de-sac also offers a convenient port of entry into the peritoneal cavity for sterilization procedures. *Advantages include less patient preparation (e.g., bladder catheter-ization), the absence of abdominal incision, and potentially less pain for the patient, with an earlier return to routine activity.* Contraindications include suspicion of major pelvic adhesions, enlarged uterus, and inability to place the patient in the lithotomy position. One major disadvantage is the need for adequate vaginal surgical training to minimize potential complications, such as cellulitis, pelvic abscess, hemorrhage, proctotomy, or cystotomy.

## Hysteroscopy

*Transcervical approaches to sterilization include **hysteroscopy** and involve gaining access to the fallopian tubes through the cervix.* The only currently available hysteroscopic steriliza-tion method involves the placement of a **titanium-Dacron spring device** directly into the tubal ostia bilaterally. The inserts stimulate a tissue reaction that ultimately leads to

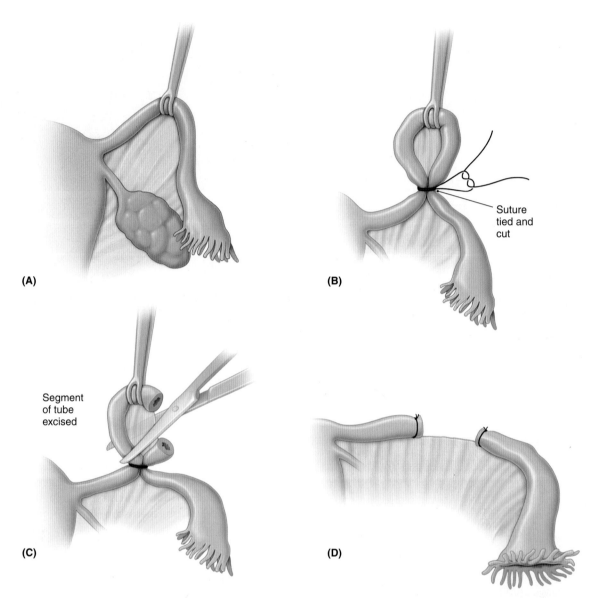

**FIGURE 25.4.** Pomeroy technique. (A) A segment of the tube is elevated. (B) A suture is tied, forming a loop in the tube. (C) The loop is excised. (D) A 1- to 2-cm gap forms between the ends of the cut tube when healing is complete.

tubal occlusion. Patients are instructed to use an additional form of contraception for 3 months after the procedure, until the efficacy of the device can be proven with **hysterosalpingography.** Contraindications include nickel or contrast allergies, active pelvic infection, and suspected pregnancy. *Patients should be pretreated with either depomedroxyprogesterone (DMPA) or continuous combined oral contraceptive pills, which ensures a thin endometrial lining, enhances visualization, and improves the success rate of the procedure.* This procedure can be used for obese patients who may otherwise not be suitable candidates for laparoscopic tubal ligation due to their body habitus. The efficacy for this procedure has been reported to be as great as 99.8%.

## Side Effects and Complications

No surgically-based technology is free of the possibility of complications or side effects. Infection, bleeding, injury to surrounding structures, or anesthetic complications may occur with any of the techniques discussed in this chapter. The overall fatality rate attributed to sterilization is about 1–4 per 100,000 procedures, significantly lower than that for childbearing in the United States, estimated at about 10 per 100,000 births.

*Although pregnancy after sterilization is uncommon, there is substantial risk that any post-sterilization pregnancies will be ectopic.* The risk varies with the type of procedure and the age of the patient. Ectopic pregnancy occurs after tubal ligation more commonly after cautery than after mechanical tubal occlusion, probably because of microscopic fistulae in the coagulated segment connecting to the peritoneal cavity. Overall, the 10-year cumulative probability of ectopic pregnancy after tubal ligation is 7.3 per 1000 procedures.

## Noncontraceptive Benefits

Patients who undergo a tubal ligation not only gain effective contraception; they also benefit from a decreased lifetime risk of ovarian cancer. The mechanism for this risk reduction is unknown at this time. Although tubal sterilization has not been shown to protect against sexually transmitted diseases (STDs), it may offer some protection against pelvic inflammatory disease.

## REVERSAL OF TUBAL LIGATION

Reversal of tubal ligation by microsurgical techniques is most successful when minimal damage is done to the smallest length of the fallopian tube (e.g., Hulka clip, Filshie clip, or Falope ring)—in some series approaching 50% to 75%. In most cases, however, rates of 25% to 50% are more reasonable expectations, so that many specialists in infertility recommend the use of assisted reproductive technology (e.g., in vitro fertilization) rather than attempts at tubal ligation reversal with the attendant low success rates and increased risk of tubal ectopic pregnancy.

*A patient who has undergone tubal reversal and becomes pregnant is presumed to have an ectopic pregnancy until intrauterine pregnancy is established.*

## THE DECISION FOR STERILIZATION

The decision for sterilization is an important one and the patient should be fully informed about the procedure and its risks, effectiveness, and long-term implications (Box 25.1). Components of presterilization counseling should include:

---

**BOX 25.1**
### Risk Indicators for Regret About Decision for Sterilization

Age younger than 25 years at the time of sterilization
Less access to, information about, or support for other contraceptive method use
Incomplete or inadequate information about the procedure
Making the decision under pressure from a spouse or because of medical indications

---

- Permanent nature of the procedure
- Alternative methods available, including male sterilization
- Reasons for choosing sterilization
- Screening for risk indicators for regret
- Details of the procedure, including risks and benefits
- The possibility of failure, including ectopic pregnancy
- The need to use condoms for protection against sexually transmitted diseases, including HIV
- Completion of informed consent process
- Local regulations regarding interval from time of consent to procedure

*Despite careful counseling, approximately 10% to 15% of patients who undergo sterilization subsequently report regret, although only 1% actually request reversal of the procedure.*

## SUGGESTED READINGS

American College of Obstetricians and Gynecologists. Benefits and risks of sterilization. ACOG Practice Bulletin No. 46. *Obstet Gynecol.* 2003;102(3):647–658.

American College of Obstetricians and Gynecologists. *Guidelines for Women's Health Care: A Resource Manual.* 3rd ed. Washington, D.C.: ACOG; 2007.

American College of Obstetricians and Gynecologists. Multifetal pregnancy reduction. ACOG Committee Opinion No. 371. *Obstet Gynecol.* 2007;110(1):217–220.

American College of Obstetricians and Gynecologists. Patient Education pamphlet, "Sterilization by Laparoscopy." AP035, Washington, DC: ACOG: 2003.

American College of Obstetricians and Gynecologists. Patient Education pamphlet, "Sterilization for Women and Men." AP011, Washington, DC: ACOG: 2005.

# 26 Vulvovaginitis

Students should be able to discuss the evaluation and management of vulvovaginitis.

V ulvovaginitis is the spectrum of conditions that cause vaginal or vulvar symptoms such as itching, burning, irritation, and abnormal discharge. Vaginal and vulvar symptoms are among the most common reasons for patient visits to obstetrician–gynecologists. Symptoms may be acute or subacute, and may range in intensity from mild to severe. Vulvovaginitis may have important consequences in terms of discomfort and pain, days lost from school or work, sexual functioning, and self-image. Depending on etiology, vulvovaginitis may also be associated with adverse reproductive outcomes in pregnant and nonpregnant women.

Vulvovaginitis has a broad differential diagnosis, and successful treatment frequently depends on accurately identifying its cause. The most common causes of vaginitis are bacterial vaginosis (22%–50% of symptomatic women), vulvovaginal candidiasis (17%–39%), and trichomoniasis (4%–35%). Common vaginal infections often present with characteristic patterns (Table 26.1). The vulva and vagina are also sites of symptoms and lesions of several sexually transmitted infections, such as herpes genitalis, human papillomavirus, syphilis, chancroid, granuloma inguinale, lymphogranuloma venereum, and molluscum contagiosum (see Chapter 27, Sexually Transmitted Diseases). It is estimated that up to 70% of women with vaginitis remain undiagnosed. In this undiagnosed group, symptoms may be caused by a broad array of conditions, including atrophic vaginitis, various vulvar dermatologic conditions, and vulvodynia.

Although sexually transmitted and other infections are common etiologies of vulvovaginitis, the patient's history and symptoms may point to chemical, allergic, or other noninfectious causes. Evaluation of women with vulvovaginitis should include a focused history about the entire spectrum of vaginal symptoms, including change in discharge, vaginal malodor, itching, irritation, burning, swelling, dyspareunia, and dysuria. Questions about the location of symptoms (vulva, vagina, anus), duration, the relation to the menstrual cycle, the response to prior treatment including self-treatment and douching, and a sexual history can yield important insights into the likely etiology. In patients with vulvar symptoms, the physical examination should begin with a thorough evaluation of the vulva. However, evaluation may be compromised by patient self-treatment with nonprescription medications.

A variety of laboratory tests are available to aid in diagnosing the cause of vulvovaginitis. Samples obtained during speculum examination can be tested for vaginal pH, amine ("whiff") test, and saline (wet mount) and 10% potassium hydroxide (KOH) microscopy. Tests for diagnosing vaginal infection, such as rapid tests for enzyme activity from bacterial vaginosis-associated organisms, *Trichomonas vaginalis* antigen, and point-of-care testing for DNA of *Gardnerella vaginalis*, *Trichomonas vaginalis*, and *Candida* species are also available, although the role of these tests in the proper management of patients with vulvovaginitis is unclear. Depending on risk factors, DNA amplification tests can be obtained for *Neisseria gonorrhoeae* and *Chlamydia trachomatis*.

## NORMAL VULVOVAGINAL ECOSYSTEM

The vulva and vagina are covered by stratified squamous epithelium. The vulva contains hair follicles and sebaceous, sweat, and apocrine glands, whereas the epithelium of the vagina is nonkeratinized and lacks these specialized elements. After puberty, with maturation of the epithelial cells that occurs with estrogen stimulation, increased levels of glycogen in the vaginal tissues favor the growth of lactobacilli in the genital tract. These bacteria break down glycogen to lactic acid, lowering the pH from the 6 to 8 range, which is common before puberty and after menopause, to the normal vaginal pH range of 3.5 to 4.7 in the reproductive-aged woman. In addition to lactobacilli, a wide range of other aerobic and anaerobic bacteria are

**TABLE 26.1  Diagnosis and Treatment of Physiologic Vaginal Secretions and Common Vaginal Infections**

| Characteristic | Normal | Bacterial Vaginosis (BV) | Candidiasis | Trichomoniasis |
|---|---|---|---|---|
| **Common symptoms** | None | - Discharge<br>- Odor that gets worse after intercourse; may be asymptomatic | - Itching<br>- Burning<br>- Irritation<br>- Thick, white discharge | - Frothy discharge<br>- Bad odor<br>- Dysuria<br>- Dyspareunia<br>- Vulvar itching and burning |
| **Amount of discharge** | Small | Often increased | Sometimes increased | Increased |
| **Appearance of discharge** | - White<br>- Clear<br>- Flocculent | - Thin, Homogeneous<br>- Gray-green<br>- White<br>- Adherent | - White<br>- Curdy<br>- "Cottage cheese-like" | - Gray-green<br>- Frothy<br>- Adherent |
| **Vaginal pH** | 3.8–4.2 | >4.5 | Normal | >4.5 |
| **KOH "whiff test" (amine odor)** | Absent | Present (fishy) | Absent | Possibly present (fishy) |
| **Microscopic appearance** | - Normal squamous epithelial cells<br>- Numerous lactobacilli | - Increased white blood cells<br>- Decreased lactobacilli<br>- Many clue cells | - Hyphae and buds | - Normal epithelial cells<br>- Increased white blood cells<br>- Trichomonads |
| **Treatment** | N/A | Metronidazole (oral or topical)<br>Clindamycin (oral or topical) | Topical synthetic imidazoles or oral fluconazole | Oral metronidazole or tinidazole |

KOH = potassium hydroxide.

normally found in the vagina at concentrations of $10^8$ to $10^9$ colonies per mL of vaginal fluid. Because the vagina is a potential space, not an open tube, a ratio of 5:1 anaerobic: aerobic bacteria is normal.

Discharge from the vagina is normal; therefore, not all discharges from the vagina indicate infection. This distinction is important to the diagnostic process. Vaginal secretions arise from several sources. The majority of the liquid portion consists of mucus from the cervix. A small amount of moisture is contributed by endometrial fluid, exudates from accessory glands such as the Skene and Bartholin glands, and from vaginal transudate. Exfoliated squamous cells from the vaginal wall give the secretions a white to off-white color and provide some increase in consistency. The action of the indigenous vaginal flora also can contribute to the secretion. These components together constitute the normal vaginal secretions that provide the physiologic lubrication that prevents drying and irritation. The amount and character of this mixture vary under the influence of many factors, including hormonal and fluid status, pregnancy, immunosuppression, and inflammation. Asymptomatic women produce approximately 1.5 g of vaginal fluid per day. Normal vaginal secretions have no odor.

## BACTERIAL VAGINOSIS (BV)

Bacterial vaginosis (BV) is a polymicrobial infection characterized by a lack of hydrogen peroxide-producing lactobacilli and an overgrowth of facultative anaerobic organisms including *G. vaginalis*, *Mycoplasma hominis*, *Bacteroides* species, *Peptostreptococcus* species, *Fusobacterium* species, *Prevotella* species, and *Atopobium vaginae*.

Women with BV generally complain of a "musty" or "fishy" odor with an increased thin gray-white to yellow discharge. The discharge may cause mild vulvar irritation in approximately 25% of the cases. The vaginal discharge is mildly adherent to the vaginal wall and has a pH greater than 4.5.

Microscopic examination made under saline wet mount shows a slight increase in white blood cells, clumps of bacteria, loss of normal lactobacilli, and characteristic "clue cells" (Fig. 26.1). These are epithelial cells with numerous coccoid bacteria attached to their surface, which makes their borders appear indistinct and their cytoplasm resemble "ground glass." Because the bacteria that cause BV are part of the normal vaginal flora, the mere presence of these organisms is not diagnostic. The diagnosis of BV

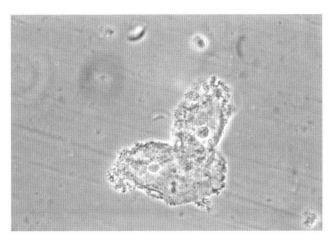

FIGURE 26.1. Clue cells. Clue cells are epithelial cells with clumps of bacteria clustered on their surfaces. Clue cells indicate the presence of a vaginal bacterial infection. CDC/M. Rein.

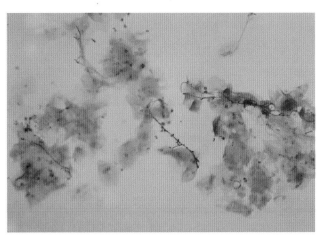

FIGURE 26.2. *Candida albicans.* Branching hyphae are present among epithelial cells in this Gram stain of a vaginal smear. CDC/Dr. Stuart Brown.

is defined by any three of the following four criteria: (1) abnormal gray discharge, (2) pH greater than 4.5, (3) positive "whiff test," and (4) the presence of clue cells.

BV may be treated with oral or topical metronidazole or oral or topical clindamycin. Symptomatic pregnant women can also be treated with these medications, as neither drug has been shown to have teratogenic effects. Some studies have shown that screening for and treatment of BV in women with high-risk pregnancies may reduce the incidence of premature rupture of membranes (PROM) and preterm delivery. However, studies do not confirm that universal BV screening and treatment in asymptomatic pregnant women helps prevent adverse outcomes. In nonpregnant women, BV has been associated with other infections, including pelvic inflammatory and postoperative infections. It has also been associated with an increased risk of acquisition of human immunodeficiency virus (HIV) and herpes simplex virus (HSV). Although preoperative BV treatment may help prevent complications stemming from postoperative infection, treatment for BV has not been shown to decrease the risk of the HIV or HSV infection.

## Vulvovaginal Candidiasis

**Vulvovaginal candidiasis** is caused by ubiquitous airborne fungi. Approximately 90% of these infections are caused by *Candida albicans* (Fig. 26.2). The remaining cases are caused by *Candida glabrata*, *Candida tropicalis*, or *Torulopsis glabrata*. Candida infections generally do not coexist with other infections and are not considered to be sexually transmitted, although 10% of male partners have concomitant penile infections. Candidiasis is more likely to occur in women who are pregnant, diabetic, obese, immunosuppressed, on oral contraceptives or corticosteroids, or have had broadspectrum antibiotic therapy. Practices that keep the vaginal

area warm and moist, such as wearing tight clothing or the habitual use of panty liners, may also increase the risk of Candida infections.

The most common presenting complaint for women with candidiasis is itching, although up to 20% of women may be asymptomatic. Burning, external dysuria, and dyspareunia are also common. The vulva and vaginal tissues are often bright red in color, and excoriation is not uncommon in severe cases. A thick, adherent "cottage cheese" discharge with a pH of 4 to 5 is generally found. This discharge is odorless.

Multiple studies conclude that a reliable diagnosis cannot be made on the basis of history and physical examination alone. Over-the-counter (OTC) treatments are safe and effective, but any woman who does not respond to OTC treatment or who has a recurrence soon after treatment should be seen by a physician for a definitive diagnosis. Patients who have self-administered treatment with OTC medications should be advised to stop treatment three days before their office visit. Diagnosis requires either visualization of blastospores or pseudohyphae on saline, or 10% KOH microscopy, or a positive culture in a symptomatic woman. The diagnosis can be further classified as uncomplicated or complicated vulvovaginal candidiasis (Box 26.1). Latex agglutination tests may be of particular use for non-*Candida albicans* strains, because they do not demonstrate the pseudohyphae on wet prep.

Treatment of candida infections is primarily with the topical application of one of the synthetic imidazoles, such as miconazole, clotrimazole, butoconazole, or terconazole in cream or suppository form placed intravaginally. Short-term oral therapy with low-dose (150 mg) fluconazole has become widely used. Pregnant women should be treated with topical agents due to the increased risk of birth defects associated with high doses (400 to 800 mg) of fluconazole.

Although these agents are associated with high cure rates, approximately 20% to 30% of patients experience recurrences one month after treatment. Weekly therapy with fluconazole for six months has been shown to be effective in preventing recurrent candidiasis in 50% of women. Intermittent therapy with topical agents (weekly or twice weekly) can also be used for prevention. *T. glabrata* is resistant to all azoles and may respond to therapy with intravaginal boric acid capsules or gentian violet. Patients with frequent recurrences should be carefully evaluated for possible risk factors such as diabetes or autoimmune disease. Prophylactic local therapy with an antifungal agent should be considered when systemic antibiotics are prescribed.

## Trichomonas Vulvovaginitis

*T. vaginalis* is a flagellate protozoan that lives only in the vagina, Skene ducts, and male or female urethra. The infection can be transmitted by sexual contact, but can also occur via fomites, and the organism has been known to survive in swimming pools and hot tubs. Trichomoniasis is associated with pelvic inflammatory disease (PID), endometritis, infertility, ectopic pregnancy, and preterm birth, and it often coexists with other sexually transmitted diseases and BV. It has also been shown to facilitate HIV transmission.

Symptoms of trichomonas infection vary from mild to severe and may include vulvar itching or burning, copious discharge with rancid odor, dysuria, and dyspareunia. Although not present in all women, the discharge associated with trichomonas infections is generally "frothy," thin, and yellow-green to gray in color, with a pH above

4.5. Examination may reveal edema or erythema of the vulva. Petechiae, or strawberry patches, are classically described as present in the upper vagina or on the cervix, but are actually found in only about 10% of affected patients. A significant number of women with trichomoniasis are asymptomatic.

The diagnosis is confirmed by microscopic examination of vaginal secretions suspended in normal saline. This wet smear will show large numbers of mature epithelial cells, white blood cells (WBCs), and the trichomonas organism (Fig. 26.3). A point-of-care test for trichomonas antigens, the OSOM Trichomonas Rapid Test, has a sensitivity of 88.3% and specificity of 98.8% compared with culture. Women diagnosed with trichomoniasis should also undergo screening for other STDs, especially gonorrhea and chlamydia.

Treatment of trichomonas infections is with oral metronidazole or tinidazole. Treating sexual partners of women with trichomoniasis is recommended, and individuals undergoing treatment should avoid unprotected intercourse. Abstinence from alcohol use when taking metronidazole is necessary to avoid a possible disulfiram-like reaction. Trichomoniasis has been associated with preterm delivery, PROM, and low birth weight. Pregnant patients should be treated, and metronidazole is considered safe for use during pregnancy. However, treatment may not prevent these pregnancy complications.

Although follow-up examination of patients with trichomoniasis for test of cure is often advocated, they are usually not cost-effective, except in the rare patient with a history of frequent recurrences. In these patients, reinfection or poor compliance must be considered as well as the possibility of infection with more than one agent or other underlying disease. Infections with metronidazole-resistant *T. vaginalis* have been reported. Although absolute resistance is rare, relative resistance may be as high as 5%. These infections are treated with high doses of tinidazole.

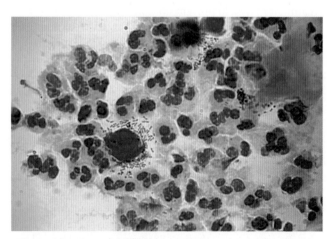

FIGURE 26.3. Trichomonads. The flagella of this parasite can be clearly seen in this image. CDC.

## OTHER CAUSES OF VULVOVAGINITIS

**Atrophic vaginitis** is defined as atrophy of the vaginal epithelium due to diminished estrogen levels. Although more common in postmenopausal women, atrophic vaginitis can be observed in younger premenopausal women. Estrogen status plays a crucial role in determining the normal state of the vagina. When estrogen levels decrease, there is loss of cellular glycogen with resulting loss of lactic acid. In the prepubertal and postmenopausal states, the vaginal epithelium is thinned, and the pH of the vagina usually is elevated (4.7 or greater). Loss of elasticity in the connective tissue may also occur, resulting in shortening and narrowing of the vagina. The urinary tract may also be affected and may demonstrate atrophic changes. Patients with atrophic vaginitis may have an abnormal vaginal discharge, dryness, itching, burning, or dyspareunia. Typical urinary symptoms include urgency, frequency, recurrent urinary tract infections, and incontinence. Atrophic vaginitis is treated with topical or oral estrogen therapy.

**Desquamative inflammatory vaginitis** is generally seen in perimenopausal and postmenopausal women, and is characterized by purulent discharge, exfoliation of epithelial cells with vulvovaginal burning and erythema, relatively little lactobacilli and overgrowth of gram-positive cocci; usually streptococci are seen. Vaginal pH is greater than 4.5. Initial therapy is clindamycin cream 2%, applied daily for 14 days.

## SUGGESTED READINGS

American College of Obstetricians and Gynecologists. Vaginitis. ACOG Practice Bulletin No. 72. *Obstet Gynecol.* 2006;107(5): 1195–1206.

Galask R, Elas DE. Vulvovaginitis. In: *Precis, Gynecology.* 3rd ed. Washington, DC: American College of Obstetricians and Gynecologists; 2006:54–64.

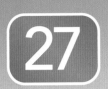

CHAPTER

# 27 Sexually Transmitted Diseases

This chapter deals primarily with APGO Educational Topic:

**Topic 36:** Sexually Transmitted Infections and Urinary Tract Infections

Students should be able to discuss diagnosis, evaluation, and management of the common sexually transmitted infections.

**S**exually transmitted diseases (STDs) are one of the most common gynecologic problems in sexually active women. STDs can be transmitted by oral, vaginal, or anal sex. The transmission of an STD may have varied consequences, including infertility, cancer, and even death. STDs are the most common cause of preventable infertility and are strongly associated with ectopic pregnancy. Sexually transmitted infections may increase the risk of HIV acquisition; preventing STDs is therefore an important strategy in preventing HIV infections. STDs can also take an individual toll, resulting in pain, discomfort, and strain on personal relationships.

Most STDs require skin-to-skin contact or exchange of body fluids for transmission. Anal sex poses a particularly high risk, because tissues in the rectum break easily, and organisms can be transmitted through these breaks. Several STDs can be transmitted through oral-genital contact. Some patients may not consider this type of sexual contact at-risk behavior, or may not consider themselves sexually active when engaging in this behavior.

*Assessment for STDs should be a routine part of women's healthcare.*

## GENERAL DIAGNOSTIC PRINCIPLES

Many sexually transmitted infections are asymptomatic in women or are asymptomatic during the initial stages of the infection. *The signs and symptoms of many STDs may be characterized by genital ulcers or infection of the cervix (cervicitis), urethra (urethritis), or both* (Table 27.2). Because 20% to 50% of patients with one STD have a coexisting infection, when one infection is confirmed, other infections must be suspected.

Because of the variations in signs and symptoms and the asymptomatic presentation of STDs, a thorough sexual history and physical examination are essential in detecting the presence of an STD. The findings obtained through a systematic physical assessment, combined with the patient's history, usually help make the proper diagnosis. The inguinal region should be evaluated for rashes, lesions, and adenopathy. The vulva, perineum, and perianal areas should be inspected for lesions or ulcerations, and palpated for thickening or swelling. The Bartholin glands, Skene ducts, and urethra should be evaluated, as these are frequent sites of gonorrheal infection. In patients with urinary symptoms, the urethra should be gently milked to express any discharge. The vagina and cervix should be inspected for lesions and abnormal discharge. If a patient engages in anal intercourse, the rectum should be considered a potential site for infection. For completeness, the oral cavity as well as the cervical and other lymph nodes should be evaluated, if appropriate, based upon the patient's modes of sexual expression.

## SCREENING

*STD screening for nonpregnant women depends on the age of the patient and assessment of risk factors (Box 27.1).*

The diagnosis of certain STDs should also prompt screening for other sexually transmitted infections. When a patient is diagnosed with cervicitis, she should also be screened for PID, chlamydial infection, gonorrhea, bacterial vaginosis, and trichomoniasis and treated, if necessary. A woman diagnosed with PID should be tested for chlamydial infection, gonorrhea, and HIV.

## PREVENTION

Prevention of STDS involves educating patients about delaying sexual activity, limiting the number of sexual

## BOX 27.1
### ACOG STD Screening Recommendations

**Routine Screening:**

- Sexually active women 25 years and younger should be routinely screened for chlamydial infection.
- All sexually active adolescents should be routinely screened for gonorrhea.
- Women with developmental disabilities should be screened for STDs.
- HIV screening is recommended for all women who are or ever have been sexually active. (Physicians should be aware of and follow their states' HIV screening requirements.)

**Screening Based On Risk Factors:**

- Women with a history of multiple sexual partners or a sexual partner with multiple contacts, sexual contact with culture-proved STDs, a history of repeated episodes of STDs, or attendance at clinics for STDs should be regularly screened for STDs.
- Asymptomatic women aged 26 and older who are at high risk for infection should be routinely screened for chlamydial infection and gonorrhea.

American College of Obstetricians and Gynecologists. *Guidelines for Women's Health Care: A Resource Manual.* 3rd ed. Washington, DC: American College of Obstetricians and Gynecologists; 2007:201.

## SPECIFIC INFECTIONS

Tables 27.1 and 27.2 summarize the prevalence, signs and symptoms, evaluation, and special considerations of the most common STDs according to whether they present as genital ulcers or cervicitis. Treatment protocols change frequently, and the most current guidelines can be found on the Centers for Disease Control and Prevention Web site (www.cdc.gov).

### Chlamydia Trachomatis

*Chlamydia trachomatis* is a gram-negative obligate intracellular bacterium that lacks the metabolic and biochemical ability to produce adenosine triphosphate (ATP) and preferentially infects columnar epithelial cells. Chlamydial infection is the most frequently reported infectious disease in the United States. In 2006, over one million cases were reported to the Centers for Disease Control and Prevention. Despite the high number of reported cases, most cases of chlamydial infection are unreported. It is estimated that over 1.7 million cases of chlamydial infections remain undiagnosed each year. *If untreated, up to 40% of women with chlamydia will develop* **pelvic inflammatory disease (PID),** *which can result in significant complications, including ectopic pregnancy, chronic pelvic pain, and infertility.* Chlamydial infections are also responsible for nongonococcal urethritis and inclusion conjunctivitis. Because of the serious consequences of untreated infection, it is recommended that all sexually active women under the age of 25 should be screened annually. Older women with risk factors, such as multiple sexual partners or a new partner, should also receive annual screening.

### DIAGNOSIS

Chlamydial infection is often asymptomatic. Signs and symptoms are often subtle and nonspecific, and may include abnormal vaginal discharge and vaginal bleeding. **Cervicitis,** characterized by a mucopurulent discharge from the cervix and eversion or ectropion of the cervix that results in intermittent cervical bleeding, may also suggest the diagnosis (Fig. 27.1). Ascending infection causes mild **salpingitis** (infection of the fallopian tubes) with insidious symptoms. Once salpingitis is established, it may remain active for many months, with increasing risk for tubal damage. *Because chlamydia is also frequently found in conjunction with* Neisseria gonorrhoeae *infection, any patient with known or suspected gonorrhea infection should also be evaluated for chlamydia.*

Laboratory testing for chlamydial infection is accomplished by culture, direct immunofluorescence, enzyme immunoassay (EIA), nucleic acid hybridization tests, and nucleic acid amplification tests (NAATs) of endocervical swab specimens. NAATs are the most sensitive tests for endocervical swab specimens and are FDA-approved for

partners, and the use of condoms. For some STDs, immunizations are available to reduce or prevent transmission, including human papillomavirus (HPV) and hepatitis B (see Chapter 2, The Obstetrician-Gynecologist's Role in Screening and Preventive Care).

Patient notification is an important part of prevention. When an STD is diagnosed, the patient's sexual partner(s) should also be evaluated. In the United States, cases of gonorrhea, chlamydial infection, and syphilis must be reported to local health departments. Treatment of male sexual partners is important in the prevention of reinfection with certain STDs. *In* **expedited partner therapy,** *a patient's sexual partner receives drug therapy for an STD without undergoing physical evaluation or testing.* Although in most cases this form of therapy does not result in adverse reactions, it can pose a significant risk. Sexual partners should always be encouraged to seek medical evaluation on their own. In some states, expedited partner therapy is prohibited or restricted; therefore, it is important for the clinical staff to be familiar with all local laws and regulations.

| TABLE 27.1 | Diseases Characterized by Genital Ulcers |
|---|---|

- Differential diagnosis: genital herpes, syphilis, chancroid, and nonsexually transmitted infections
- Diagnosis: history and physical examination frequently inaccurate; all patients should be tested for syphilis and herpes; consideration given to chancroid

|  | Herpes | Syphilis | Chancroid | Granuloma Inguinale | Lymphogranuloma Venereum (LGV) |
|---|---|---|---|---|---|
| Prevalence | • At least 50 million persons in the United States have HSV infection | • Decreasing; more prevalent in metropolitan areas | • Usually in discrete outbreaks—high rates of HIV coinfection | • Occurs rarely in the United States; endemic in India, Papua New Guinea, central Australia, western Africa | • Unknown in the United States |
| Presentation | • Classic presentation of vesicles/ulcers absent in many cases<br>• Many women with either HSV-1 or HSV-2 infection are asymptomatic.<br>• Recurrences much less common with HSV-1; important fact for counseling | • Primary: ulcer or chancre<br>• Secondary: skin rash, lymphadenopathy, mucocutaneous lesions<br>• Tertiary: cardiac or ophthalmic manifestations, auditory abnormalities, gummatous lesions<br>• Latent: no symptoms, diagnosed by serology | • Combination of a painful genital ulcer and tender suppurative inguinal adenopathy | • Raised, red lesions that bleed easily | • Self-limited vesicle or ulcer at site of infection (sometimes)<br>• Inguinal or femoral lymphadenopathy |
| Diagnosis | • Clinical diagnosis should be confirmed by laboratory testing.<br>• Isolation of HSV in cell culture is the preferred virologic test.<br>• Viral culture isolates should be typed to determine if HSV-1 or HSV-2 is the cause of the infection.<br>• The serologic type-specific glycoprotein G-based assays should be specifically requested when serology is performed. | • Dark-field examinations and direct fluorescent antibody tests of lesion exudate or tissue are the definitive methods for diagnosing early syphilis.<br>• Presumptive diagnosis is possible with nontreponemal tests (VDRL and RPR) and treponemal tests (eg, FTA-ABS and TP-PA).<br>• The use of only one type of serologic test is insufficient; false-positive nontreponemal test results are sometimes associated with medical conditions unrelated to syphilis. | • Culture media and PCR testing not readily available<br>• Probable diagnosis: patient with ulcers, no evidence of syphilis, typical chancroid presentation, and diagnostic tests negative for herpes | • Clinical suspicion<br>• Wright or Giemsa-stained smears or biopsies of granulation tissue; presence of dark-staining Donovan bodies is diagnostic | • Clinical suspicion<br>• Exclusion of other causes<br>• Positive test for causative agent (C. trachomatis) |

FTA-ABS indicates fluorescent treponemal antibody absorbed; HIV, human immunodeficiency virus; HSV, herpes simplex virus; PCR, polymerase chain reaction; RPR, rapid plasma reagin; TP-PA, T pallidum particle agglutination; VDRL, Venereal Disease Research Laboratory.
Data from Workowski KA, Berman SM. Sexually transmitted diseases treatment guidelines 2006. *MMWR Recomm Rep.* 2006;55(RR-11):1–94. Table modified from American College of Obstetricians and Gynecologists. *Guidelines for Women's Health Care: A Resource Manual.* 3rd ed. Washington, DC: ACOG; 2007:205.

TABLE
27.2  Diseases Characterized by Cervicitis or Urethritis

| | Chlamydial Infection | Gonorrhea |
|---|---|---|
| Prevalence | • Most frequently reported infectious disease in the United States<br>• Highest prevalence in persons 25 years and younger | • Estimated 600,000 new infections in the United States each year<br>• Prevalence varies widely among communities and populations.<br>• Women younger than 25 years are at highest risk. |
| Presentation | • Asymptomatic infection common<br>• Other presentations: mucopurulent cervicitis, abnormal vaginal discharge, irregular intermenstrual vaginal bleeding | • Frequently asymptomatic |
| Evaluation | • All sexually active women 25 years and younger should be screened annually.<br>• Urogenital infection in women can be diagnosed by testing urine or swab specimens collected from the endocervix or vagina.<br>• Culture, direct immunofluorescence, EIA, nucleic acid hybridization tests, and NAATs are available for the detection of Chlamydia trachomatis on endocervical swab specimens.<br>• NAATs are the most sensitive tests for endocervical swab specimens and are FDA-cleared for use with urine, and some tests are cleared for use with vaginal swab specimens.<br>• ACOG recommends consideration of urine screening for adolescents reluctant to have pelvic examination or seen where pelvic examination is not feasible. | • Testing appropriate in patients at high risk for STDs<br>• ACOG recommends annual screening for gonorrhea in sexually active adolescents.<br>• Pharyngeal and anorectal infections should be considered based on sexual practices elicited during the sexual history.<br>• Consider urine screening when adolescents are reluctant to have pelvic examination or are seen where pelvic examination is not feasible. |
| Special considerations | • Persons treated for chlamydial infection should be instructed to abstain from sexual intercourse for 7 days after single-dose therapy or until completion of a 7-day regimen, and be instructed to abstain from sexual intercourse until all of their sex partners are treated.<br>• Test of cure (repeated testing 3–4 weeks after completing therapy) is not recommended for persons treated with the recommended or alternative regimens, unless therapeutic compliance is in question, symptoms persist, or reinfection is suspected.<br>• Because of high rates of reinfection, consider advising all women with chlamydial infection to be retested approximately 3 months after treatment and encourage retesting for all women treated for chlamydial infection whenever they next seek medical care within the following 3–12 months. | • Patients with gonorrhea should be treated routinely for chlamydial infection unless it has been excluded by NAAT.<br>• Consider advising all patients with gonorrhea to be retested 3 months after treatment. If patients do not seek retesting in 3 months, encourage retesting whenever these patients seek medical care within the following 12 months. |

ACOG, American College of Obstetricians and Gynecologists; CDC, Centers for Disease Control and Prevention; EIA, enzyme immunoassay; FDA, Food and Drug Administration; NAAT, nucleic acid amplification test; STD, sexually transmitted disease.
Data from Workowski KA, Berman SM. Sexually transmitted diseases treatment guidelines 2006. *MMWR Recomm Rep.* 2006;55(RR-11):1–94. http://www.cdc.gov/mmwr/preview/mmwrhtml/rr5511a1.htm. Accessed October 20, 2008.
Table modified from American College of Obstetricians and Gynecologists. *Guidelines for Women's Health Care: A Resource Manual.* 3rd ed. Washington, DC: ACOG; 2007:206–207.

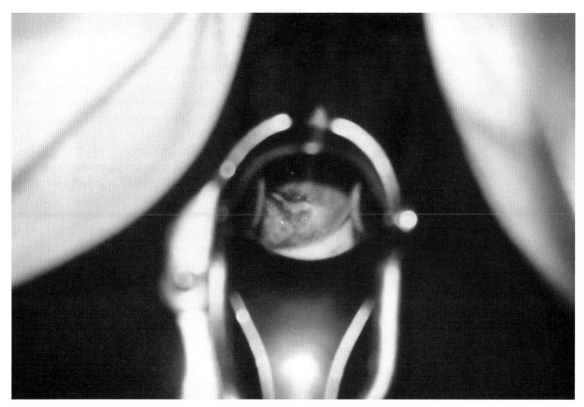

FIGURE 27.1. Cervicitis. Mucopurulent discharge from the cervix and eversion or ectropion of the cervix that results in intermittent cervical bleeding are suggestive of cervicitis, which may be caused by chlamydia or gonorrheal infection. (Centers for Disease Control, Atlanta, GA; 1970).

use with vaginal swab specimens. Adolescents who are reluctant to undergo a pelvic examination or who receive care where pelvic examination is not possible can be tested with urine screening.

## Treatment

Chlamydia is treated with antibiotics including azithromycin or doxycycline. Alternative antibiotic therapies include erythromycin base, erythromycin ethylsuccinate, ofloxacin, or levofloxacin. Although erythromycin is an alternative treatment option, gastrointestinal side effects may be significant.

*Patients with persistent symptoms, who are suspected to be noncompliant with treatment, or who may have become re-infected should be have a **test of cure** performed (repeated testing) 3 to 4 weeks after initial treatment is completed.*

Because of the high rates of reinfection, all women with chlamydial infection should be advised to be retested 3 months after treatment. Retesting for these women should also be encouraged whenever they seek medical care in the following 3 to 12 month. Persons undergoing treatment for chlamydia should be instructed to abstain from sexual intercourse until treatment is completed and all of their sexual partners are treated.

## *Neisseria gonorrhoeae* (Gonorrhea)

Infections with *N. gonorrhoeae*, a gram-negative intracellular diplococcus, are the second most common STD in the United States. It is estimated that 600,000 new cases of gonorrhea occur each year in the United States, and less than half of them are reported to the Centers for Disease Control. The emergence of **antimicrobial-resistant strains,** an increased frequency of asymptomatic infections, and changing patterns of sexual behavior have all contributed to a rise in its incidence. *The highest rates of infection are seen in adolescents and young adults.* N. gonorrhoeae infection can lead to PID with its concurrent risks of infertility caused by adhesion formation, tubal damage, and hydrosalpinx formation. Studies also suggest that infection with N. gonorrhoeae may facilitate transmission of HIV. Infections with *N. gonorrhoeae* are easily acquired by women and can affect the genital tract, rectum, and pharynx. Gonorrhea is considered a reportable disease in all states, and sexual partners of infected individuals must be tested and treated.

## DIAGNOSIS

Signs and symptoms appear within 3 to 5 days of infection, but asymptomatic infections are common in both men and women. In men, infection is characterized by **urethritis,** a mucopurulent or purulent discharge from the urethra. *In women, signs and symptoms are often mild enough to be overlooked, and can include purulent discharge from the urethra, Skene duct, cervix, vagina, or anus.* Anal intercourse is not always a prerequisite to anal infection. A greenish or yellow discharge from the cervix indicative of cervicitis should alert the physician to the possibility of either *N. gonorrhoeae* or *C. trachomatis* infection. Infection of the Bartholin glands is frequently encountered and can lead to secondary infections, abscesses, or cyst formation. When the gland becomes full and painful, incision and drainage are appropriate.

The laboratory diagnosis of *N. gonorrhoeae* infection in women is made by testing endocervical, vaginal, or urine specimens. Specimens can be tested by culture, nucleic hybridization, or NAAT. Culture is the most widely used testing modality for specimens obtained from the pharynx or rectum, as there are no nonculture tests that are FDA-approved for the testing of these specimens. Male urethral specimens may be tested by Gram-stain in symptomatic men, but are not recommended as definitive testing for women or asymptomatic men.

> *All patients who are tested for gonorrhea should also be tested for other STDS, including chlamydia, HIV, and syphilis.*

## TREATMENT

Aggressive therapy for patients with either suspected or confirmed *N. gonorrhoeae* should be undertaken to prevent the serious sequelae of untreated disease. Because of the emergence of quinolone-resistant strains of *N. gonorrhoeae*, these antimicrobials are no longer used for the treatment of these infections. Antimicrobials currently used for therapy are ceftriaxone, cefixime, or ciprofloxacin. Due to the high likelihood of concurrent chlamydial infection, patients should be treated for chlamydia as well, if chlamydial infection is not ruled out by nucleic acid amplification test (NAAT).

## Pelvic Inflammatory Disease

**Pelvic inflammatory disease** (PID) represents the most serious form of sexually transmitted disease. It involves infection of the upper genital tract (endometrium, fallopian tubes, ovaries, and pelvic peritoneum) as a result of direct spread of pathogenic organisms along mucosal surfaces after initial infection of the cervix. The predominant organisms responsible for PID are *C. trachomatis* and *N. gonor-*

*rhoeae*. Other organisms that have been isolated from the fallopian tubes of patients with PID include *Mycoplasma, Streptococcus, Staphylococcus, Haemophilus, Escherichia coli, bacteroides, Peptostreptococcus, Clostridium,* and *Actinomyces.*

Timing of cervical infection in relation to the menstrual cycle is important; the endocervical mucus resists upward spread, especially during the progesterone-dominant part of the cycle. Oral contraceptives mimic this effect, which explains in part their action in limiting PID. The presence of motile sperm or strings from intrauterine contraceptives (IUC) can allow penetration of organisms through this protective barrier. Tubal ligation usually provides a barrier to spread, although in some cases small micro-channels facilitate continued spread. The relative mobility of the fallopian tube probably contributes to the rapid and widespread extension of infection.

## RISK FACTORS

*The greatest risk factor for PID is prior PID.* Adolescence, having multiple sexual partners, not using condoms, and infection with any of the causative organisms are important risk factors. Between 10% and 40% of women with untreated chlamydial or gonorrheal infections of the cervix will develop acute PID. *The importance of early diagnosis and treatment of PID lies in its prevention of infertility and ectopic pregnancy.* Infertility results from scarring of damaged fallopian tubes and intraperitoneal adhesions, and occurs in approximately 15% of patients after a single episode of salpingitis, increasing to 75% after three or more episodes. The risk of ectopic pregnancy is increased 7 to 10 times in women with a history of salpingitis.

## DIAGNOSIS

Findings in PID are often nonspecific, and patients presenting with these symptoms should be differentiated from those with ectopic pregnancy, septic incomplete abortions, acute appendicitis, diverticular abscesses, and adnexal torsion. Patients with PID may also present with only mild, nonspecific symptoms, such as vaginal discharge or intermittent vaginal bleeding. More pronounced signs and symptoms include muscular guarding, cervical motion tenderness, or rebound tenderness. A purulent cervical discharge is often seen, and the adnexa are usually moderately to exquisitely tender with a mass or fullness potentially palpable. Fever or chills may also be present and the white blood cell count is usually elevated (Box 27.2). Peritoneal involvement can also include **perihepatitis (Fitz-Hugh-Curtis syndrome)**. Perihepatitis consists of inflammation leading to localized fibrosis and scarring of the anterior surface of the liver and adjacent peritoneum. It is probably caused by chlamydial infection more often than by gonorrheal infection, with which it was originally described

## BOX 27.2
### Clinical Criteria for Diagnosis of Acute Salpingitis

All 3 of the following are necessary:
1. Abdominal tenderness with/without rebound
2. Adnexal tenderness
3. Cervical motion tenderness

PLUS

1 or more of the following:
1. Gram stain of endocervix positive for gram-negative, intracellular diplococci
2. Temperature ≥38°C
3. WBC >10,000
4. Pus on culdocentesis or laparoscopy
5. Pelvic abscess on bimanual exam or sonogram

WBC = white blood cell

(Fig. 27.2). In severe cases or in patients with one or more prior episodes of PID, **tuboovarian abscesses (TOA)** may form. Patients with TOA are acutely ill, often presenting with high fever, tachycardia, severe pelvic and abdominal pain, and nausea and vomiting.

*Because PID may not be associated with specific signs and symptoms, empiric treatment for PID is recommended for sexually active young women who appear to have no other cause of illness and who are found to have uterine tenderness, adnexal tenderness, or cervical motion tenderness on pelvic examination.* Women who are diagnosed with PID should also undergo testing for chlamydial, HIV, or gonorrheal infection.

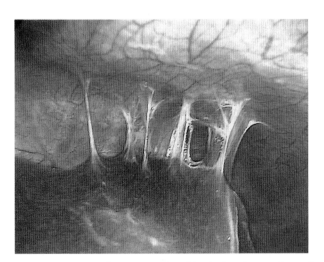

FIGURE 27.2. Perihepatitis (Fitz-Hugh-Curtis syndrome). Adhesions between the liver and diaphragm are evidence of perihepatitis caused by chlamydial infection. (From Overton C, Davis C, McMillan L, Shaw RW. *An Atlas of Endometriosis.* 3rd ed. London: Informa UK; 2007:9.4).

## TREATMENT

Patients with mild or moderate cases of PID can be managed with an oral antibiotic regimen; however, many patients require hospitalization for adequate care. The decision for hospitalization should be individualized and based on certain criteria (Box 27.3). Hospitalization allows for the administration of high-dose intravenous antibiotic therapy with an antimicrobial spectrum that covers aerobic and anaerobic organisms. In the case of TOA, surgical drainage or even hysterectomy, depending on the reproductive status and desires of the patient, may be warranted in patients who do not respond to an aggressive course of parenteral antibiotics. Rupture of a TOA with septic shock is a life-threatening complication with mortality approaching 10%. These patients must be treated surgically.

## Genital Herpes

**Genital herpes** is caused by infection with the herpes simplex virus (HSV), a DNA virus. This condition affects more than 50 million persons in the United States, and as many as 75% of primary infections go unrecognized by either patient or provider. Herpes simplex infections are highly contagious. There are two types of HSV—HSV-1, which is associated with cold sore lesions of the mouth but may also cause genital lesions, and HSV-2. Most HSV genital infections are caused by HSV-2, but genital HSV-1 infections are becoming increasingly common, particularly among adolescent and young women. *Up to 80% of new genital infections among women may be due to HSV-1, with the highest rates occurring in adolescents and young adults.* Women infected with HSV-1 remain at risk for acquiring HSV-2 infection.

## BOX 27.3
### Suggested Criteria for Hospitalization for Pelvic Inflammatory Disease

- Surgical emergencies (e.g., appendicitis) cannot be excluded.
- The patient is pregnant.
- The patient does not response clinically to oral antimicrobial therapy.
- The patient is unable to follow or tolerate an outpatient oral regimen.
- The patient has a severe illness, nausea and vomiting, or high fever.
- The patient has a tuboovarian abscess.

Workowski KA, Berman SM. Sexually transmitted diseases treatment guidelines, 2006. *MMWR Recomm Rep.* 2006;55 (RR-11):1–94. http://www.cdc.gov/mmwr/preview/mmwrhtml/rr5511a1.htm. Accessed October 20, 2008.

## DIAGNOSIS

First episode infections, which represent new acquisition of HSV, usually are most severe, and recurrent infections may be milder. *First episode infections often are accompanied by systemic symptoms, including a prominent flu-like syndrome and frequent neurologic involvement, which occur within 2 to 3 days following infection.* Painful vesicular and ulcerated lesions appear on the vulva, vagina, cervix, or perineal and perianal skin, often extending onto the buttocks, 3 to 7 days after exposure and usually resolving in approximately 1 week (Fig. 27.3). These vesicles lyse and progress to shallow, painful ulcers with a red border. The lesions of herpes simplex infections are distinguishable from the ulcers found in chancroid, syphilis, or granuloma inguinale by their appearance and extreme tenderness. Dysuria caused by vulvar lesions or urethral and bladder involvement may lead to urinary retention. Patients with primary lesions may require hospitalization for pain control or management of urinary complications. Aseptic meningitis with fever, headache, and meningismus occurs in some patients 5 to 7 days after the appearance of the genital lesions.

After primary infection, the HSV migrates via nerve fibers to remain dormant in the dorsal root ganglia. Recurrences are triggered by unknown stimuli, resulting in the virus traveling down the nerve fiber to the affected area. *Recurrent lesions are usually milder in severity than lesions associated with primary infection and persist for a shorter duration, generally lasting 2 to 5 days.* Recurrent lesions may be unilat-

eral rather than bilateral and present as fissures or vulvar irritation, as opposed to being vesicular in appearance. Infections with HSV-1 are less likely to cause recurrences than HSV-2, a fact that should be considered when a patient is considering suppressive therapy.

Most HSV-1 and HSV-2 infections are asymptomatic in women. *The classic presentation of a painful cluster of vesicles and ulcers occurs in a small proportion of women, and most women will have atypical lesions, such as abrasions, fissures, or itching without obvious lesions.* Viral shedding can occur for up to 3 weeks after lesions appear. Definitive diagnosis must be confirmed with reliable laboratory testing.

The laboratory test used most often has been viral culture. Culture is highly specific; however, it is not very sensitive, with a false-negative rate of 25% with primary infection and as high as 50% in a recurrent infection. PCR testing has a higher sensitivity and will most likely replace culture in the future as the definitive test for HSV infection. In addition to viral detection methods, the detection of type-specific antibodies to HSV-1 and HSV-2 also can help to establish the diagnosis. These tests may yield false-negative test results when administered in the early stages of infection, as the median time from infection to seroconversion is 22 days. Approximately 20% of patients may remain seronegative after 3 months, particularly if they have received antiviral therapy. Type-specific testing may be useful in the following scenarios: (1) recurrent genital or atypical symptoms with negative HSV cultures, (2) clinical diagnosis of genital herpes in the absence of laboratory diagnosis, and (3) a partner with genital herpes.

## TREATMENT

**Antiviral drugs** are the mainstay of treatment. Oral medication can reduce the duration of viral shedding and shorten the initial symptomatic disease course, but it does not affect the long-term course of the disease. Treatments for first episode genital herpes include acyclovir, famciclovir, or valacyclovir. Treatment is usually prescribed for 7 to 10 days, but can be given longer if new lesions persist. These therapies do not decrease the likelihood of recurrence. Lesions should be kept clean and dry. In addition, analgesics should be provided as needed (e.g., acetaminophen or ibuprofen). Warm water baths often are helpful during the first few days. Topical lidocaine also is occasionally beneficial, but it can result in local allergic reactions. Severe episodes may require hospitalization for parenteral analgesia and intravenous antiviral therapy. Such therapy is generally recommended for immunosuppressed or otherwise compromised patients.

Recurrences may also be treated with oral antiviral therapy. *Episodic therapy decreases the duration of the episode (lesion, pain, and viral shedding) and is most effective when the patient initiates the therapy at prodrome, or at the beginning of the episode.* Treatment regimens for recurrences are usu-

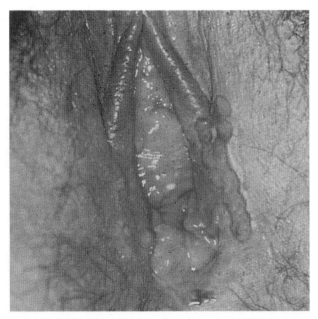

FIGURE 27.3. Genital herpes. The linear appearance of these painful herpetic erosions on the labia is a result of coalescence of several closely grouped vesicles. (Courtesy of Barbara Romanowski, MD. In Morse SA, Ballard RC, Homes KK, Moreland AA. *Atlas of Sexually Transmitted Diseases and AIDS.* Philadelphia, PA: Mosby/Elsevier; 2003:13.12.)

ally of a shorter duration than those administered for first episodes (3 to 5 days). Episodic therapy is recommended for patients with infrequent symptomatic recurrences. *Suppressive therapy for genital herpes (in which the medication is taken daily) prevents approximately 80% of recurrences and results in a 48% reduction in viral transmission between sexual partners as a result of decreased viral shedding. It may be most effective for patients with frequent occurrences.* It should also be recommended for women with HSV-2 whose sexual partner does not have HSV or who has HSV-1 infection. Such discordant couples should also be advised that consistent use of condoms decreases, but does not eliminate the risk of transmission.

Pregnant women with a history of genital herpes should be carefully screened throughout the prenatal course for evidence of outbreaks. *Cesarean delivery is indicated for women with active lesions or a typical herpetic prodrome at the time of delivery to prevent neonatal transmission.*

## Human Papillomavirus

**Human papillomavirus** (HPV) is extremely common, occurring in up to 80% of sexually active women by age 50. Transmission occurs through contact with infected genital skin, mucous membranes, or body fluids from a partner with either overt or subclinical HPV infections. HPV is species-specific and only infects humans. Most infections are transient, but the proportion of women whose infections resolve decreases with age. Unlike other STDs, sequelae of HPV infection may take years to develop. More than 100 HPV subtypes have been identified, with at least 40 identified in genital infections. HPV viral types are routinely classified into low-risk and high-risk categories. *Low-risk subtypes, such as 6 and 11, are typically associated with genital condyloma. High-risk subtypes, such as 16, 18, 31, 33, and 45, are so classified because of their association with cervical dysplasia and cervical cancer.* Of the high-risk subtypes, HPV 16 and 18 together account for approximately two-thirds of cervical cancer cases, whereas low-risk HPV subtypes rarely lead to cancer.

## CONDYLOMA ACUMINATA

**Condyloma acuminata** (genital or venereal warts) are soft, fleshy growths that may arise from the vulva, vagina, cervix, urethral meatus, perineum, and anus (Fig. 27.4). They may occasionally also be found on the tongue or oral cavity. These distinctive lesions may be single or multiple and generally cause few symptoms. They are often accompanied by other STDs. Because HPV is spread by direct skin-to-skin contact, symmetrical lesions across the midline are common.

The diagnosis of condyloma acuminata is based on physical examination, but may be confirmed through biopsy of the warts. Thorough inspection of the external

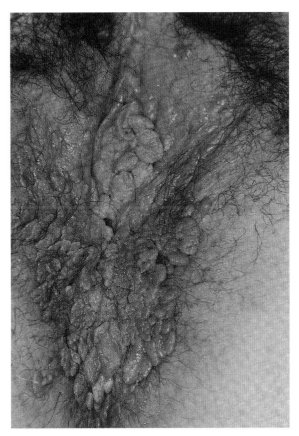

FIGURE 27.4. Condyloma acuminata. (From Wilkinson EJ, Stone IK. *Atlas of Vulvar Disease*. Baltimore, MD: Williams & Wilkins; 2003:9.3.)

genitalia and anogenital region should be performed during the routine gynecologic examination, especially in patients with known cervical or vaginal lesions. Because the condyloma lata of syphilis may be confused with genital warts, the clinician must be able to distinguish the two types of lesions in patients at high risk for both infections (see Fig. 27.5 photo of syphilis).

Management options include chemical treatments, cautery, and immunologic treatments. Patient-applied products include podofilox and imiquimod; these treatments should not be used during pregnancy. Treatments that are administered by a healthcare provider include application of trichloroacetic acid, application of podophyllin resin in tincture of benzoin, cryosurgery, surgical excision, laser surgery, or intralesional interferon injections. Lesions exceeding 2 cm respond best to cryotherapy, cautery, or laser treatment.

Lesions are more resistant to therapy in patients who are pregnant, have diabetes, smoke, or are immunosuppressed. In patients with extensive vaginal or vulvar lesions, delivery via cesarean section may be required, to avoid extensive vaginal lacerations and problems with suturing tissues with these lesions. Cesarean delivery also decreases the possibility of transmission to the infant, which can cause subsequent development of laryngeal papillomata, although the risk is small and is not considered an indication for cesarean delivery.

## CERVICAL DYSPLASIA

*The relationship between infection by high-risk subtypes and cervical dysplasia and cancer is now well-established.* The diagnosis and management of these conditions is covered in Chapter 43, Cervical Neoplasia and Carcinoma. *A quadrivalent* **HPV vaccine** *protects against HPV genotypes 6, 11, 16, and 18 (the strains of HPV that cause 90% of genital warts and 70% of cervical cancers).* Additional vaccines are also being investigated.

*ACOG currently recommends that all girls and women aged 9 to 26 years be immunized against HPV.* The vaccine is a protective tool and is not a substitute for cancer screening; women should be advised to follow current cervical cytologic screening guidelines regardless of their vaccination status.

## Syphilis

In the United States, the incidence of syphilis declined steadily in the 1990s and reached its lowest rate in 2000. Beginning in 2001, the rate of syphilis began to increase, especially among men who have sex with men. Rates in women also increased, although not as steeply. Between 2005 and 2006, the number of reported syphilis cases increased 11.8%. Between 2001 and 2008, the overall increase in cases of syphilis was 76%. In addition, after a 14-year decline, the rate of congenital syphilis increased 3.7% between 2005 and 2006. This increase may relate to the increase in the rate of syphilis that has occurred in past several years. One reason suggested for the rise in syphilis rates overall is the increasing use of nonpenicillin antibiotics to treat penicillin-resistant gonorrhea; in the past, penicillin treatment of gonorrhea provided treatment for coexisting syphilis.

**Treponema pallidum,** the causative organism of syphilis, is one of a small group of spirochetes that are virulent in humans. *Because this motile anaerobic spirochete can rapidly invade intact moist mucosa, the most common sites of entry for women are the vulva, vagina, and cervix.* Transplacental spread may occur at any time during pregnancy and can result in congenital syphilis (see Chapter 15, Infectious Diseases in Pregnancy).

### DIAGNOSIS

Syphilis can be a long-term disease with several stages. *Primary syphilis, the first stage of the disease, is characterized by the appearance of a* **chancre** *at the site of entry approximately 10 to 60 days after infection with* T. pallidum. The chancre has a firm, punched-out appearance and has rolled edges

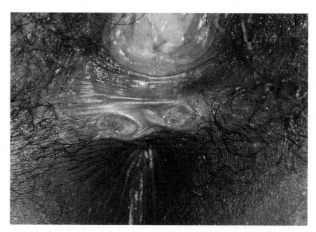

FIGURE 27.5. Syphilis chancres. Note the punched-out appearance and rolled edges. (From Wilkinson EJ, Stone IK. *Atlas of Vulvar Disease.* Baltimore, MD: Williams & Wilkins; 2003:8.46.)

(Fig. 27.5). Because it is small and painless, the chancre may be missed during routine physical examination. Adenopathy or other mild systemic symptoms may also be present. The chancre heals spontaneously within 3 to 6 weeks. Serologic-testing results at this stage of syphilis generally are negative.

Four to 8 weeks after the primary chancre appears, manifestations of **secondary syphilis** develop. *This stage is characterized by a skin rash that often appears as rough, red or brown lesions on the palms of the hands and soles of the feet.* Other symptoms include lymphadenopathy, fever, headache, weight loss, fatigue, muscle aches, and patchy hair loss. Highly infective secondary eruptions, called mucocutaneous mucous patches, occur in 30% of patients during this stage. In moist areas of the body, flat-topped papules may coalesce, forming condyloma lata (Fig. 27.6). These may be distinguished from venereal warts by their broad base and flatter appearance.

*In untreated individuals, this stage also resolves spontaneously in 2 to 6 weeks, and the disease enters the* **latent phase.** During the latent stage, the patient has no signs or symptoms of the disease, although serologic tests are positive. In the late or **tertiary** stages of the disease, transmission of the infection is unlikely, except via blood transfusion or placental transfer. However, severe damage to the central nervous and cardiovascular systems develop, along with ophthalmic and auditory abnormalities. Destructive, necrotic, granulomatous lesions, called **gummas,** may develop 1 to 10 years after infection.

### DIAGNOSIS

Syphilis is determined by identifying motile spirochetes on dark-field microscopic examination and direct fluorescent antibody tests of material from primary or secondary

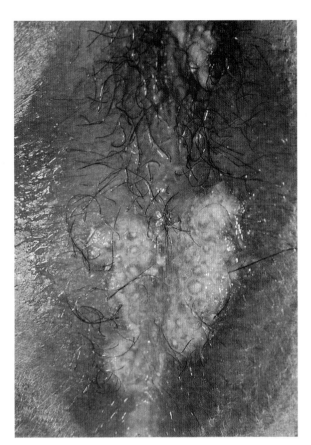

FIGURE 27.6. Condyloma lata in a patient with syphilis. (From Wilkinson EJ, Stone IK. *Atlas of Vulvar Disease.* Baltimore, MD: Williams & Wilkins; 2003:8.47.)

lesions or lymph node aspirates. Presumptive diagnosis is possible with nontreponemal tests (the Venereal Disease Research Laboratory [VDRL] and rapid plasma reagin [RPR]) and treponemal tests (e.g., fluorescent treponemal antibody absorption [FTA-ABS] and *Treponema pallidum* particle agglutination [TP-PA]) [Box 27.4]. *The use of only*

---

### BOX 27.4
### Types of Serologic Tests for Syphilis

**Nontreponemal:**
Venereal Disease Research Laboratory (VDRL)
Rapid plasma reagin (RPR) card test
Automated reagin test

**Treponemal:**
Fluorescent treponemal antibody absorption (FTA-ABS)
*Treponema pallidum* particle agglutination (TP-PA)
Microhemagglutination assay for antibodies to *Treponema pallidum* (MHA-TP)

---

*one serologic test is insufficient; false-positive nontreponemal test results are sometimes associated with medical conditions unrelated to syphilis.* A woman with a positive treponemal test will usually have this positive result for life, irrespective of treatment or activity of the disease. When neurosyphilis is suspected, a lumbar puncture, with a VDRL performed on the spinal fluid, is required.

### TREATMENT

Syphilis is treated with benzathine penicillin G. The patient should be followed by quantitative VDRL titers and examinations at 3, 6, and 12 months, and should abstain from sexual intercourse until lesions are completely healed.

## Human Immunodeficiency Virus and AIDS

**AIDS** is the advanced manifestation of infection by the human immunodeficiency virus (HIV), an RNA retrovirus. The virus targets "helper" T cells (those with the CD4 marker) and monocytes. Depletion of these CD4 cells is an important manifestation of HIV infection. Two types of HIV have been identified. HIV-1 is the most common type in the United States, while HIV-2 is more common in West African countries. The progression of HIV-1 infection varies from individual to individual. In addition to depletion in the number of CD4 cells, HIV-1 may weaken the immune function of these cells. Both lead to immune-system compromise that leaves the body vulnerable to serious, often life-threatening infections from other bacteria, viruses, and parasites.

It is estimated that 1.2 million individuals in the United States are living with HIV or AIDS. AIDS is now one of the top five causes of death in reproductive-age women. The proportion of all AIDS cases reported among adult and adolescent women in the United States has more than tripled, from 7% in 1985 to 27% in 2004. AIDS is the third leading cause of death in black women of ages 24 to 44 years, and the fourth leading cause of death in Hispanic women in the same age group. *The three primary methods of contracting the virus are: (1) intimate sexual contact, (2) use of contaminated needles or blood products, and (3) perinatal transmission from mother to child.* HIV transmission in pregnancy has been greatly reduced as a result of routine screening in the first trimester as well as aggressive therapy at the time of delivery. Viral loads are calculated at the time of labor and most infants born to HIV-infected mothers are delivered via cesarean birth.

The screening test for AIDS is an enzyme-linked immunosorbent assay (ELISA) that tests for antibodies against HIV. Although rare, false-positive tests are possible and are more common in multiparous women and women taking oral contraceptives. Confirmation is achieved with the more specific Western blot technique.

Management of HIV focuses on prevention and chemotherapy. Prevention emphasizes use of latex condoms and safe sex practices. Drug therapy for HIV infection includes various classes of anti-HIV drugs, including the nucleoside reverse transcriptase inhibitors (NRTIs) such as zidovudine, nonnucleoside reverse transcriptase inhibitors (NNRTIs), and protease inhibitors. Monotherapy is not advocated because of development of drug resistance. Instead, highly active antiretroviral therapy (HAART) consisting of at least three agents has been recommended.

## Other Sexually Transmitted Diseases

STDs that are less common in the United States include **granuloma inguinale** and **lymphogranuloma venereum (LGV),** both of which can present with genital ulcers. *C. trachomatis* serovars L1, L2, and L3 cause LGV, a disease that has increased in prevalence in the Netherlands and other European countries. When transmitted via vaginal intercourse, LGV presents with inguinal or femoral lymphadenopathy in women. When transmitted anally, symptoms of anal bleeding, purulent anal discharge, constipation, and anal spasms may occur. A self-limiting genital or rectal vesicle or papule sometimes forms at the site of entry of the bacterium. *LGV is a systemic infection that, if untreated, can cause secondary infection of rectal or anal lesions, which may lead to abscesses or fistulas.*

**Granuloma inguinale** is caused by sexual transmission of the bacterium *Klebsiella granulomatis.* Rare in the United States, it is endemic in Papua New Guinea, central Australia, India, and western Africa. The lesions are vascular and bleed easily on contact. The disease is diagnosed clinically and can be confirmed by special stains of specimens taken from the lesions or from biopsy.

***Chancroid,*** *another STD characterized by genital ulcers, usually occurs in discrete outbreaks.* Ten percent of individuals diagnosed with chancroid are also infected with HSV or *T. pallidum.* It is also a cofactor for HIV transmission. The causative bacterium, *Haemophilus ducreyi,* is difficult to culture. PCR is often used to confirm the diagnosis, which is made by clinical criteria and ruling out syphilis and HSV through testing of the ulcer secretion.

***Molluscum contagiosum*** *is a highly contagious viral skin infection that can be transmitted through sexual contact.* It is characterized by small, painless papules that appear on the genital region, inner thighs, and buttocks. The papules usually resolve spontaneously within six months to one year. Antiviral drugs or topical preparations are used to treat the disease and prevent transmission.

Parasitic infections include **pediculosis pubis (pubic lice)** and **scabies.** Pubic lice are usually transmitted by sexual contact; some cases in which the lice have been transmitted through contact with infested clothing or bedding have been reported. Scabies can also be transmitted via these routes. The predominant symptom of both conditions is itching of the pubic area. Pubic lice or nits can sometimes be detected on pubic hair. Itching due to scabies infection may be delayed several weeks, as the individual becomes sensitized to the antigens released by the parasites; however, itching may occur within 24 hours following reinfection. Pubic lice and scabies are treated with topical medications. Lindane is not recommended as a first-line treatment due to its toxicity.

## SUGGESTED READINGS

American College of Obstetricians and Gynecologists. Cervical cytology screening. ACOG Practice Bulletin No. 45. *Obstet Gynecol.* 2003;102(2):417–427.

American College of Obstetricians and Gynecologists. *Guidelines for Women's Health Care: A Resource Manual.* 3rd ed. Washington, DC: American College of Obstetricians and Gynecologists; 2007: 197–216.

American College of Obstetricians and Gynecologists. Gynecologic herpes simplex virus infections. ACOG Practice Bulletin No. 57. *Obstet Gynecol.* 2004;104(5):1111–1117.

American College of Obstetricians and Gynecologists. Human immunodeficiency virus. ACOG Committee Opinion No. 389. *Obstet Gynecol.* 2007;110(6):1473–1478.

American College of Obstetricians and Gynecologists. Human papillomavirus. ACOG Practice Bulletin No. 61. *Obstet Gynecol.* 2005;105(4):905–918.

American College of Obstetricians and Gynecologists. Sexually transmitted diseases in adolescents. ACOG Committee Opinion No. 301. *Obstet Gynecol.* 2004;104(4):891–898.

Centers for Disease Control and Prevention. *Trends in Reportable Sexually Transmitted Diseases in the United States, 2006: National Surveillance Data for Chlamydia, Gonorrhea, and Syphilis.* Atlanta, GA: Centers for Disease Control and Prevention; 2007.

Workowski KA, Berman SM. Sexually transmitted diseases treatment guidelines, 2006. *MMWR Recomm Rep.* 2006;55(RR-11):1–94. http://www.cdc.gov/mmwr/preview/mmwrhtml/rr5511a1.htm. Accessed October 20, 2008.

# 28 Pelvic Support Defects, Urinary Incontinence, and Urinary Tract Infection

This chapter deals primarily with APGO Educational Topic:

**Topic 37:** Pelvic Relaxation and Urinary Incontinence

Students should be able to discuss the types of pelvic relaxation, urinary incontinence, and urinary tract infection as well as their causes and presentations, evaluation, and management (behavioral, medical, or surgical).

## PELVIC SUPPORT DEFECTS

**Pelvic support defects** comprise a variety of conditions related to loss of connective tissue support surrounding the reproductive tract organs, including loss of uterine support, paravaginal tissue support, bladder wall and urethrovesical angle support, and support overlying the distal rectum. **Pelvic organ prolapse** is a disorder in which organs have lost their support and descend through the urogenital hiatus. *Patients with pelvic support disorders present in many different and often subtle ways.* To identify patients who would benefit from therapy, the physician should be familiar with the types of pelvic support defects and the approach to the patient with symptoms suggestive of these problems.

*Although not exclusively a condition of advancing age, pelvic support defects are more common among women of this group, as tissues become less resilient and accumulated stresses have an additive effect.* Possible risk factors include genetic predisposition, parity (particularly vaginal birth), menopause, advancing age, prior pelvic surgery, connective tissue disorders, and factors associated with elevated intra-abdominal pressure (e.g., obesity, chronic constipation with excessive straining). Loss of pelvic support can have both medical and social implications that necessitate evaluation and intervention. Signs and symptoms of these disorders include urinary or fecal loss or retention; vaginal pressure or heaviness; abdominal, low back, vaginal, or perineal pain or discomfort; a mass sensation; difficulty walking, lifting, or sitting; cervical hypertrophy, excoriation, ulceration, or bleeding; difficulty with sexual relations; and stress or fear related to anxiety about the problem. Life-threatening symptoms, such as ureteral obstruction, systemic infection, incarceration, and evisceration, are uncommon. *Most women who are identified as having a pelvic support defect on physical examination are not clinically affected, and physical findings are not well-correlated with specific pelvic symptoms.*

## Causes

The pelvic organs are supported by a complex interaction of muscles (levator muscles), fasciae (urogenital diaphragm, endopelvic fascia), and ligaments (uterosacral and cardinal ligaments). Each of these structures can lose its ability to provide support through birth trauma; chronic elevations of intra-abdominal pressure, e.g., in obesity, chronic cough, or repetitive heavy lifting; intrinsic weaknesses; or atrophic changes caused by aging or estrogen loss. For many years, pelvic support disorders were believed to result solely from attenuation or stretching of pelvic connective tissue.

*Recently, investigators have shown that breaks or tears of site-specific connective tissue result in identifiable anatomic defects in the connective tissue network.*

## Types

Loss of adequate support for the pelvic organs may be manifest by descent or prolapse of the uterus, urethra (urethral detachment or **urethrocele**), bladder (**cystocele**), or rectum (**rectocele**). A true hernia at the top of the vagina allowing the small bowel to herniate through (**enterocele**) can also occur. These anatomic defects are illustrated in Figure 28.1.

A useful concept that can help in understanding these disorders is to visualize the anterior vaginal wall as a hammock. With good support, the hammock is pulled tight, allowing the bladder to rest on the hammock. When support is lost, the hammock sinks, as if someone were now sitting in the hammock. The bladder now forces the anterior vaginal wall down and out, creating an anterior wall defect or cystocele. A similar force occurs in creating a rectocele, a posterior wall defect. The posterior vaginal wall loses the lateral support, and thus the pressure from the rectum forces the posterior vaginal wall in an upward

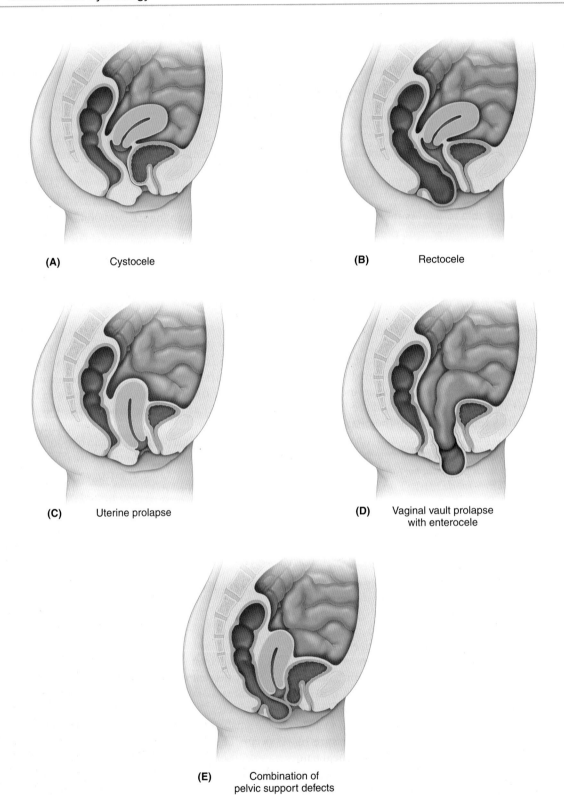

(A)    Cystocele

(B)    Rectocele

(C)    Uterine prolapse

(D)    Vaginal vault prolapse
       with enterocele

(E)    Combination of
       pelvic support defects

FIGURE 28.1. Pelvic support defects. (A) Cystocele. (B) Rectocele. (C) Uterine prolapse. (D) Uterine prolapse with enterocele. (E) Combination of defects. (Used with permission from the American College of Obstetricians and Gynecologists.)

direction. Loss of support for the uterus can lead to varying degrees of uterine prolapse. When the cervix descends beyond the vulva, it is termed **procidentia.** Loss of tissue support can also result in prolapse of the vaginal vault in patients who have had a hysterectomy. *Although loss of support may affect any of the pelvic organs individually, multiple organ involvement is most common.*

## Evaluation

The evaluation of patients with pelvic relaxation is based on the history and physical examination. *A comprehensive physical examination includes the evaluation of specific sites and measurements that aid in classifying the severity of prolapse and allows for planning of treatment options.* Specific sites to be evaluated include the urethra, vagina (including the anterior and posterior vaginal walls, paravaginal wall, and vaginal apex), perineum, and anal sphincter. A common classification scheme used to describe pelvic support defects involves the use of specific measurements that are recorded during the physical examination that have been quantified into stages (Fig. 28.2):

* Stage 0: No prolapse. The cervix (or vaginal cuff, if the patient has had a hysterectomy) is at least as high as the vaginal length.
* Stage I: The leading part of the prolapse is more than 1 cm above the hymen.
* Stage II: The leading edge is less than or equal to 1 cm above or below the hymen.
* Stage III: The leading edge is more than 1 cm beyond the hymen, but less than or equal to the total vaginal length.
* Stage IV: Complete eversion.

A common complaint of patients with a cystocele or urethrocele is urinary incontinence. As the bladder loses its support, the mobility of the urethra increases, and it pulls away from the pubic symphysis when the patient performs the Valsalva maneuver. *Incontinence does not occur in all patients, and the degree of incontinence is often not commensurate with the degree of pelvic relaxation.* The extent of urethral hypermobility is assessed by the **Q-tip test.** With the patient in the lithotomy position, a cotton-tipped swab lubricated with lidocaine jelly is placed into the bladder and pulled back until resistance is met. Once placed, the patient is asked to bear down. If there is urethral hypermobility, the urethral-vesicular junction (UVJ) deflects downward, thus causing the swab to rise. An angle greater than 30 degrees is considered a positive test. The Q-tip test does not predict incontinence, but provides more detail to the physical examination. It may also be used to predict the success of treatment options that work by stabilizing the urethra.

Some patients with Stage III or IV prolapse may not present with incontinence, but have experienced it in the past. These patients may have a kinked urethra that prevents complete urination. The medical issue of great-est concern for a patient with significant prolapse is hydronephrosis or hydroureter, although this condition is uncommon. The insertion of the ureter into the trigone kinks the trigone, and urine begins to back up into the collecting system. A renal ultrasound is helpful to evaluate this scenario.

Most pelvic relaxation disorders are the result of structural failure of the tissues involved, but other contributing factors should be considered in the complete care of the patient. Questions that should be asked include the following:

* Has there been a change in intra-abdominal pressure? If yes, what is the cause?
* Does the patient have a chronic cough that has precipitated her symptoms?
* Is a neurologic process (such as diabetic neuropathy) complicating the patient's presenting complaint?

Each of these issues should be considered prior to the selection of a diagnostic or therapeutic plan.

## Differential Diagnosis

The presumptive diagnosis of a pelvic support defect is based on the evaluation of the structural integrity of pelvic support by physical examination. Other processes that may be considered include urinary tract infection, which may lead to urgency and urethral diverticulum or Skene gland abscesses, which may mimic a cystourethrocele and, in the case of diverticula, may be a source of incontinence. These conditions can be identified by the patient's symptoms, careful "milking" of the urethra, or cystoscopy. It is occasionally difficult to differentiate between a high rectocele and an enterocele. This distinction may be facilitated through rectal examination or the identification of the small bowel in the hernia sac. It is common for the diagnosis of an enterocele not to be established until surgical repair is undertaken.

In patients who have had a history of recent pelvic surgery or radiation, fistulae between the vagina and the bladder (vesicovaginal), urethra (urethrovaginal), or ureter (ureterovaginal) should also be considered. Fistulae should also be considered in patients who present with involuntary loss of urine. A communication between the bladder and the uterus (vesicouterine) may also be found on rare occasions. A fistula also may occur between the rectum and vagina (rectovaginal fistula), resulting in the passage of flatus or feces from the vagina (Fig. 28.3).

## Treatment

Women with prolapse who are asymptomatic or mildly symptomatic can be observed at regular intervals, unless new, bothersome symptoms develop. *The option of non-surgical management should be discussed with all women with*

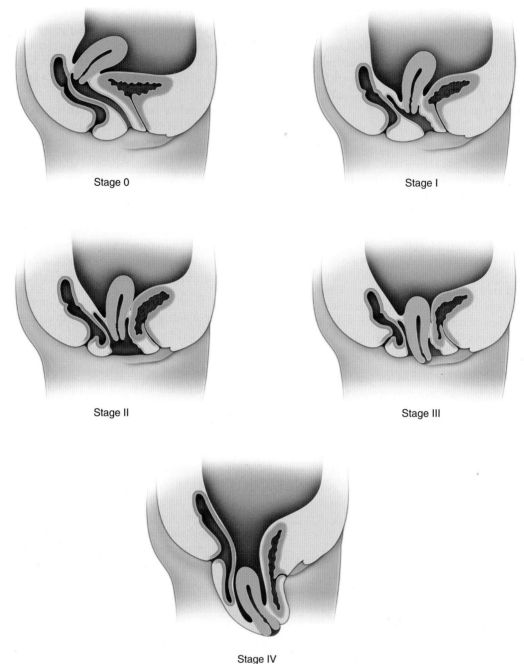

Stage 0

Stage I

Stage II

Stage III

Stage IV

FIGURE 28.2. Pelvic relaxation classified by stage.

*prolapse.* Nonsurgical alternatives include pessaries, pelvic floor exercises, and symptom-directed management. A variety of surgical procedures can also be considered.

**Pessaries** can be used in any situation when a woman prefers a nonsurgical alternative. Pessaries can be fitted in most women with prolapse, regardless of prolapse stage or site of predominant prolapse, and are used by 75% of urogynecologists as first-line therapy for prolapse. Pessary devices are available in various shapes and sizes, and can be categorized as supportive (such as a ring pessary) or space-occupying (such as a donut pessary). Pessaries com-

monly used for prolapse include ring pessaries (with and without support) and Gellhorn, donut, and cube pessaries.

Surgical treatments for prolapse include hysterectomy, uterosacral or sacrospinous ligament fixation by the vaginal approach, or sacral hysteropexy (abdominal attachment of the lower uterus or upper vagina to the sacral promontory with synthetic mesh) by the abdominal approach. **Colpocleisis** (complete obliteration of the vaginal lumen) can be offered to women who are at high risk for complications with reconstructive procedures and who do not desire vaginal intercourse.

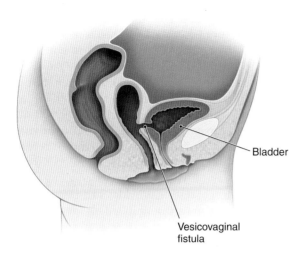

FIGURE 28.3. Fistula. (Used with permission from the American College of Obstetricians and Gynecologists.)

Many women with advanced prolapse, particularly prolapse involving the anterior vagina, will not have symptoms of urinary incontinence. Some of these women will become incontinent after prolapse surgery.

*Clinicians should discuss with women the potential risks and benefits of performing a prophylactic anti-incontinence procedure at the time of prolapse repair.*

## URINARY INCONTINENCE

The prevalence of urinary incontinence appears to increase gradually during young adult life, has a broad peak around middle age, and then steadily increases in the elderly. Urinary incontinence has been shown to affect women's social, clinical, and psychologic well-being. It is estimated that less than one half of all incontinent women seek medical care, even though the condition can often be treated.

## Types

Several types of urinary incontinence have been identified, and a patient may have more than one type (Table 28.1).

### DETRUSOR OVERACTIVITY (URGE INCONTINENCE)

The normal voiding "reflex" is initiated when stretch receptors within the **detrusor muscle,** the layer of muscle that lines the interior bladder wall, send a signal to the brain. The brain then decides if it is socially acceptable to void. The detrusor muscle contracts, elevating the bladder pressure to exceed the urethral pressure. The external urethral sphincter, under voluntary control, relaxes, and voiding is completed.

Normally, the detrusor muscle allows the bladder to fill in a low-resistance setting. The volume increases within the bladder, but the pressure within the bladder remains low. Patients with an overactive detrusor muscle have uninhibited detrusor contractions. These contractions cause a rise in the bladder pressure that overrides the urethral pressure, and the patient will leak urine without evidence of increased intra-abdominal pressure. Idiopathic detrusor overactivity has no organic cause, but has a neurogenic component.

*A patient with detrusor overactivity presents with the feeling that she must run to the bathroom frequently and urgently.* This may or may not be associated with nocturia. These symptoms may occur after bladder surgery to correct stress incontinence or after extensive bladder dissection during pelvic surgery.

| TABLE 28.1 | Characteristics of Urinary Incontinence | | |
|---|---|---|---|
| Characteristic | Stress Incontinence | Urge Incontinence | Overflow Incontinence |
| Associated symptoms | None (occasional pelvic pressure) | Urgency, nocturia | Fullness, pressure, frequency |
| Amount of loss | Small, spurt | Large, complete emptying | Small, dribbling |
| Duration of loss | Brief, corresponds to stress | Moderate, several seconds | Often continuous |
| Associated event | Cough, laugh, sneeze, physical activity | None, change in position, running water | None |
| Position | Upright, sitting; rare when supine or asleep | Any | Any |
| Cause | Structural (cystocele, urethrocele) | Loss of bladder inhibition | Obstruction, loss of neurologic control |

## STRESS URINARY INCONTINENCE

Normal physiology and anatomy allow for increased abdominal pressure to be transmitted along the entire urethra. In addition, the endopelvic fascia that extends beneath the urethra allows for the urethra to be compressed against the endopelvic fascia, thus maintaining a closed system and maintaining the bladder neck in a stable position. In patients with stress incontinence, increased intra-abdominal pressure is transmitted to the bladder, but not to the urethra (specifically, the urethral–vesical junction [UVJ]), due to loss of integrity of the endopelvic fascia. The bladder neck descends, the bladder pressure is elevated above the intra-urethral pressure, and urine is lost. *Patients with stress incontinence present with loss of urine during activities that cause increased intra-abdominal pressure, such as coughing, laughing, or sneezing.*

## MIXED INCONTINENCE

*Some patients may have symptoms of both urge incontinence and stress incontinence.* These patients experience urine leakage during coughing, laughing, or sneezing; the increased intra-abdominal pressure that occurs during these activities causes the UVJ to descend and also stimulates the detrusor to contract. This clinical scenario may be treated as stress or as detrusor instability, although it is not clear which approach offers a better outcome.

## OVERFLOW INCONTINENCE

In this form of incontinence, the bladder does not empty completely during voiding due to an inability of the detrusor muscle to contract. This may occur because of an obstruction of the urethra or a neurologic deficit that causes the patient to lose the ability to perceive the need to void. Urine leaks out of the bladder when the bladder pressure exceeds the urethral pressure. *These patients experience continuous leakage of small amounts of urine.*

## Evaluation

Patients with urinary incontinence should undergo a basic evaluation that includes a history, physical examination, direct observation of urine loss, measurement of postvoid residual volume, urine culture, and urinalysis. These tests and examinations are performed to rule out urinary tract infection, neuromuscular disorders, and pelvic support defects, all of which are associated with urinary incontinence. The patient should also be asked about her fluid intake, the relationship of her symptoms to fluid intake and activity, and medications. A voiding diary may be helpful in this evaluation process.

Urodynamic testing may also be useful. These tests measure the pressure and volume of the bladder as it fills and the flow rate as it empties. In **single-channel uro-dynamic testing,** the patient voids, and the volume is recorded. A urinary catheter is then placed and the postvoid residual (PVR) urine is recorded. The bladder is filled in a retrograde fashion. The patient is asked to note the first sensation that her bladder is being filled. She then is asked to note when she has a desire to void, and when she can no longer hold her urine. Normal values are: 100–150 cc for first sensation, 250 cc for first desire to void, and 500–600 cc for maximum capacity. In **multichannel urodynamic testing,** a transducer is placed in the vagina or rectum to measure intra-abdominal pressure. A transducer is placed in the bladder, and EMG pads are placed along the perineum. This form of testing provides an assessment of the entire pelvic floor, and an uninhibited bladder contraction can be clearly documented.

**Cystourethroscopy** may be used in the evaluation of urinary incontinence. In this procedure, a slender, lighted scope is introduced into the bladder. Cystourethroscopy can help to identify bladder lesions and foreign bodies, as well as urethral diverticula, fistulas, urethral strictures, and intrinsic sphincter deficiency. It frequently is used as part of the surgical procedures to treat incontinence.

## Treatment

There are many options for treatment. Often, treatments are more effective when used in combination.

## NONSURGICAL TREATMENT OPTIONS

Lifestyle interventions that may help modify incontinence include weight loss, caffeine reduction and fluid management, reduction of physical forces (e.g., work, exercise), cessation of smoking, and relief of constipation. Pelvic muscle training (Kegel exercises) can be extremely effective in treating some forms of incontinence, especially stress incontinence. The exercises work to strengthen the pelvic floor and thus decrease the degree of urethral hypermobility. The patient is instructed to repeatedly tighten her pelvic floor muscles as though she were voluntarily stopping a urine stream. Biofeedback techniques and weighted vaginal cones are available to assist patients in learning the proper technique. *When performed correctly, these exercises have success rates of about 85%.* Success is defined as a decreased number of episodes of incontinence. However, once the patient stops the exercise regimen, she will revert to her original status. Other treatments for stress incontinence include various pessaries and continence tampons that can be placed vaginally to aid in urethral compression.

Behavioral training is aimed at increasing the patient's bladder control and capacity by gradually increasing the amount of time between voids. This type of training is most often used to treat urge incontinence, but may also be successful in treating stress incontinence and mixed incontinence. It may be augmented by biofeedback.

*A number of other pharmacologic agents appear to be effective for treating frequency, urgency, and urge incontinence.* However, the response to treatment often is unpredictable, and side effects are common with effective doses. Generally, drugs improve detrusor overactivity by inhibiting the contractile activity of the bladder. These agents can be broadly classified into anticholinergic agents, tricyclic antidepressants, musculotropic drugs, and a variety of less commonly used drugs.

## Surgical Therapy

Many surgical treatments have been developed for stress urinary incontinence, but only a few—**retropubic colposuspension** and **sling procedures**—have survived and evolved with enough supporting evidence to make recommendations (Figs. 28.4 A and B). The aim of retropubic colposuspension is to suspend and stabilize the anterior vaginal wall and, thus, the bladder neck and proximal urethra, in a retropubic position. This prevents their descent and allows for urethral compression against a stable suburethral layer. In the **Burch procedure,** which can be performed abdominally or laparoscopically, two or three nonabsorbable sutures are placed on each side of the midurethra and bladder neck. Another procedure uses tension-free tape placed at the midurethra to raise the urethra back into place. This procedure can be done through the vagina. The success of tension-free vaginal tape has led to the introduction of similar products with modified methods of midurethral sling placement (retropubic "top-down" and transobturator). **Bulking agents,** such as collagen, carbon-coated beads, and fat, are used for the treatment of urodynamic stress incontinence with intrinsic sphincter deficiency (Fig. 28.4C). They are injected transurethrally or periurethrally in the periurethral tissue around the bladder neck and proximal urethra. They provide a "washer" effect around the proximal urethra and the bladder neck. These agents usually are used as second-line therapy after surgery has failed, when stress incontinence persists with a nonmobile bladder neck, or among older, debilitated women for whom any form of operative treatment may be hazardous.

Success rates vary depending on the skill of the surgeon and the technique used. Tension-free vaginal tape and the Burch suspension have success rate at five years of 85%. *Preoperative counseling should include not only the risks of the procedures, but also the goals.* The patient must understand that the procedure may not allow her to be completely continent, as overcorrection (making the sling too tight) may lead to urinary retention. In addition, studies only show 5-year data; thus, surgery should not be presented as a permanent solution. *One study of women who underwent Burch colposuspension found that the cure rate of stress incontinence gradually decreased over 10–12 years, reaching a plateau at 69%.* Approximately 10% of patients required at least one additional surgery to cure their stress incontinence.

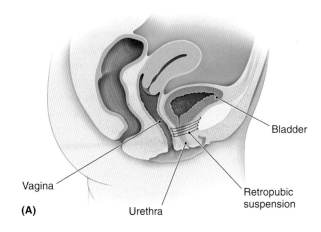
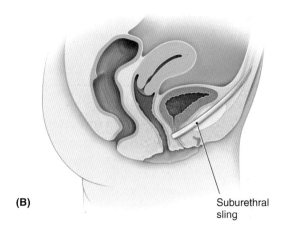
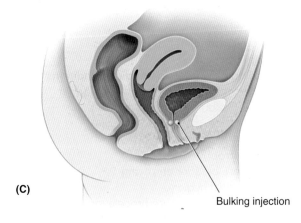

FIGURE 28.4. Surgical procedures for the treatment of incontinence. (A) Retropubic colposuspension. (B) Sling procedure. (C) Bulking agents. (Used with permission from the American College of Obstetricians and Gynecologists.)

## URINARY TRACT INFECTIONS

*An estimated 11% of U.S. women report at least one physician-diagnosed* **urinary tract infection (UTI)** *per year, and the lifetime probability that a woman will have a UTI is 60%.* Most UTIs in women ascend from bacterial contamination of the urethra. Except in patients with tuberculosis or in immunosuppressed patients, infections are rarely acquired by hematogenous or lymphatic spread. The relatively short female urethra, exposure of the meatus to vestibular and rectal pathogens, and sexual activity that may induce trauma or introduce other organisms, all increase the potential for infection (Box 28.1). *Estrogen deficiency also causes a decrease in urethral resistance to infection, which contributes to ascending contamination.* This increased susceptibility may explain the 20% prevalence of asymptomatic bacteriuria in women over the age of 65.

*Of first infections, 90% are caused by Escherichia coli.* The remaining 10% to 20% of UTIs are caused by other microorganisms, occasionally colonizing the vagina and periurethral area. *Staphylococcus saprophyticus* frequently causes lower UTIs. *Proteus, Pseudomonas, Klebsiella,* and *Enterobacter* species all have been isolated in women with cystitis or pyelonephritis, and these frequently are associated with structural abnormalities of the urinary tract, indwelling catheters, and renal calculi. *Enterococcus* species also have been isolated in women with structural abnormalities. Gram-positive isolates, including group B streptococci, are increasingly isolated along with fungal infections in women with indwelling catheters.

### Clinical History

Patients with **lower UTIs** typically present with symptoms of frequency, urgency, nocturia, or dysuria. The symptoms found vary somewhat with the site of the infection. Symptoms caused by irritation of the bladder or trigone include urgency, frequency, and nocturia. Irritation of the urethra leads to frequency and dysuria. Some patients may report suprapubic tenderness or urethral or bladder-base tenderness. Fever is uncommon in women with uncomplicated lower UTI. **Upper UTI** or acute pyelonephritis frequently occurs with a combination of fever and chills, flank pain, and varying degrees of dysuria, urgency, and frequency (Box 28.2).

### Laboratory Evaluation

The evaluation of the patient suspected of having a urinary tract infection should include a urinalysis.

---

**BOX 28.1**
**Risk Factors for Urinary Tract Infection**

**Premenopausal Women**
- History of urinary tract infection
- Frequent or recent sexual activity
- Diaphragm contraception use
- Use of spermicidal agents
- Increasing parity
- Diabetes mellitus
- Obesity
- Sickle cell trait
- Anatomic congenital abnormalities
- Urinary tract calculi
- Neurologic disorders or medical conditions requiring indwelling or repetitive bladder catheterization

**Postmenopausal Women**
- Vaginal atrophy
- Incomplete bladder emptying
- Poor perineal hygiene
- Rectocele, cystocele, urethrocele, or uterovaginal prolapse
- Lifetime history of urinary tract infection
- Type 1 diabetes mellitus

(From American College of Obstetricians and Gynecologists. Treatment of urinary tract infections in nonpregnant women. ACOG Practice Bulletin No. 91. *Obstet Gynecol.* 2008; 111(3): 785–794.)

---

**BOX 28.2**
**Urinary Tract Infections: Key Definitions**

- *Asymptomatic bacteriuria:* considerable bacteriuria in a woman with no symptoms
- *Cystitis:* infection that is limited to the lower urinary tract and occurs with symptoms of dysuria and frequent and urgent urination and, occasionally, suprapubic tenderness
- *Acute pyelonephritis:* infection of the renal parenchyma and pelvicaliceal system accompanied by significant bacteriuria, usually occurring with fever and flank pain
- *Relapse:* recurrent UTI with the same organism after adequate therapy
- *Reinfection:* recurrent UTI caused by bacteria previously isolated after treatment and a negative intervening urine culture result, or a recurrent UTI caused by a second isolate.

(From: American College of Obstetricians and Gynecologists. Treatment of urinary tract infections in nonpregnant women. ACOG Practice Bulletin No. 91. *Obstet Gynecol.* 2008; 111(3): 785–794.)

*The initial treatment of a symptomatic lower UTI with pyuria or bacteriuria does not require a urine culture.*

However, if clinical improvement does not occur within 48 hours or, in the case of recurrence, a urine culture is useful to help tailor treatment.

*A urine culture should be performed in all cases of upper UTIs.*

Urine for these studies is obtained through a "clean-catch midstream" sample, which involves cleansing the vulva and catching a portion of urine passed during the middle of uninterrupted voiding. Urine obtained from catheters or suprapubic aspiration may also be used. A standard urinalysis will detect pyuria, defined as 10 leukocytes per milliliter, but pyuria alone is not a reliable predictor of infection. However, pyuria and bacteriuria together on microscopic examination results markedly increase the probability of UTI.

"Dipstick" tests for infection based on the detection of leukocyte esterase are useful as screening tests. However, women with negative test results and symptoms should have a urine culture or urinalysis or both performed, because false-negative results are common.

Cultures of urine samples that show colony counts of more than 100,000 for a single organism generally indicate infection. Colony counts as low as 10,000 for *E. coli* are associated with infection when symptoms are present. If a culture report indicates multiple organisms, contamination of the specimen should be suspected.

## Treatment

Once infection is confirmed by urinalysis or culture, antibiotic therapy should be instituted.

*Recent data have shown that 3 days of therapy is equivalent in efficacy to longer durations of therapy, with eradication rates exceeding 90%.*

Recommended agents for the 3-day therapy include trimethoprim-sulfamethoxazole, trimethoprim, ciprofloxacin, levofloxacin, and gatifloxacin.

In cases of acute pyelonephritis, treatment should be initiated immediately. The choice of drug should be based on knowledge of resistance in the community. Once the urine and susceptibility culture results are available, therapy is altered as needed. *Most women can be treated on an outpatient basis initially or given intravenous fluids and one parenteral dose of an antibiotic before being discharged and given a regimen of oral therapy.* Patients who are severely ill, have

complications, are unable to tolerate oral medications or fluids, or who the clinician suspects will be noncompliant with outpatient therapy should be hospitalized and receive empiric broad-spectrum parenteral antibiotics.

Women with frequent recurrences and prior confirmation by diagnostic tests and who are aware of their symptoms may be empirically treated without recurrent testing for pyuria. *Management of recurrent UTIs should start with a search for known risk factors associated with recurrence.* These include frequent intercourse, long-term spermicide use, diaphragm use, a new sexual partner, young age at first UTI, and a maternal history of UTI. Behavioral changes, such as using a different form of contraception instead of spermicide, should be advised. The first-line intervention for the prevention of the recurrence of cystitis is prophylactic or intermittent antimicrobial therapy. For women with frequent recurrences, continuous prophylaxis with once-daily treatment with nitrofurantoin, norfloxacin, ciprofloxacin, trimethoprim, trimethoprim–sulfamethoxazole, or another agent has been shown to decrease the risk of recurrence by 95%. Drinking cranberry juice has been shown to decrease symptomatic UTIs, but the length of therapy and the concentration required to prevent recurrence long-term are not known.

*Recurrence is most common in postmenopausal women; the hypoestrogenic state with associated genitourinary atrophy likely contributes to the increased prevalence.* Oral and vaginal exogenous estrogens have been studied with varying results.

*Screening for and treatment of asymptomatic bacteriuria is not recommended in nonpregnant, premenopausal women.* Specific groups for whom treatment of asymptomatic bacteriuria is recommended include all pregnant women, women undergoing a urologic procedure in which mucosal bleeding is anticipated, and women in whom catheter-acquired bacteriuria persists 48 hours after catheter removal. Treatment of asymptomatic bacteriuria in women with diabetes mellitus, older institutionalized patients, older patients living in a community setting, patients with spinal cord injuries, or patients with indwelling catheters is not recommended.

## SUGGESTED READINGS

Julian TM. Pelvic support defects: diagnosis and nonsurgical management. In: American College of Obstetricians and Gynecologists. *Precis: Gynecology.* 3rd ed. Washington, DC: American College of Obstetricians and Gynecologists; 2006: 65–74.

Rosenblatt PL. Pelvic support defects: surgical management. In: American College of Obstetricians and Gynecologists. *Precis: Gynecology.* 3rd ed. Washington, DC: American College of Obstetricians and Gynecologists; 2006:75–84.

American College of Obstetricians and Gynecologists. Treatment of urinary tract infections in nonpregnant women. ACOG Practice Bulletin No. 91. *Obstet Gynecol.* 2008;111(3):785–94.

American College of Obstetricians and Gynecologists. Urinary incontinence in women. ACOG Practice Bulletin No. 63. *Obstet Gynecol.* 2005;105(6):1533–1545.

# 29 Endometriosis

This chapter deals primarily with APGO Educational Topic:

Topic 38: Endometriosis

Students should be able to describe the theories of the pathogenesis of endometriosis as well as the signs and symptoms, evaluation, and medical and surgical management of endometriosis. They should also be able to explain the relationship between infertility and endometriosis, how to evaluate and manage the combined problem, and the relationship between endometriosis and chronic pelvic pain.

**E**ndometriosis is the presence of endometrial glands and stroma in any extrauterine site, and may be suspected based on history, symptoms, and physical examination as well as laboratory and imaging information. Like the endometrial tissue from which it is derived, endometriosis implants and cysts respond to the hormonal fluctuations of the menstrual cycle. Laparotomy or laparoscopy may reveal lesions consistent with endometriosis, but because lesions may be small or atypical or caused by pathology other than endometriosis, *only proven tissue biopsy diagnosis is diagnostic.* Many women with endometriosis are asymptomatic, and diagnosis is confirmed only when surgery is performed for other indications.

It is estimated that 7% to 10% of women in the general population have endometriosis. Pelvic endometriosis is present in 6% to 43% of women undergoing sterilization, 12% to 32% of women undergoing laparoscopy for pelvic pain, and 21% to 48% of women undergoing laparoscopy for infertility. Endometriosis usually occurs in women of reproductive age, and is less frequently found in postmenopausal women. Endometriosis occurs more often in women who have never had children.

Some evidence suggests that endometriosis may have a genetic component. Women with first-degree relatives with endometriosis have nearly a 10-fold increased risk of developing endometriosis. The proposed mechanism of inheritance is polygenic and multifactorial.

## PATHOGENESIS

The exact mechanisms by which endometriosis develops are not clearly understood. Three major theories are commonly cited.

1. Direct implantation of endometrial cells, typically by means of **retrograde menstruation.** This mechanism is consistent with the occurrence of pelvic endometriosis and its predilection for the ovaries and pelvic peritoneum, as well as for sites such as an abdominal incision or episiotomy scar. Direct implantation is commonly referred to as Sampson's theory because of his experimental work that showed the possibility of such a mechanism.
2. **Vascular and lymphatic dissemination** of endometrial cells (Halban's theory). Distant sites of endometriosis can be explained by this process (i.e., endometriosis in locations such as lymph nodes, the pleural cavity, and kidney).
3. **Coelomic metaplasia** of multipotential cells in the peritoneal cavity (Meyer's theory) states that, under certain conditions, these cells can develop into functional endometrial tissue. This could even occur in response to the irritation caused by retrograde menstruation. The early development of endometriosis in some adolescents before the onset of menstruation lends credence to this theory.

It is probable that more than one theory is necessary to explain the diverse nature and locations of endometriosis. Underlying all these possibilities is a yet undiscovered immunologic factor that would explain why some women develop endometriosis whereas others with similar characteristics do not.

## PATHOLOGY

Endometriosis is found on the ovaries in most patients and is typically bilateral. Other common pelvic structures involved include the pouch of Douglas (particularly the uterosacral ligaments and rectovaginal septum), the round ligament, the fallopian tubes, and the sigmoid colon (Fig. 29.1 and Table 29.1). On rare occasions, distant endometriosis is found in abdominal surgical scars, the umbilicus, and various organs outside the pelvic cavity.

*The gross appearance of endometriosis varies considerably and includes the following forms:*

- Small (1-mm), clear or white lesions
- Small, dark red ("mulberry") or brown ("powder burn") lesions
- Cysts filled with dark-red or brown hemosiderin-laden fluid ("chocolate" cysts)
- Dark-red or blue "domes" that may reach 15–20 cm in size

Reactive fibrosis frequently surrounds these lesions, which gives a puckered appearance. More advanced disseminated disease causes further fibrosis and may result in dense adhesions.

## SIGNS AND SYMPTOMS

*Women with endometriosis demonstrate a wide variety of symptoms.* The nature and severity of symptoms may not match either the location or extent of the disease. Women with grossly extensive endometriosis may have few symptoms, whereas those with minimal gross endometriosis may have severe pain. *Endometriosis may also be asymptomatic.* The pain associated with endometriosis is thought to depend more upon the depth of invasion of the implants rather than on the number or extent of the superficial implants. *The classic symptoms of endometriosis include progressive* **dysmenorrhea** *and deep* **dyspareunia.** Some patients experience chronic, unremitting pelvic discomfort along with dysmenorrhea and dyspareunia. Chronic pelvic pain may be related to the adhesions and pelvic scarring found in association with endometriosis.

Dysmenorrhea caused by endometriosis is not directly related to the amount of visible disease. In many women with endometriosis, the dysmenorrhea worsens over time. Endometriosis should be considered a possible etiology in patients who present with dysmenorrhea that does not respond to oral contraceptives or nonsteroidal anti-inflammatory agents (NSAIDs). Dyspareunia is often associated with uterosacral or deep posterior cul-de-sac involvement with endometriosis. The dyspareunia is typically reported on deep penetration, although there is no correlation between dyspareunia and the extent of endometriosis.

*Infertility is more frequent in women with endometriosis, although a cause-and-effect relationship has not been established.* With extensive disease, pelvic scarring and adhesions that distort pelvic anatomy may cause infertility, but the cause of infertility in women with minimal endometriosis is unclear. Prostaglandins and autoantibodies have been implicated, but these relationships remain unproven. In

FIGURE 29.1. Locations of endometriosis implants.

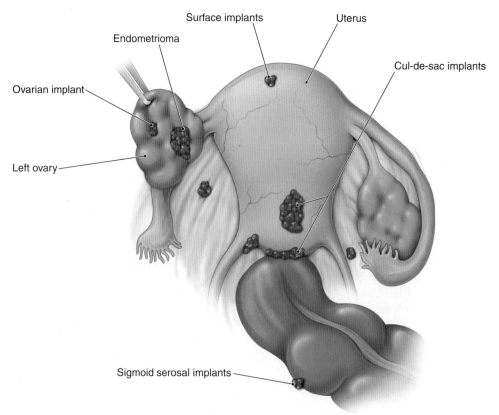

| TABLE 29.1 Sites of Endometriosis | |
|---|---|
| Site | Frequency (percentage of patients) |
| Most common<br>• Ovary (often bilateral)<br>• Pelvic peritoneum over the uterus<br>• Anterior and posterior cul-de-sacs<br>• Uterosacral ligaments<br>• Fallopian tubes<br>• Pelvic lymph nodes | 60 |
| Infrequent<br>• Rectosigmoid<br>• Other GI tract sites<br>• Vagina | 10–15 |
| Rare<br>• Umbilicus<br>• Episiotomy or surgical scars<br>• Kidney<br>• Lungs<br>• Arms<br>• Legs<br>• Nasal mucosa | 5 |

some cases, infertility may be the only complaint, and endometriosis is discovered at the time of laparoscopic evaluation as part of the infertility workup. The presence of endometriosis in asymptomatic infertility patients varies between 30% and 50%.

Other, less-common symptoms of endometriosis include gastrointestinal symptoms, such as rectal bleeding and **dyschezia** (painful bowel movements) in patients with endometrial implants on the bowel and urinary symptoms such as hematuria in patients with endometrial implants on the bladder or ureters. Occasionally, patients may present with an acute abdominal emergency, which may be associated with the rupture or torsion of an endometrioma.

Pelvic examination may reveal the "classic" sign of uterosacral nodularity associated with endometriosis, but it is often absent even when substantial gross endometriosis is discovered at surgery. The uterus may be relatively fixed and retroflexed in the pelvis because of extensive adhesions. Ovarian endometriomas may be tender, palpable, and freely mobile in the pelvis, or adhered to the posterior leaf of the broad ligament, the lateral pelvic wall, or in the posterior cul-de-sac (see Fig. 29.2).

## DIFFERENTIAL DIAGNOSIS

Depending on the symptoms, the differential diagnosis will change. In patients with chronic abdominal pain, diagnoses such as chronic pelvic inflammatory disease, pelvic adhe-

sions, gastrointestinal dysfunction, and other etiologies of chronic pelvic pain should be considered. In patients with dysmenorrhea, both primary dysmenorrhea and secondary dysmenorrhea should be considered. In patients with dyspareunia, differential diagnoses include chronic pelvic inflammatory disease, ovarian cysts, and symptomatic uterine retroversion. Sudden abdominal pain may be caused by a ruptured endometrioma as well as by ectopic pregnancy, acute pelvic inflammatory disease, adnexal torsion, and rupture of a corpus luteum cyst or ovarian neoplasm.

## DIAGNOSIS

Endometriosis should be suspected in patients with the previously described symptoms. Many symptomatic women have normal findings on pelvic examination. *The diagnosis of endometriosis can be substantiated only by direct visualization during laparoscopy or laparotomy confirmed by tissue biopsy.* The presence of two or more of the following histologic features is used as the threshold criteria for the diagnosis by a pathologist:

- Endometrial epithelium
- Endometrial glands
- Endometrial stroma
- Hemosiderin-laden macrophages

Because tissue confirmation of the diagnosis of endometriosis requires a surgical procedure, investigators have searched for a noninvasive alternative. Increased serum CA-125 levels have been correlated with moderate to severe endometriosis. However, because CA-125 levels may be elevated in many conditions, the clinical utility of using it as a diagnostic marker is limited.

Imaging studies, such as ultrasonography, magnetic resonance imaging, and computed tomography appear to be useful only in the presence of a pelvic or adnexal mass. Ultrasonography may be used to visualize ovarian endometriomas, which typically appear as cysts containing low-level, homogeneous internal echoes consistent with old blood. Magnetic resonance imaging may detect deeply infiltrating endometriosis that involves the uterosacral ligaments and the cul-de-sac, but lacks sensitivity in detecting rectal involvement.

Once endometriosis is diagnosed, its extent and severity should be documented. The most widely accepted classification system has been established by the American Society for Reproductive Medicine (Fig. 29.3). While this classification scheme has limitations, it provides a uniform system for recording findings and comparing the results of various therapies.

## TREATMENT

Available therapies include expectant, hormonal, surgical, and combination medical-and-surgical treatment. The choice of treatment depends on the patient's individual

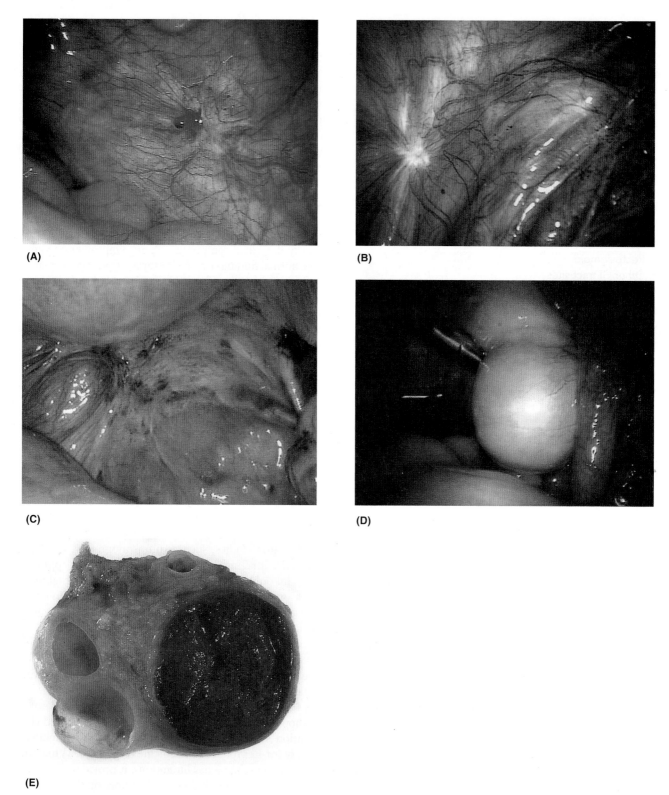

(A)

(B)

(C)

(D)

(E)

FIGURE 29.2.  Endometriosis implants. (A) Clear lesion on the ovarian fossa; (B) white endometriotic deposit on the left uterosacral ligament; (C) "Powder burn" lesion on the uterosacral ligaments; (D) right ovarian endometrioma; (E) chocolate cyst in an ovary containing other smaller fibrous-filled cavities. (From Overton C, Davis C, McMillan L, Shaw RW. *An Atlas of Endometriosis.* 3rd ed. London: Informa UK; 2007:3.2, 4.2, 5.3, 5.4, 9.55.)

American Society for Reproductive Medicine
Revised Classification of Endometriosis

Patient's name _____  Date _____

Stage I (minimal)    —   1–5
Stage II (mild)      —   6–15
Stage III (moderate) —   16–40      Laparoscopy _____ Laparotomy _____ Photography _____
Stage IV (severe)    —   >40        Recommended treatment _____
                                    _____
Total _____             Prognosis _____

| Peritoneum | Endometriosis | <1 cm | 1–3 cm | >3 cm |
|---|---|---|---|---|
| | Superficial | 1 | 2 | 4 |
| | Deep | 2 | 4 | 6 |
| Ovary | R  Superficial | 1 | 2 | 4 |
| | Deep | 4 | 16 | 20 |
| | L  Superficial | 1 | 2 | 4 |
| | Deep | 4 | 16 | 20 |

| | Posterior cul-de-sac obliteration | Partial | | Complete | |
|---|---|---|---|---|---|
| | | 4 | | 40 | |

| | Adhesions | <1/3 Enclosure | 1/3 – 2/3 Enclosure | >2/3 Enclosure |
|---|---|---|---|---|
| Ovary | R  Filmy | 1 | 2 | 4 |
| | Dense | 4 | 8 | 16 |
| | L  Filmy | 1 | 2 | 4 |
| | Dense | 4 | 8 | 16 |
| Tube | R  Filmy | 1 | 2 | 4 |
| | Dense | 4* | 8* | 16 |
| | L  Filmy | 1 | 2 | 4 |
| | Dense | 4* | 8* | 16 |

*If the fimbriated end of the fallopian tube is completely enclosed, change the point assignment to 16. Denote appearance of superficial implant types as red [(R), red, red-pink, flamelike, vesicular blobs, clear vesicles], white [(W), opacifications, peritoneal defects, yellow-brown], or black [(B), black, hemosiderin deposits, blue]. Denote percent of total described as R__%, W__%, and B__%. Total should equal 100%.

Additional endometriosis: _____  |  Associated pathology: _____
                                            |  _____
_____          |  _____

| To be used with normal tubes and ovaries | To be used with abnormal tubes and/or ovaries |

L                                    R    L                                    R

FIGURE 29.3. Revised American Society for Reproductive Medicine classification of endometriosis. (Reprinted from American Society for Reproductive Medicine. Revised American Society for Reproductive Medicine classification of endometriosis: 1996. *Fertility and Sterility*; 1997:67(5):817–821, with permission from the American Society for Reproductive Medicine.) *(continued on next page)*

Examples & Guidelines

Stage I (minimal)

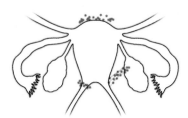

Peritoneum
    Superficial endo — 1–3 cm    -2
R. ovary
    Superficial endo — <1 cm     -1
    Filmy adhesions — <1/3       -1
Total points                      4

Stage II (mild)

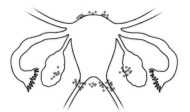

Peritoneum
    Deep endo          — >3 cm    -6
R. ovary
    Superficial endo — <1 cm      -1
    Filmy adhesions — <1/3        -1
L. ovary
    Superficial endo — <1 cm      -1
Total points                       9

Stage III (moderate)

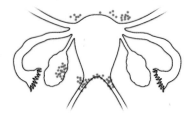

Peritoneum
    Deep endo          — >3 cm    -6
Cul-de-sac
    Partial obliteration          -4
L. ovary
    Deep endo          — 1–3 cm   -16
Total points                       26

Stage III (moderate)

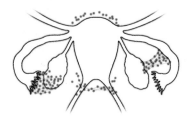

Peritoneum
    Superficial endo — >3 cm      -4
R. tube
    Filmy adhesions — <1/3        -1
R. ovary
    Filmy adhesions — <1/3        -1
L. tube
    Dense adhesions— <1/3         -16*
L. ovary
    Deep endo          — <1 cm    -4
    Dense adhesions— <1/3         -4
Total points                       30

Stage IV (severe)

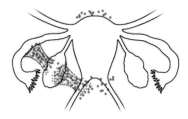

Peritoneum
    Superficial endo — >3 cm      -4
L. ovary
    Deep endo          — 1–3 cm   -32†
    Dense adhesions— <1/3         -8†
L. tube
    Dense adhesions— <1/3         -8†
Total points                       52

*Point assignment changed to 16.
†Point assignment doubled.

Stage IV (severe)

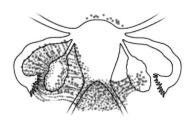

Peritoneum
    Deep endo          — >3 cm    -6
Cul-de-sac
    Complete obliteration         -40
R. ovary
    Deep endo          — 1–3 cm   -16
    Dense adhesions— <1/3         -4
L. tube
    Dense adhesions— >2/3         -16
L. ovary
    Deep endo          — 1–3 cm   -16
    Dense adhesions— >2/3         -16
Total points                       114

*Determination of the stage or degree of endometrial involvement is based on a weighted point system. Distribution of points has been arbitrarily determined and may require further revision or refinement as knowledge of the disease increases.

To ensure complete evaluation, inspection of the pelvis in a clockwise or counterclockwise fashion is encouraged. Number, size, and location of endometrial implants, plaques, endometriomas, and/or adhesions are noted. For example, five separate 0.5-cm superficial implants on the peritoneum (2.5 cm total) would be assigned 2 points. (The surface of the uterus should be considered peritoneum.) The severity of the endometriosis or adhesions should be assigned the highest score only for peritoneum, ovary, tube, or cul-de-sac. For example, a 4-cm superficial and a 2-cm deep implant of the peritoneum should be given a score of 6 (not 8). A 4-cm deep endometrioma of the ovary associated with more than 3 cm of superficial disease should be scored 20 (not 24).

In those patients with only one adnexa, points applied to disease of the remaining tube and ovary should be multiplied by two.

†Points assigned may be circled and totaled. Aggregation of points indicates stage of disease (minimal, mild, moderate, or severe).

The presence of endometriosis of the bowel, urinary tract, fallopian tube, vagina, cervix, skin, etc., should be documented under "additional endometriosis." Other pathology such as tubal occlusion, leiomyomata, uterine anomaly, etc, should be documented under "associated pathology." All pathology should be depicted as specifically as possible on the sketch of pelvic organs, and means of observation (laparoscopy or laparotomy) should be noted.

FIGURE 29.3.   *Continued*

circumstances, which include (1) the presenting symptoms and their severity, (2) the location and severity of endometriosis, and (3) the desire for future childbearing. No treatment provides a permanent cure. Total abdominal hysterectomy with bilateral salpingo-oophorectomy is associated with a 10% risk of recurrent symptoms and a 4% risk of additional endometriosis. Reasonable goals for management of endometriosis include reduction in pelvic pain, minimizing surgical intervention, and preserving fertility.

## Expectant Management

Patients can be treated expectantly (i.e., without either medical or surgical therapy) in some selected cases, including patients with limited disease whose symptoms are minimal or nonexistent or patients who are attempting to conceive. Because endometriosis responds to estrogen and progesterone, older patients with mild symptoms may opt to wait until the natural decrease in levels of these hormones that occurs with menopause.

## Medical Therapy

Because the glands and stroma of endometriosis respond to both exogenous and endogenous hormones, suppression of endometriosis is based on a medication's potential ability to induce atrophy of the endometrial tissue. This treatment approach is optimal for patients who are currently symptomatic, have documented endometriosis beyond minimal disease, or who desire pregnancy in the future. The patient should be aware that recurrence after the completion of medical therapy is common and that medical therapy does not affect adhesions and fibrosis caused by the endometriosis. Medical therapy may often be instituted empirically without a definitive surgical diagnosis of endometriosis, if the patient's symptoms are consistent with the disease and appropriate, thorough physical examination and workup have been performed to rule out other causes of pain, including gynecological, gastrointestinal, and urologic causes.

Because of their ease of administration and relatively low level of side effects, combined oral contraceptives used in conjunction with NSAIDs are often the first line of treatment for pain associated with endometriosis. *Oral contraceptive therapy induces a decidual reaction in the functioning endometriotic tissue.* Continuous therapy, in which the oral contraceptive regimen is taken continuously without the 7 days of inactive pills that induce withdrawal bleeding, can also be prescribed to prevent secondary dysmenorrhea.

*Progesterone therapy, in the form of injectable depomedroxyprogesterone acetate (DMPA) or implants, suppresses gonadotropin release and, in turn, ovarian steroidogenesis; it also directly affects the uterine endometrium and endometrial implants.* DMPA has been associated with an increased risk of bone mineral loss and its use should be weighed against

a woman's existing risk factors for osteoporosis (see Chapter 24, Contraception).

Danazol is a medication that suppresses both luteinizing hormone (LH) and follicle-stimulating hormone (FSH) midcycle surges. In the absence of LH and FSH stimulation, the ovary no longer produces estrogen, which induces amenorrhea and endometrial atrophy. Side effects of danazol, which occur in a minority of patients, are related to its hypoestrogenic and androgenic properties and include acne, spotting and bleeding, hot flushes, oily skin, growth of facial hair, decreased libido, and atrophic vaginitis, and deepening of the voice. Some of these side effects do not resolve with the discontinuation of therapy. Lipoprotein metabolism is also altered; serum high-density lipoprotein (HDL) levels increase significantly while low-density lipoprotein (LDL) levels decrease.

Comparable symptom relief can be achieved with fewer effects using gonadotropin-releasing hormone (GnRH) agonists. *GnRH agonists down-regulate the pituitary gland and cause marked suppression of LH and FSH.* However, the side effects are less severe than those of danazol, because androgenic side effects are eliminated. However, the hypoestrogenic effect produced by GnRH agonists may cause hot flushes and night sweats and a slight increase in the risk of bone density loss. If a patient develops side effects while taking a GnRH agonist, if the therapy is required for longer than 6 months, or if repeated treatments are required, **add-back therapy** consisting of low-dose combination oral contraceptives or medroxyprogesterone should be considered. Add-back therapy is often started with GnRH agonist therapy, because it does not affect the drug's control of pelvic pain and mitigates the vasomotor and bone density side effects.

## Surgical Therapy

*The surgical management of endometriosis can be classified as either conservative or extirpative.* Conservative surgery includes excision, cauterization, or ablation (by laser or electrocoagulation) of visible endometriotic lesions and preservation of the uterus and other reproductive organs to allow for a possible future pregnancy. Conservative surgery is often undertaken at the time of the initial laparoscopy performed for pain or infertility. If extensive disease is found, conservative surgery involves lysis of adhesions, removal of active endometriotic lesions, and possibly reconstruction of reproductive organs. Success rates of conservative surgery appear to correlate with the severity of the disease at the time of surgery as well as with the skill of the surgeon. Medical therapy can be instituted before surgery to reduce the amount of endometriosis, and after surgery to facilitate healing and prevent recurrence. Pregnancy rates following electrical energy or argon laser range from 34% to 75%. Pregnancy rates after carbon dioxide laser vaporization range from 25% to 100%

for stage 2 disease, from 19% to 66% for stage 3 disease, and from 25% to 50% for stage 4 disease.

*Extirpative surgery for endometriosis is reserved only for cases in which the disease is so extensive that conservative medical or surgical therapy is not feasible, or when the patient has completed her family and wishes definitive therapy.* Definitive surgery includes total abdominal hysterectomy, bilateral salpingo-oophorectomy, lysis of adhesions, and removal of endometriotic implants. One or both ovaries may be spared if they are uninvolved and the endometriosis can be resected completely. Approximately one-third of women treated conservatively will have recurrent endometriosis and require additional surgery within 5 years. Ovarian conservation at the time of hysterectomy carries an increased risk of recurrent endometriosis requiring additional surgery. After bilateral oophorectomy, estrogen therapy may be initiated immediately, with little risk of reactivating residual disease.

## SUGGESTED READINGS

American College of Obstetricians and Gynecologists. Medical management of endometriosis. ACOG Practice Bulletin No. 11. *Obstet Gynecol.* 1999;49(6):1–4.

Schenken RS. Endometriosis. *Precis, an Update in Obstetrics and Gynecology: Reproductive Endocrinology.* 3rd ed. Washington, DC: American College of Obstetricians and Gynecologists; 2007: 131–139.

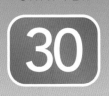

# 30 Dysmenorrhea and Chronic Pelvic Pain

Topic 46: Dysmenorrhea

Topic 39: Chronic Pelvic Pain

Students should be able to define primary and secondary dysmenorrhea and describe the evaluation and management of each. Students should be able to define chronic pelvic pain and list its possible causes. They should also be able to describe an approach to the diagnosis and management of chronic pelvic pain, including the psychosocial issues associated with chronic pelvic pain.

D ysmenorrhea is defined as painful menstruation that prevents a woman from performing normal activities. It may also be accompanied by other symptoms, including diarrhea, nausea, vomiting, headache, and dizziness. Dysmenorrhea may be caused by a clinically identifiable cause (**secondary dysmenorrhea**) or by an excess of prostaglandins, leading to painful uterine muscle activity (**primary dysmenorrhea**). The term **chronic pelvic pain** refers to noncyclic pelvic pain (not solely associated with menstruation) that lasts for 6 months or more.

For most patients, diagnosis of dysmenorrhea or chronic pelvic pain is made by careful evaluation through history and physical examination. In some instances, evaluation using other modalities, including laparoscopy, may be needed. Once the diagnosis is established, therapies may be instituted.

## DYSMENORRHEA

*Primary and secondary dysmenorrhea are a source of recurrent disability for a significant number of women in their early reproductive years.* It is uncommon for primary dysmenorrhea to occur during the first three to six menstrual cycles, when regular ovulation is not yet well-established. The incidence of primary dysmenorrhea is greatest in women in their late teens to early 20s and declines with age. Secondary dysmenorrhea becomes more common as a woman ages, because it accompanies the rising prevalence of causal factors. Childbearing does not affect the occurrence of either primary or secondary dysmenorrhea.

## Etiology

Primary dysmenorrhea is caused by excess **prostaglandin $F_{2\alpha}$** produced in the endometrium. Prostaglandin production in the uterus normally increases under the influence of progesterone, reaching a peak at, or soon after, the start of menstruation. With the onset of menstruation, formed prostaglandins are released from the shedding endometrium. Prostaglandins are potent smooth-muscle stimulants that cause intense uterine contractions, resulting in intrauterine pressures that can exceed 400 mm Hg and baseline intrauterine pressures in excess of 80 mm Hg. Prostaglandin $F_{2\alpha}$ also causes contractions in smooth muscle elsewhere in the body, resulting in nausea, vomiting, and diarrhea (Table 30.1). In addition to the increase in prostaglandins from endometrial shedding, necrosis of endometrial cells provides increased substrate arachidonic acid from cell walls for prostaglandin synthesis. Besides prostaglandin $F_{2\alpha}$, prostaglandin $E_2$ is also produced in the uterus. Prostaglandin $E_2$, a potent vasodilator and inhibitor of platelet aggregation, has been implicated as a cause of primary menorrhagia.

Secondary dysmenorrhea is caused by structural abnormalities or disease processes that occur outside the uterus, within the uterine wall, or within the uterine cavity (Box 30.1). Common causes of secondary dysmenorrhea include **endometriosis** (the presence of ectopic endometrial tissue outside of the uterus), **adenomyosis** (the presence of ectopic endometrial tissue within the myometrium), adhesions, **pelvic inflammatory disease,** and **leiomyomata** (uterine fibroids).

| TABLE 30.1 | Pain and Associated Systemic Symptoms in Primary Dysmenorrhea | |
|---|---|---|
| **Symptom** | | **Estimated Incidence (%)** |
| Pain: spasmodic, colicky, labor-like; sometimes described as an aching or heaviness in lower middle abdomen; may radiate to the back and down the thighs; starts at onset of menstruation; lasts hours to days | | 100 |
| Associated symptoms | | |
| Nausea and emesis | | 90 |
| Tiredness | | 85 |
| Nervousness | | 70 |
| Dizziness | | 60 |
| Diarrhea | | 60 |
| Headache | | 50 |

## Diagnosis

Patients with primary dysmenorrhea present with recurrent, month-after-month, spasmodic lower abdominal pain that occurs on the first 1 to 3 days of menstruation. **Dyspareunia** is generally not found in patients with primary dysmenorrhea and, if present, should suggest a secondary cause.

## BOX 30.1
### Causes of Secondary Dysmenorrhea

**Extrauterine Causes**
Endometriosis

**Tumors (Benign, Malignant)**
Inflammation
Adhesions
Psychogenic (rare)
Nongynecologic causes

**Intramural Causes**
Adenomyosis
Leiomyomata

**Intrauterine Causes**
Leiomyomata
Polyps
Intrauterine contraceptive devices
Infection
Cervical stenosis and cervical lesions

## SYMPTOMS

In patients with primary dysmenorrhea, the pain is often diffusely located in the lower abdomen and suprapubic area, with radiation around or through to the back. The pain is described as "coming and going" or similar to labor. The patient often illustrates her description with a fist opening and closing. This pain is frequently accompanied by moderate to severe nausea, vomiting, and/or diarrhea. Fatigue, low backache, and headache are also common. Patients often assume a fetal position in an effort to gain relief, and many report having used a heating pad or hot water bottle in an effort to decrease their discomfort.

In patients with secondary dysmenorrhea, the pain often lasts longer than the menstrual period. It may start before menstrual bleeding begins, become worse during menstruation, then persist after menstruation ends. Secondary dysmenorrhea often starts later in life than primary dysmenorrhea.

## HISTORY

The specific complaints that an individual patient has are determined by the underlying abnormality. Therefore, a careful medical history often suggests the underlying problem and helps direct further evaluations. Complaints of heavy menstrual flow, combined with pain, suggest uterine changes such as adenomyosis, leiomyomata, or polyps. Pelvic heaviness or a change in abdominal contour should raise the possibility of large leiomyomata or intraabdominal neoplasia. Fever, chills, and malaise suggest infection. A coexisting complaint of infertility may suggest endometriosis or chronic pelvic inflammatory disease.

## ASSESSMENT

*For patients with dysmenorrhea, the physical examination is directed toward uncovering possible causes of secondary dysmenorrhea.* A pelvic examination may reveal asymmetry or irregular enlargement of the uterus, suggesting leiomyomata or other tumors. Uterine leiomyomata are easily recognizable on bimanual exam by their smooth contour and rubbery solid consistency. Adenomyosis may cause a tender, symmetrically enlarged, "boggy" uterus. This diagnosis is supported by exclusion of other causes of secondary dysmenorrhea, but definitive diagnosis can be made only by histologic examination of a hysterectomy specimen. Painful nodules in the posterior cul-de-sac and restricted motion of the uterus should suggest endometriosis (see Chapter 29, Endometriosis). Restricted motion of the uterus is also found in cases of pelvic scarring from adhesions or inflammation. Thickening and tenderness of the adnexal structures caused by inflammation may suggest this diagnosis as the cause of secondary dysmenorrhea. Cultures of the cervix for *Neisseria gonorrhoeae* and *Chlamydia trachomatis* should be obtained if infection is suspected. In some patients, a final diagnosis may not be established without invasive procedures, such as laparoscopy.

In evaluating the patient thought to have primary dysmenorrhea, the most important differential diagnosis is that of secondary dysmenorrhea. Although the patient's history is often characteristic, primary dysmenorrhea should not be diagnosed without a thorough evaluation to eliminate other possible causes.

*Physical finding of patients with primary dysmenorrhea should be normal.*

There should be no palpable abnormalities of the uterus or adnexa, and no abnormalities should be found on speculum or abdominal examinations. Patients examined while experiencing symptoms often appear pale and "shocky," but the abdomen is soft and nontender, and the uterus is normal.

## Therapy

*Primary dysmenorrhea is an appropriate diagnosis for patients with dysmenorrhea in whom no other clinically identifiable cause is apparent.* Patients with primary dysmenorrhea generally experience exceptional pain relief through the use of **nonsteroidal anti-inflammatory drugs (NSAIDs),** which are prostaglandin-synthetase inhibitors. Ibuprofen, naproxen, and mefenamic acid are commonly prescribed NSAIDs for primary dysmenorrhea. For a time, cyclo-oxygenase inhibitors (COX-2 inhibitors) were becoming the NSAID of choice because of their targeted action. However, these drugs are now rarely used because of their potential association with life-threatening cardiovascular and gastrointestinal effects. Recent studies suggest that continuous low-level topical heat therapy can provide pain relief comparable to that offered by NSAID therapy without the systemic side effects that may occur with these drugs.

Therapy with nonsteroidal anti-inflammatory agents is generally so successful that, if some response is not evident, the diagnosis of primary dysmenorrhea should be reevaluated. Other useful components of therapy for primary dysmenorrhea include the application of heat; exercise; psychotherapy and reassurance; and, on occasion, endocrine therapy, i.e., oral contraceptives to induce anovulation (see Chapter 24, Contraception).

In the rare patient who does not respond to medical and other therapy and whose pain is so severe as to be incapacitating, **presacral neurectomy** may be a consideration. The procedure involves surgical disruption of the "presacral nerves," the superior hypogastric plexus, which is found in the retroperitoneal tissue from the fourth lumbar vertebra to the hollow over the sacrum. The risk of intraoperative complications, including injury to adjacent

vascular structures and long-term sequelae such as chronic constipation, limit the use of this surgical procedure.

For secondary dysmenorrhea, when a specific diagnosis is possible, therapy directed at the underlying condition is most likely to succeed. Specific treatments for many of these diagnoses are discussed in their respective chapters. When definitive therapy cannot be used—for example, in the case of a patient with adenomyosis who wishes to preserve fertility—symptomatic therapy in the form of analgesics or modification of the menstrual cycle may be effective.

**Combined oral contraceptives** can be useful in patients who do not desire childbearing and who do not have contraindications to their use. They work by suppressing ovulation and stabilizing estrogen and progesterone levels, with a resultant decrease in endometrial prostaglandins and spontaneous uterine activity. Oral contraceptives may be taken in the traditional 28-day cycle, or in an extended fashion that increases the interval between menses.

## CHRONIC PELVIC PAIN

Chronic pelvic pain is a common disorder that represents significant disability and utilization of resources. Estimates suggest that 15% to 20% of women aged 18 to 50 years have chronic pelvic pain that lasts longer than 1 year. Although there is no generally accepted definition of chronic pelvic pain, *one proposed definition is noncyclic pain lasting for more than 6 months that localizes to the anatomic pelvis, anterior abdominal wall at or below the umbilicus, the lumbosacral back, or the buttocks and is of sufficient severity to cause functional disability or lead to medical care.* Chronic pelvic pain may be caused by diseases of the reproductive, genitourinary, and gastrointestinal tracts (Box 30.2 and Table 30.2). Other potential somatic sources of pain include the pelvic bones, ligaments, muscles, and fascia. Sometimes there is no clear etiology for the pain.

## Assessment

The successful evaluation and treatment of chronic pelvic pain requires time and a patient, caring physician. The taking of the history and physical examination is a time in which the physician may both gather information and establish a trusting rapport. Effective management of this disease is dependent on a good doctor–patient relationship, and the therapeutic effects of the relationship itself should not be overlooked.

As with the evaluation of any pain, attention must be paid to the description and timing of the symptoms involved. The history should include a thorough medical, surgical, menstrual, and sexual history. Inquiries should be made into the patient's home and work status, social history, and family history (past and present). The patient should be questioned about sleep disturbances and other signs of depression, as well as a past history of physical and

BOX 30.2
**Gynecologic Conditions That May Cause or Exacerbate Chronic Pelvic Pain, by Level of Evidence**

**Level A\***
- Endometriosis[†]
- Gynecologic malignancies (especially late stage)
- Ovarian retention syndrome (residual ovary syndrome)
- Ovarian remnant syndrome
- Pelvic congestion syndrome
- Pelvic inflammatory disease[†]
- Tuberculous salpingitis

**Level B[‡]**
- Adhesions[†]
- Benign cystic mesothelioma
- Leiomyomata[†]
- Postoperative peritoneal cysts

**Level C[§]**
- Adenomyosis
- Atypical dysmenorrhea or ovulatory pain
- Adnexal cysts (nonendometriotic)
- Cervical stenosis
- Chronic ectopic pregnancy
- Chronic endometritis
- Endometrial or cervical polyps
- Endosalpingiosis
- Intrauterine contraceptive device
- Ovarian ovulatory pain
- Residual accessory ovary
- Symptomatic pelvic relaxation (genital prolapse)

*Level A: good and consistent scientific evidence of causal relationship to chronic pelvic pain.
[†]Diagnosis frequently reported in published series of women with chronic pelvic pain.
[‡]Level B: limited or inconsistent scientific evidence of causal relationship to chronic pelvic pain.
[§]Level C: causal relationship to chronic pelvic pain based on expert opinions.
From American College of Obstetricians and Gynecologists. Chronic pelvic pain. ACOG Practice Bulletin No. 51. *Obstet Gynecol.* 2004;103(3):589–605.

ized, the patient will point to a specific location with a single finger; if the pain is diffuse, the patient will use a sweeping motion of the whole hand. Maneuvers that duplicate the patient's complaint should be noted, but undue discomfort should be avoided to minimize guarding, which would limit a thorough examination.

*Many of the same conditions that cause secondary dysmenorrhea may cause chronic pain states.* As in the evaluation of patients with dysmenorrhea, cervical cultures should be obtained if infection is suspected. For most patients, a reasonably accurate differential diagnosis can be established through the history and physical examination. The wide range of differential diagnoses possible in chronic pelvic pain lends itself to a multidisciplinary approach, which might include psychiatric evaluation or testing. Consultation with social workers, physical therapists, gastroenterologists, anesthesiologists, orthopaedists, and others should be considered. The use of imaging technologies or laparoscopy may also be required to determine a diagnosis. However, in approximately one-third of patients with chronic pelvic pain who undergo laparoscopic evaluation, no identifiable cause is found. However, two-thirds of these patients have potential causes identified where none was apparent before laparoscopy.

The evaluation should begin with the presumption that there is an organic cause for the pain. Even in patients with obvious psychosocial stress, organic pathology can and does occur. Only when other reasonable causes have been ruled out should psychiatric diagnoses such as somatization, depression, or sleep and personality disorders be entertained.

## Conditions That Increase the Risk of Chronic Pelvic Pain

Common disorders in women with chronic pelvic pain are pelvic inflammatory disease, irritable bowel syndrome, interstitial cystitis, endometriosis, and adhesions. However, it is sometimes difficult to pinpoint a specific cause of chronic pelvic pain, and many women with chronic pelvic pain have more than 1 disease that might lead to pain.

## Pelvic Inflammatory Disease

*Approximately 18% to 35% of women who have had pelvic inflammatory disease will develop chronic pelvic pain.* The exact mechanism is unknown, but may involve chronic inflammation, adhesive disease, and the coexistence of psychosocial factors. Pelvic inflammatory disease is discussed in more detail in Chapter 27, Sexually Transmitted Diseases.

### IRRITABLE BOWEL SYNDROME

**Irritable bowel syndrome (IBS)** occurs in 50% to 80% of women with chronic pelvic pain. The diagnosis of IBS

sexual abuse. Studies have found a significant correlation between a history of abuse and chronic pain. If a history of abuse is obtained, the patient should also be screened for any current physical or sexual abuse.

Physical examination of patients with chronic pain is directed toward uncovering possible causative pathologies. The patient should be asked to indicate the location of the pain as a guide to further evaluation and to provide some indication of the character of the pain. If the pain is local-

| TABLE 30.2 | Nongynecologic Conditions That May Cause or Exacerbate Chronic Pelvic Pain, by Level of Evidence |

| Level of Evidence | Urologic | Gastrointestinal | Musculoskeletal | Other |
|---|---|---|---|---|
| Level A* | Bladder malignancy | Carcinoma of the colon | Abdominal wall myofascial pain (trigger points) | Abdominal cutaneous nerve entrapment in surgical scar |
| | Interstitial cystitis[†] | Constipation | Chronic coccygeal or back pain[†] | Depression[†] |
| | Radiation cystitis | Inflammatory bowel disease | Faulty or poor posture | Somatization disorder |
| | Urethral syndrome | Irritable bowel syndrome[†] | Fibromyalgia | |
| | | | Neuralgia of iliohypogastric, ilioinguinal, and/or genitofemoral nerves | |
| | | | Pelvic floor myalgia (levator ani or piriformis syndrome) | |
| | | | Peripartum pelvic pain syndrome | |
| Level B[‡] | Uninhibited bladder contractions (detrusor dyssynergia) | — | Herniated nucleus pulposus | Celiac disease |
| | Urethral diverticulum | | Low back pain[†] | Neurologic dysfunction |
| | | | Neoplasia of spinal cord or sacral nerve | Porphyria |
| | | | | Shingles |
| | | | | Sleep disturbances |
| Level C[§] | Chronic urinary tract infection | Colitis | Compression of lumbar vertebrae | Abdominal epilepsy |
| | Recurrent, acute cystitis | Chronic intermittent bowel obstruction | Degenerative joint disease | Abdominal migraine |
| | Recurrent, acute urethritis | Diverticular disease | Hernias: ventral, inguinal, femoral, spigelian | Bipolar personality disorders |
| | Stone/urolithiasis | | Muscular strains and sprains | Familial Mediterranean fever |
| | | | Rectus tendon strain | |
| | Urethral caruncle | | Spondylosis | |

*Level A: good and consistent scientific evidence of causal relationship to chronic pelvic pain.
[†]Diagnosis frequently reported in published series of women with chronic pelvic pain.
[‡]Level B: limited or inconsistent scientific evidence of causal relationship to chronic pelvic pain.
[§]Level C: causal relationship to chronic pelvic pain based on expert opinions.
Data from Howard FM. Chronic pelvic pain. *Obstet Gynecol.* 2003;101(3):594–611.
From American College of Obstetricians and Gynecologists. Chronic pelvic pain. ACOG Practice Bulletin No. 51. *Obstet Gynecol.* 2004;103(3):589–605.

is defined by the **Rome II criteria:** abdominopelvic pain for 12 weeks (not necessarily consecutive) in the preceding 12 months that cannot be explained by known disease, having at least two of the following features: (1) relieved with defecation, (2) onset associated with a change in the frequency of bowel movements (diarrhea or constipation), or (3) onset associated with a change in the form of stool (loose, watery, with mucus, or pellet-like). IBS is often usefully subcategorized for purposes of treatment depending on the predominant complaint: pain, diarrhea, constipation, or alternating constipation and diarrhea. The pathophysiology of the syndrome is not clearly identified, but factors proposed to be involved include altered bowel motility, visceral hypersensitivity, psychosocial factors (especially stress), an imbalance of neurotransmitters (especially serotonin), and infection (often indolent or subclinical). A history of childhood sexual or physical abuse is highly correlated with the severity of symptoms experienced by those with IBS.

### INTERSTITIAL CYSTITIS

**Interstitial cystitis** is a chronic inflammatory condition of the bladder that is often characterized by pelvic pain, urinary urgency and frequency, and dyspareunia. The proposed etiology is a disruption of the **glycosaminoglycan**

layer that normally coats the mucosa of the bladder. The interstitial cystitis symptom index predicts the diagnosis of interstitial cystitis and may be used to help determine whether cystoscopy is indicated. Further evaluation can be done with bladder distention with water or intravesical potassium sensitivity testing.

## THERAPY

*Patients with chronic pelvic pain offer a therapeutic challenge.* If possible, care should be directed at a specific cause. The use of analgesics should be on a fixed time schedule that is independent of symptoms.

Suppression of ovulation may be useful as either a therapeutic modality or as a diagnostic tool to assist in ruling out ovarian or cyclic processes. Gonadotropin-releasing hormone **(GnRH) agonists** cause a central down-regulation of the ovarian hormones and have been used in the treatment of endometriosis. These agents may also help relieve some of the symptoms of IBS, interstitial cystitis, and pelvic congestion syndrome (in which engorged pelvic blood vessels are purported to cause pelvic aching and pain).

Patients with symptoms characteristic of IBS or infection should be referred to a gastroenterologist for further evaluation. Use of a food diary to identify and eliminate foods that are associated with symptoms, combined with the nurturing physician–patient relationship to avoid "doctor shopping" and episodic care, are the mainstays of treatment. The limiting of caffeine, alcohol, fatty foods, and gas-producing vegetables is often helpful. Lactose or wheat gluten intolerance may be identified by the diary. If constipation is a major symptom, the consumption of 20 to 30 g of fiber or the use of osmotic laxatives such as lactulose is often useful. When diarrhea is a major symptom, antidiarrheals can be useful. Gas pain and cramping may be treated with antispasmodics such as dicyclomine and hyoscyamine.

Treatments for interstitial cystitis include dietary modification, intravesical agents, and oral agents aimed at decreasing inflammation and pain signals. As with IBS, caffeine, alcohol, artificial sweeteners, and acidic foods should be eliminated. **Dimethyl sulfoxide (DMSO)** is the only drug approved for direct bladder instillation to treat interstitial cystitis, although many physicians treat with a "cocktail" of anti-inflammatory and analgesic medications. Oral agents include antihistamines, tricyclic antidepressants, and **pentosan polysulfate,** a glycosaminoglycan analogue that may help reestablish the disrupted mucosa of the bladder.

Surgical therapies, such as **hysterectomy,** should be performed only after nongynecologic causes have been ruled out. Hysterectomy is very effective is relieving pain arising from the uterus and may also improve symptoms in women without identifiable uterine pathology. Alternate treatment modalities, such as transcutaneous electrical nerve stimulation (TENS), biofeedback, nerve blocks, laser ablation of the uterosacral ligaments, and presacral neurectomy may be used, as appropriate. Adding psychotherapy to medical treatment of chronic pelvic pain appears to improve response over that of medical treatment alone and should be considered. In some cases, the goal in treatment may not be a cure, that is, elimination of the chronic pain, but rather successful management of the symptoms to allow maximal function and quality of life.

## FOLLOW-UP

Patients being treated for pelvic pain (dysmenorrhea or chronic pain states) should be carefully monitored for success and the possibility of complications from the therapy. Patients on oral contraceptives for the first time should be asked to return for follow-up after 2 months and again after 6 months. Once successful therapy is established, routine periodic health maintenance visits should continue. Patients with chronic pelvic pain should be encouraged to return for follow-up on a periodic basis, rather than only when pain is present, thus avoiding reinforcing pain behavior as a means to an end.

## SUGGESTED READINGS

American College of Obstetricians and Gynecologists. Chronic pelvic pain. ACOG Practice Bulletin No. 51. *Obstet Gynecol.* 2004;103(3):589–605.

American College of Obstetricians and Gynecologists. Endometriosis in adolescents. ACOG Committee Opinion No. 310. *Obstet Gynecol.* 2005;105(4):921–927.

American College of Obstetricians and Gynecologists. *Guidelines for Women's Health Care: A Resource Manual.* 3rd ed. Washington, D.C.: ACOG; 2007.

American College of Obstetricians and Gynecologists. Medical management of endometriosis. ACOG Practice Bulletin No. 11. *Obstet Gynecol.* 1999;94(6):1–14.

# Disorders of the Breast

This chapter deals primarily with APGO Educational Topic:

Topic 40:   Disorders of the Breast

Students should understand the evaluation of common symptoms associated with the breast.

D iseases of the breast encompass a diverse spectrum of pathology, from benign breast disease to breast cancer. It is imperative that women's healthcare providers understand the evaluation, treatment, and surveillance of breast-related complaints. Providers must ensure appropriate breast cancer screening for all patients, whether at high or low risk. In order to properly evaluate, treat, and follow breast-related complaints, a multidisciplinary approach is often necessary. *Although referral to a specialist is sometimes necessary, the obstetrician-gynecologist is often the first person a woman consults for breast-related signs and symptoms.*

## ANATOMY

The adult female breast is actually a modified sebaceous gland, located within the superficial fascia of the chest wall (Fig. 31.1). Histologically, the breast is composed primarily of lobules or glands, milk ducts, connective tissue, and fat. The relative amounts of these tissue types vary considerably with age. In younger women, the breast consists predominantly of glandular tissue. With age, the glands involute and are replaced by fat, a process accelerated by menopause. Differences in palpable consistency and in radiographic density between the glands and fat are key components of breast cancer detection programs.

Architecturally, the breast is organized into 12 to 20 lobes, with a disproportionate amount of the glandular or lobular tissue in the upper outer quadrants of each breast. This disproportionate distribution of glandular tissue accounts for why breast cancer most commonly arises in the upper outer quadrant. The lobules consist of clusters of secretory cells arranged in an alveolar pattern and surrounded by myoepithelial cells. These glands drain into a series of collecting milk ducts that course through the breast, ultimately coalescing into approximately five to

ten collecting ducts that lead to and drain at the nipple. Typically, cancer begins at these terminal duct-lobular units of the breast and follows the path of those ducts.

Congenital anomalies of the breast can include absence of the breast as well as accessory breast tissue located anywhere along the "milk lines," which extend from the axilla to the groin in the fetus. Extra nipples (**polythelia**) are more common than true accessory breasts (**polymastia**).

The breast has a rich blood supply and lymphatic system, which support milk production and overall breast health. The blood supply comes from perforating branches of the internal mammary artery, the lateral thoracic artery, the thoracodorsal artery, the thoracoacromial artery, and various intercostal perforating arteries. The lymphatic vessels lead to several superficial and deep nodal chains throughout the trunk and neck, including those located in the axilla, deep to the pectoralis muscles, and caudal to the diaphragm (Fig. 31.2). The ipsilateral lymph node and occasionally the internal mammary nodes are the most common route of metastasis.

*Breast tissue is very sensitive to hormonal changes, especially the glandular cells.* The transition from the immature, pediatric breast to the mature, adult breast is orchestrated by the changes in circulating levels of estrogen and progesterone that accompany puberty. **Estrogen** is primarily responsible for the growth of adipose tissue and lactiferous ducts. Conversely, **progesterone** stimulation leads to lobular growth and alveolar budding.

## EVALUATION OF BREAST SIGNS AND SYMPTOMS

A timely evaluation of the patient who presents with a breast complaint is important if for no other reason than to relieve patient anxiety. A systematic approach to evaluating a breast-related complaint will efficiently yield the proper diagnosis.

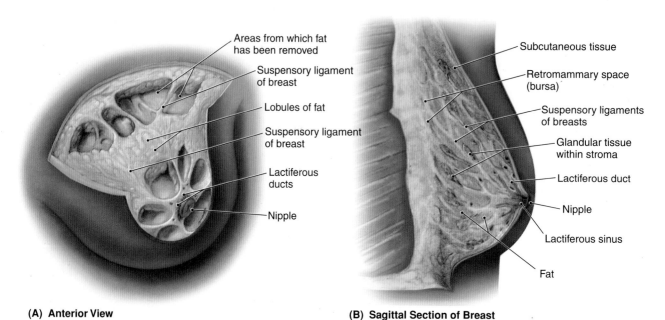

**(A) Anterior View**

- Areas from which fat has been removed
- Suspensory ligament of breast
- Lobules of fat
- Suspensory ligament of breast
- Lactiferous ducts
- Nipple

**(B) Sagittal Section of Breast**

- Subcutaneous tissue
- Retromammary space (bursa)
- Suspensory ligaments of breasts
- Glandular tissue within stroma
- Lactiferous duct
- Nipple
- Lactiferous sinus
- Fat

FIGURE 31.1. Anatomy of the breast. (From Agur A, Dalley AF. *Grant's Atlas of Anatomy*. 12th ed. Baltimore, MD: Lippincott Williams & Wilkins: 2008:5.)

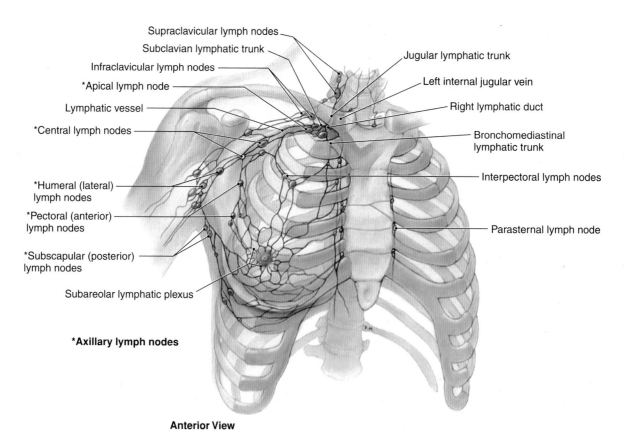

- Supraclavicular lymph nodes
- Subclavian lymphatic trunk
- Infraclavicular lymph nodes
- *Apical lymph node
- Lymphatic vessel
- *Central lymph nodes
- *Humeral (lateral) lymph nodes
- *Pectoral (anterior) lymph nodes
- *Subscapular (posterior) lymph nodes
- Subareolar lymphatic plexus

- Jugular lymphatic trunk
- Left internal jugular vein
- Right lymphatic duct
- Bronchomediastinal lymphatic trunk
- Interpectoral lymph nodes
- Parasternal lymph node

**\*Axillary lymph nodes**

**Anterior View**

FIGURE 31.2. Lymphatic drainage of the breast. (From Agur A, Dalley AF. *Grant's Atlas of Anatomy*. 12th ed. Baltimore, MD: Lippincott Williams & Wilkins; 2008:9.)

*The two most common presenting complaints related to the breast are pain and concern about a mass.* Gynecologists should be aware of the different etiologies of breast pain and be able to offer reassurance, follow-up, and potential treatment. One study has found that breast cancer was diagnosed in 6% of patients with breast complaints (most commonly a mass). Therefore, it is important that breast signs and symptoms be properly evaluated.

## Patient History

The patient interview is considered the single most important step in the initial evaluation of any disease process. In the case of complaints related to the breast, questions that will aid in deciding the next step include the location of complaints, duration of symptoms, how it was first discovered, presence or absence of nipple discharge, any changes in size, and association with menstrual cycle. *In addition, the clinician should ask about the presence of risk factors that would increase the likelihood of malignancy* (Box 31.1).

## Physical Examination

A complete breast exam should evaluate both breasts in a systematic fashion, both axillae, and the entire chest wall.

*The best time to perform a breast exam is in the follicular phase of the menstrual cycle.*

If the initial exam fails to yield a dominant mass, the options (based on the patient's risk factors) include either performing a repeat exam in 3 months or referral to a specialized breast care clinic.

## Diagnostic Testing

After performing a complete history and physical examination, a number of modalities can be used to help locate and characterize a breast mass.

### MAMMOGRAPHY

**Mammography** is an x-ray technique used to study the breast.

*Mammography is able to detect lesions approximately 2 years before they become palpable (Fig. 31.3).*

Mammography can be done either as a screening or a diagnostic test. During a screening mammogram, the patient stands or sits in front of the x-ray machine. Two smooth plastic plates are placed around the breast and subsequently compressed to allow for complete visualization of the tissue. *A standard four-image screening mammogram involves two craniocaudal and two mediolateral images.* The images are evaluated for defects suspicious of cancer, microcalcifications, distortion of the normal architecture, and any discrete nonpalpable lesion. *Lobular carcinoma is more difficult to detect with routine screening mammography.*

In collaboration with the National Cancer Institute and the FDA, the American College of Radiology has standardized the reporting of mammographic results through a system known as the Breast Imaging Reporting and Data System (BI-RADS®). This system helps clearly

---

**BOX 31.1**
**Risk factors for Breast Cancer**

- Age
- Personal history of breast cancer
- History of atypical hyperplasia (ductal or lobular) on past biopsies
- Inherited genetic mutations
- First-degree relatives with breast or ovarian cancer diagnosed at an early age
- Early menarche (age >12 years)
- Late cessation of menses (age >55 years)
- No term pregnancies
- Late age at first live birth (>30)
- Never breastfed
- Alcohol consumption
- Recent oral contraceptive use
- Use of hormone therapy
- Personal history of endometrial, ovarian, or colon cancer
- Jewish heritage

---

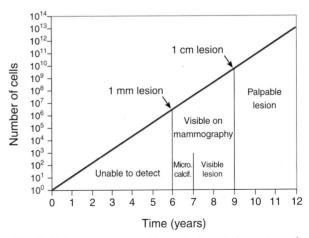

FIGURE 31.3. Mammographic and clinical detection of a breast mass. With a presumed doubling time of 100 days, breast cancer may be detected by mammography significantly earlier than it can be identified clinically. Micro calcif. = microcalcification.

| TABLE 31.1 | American College of Radiology Breast Imaging Reporting and Data System (BI-RADS) | |
|---|---|---|
| **BI-RADS Classification** | **Summary Recommendations** | **Explanation** |
| 0 | Need additional imaging evaluation | A mammogram with a lesion which needs additional imaging, such as spot compression films, magnifications, or additional views |
| 1 | Negative | Breast appears normal |
| 2 | Benign findings | Negative mammogram but interpreter wishes to describe a finding |
| 3 | Probably benign finding | A mammogram with a lesion highly likely to be benign. Follow-up is suggested to establish mammographic stability. |
| 4 | Suspicious abnormality | A concerning lesion with a definite probability of being malignant; recommend biopsy |
| 5 | Highly suggestive of malignancy | A lesion with a high probability of being cancer—appropriate referral to a breast surgeon is needed |
| 6 | Known biopsy proven malignancy | Appropriate action should be taken. |

communicate the final assessment and recommendations to referring physicians (Table 31.1).

*A diagnostic mammogram is done to supplement an abnormal screening mammogram.* In women older than 40 years of age, mammography is often used as the first-line study in evaluating a patient presenting with a breast mass, even if not palpable on clinical breast examination. Spot compressions and magnified views are used to further localize any lesions, along with providing dimensions of the surrounding tissue (Fig. 31.4). *The contralateral breast should also be imaged in cases of a clinically apparent mass. If possible, the lymph nodes are also imaged to search for unrecognized abnormalities.*

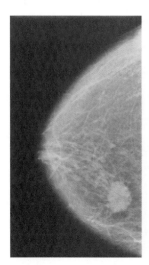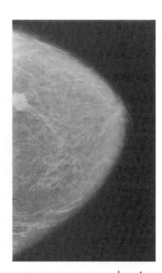

FIGURE 31.4. Bilateral film screen mammograms showing typical carcinoma in each breast, illustrating the importance of bilateral mammography in the workup of a clinically apparent mass. (Berek JS, Hacker NF. *Practical Gynecologic Oncology.* 4th ed. Philadelphia, PA: Lippincott Williams & Wilkins; 2005:630.)

### ULTRASONOGRAPHY

Ultrasonography has come to play an important role in the evaluation of breast lesions. It is useful in evaluating the breasts of young women and others with dense tissue, differentiating between a solid and cystic mass, and in guiding tissue core-needle biopsies. An anechoic defect found on ultrasound is consistent with a simple cyst and can be drained for symptomatic relief. *In women younger than 40 years of age, ultrasonography is the recommended initial modality to evaluate a breast mass.*

### MRI

Magnetic resonance imaging (MRI) can be a useful adjunct to diagnostic mammography. *The use of MRI for screening the general population is limited by the cost of the exam, lack of standard examination technique, and inability to detect microcalcifications.* However, MRI is being used for early detection of breast cancer in women at very high risk.

### FINE-NEEDLE ASPIRATION BIOPSY (FNAB)

**Fine-needle aspiration** is useful in determining if a palpable lump is a simple cyst. The procedure is performed in the office with the aid of local anesthesia. The suspected mass is stabilized between two fingers of one hand and aspirated using a 22-gauge to 24-gauge needle. Clear aspirated fluid does not need to undergo pathologic evaluation, and the patient may return for a clinical breast evaluation within 4 to 6 months if the mass disappears. If it reappears, the patient is managed with diagnostic mammography and ultrasonography. Bloody aspirated fluid should be evaluated pathologically, and the patient should undergo diagnostic mammography and ultrasonography.

In a **core-needle biopsy,** a large needle (14 to 16 gauge) is used to obtain samples from larger, solid breast masses. Three to six samples of tissue approximately 2 cm long are obtained and are evaluated for abnormal cells in relation to the surrounding breast tissue taken in the sample.

## Diagnosis Algorithm

If a breast mass is found through a clinical breast examination, self-examination, or historically by a patient, the clinician must clearly document the finding and assign appropriate follow-up care. Figure 31.5 presents a practical algorithm for the evaluation and follow-up of a patient with a breast mass.

## BENIGN BREAST DISEASE

**Benign breast disease** includes a large number of conditions that can significantly affect a woman's quality of life. With accurate diagnosis, many benign breast conditions can be effectively treated with medications or other measures. Women presenting with a breast mass should also be evaluated for their risk of breast cancer.

## Mastalgia

***Mastalgia,*** *or breast pain, can be divided into three categories: cyclic, noncyclic, and extramammary (nonbreast) pain.* **Cyclic mastalgia** begins with the luteal phase of the menstrual cycle and resolves after the onset of menses. The pain is generally bilateral and often involves the upper outer

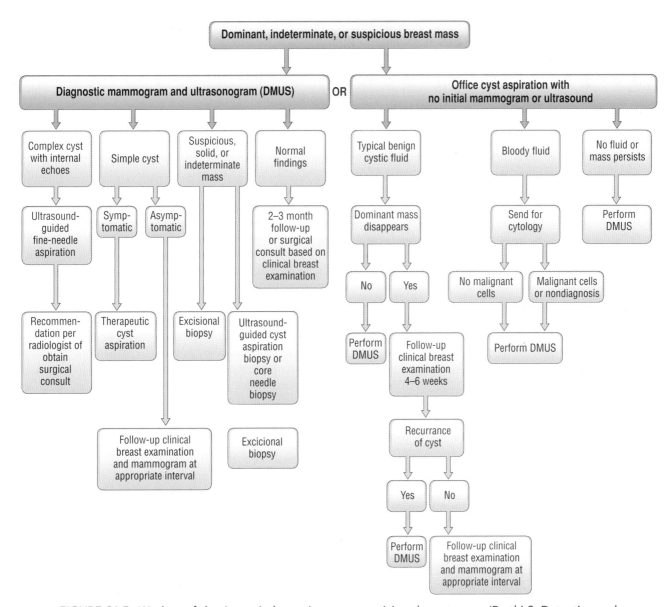

FIGURE 31.5. Workup of dominant, indeterminate, or suspicious breast mass. (Pruthi S. Detection and evaluation of a palpable breast mass. *Mayo Clin Proc.* 2001;76(6):641–647.)

quadrants of the breast. **Noncyclic mastalgia** is not associated with the menstrual cycle and includes such etiologies as tumors, mastitis, cysts, and a history of breast surgery. In some women, noncyclic mastalgia is idiopathic and no cause is found. Noncyclic pain has also been associated with some medications, including hormonal medications, antidepressants such as sertraline and amitriptyline, and antihypertensive drugs, in addition to others. If the onset of mastalgia is associated with the start of hormonal therapy, stopping or reducing the hormones may be beneficial. **Nonmammary pain** can be caused by a number of conditions, such as chest wall trauma, rib fractures, and fibromyalgia. Treatment for musculoskeletal disorders includes antiinflammatory drugs, but more serious causes of chest pain, such as angina, need to be ruled out.

*The only medication approved by the FDA for treating mastalgia is danazol, but it has significant side effects.* Other hormonal therapies that may decrease pain include bromocriptine and gonadotropin-releasing hormone agonists, but these drugs also have side effects that limit their widespread use. Lisuride maleate is a dopamine agonist that has shown pain-reducing effects, and it has fewer side effects than bromocriptine. *Selective estrogen receptor modulators, such as tamoxifen, also have a role in treating severe mastalgia.* These medications act as estrogen antagonists in the breast. Side effects of tamoxifen include an increased risk of endometrial hyperplasia and deep venous thrombosis, as well as hot flushes and vaginal bleeding. A recent study concluded that side effects are reduced when the medication is given in smaller doses.

> *Tamoxifen should be used only for cases of severe mastalgia that does not respond to other therapies.*

Some women with cyclic mastalgia have reported a decrease in pain with oral contraceptives or the injectable contraceptive medroxyprogesterone acetate.

Nonpharmacologic measures to help relieve breast pain include a properly fitting brassiere or a sports bra worn throughout the day or during exercise, weight reduction, and regular exercise. Although no studies have demonstrated the efficacy of these measures, they are worth recommending to patients and may help relieve pain.

## Nipple Discharge

Nipple discharge is usually benign, but may be an early sign of endocrine dysfunction or cancer. The color, consistency, and whether the discharge is bilateral or unilateral can yield important clues about its cause. A nonspontaneous, nonbloody, bilateral nipple discharge is usually attributed to fibrocystic changes of the breast or **ductal ectasia,** a condition characterized by dilation of the mammary ducts, periductal fibrosis, and inflammation. Ductal ectasia is seen in adolescent women as well as in perimenopausal women. Milky discharge is common during childbearing, but it can also be associated with other endocrinologic abnormalities (hyperprolactinemia or hypothyroidism) and medications (oral contraceptives and tricyclic antidepressants). Purulent discharge may indicate an infectious etiology and may be due to mastitis or a breast abscess. Green, yellow, or brown sticky discharge can be due to ductal ectasia or fibrocystic changes of the breast.

Bloody, unilateral nipple discharge may be caused by an invasive ductal carcinoma, intraductal papilloma, or an intraductal carcinoma. Patients with nipple discharge of this type usually require ductography and ductal excision. Breast ductography is an imaging technique that can reveal the location of an intraductal lesion. *A new technique that employs fiberoptic technology, fiberoptic ductoscopy (FDS), allows the direct visualization of the breast ducts, as well as sampling of ductal cells.* However, this modality is not widely available.

## Breast Masses

The most worrisome finding for patients and clinicians is an unexplained breast mass. Some characteristics of breast masses that suggest malignancy include size greater than 2 cm, immobility, poorly defined margins, firmness, skin dimpling or color changes, retraction or change in the nipple (e.g., scaling), bloody nipple discharge, and ipsilateral lymphadenopathy. The growth rate of a tumor in the breast is thought to be constant from the time of its origin. It is estimated that it takes an average of 5 years for a tumor to reach palpable size.

## Benign Breast Masses

A variety of benign breast masses are found on screening mammograms or incidentally. Table 31.2 summarizes the three morphologic categories and their associated risk of developing invasive breast cancer.

### NON-PROLIFERATIVE LESIONS

*Fibrocystic changes of the breast are a spectrum of features that can be observed in the normal breast.* Lobules of the breast may dilate and form cysts of varying sizes. The cyst walls are lined by flattened atrophic epithelium or may be modified through apocrine metaplasia. If these cysts rupture, the resulting scarring and inflammation may lead to fibrotic changes which make the breast feel firm. An increase in the number of glands with associated lobular growth is known as **adenosis.** In this case, the architecture of the lobule remains unchanged. In some lactating women, a palpable lactation adenoma may arise secondary to an exaggerated hormonal response.

**Simple fibroadenomas** are common tumors found in women in their late teens and early twenties. These masses are solid, round, rubbery, and mobile on examination.

| TABLE 31.2 Benign Breast Lesions | |
|---|---|
| **Pathologic Lesion** | **Relative Risk of Developing Invasive Breast CA** |
| <u>Non-proliferative</u> | 1.0 |
| Fibrocystic changes | |
| Cysts | |
| Fibrosis | |
| Adenosis | |
| Lactational adenomas | |
| Fibroadenomas | |
| <u>Proliferative without atypia</u> | 1.5–2.0 |
| Epithelial hyperplasia | |
| Sclerosing adenosis | |
| Complex sclerosing lesions (radial scar) | |
| Papillomas | |
| <u>Proliferative with atypia</u> | 8.0–10.0 |
| Lobular carcinoma in situ | |
| Ductal carcinoma in situ | |

Modified from Kumar V, Abbas AK, Nelson F, eds. *Robbins and Cotran Pathologic Basis of Disease.* 7th ed. Philadelphia, PA: Elsevier Saunders; 2005. CA = Cancer.

The tumors do have structural and glandular components in the mass. Although they do not have malignant potential, they can enlarge in pregnancy and cause discomfort.

## PROLIFERATIVE LESIONS WITHOUT ATYPIA

These lesions are commonly found on mammography and do not usually cause a palpable mass. Histologically, they represent proliferation of cells of the ductal or lobular epithelium. The cells themselves are normal, i.e., nonmalignant.

In a normal breast, only myoepithelial cells and a single layer of luminal cells rest on the basement. If there are more than 2 cell layers, the abnormality is known as **epithelial hyperplasia.** If there is increased fibrosis within the expanded lobule, with distortion and compression of the epithelium, the lesion is termed **sclerosing adenosis.** A **radial scar** (or complex sclerosing lesion) is a nidus of tubules entrapped in a densely hyalinized stroma surrounded by radiating arms of epithelium. The lesion mimics an invasive carcinoma. Finally, **papillomas** are intraductal growths composed of abundant stroma and lined by both luminal and myoepithelial cells. Solitary intraductal papillomas are found in the major lactiferous ducts of women, typically between the ages of 30 and 50, and cause a serous or serosanguineous drainage.

## PROLIFERATIVE LESIONS WITH ATYPIA

*When malignant cells replace the normal epithelium lining the ducts or lobules, the lesion is known as a carcinoma in situ.* The basement membrane remains intact and, therefore, the cells cannot metastasize.

There are two major types of carcinoma in situ: **lobular carcinoma in situ (LCIS)** and **ductal carcinoma in situ (DCIS).** LCIS is characterized by obliteration of the lumina of the glandular acini by a uniform population of small, atypical cells. In DCIS, the ducts are filled with atypical epithelial cells. Women with DCIS are at increased risk of developing invasive cancer or a recurrence of the DCIS lesion. For these reasons, DCIS should be evaluated with core-needle biopsy followed by surgical biopsy or excision. Management of LCIS and its related condition, atypical lobular hyperplasia, consists of excisional biopsy. *Following treatment of both LCIS and DCIS, preventive therapy with selective estrogen receptor modulators such as tamoxifen has been shown to reduce the risk of invasive breast cancer in these patients.*

# BREAST CANCER

*Breast cancer is the second most common malignancy in women, ranking only behind skin cancer.* In addition, it is the second leading cause of cancer-related death in women. According to the National Cancer Institute, there were 178,500 new cases and approximately 40,500 deaths related to breast cancer in 2007. The steady increase in the incidence of breast cancer can be attributed to the increased use of mammography screening, which has enabled the detection of smaller invasive lesions and the earlier diagnosis of in-situ lesions. Advances in treatment have also helped maintain the downward trend in overall breast cancer mortality.

Nevertheless, breast cancer is a serious health concern in the United States. It is estimated that the United States spends approximately $8.1 billion annually on treating breast cancer. The lifetime risk of developing breast cancer in the United States is approximately 12.5% (1 in 8), while the lifetime risk of dying from breast cancer is 3.6% (1 in 28).

## Risks Factors

Numerous studies have documented factors that increase the relative risk for breast cancer (see Box 31.1).

### AGE AND RACE

*Age is the single largest risk factor for developing breast cancer.* A majority of breast cancer cases occur in women over the age of 50. Stratified studies relate risk with age (by decades), and show that the risk for developing breast cancer increases as a woman gets older. For example, a woman has a 1.4% chance of being diagnosed with breast cancer between the ages of 40 and 49, compared to 3.7% between the ages of 60 and 69. When stratified by race, white women are more likely to be diagnosed with breast cancer compared to age-matched women of Latin, Asian, or African American descent.

### FAMILY HISTORY AND GENETICS

Women who have first-degree relatives (parent, sibling, or offspring) with breast cancer have a higher risk than the general population.

> *If a woman before the age of 40 is diagnosed with breast cancer, evaluating for genetic mutations that predispose individuals to cancer is reasonable.*

The two most commonly discussed genetic mutations linked to breast cancer are the BRCA1 and BRCA2 gene mutations.

**BRCA1** is a gene located on the 17q21 chromosome. This mutation is associated with nearly half of the early-onset breast cancers and approximately 90% of hereditary ovarian cancers. **BRCA2** is a gene located on the 13q12–13 chromosome. This mutation has a lower incidence of early-onset breast cancers (35%) and much lower risk of ovarian cancer, compared to BRCA1.

### REPRODUCTIVE AND MENSTRUAL HISTORY

In general, women who have an early age of menstrual onset (before the age of 12) and transition through menopause after age 55 are at increased risk of breast cancer. Delayed childbearing and nulliparity also increase the chance of breast cancer.

### RADIATION EXPOSURE

Breast tissue of young women (along with the bone marrow and infant thyroid) is highly susceptible to the cancer-causing effects of ionizing radiation. Women who have received a sufficiently large dose of radiation (radiation therapy to treat Hodgkin disease or an enlarged thymus gland) are at risk for radiation-induced breast cancer. The relationship between dose of radiation and risk of cancer is directly linear, although the threshold is unclear. Thus far, epidemiologic studies have not detected a significant increase in cancer risk below a cumulative dose of about 20 cGy. To put this dose into perspective, a typical mammogram results in a breast tissue dose of about 0.3 cGy. The time needed for a radiation-induced lesion to develop is about 5 to 10 years from exposure.

### BREAST CHANGES

It is believed that women with dense breast tissue are at increased risk for breast cancer. In addition, histologic biopsies finding atypical hyperplasia or lobular carcinoma in situ greatly increase the risk for breast cancer.

### OTHER FACTORS

*Being overweight after menopause has been linked to an increased risk for breast cancer.* A possible mechanism in this relationship is that the increased peripheral conversion of androstenedione to estrone stimulates breast cancer development. Lack of exercise throughout life is linked to the increased risk of breast cancer through the associated risk of obesity.

*Women who consume 2 to 4 alcoholic drinks per week have a 30% greater risk of dying from breast cancer than women who never drink.* The exact mechanism of action is unclear, but researchers speculate that alcohol consumption stimulates the growth and progression of breast cancer by inducing angiogenesis and increasing the expression of vascular endothelial growth factor (VEGF).

## Breast Cancer Risk Assessment Tool: The Gail Model

The National Cancer Institute (NCI) has developed a computer-based tool to allow clinicians to estimate a woman's risk of developing invasive breast cancer over the next 5 years and in their lifetime (up to age 90). *The tool is based on a mathematical model of breast cancer risk calculation called the Gail Model.* Seven risk factors are used in the calculations: a history of LCIS or DCIS, age, age at onset of menstruation, age at time of the first live birth, number of first-degree relatives with breast cancer, history of breast biopsy, and race/ethnicity. The usefulness of the Gail model is limited in patients with second-degree relatives with breast cancer (eg, paternal transmission) and is falsely increased in patients with multiple breast biopsies.

Women at high risk, defined as a 5-year risk of 1.7% or more, can be referred for possible prophylactic therapy. *Current prophylactic options include chemoprevention with the selective estrogen receptor modulators tamoxifen and raloxifene, and prophylactic mastectomy.* Since all of the options are associated with significant side effects, individualized risk assessment should be performed to determine whether a patient is a candidate for breast cancer risk reduction and, if so, which option is best.

## Histologic Types of Breast Cancer

Malignant tumors of the breast may arise from any of the major components of the breast. *The American Joint Committee on Cancer classifies most breast malignancies into one of three histologic categories according to their corresponding cells of origin: ductal, lobular, and nipple.* Seventy to eighty percent of breast cancers are invasive ductal carcinomas. These are most common among women in their 50s and have a tendency to spread to regional lymph nodes. Invasive lobular carcinomas comprise 5% to 50% of breast cancers. This type is often multifocal and bilateral. Table 31.3 summarizes the differences between the two processes. Paget disease of the nipple presents as a superficial skin lesion similar to eczema.

## Breast Cancer Staging

The American Joint Committee on Cancer stages breast malignancies according to the TNM system that describes characteristics of the primary *t*umor, involvement of regional lymph *n*odes, and distant *m*etastasis. Surgical stage helps determine the appropriate types of therapy (Tables 31.4 and 31.5).

| TABLE 31.3 | Major Differences between DCIS and LCIS | |
|---|---|---|
| | **DCIS** | **LCIS** |
| Structure Involved | Ducts | Lobules |
| Type of subsequent cancer | Ductal | Ductal or lobular |
| Breast at risk for invasive cancer | Ipsilateral breast | Either breast |
| Laterality | Unilateral | Often bilateral |
| Number of sites of origin | Unicentric | Multicentric |

In addition to stage, receptor status is another important indicator of breast cancer prognosis. *Expression of estrogen or progesterone receptors positively affects prognosis.* The **Her2/neu (or c-erb-B2)** is an oncogene encoding a membrane-bound growth-factor receptor. Overexpression confers a poor prognosis and is noted in 20% to 30% of invasive ductal cancers.

## Breast Cancer Treatment

Breast cancer poses both a local regional risk (i.e., to the breast and regional lymph nodes) and a systemic risk. *The surgical treatment is **lumpectomy (breast conservation therapy)** or **mastectomy.*** Both procedures are aimed at achieving local control. Mastectomy is removal of all breast tissue and the nipple areolar complex with preservation of the pectoralis muscles. A modified radical mastectomy also includes removal of the axillary lymph nodes. Radiation therapy is used in conjunction with mastectomy for later stages of breast cancer, and to accompany lumpectomy and partial mastectomy for early stages of breast cancer. Radiation is an essential component of lumpectomy. This combination yields outcomes that are equal to those of radical mastectomy.

*Breast reconstruction should be an option for all women who desire it.* Reconstruction can be achieved by several methods, including the insertion of a saline implant under the pectoral muscle or by using a rectus muscle to replace the lost tissue. To prepare for a saline implant, a tissue expander is placed beneath the muscle. Saline is injected into the expander over a period of weeks to months until the space is large enough to accommodate the implant. Breast reconstruction can take place immediately after surgery, or it can be delayed for several months. Radiation therapy can be given if breast reconstruction has taken place.

**Adjuvant (systemic) therapy** is used in the treatment of all stages of breast cancer, regardless of lymph node status. *Adjuvant therapy includes chemotherapeutic drugs that kill cancer cells and hormonal therapies such as tamoxifen that act as*

## TABLE 31.4    Breast Cancer Staging

**Primary Tumor (T)**
- TX Primary tumor cannot be assessed
- T0 No evidence of primary tumor
- Tis Carcinoma in situ; intraductal carcinoma, lobular carcinoma in situ,
  - or Paget disease of the nipple with no tumor
- T1 Tumor 2 cm or less in greatest dimension
  - T1a 0.5 cm or less in greatest dimension
  - T1b More than 0.5 cm but not more than 1 cm in greatest dimension
  - T1c More than 1 cm but not more than 2 cm in greatest dimension
- T2 Tumor more than 2 cm but not more than 5 cm in greatest dimension
- T3 Tumor more than 5 cm in greatest dimension
- T4 Tumor of any size with direct extension to chest wall or skin
  - T4a Extension to chest wall
  - T4b edema (including peau d'orange) or ulceration of the skin of the breast or satellite skin nodules confined to the same breast
  - T4c Both (T4a and T4b)
  - T4d Inflammatory carcinoma (see the definition of inflammatory carcinoma in the introduction)

*Note: Paget disease associated with a tumor is classified according to the size of the tumor.*

**Regional Lymph Nodes (N)**
- NX Regional lymph nodes cannot be assessed (e.g., previously removed)
- N0 No regional lymph node metastasis
- N1 Metastasis to movable ipsilateral axillary lymph node(s)
- N2 Metastasis to ipsilateral axillary lymph node(s) fixed to one another or to other structures
- N3 Metastasis to ipsilateral internal mammary lymph node(s).

**Pathologic classification (pN)**
- pNX Regional lymph nodes cannot be assessed (e.g., previously removed, or not removed for pathologic study)
- pN0 No regional lymph node metastasis
- pN1 Metastasis to movable ipsilateral axillary lymph node(s)
- pN1a Only micrometastasis (none larger than 0.2 cm)
- pN1b Metastasis to lymph node(s), any larger than 0.2 cm
- pN1bi Metastasis in one to three lymph nodes, any more than 0.2 cm and all less than 2 cm in greatest dimension
- pN1bii Metastasis to four or more lymph nodes, any more than 0.2 cm and all less than 2 cm in greatest dimension
- pN1biii Extension of tumor beyond the capsule of a lymph node metastasis less than 2 cm in greatest dimension
- pN1biv Metastasis to a lymph node 2 cm or more in greatest dimension
- pN2 Metastasis to ipsilateral axillary lymph nodes that are fixed to one another or to other structures
- pN3 Metastasis to ipsilateral internal mammary lymph node(s)

**Distant metastasis (M)**
- MX Presence of distant metastasis cannot be assessed
- M0 No distant metastasis
- M1 Distant metastasis (includes metastasis to ipsilateral supraclavicular lymph node[s])

**AJCC Stage Groupings**
**Stage 0**
- Tis, N0, M0

**Stage I**
- T1*, N0, M0

**Stage IIA**
- T0, N1, M0
- T1*, N1, M0
- T2, N0, M0

**Stage IIB**
- T2, N1, M0
- T3, N0, M0

**Stage IIIA**
- T0, N2, M0
- T1*, N2, M0
- T2, N2, M0
- T3, N1, M0
- T3, N2, M0

**Stage IIIB**
- T4, N0, M0
- T4, N1, M0
- T4, N2, M0

**Stage IIIC****
- Any T, N3, M0

**Stage IV**
- Any T, Any N, M1

*T1 includes T1mic.
**Stage IIIC breast cancer includes patients with any T stage who have pN3 disease. Patients with pN3c disease are considered inoperable.
American Joint Committee on Cancer. *AJCC Cancer Staging Manual*. 6th ed. New York, NY: Springer: 2002:171–180.

| TABLE 31.5 | Treatment of Breast Cancer by Stage | |
|---|---|---|
| **Stage** | **Surgery** | **Adjuvant Treatment** |
| 0 | Total mastectomy or breast conservation therapy (includes lumpectomy and breast irradiation) | |
| I | Total mastectomy or breast conservation therapy (includes lumpectomy and breast irradiation) ± sentinel node biopsy/axillary lymph-node dissection | Chemotherapy >1 cm ± Tamoxifen |
| II | Modified radical mastectomy or breast conservation therapy (includes lumpectomy and breast irradiation)/ axillary lymph node dissection | Chemotherapy >1 cm<br><br>± Tamoxifen<br><br>Radiation therapy of the supraclavicular nodes ± chest wall, if mastectomy performed if ≥ 4 positive nodes |
| III | Modified radical mastectomy or breast conservation therapy (includes lumpectomy and breast irradiation)/ axillary lymph node dissection | Chemotherapy ± neoadjuvant chemotherapy<br><br>± Tamoxifen<br><br>Radiation therapy of the supraclavicular nodes ± chest wall, if mastectomy performed<br><br>Radiation therapy of the breast (inflammatory breast cancer) |
| IV | Surgery for local control | ± Chemotherapy<br><br>± Hormonal agents |

Modified from Gemigani ML. Breast cancer. In: Barakat RR, Bevers MW, Gershenson DM, Hoskins WJ, eds. *The Memorial Sloan-Kettering & MD Anderson Cancer Center Handbook of Gynecologic Oncology.* 2nd ed. London: Martin Dunitz Publishers; 2002:297–319.

*estrogen antagonists.* Tamoxifen is used to treat women with estrogen receptor-positive breast cancer. It can be used in conjunction with chemotherapy. It is also given as a 5-year course of preventive treatment following surgery. **Aromatase inhibitors** (AIs) prevent the production of estrogen in postmenopausal women.

> *AIs are used to extend survival in women with metastatic cancer, as primary adjuvant therapy, and in conjunction with tamoxifen to prevent cancer recurrence.*

Another drug used to treat breast cancer is trastuzumab. It acts on membrane-bound protein produced by Her2/neu. *If a patient's cancer is found to overexpress the Her2/neu protein, trastuzumab can be given as adjuvant therapy.* Trastuzumab is associated with significant side effects, including heart failure, respiratory problems, and life-threatening allergic reactions.

Obstetrician-gynecologists are in the unique position of providing care for women who have been treated for breast cancer. For some women, the continuation of care spans many years. Once the initial treatment has been completed, the obstetrician-gynecologist often takes on the role of screening and surveillance. For the first two years, follow-up appointments occur every 3 to 6 months and then annually after that. Annual mammography and physical exams should continue indefinitely. Most breast cancer recurrence will occur within 5 years of primary therapy.

## SCREENING GUIDELINES

For the general population, breast cancer surveillance involves a combination of clinical breast examinations and radiographic imaging. In 2002, the U.S. Preventative Service Task Force (USPSTF) found insufficient evidence for or against breast self-examinations (BSE). The American College of Obstetricians and Gynecologists (2003) continues to support the practice of BSE, because of the potential ability to detect a palpable breast cancer. The value of clinical breast examination in detecting breast cancer has also been studied. Pooled data from multiple studies supports the use and effectiveness of clinical breast examination. Multiple reviews have supported the combination of clinical breast examination and mammography for breast cancer screening for women aged 50 to 69 years. ACOG supports the recommendations of the American Cancer Society, which calls for clinical breast examinations every 3 years for women aged 20 to 39, and annually thereafter.

*The value of mammography increases with age.* The USPSTF found sufficient evidence to demonstrate that mammogram screening every 1 to 3 years significantly reduced mortality from breast cancer. Controversy exists over screening intervals in younger women, where the incidence of breast cancer remains low. ACOG and the USPSTF currently recommend that mammography be performed every 1 to 2 years between ages 40 and 49, and annually thereafter.

These screening standards do not apply to women with inherited genetic mutations placing them at increased risk for developing breast cancer. *In this population, breast cancer occurs at a younger age and is missed by screening mammography nearly 50% of the time.* Current recommendations for BRCA carriers includes monthly breast self-examinations beginning at ages 18 to 20, annual clinical breast exams, and screening mammograms beginning after age 25 (or 5–10 years before the age of diagnosis in the affected relative). MRI is recommended as a supplement to mammography, not a replacement.

## SUGGESTED READINGS

American College of Obstetricians and Gynecologists. Breast concerns in the adolescent. ACOG Committee Opinion No. 350. *Obstet Gynecol.* 2006;108(5):1329–1336.

American College of Obstetricians and Gynecologists. *Detecting and Treating Breast Problems.* ACOG Patient Education Pamphlet AP026. Washington, DC: American College of Obstetricians and Gynecologists; 2004. http://www.acog.org/publications/patient_education/bp026.cfm. Accessed October 21, 2008.

American College of Obstetricians and Gynecologists. *Fibrocystic Breast Changes.* ACOG Patient Education Pamphlet AP138. Washington, DC: American College of Obstetricians and Gynecologists; 2000. http://www.acog.org/publications/patient_education/bp138.cfm. Accessed October 21, 2008.

American College of Obstetricians and Gynecologists. Role of the obstetrician-gynecologist in the screening and diagnosis of breast masses. ACOG Committee Opinion No. 334. *Obstet Gynecol.* 2006; 107(5):1213–1214.

Witkop CT. Benign breast disease. In: American College of Obstetricians and Gynecologists. *Precis, An Update in Obstetrics and Gynecology: Gynecology.* 3rd ed. American College of Obstetricians and Gynecologists; 2006:159–166.

# 32 Gynecologic Procedures

Evaluation and management of gynecologic problems frequently require performing diagnostic and therapeutic surgical procedures. Understanding the risks and benefits of such procedures is important in counseling patients about their treatment options and the reasons for having the procedures performed.

## IMAGING STUDIES

Gynecologic imaging plays an important role in the diagnostic evaluation of women for a variety of reproductive health conditions. Although the ability to image various parts and organs of the body has dramatically enhanced clinicians' diagnostic capabilities, these methods do not replace a careful and thoughtful history and physical evaluation. However, they can add more detail, which assists in both medical and surgical management. The effective use of these modalities requires that the physician be familiar with the benefits and limitations of each method.

### Ultrasonography

**Ultrasonography** remains the most common modality for evaluation of the female pelvis. It uses high-frequency sound reflections to identify different body tissues and structures. Short bursts of low-energy sound waves are sent into the body. When these waves encounter the interface between two tissues that transmit sound differently, some of the sound energy is reflected back toward the sound source. The returning sound waves are detected, and the distance from the sensor is deduced using the elapsed time from transmission to reception. An image is then created and displayed on a monitor. *Ultrasonography is safe for pregnant and nonpregnant patients.*

Most ultrasonography produces two-dimensional images. Three-dimensional studies can be used for volume calculation and to provide detail about the surfaces of particular structures. In gynecology, three-dimensional ultrasonography is especially useful in the evaluation of müllerian abnormalities (see Chapter 4, Embryology and Anatomy.) Four-dimensional ultrasonography, which shows movement, is also available.

Two kinds of probes are used in ultrasonography: transabdominal and transvaginal (Fig. 32.1). A transabdominal probe has an increased depth of penetration, which allows for the assessment of large uterine or adnexal masses. However, in obese patients, it may not allow proper imaging of pelvic structures. A transvaginal probe can be placed internally; thus, it often gives improved views of the cervix, uterus, ovaries, and tubes. Also, it has a higher frequency and shorter depth of penetration, which result in enhanced image clarity.

*One of the most valuable uses for ultrasonography in gynecology is for imaging masses.* The imaging technique helps distinguish between cystic and solid adnexal masses. Although magnetic resonance imaging (MRI) or computed tomography (CT) can also be used for evaluation of ovarian cysts, ultrasonography is far less costly; for this purpose, experts consider it superior to either MRI or CT. It is also possible to delineate leiomyoma (fibroid) size and number using ultrasonography.

Use of the endometrial stripe thickness for evaluation of postmenopausal bleeding has been studied extensively. Following menopause, the endometrium becomes atrophic and its thickness decreases, remaining relatively constant without hormonal stimulation. Ultrasonographic evaluation of the endometrial stripe involves measuring the thickest portion of the endometrial echo in the sagittal plane. An endometrial stripe thickness of 5 mm or greater should be interpreted as abnormal in postmenopausal women not taking hormone therapy. These patients should receive histologic assessment of an endometrial tissue sample to exclude endometrial carcinoma.

Saline infusion during ultrasonography **(sonohysterography, or SHG)** can aid in the visualization of the endometrial cavity and can often identify intrauterine polyps or submucosal leiomyomas (Fig. 32.2). In this technique, saline is infused via a transcervically inserted catheter. The saline acts as a contrast agent to delineate the endometrium and intracavity masses. The primary role of SHG is in the diagnosis of the cause of abnormal uterine bleeding (AUB). It is preferred over unenhanced ultrasonography in the

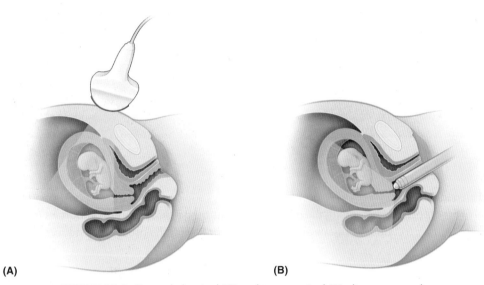

**(A)**    **(B)**

FIGURE 32.1. Transabdominal (A) and transvaginal (B) ultrasonography.

evaluation of AUB because of its increased diagnostic accuracy and greater cost-effectiveness.

## Computed Axial Tomography

**Computed axial tomography (CT or CAT)** scanning uses computer algorithms to construct cross-sectional images based on x-ray information. With the use of oral or intravenous contrast agents, CT scanning can help evaluate pelvic masses, identify lymphadenopathy, or plan radiation therapy.

CT involves slightly greater radiation exposure than a conventional single-exposure radiograph, but provides significantly more information. The radiation dose of an abdominal CT is still below that thought to cause fetal harm. Nevertheless, because of CT's increased risk of fetal effects, magnetic resonance imaging (see below) or ultrasonography should be used for imaging instead of CT, whenever possible in pregnancy.

## Magnetic Resonance Imaging

**Magnetic resonance imaging (MRI)** is based on the magnetic characteristics of various atoms and molecules in the body. Because of the variations in chemical composition of body tissues (especially the content of hydrogen, sodium, fluoride, or phosphorus), MRI can distinguish between types of tissues, such as blood and fat. This distinction is useful in visualizing lymph nodes, which are usually surrounded by fat; in characterizing adnexal masses; and in locating hemorrhage within organs. MRI is also useful for visualizing the endometrium, myometrium, and cystic structures in the ovaries. Emerging areas of clinical applicability include assessment of lesions in the breast and staging of cervical cancer.

## Breast Imaging

**Mammography** is an x-ray procedure used to screen for breast cancer. It is performed by passing a small amount of radiation through compressed breast tissue (Fig. 32.3). Because mammography has a high false-positive rate (10% per screening in postmenopausal women and as high as 20% per screening in obese or premenopausal women), additional testing may be required. Digital mammography allows better visualization of dense breast tissue than conventional mammography.

Ultrasonography is also used to evaluate cystic or solid breast masses and guide aspiration of cysts. MRI may also be used as an imaging technique for breast tissue.

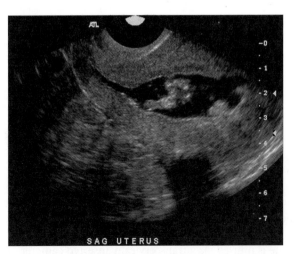

FIGURE 32.2. Sonohysterogram showing several polyps. (From Breitkopf DM. Gynecologic imaging. In: *Precis: Gynecology.* 3rd ed. Washington, DC: American College of Obstetricians and Gynecologists; 2006:17.)

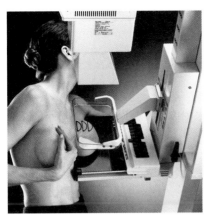

FIGURE 32.3.  Mammogram. (From *Stedman's Medical Dictionary.* 27th ed. Baltimore, MD: Lippincott Williams & Wilkins; 2000.)

## Hysterosalpingography

**Hysterosalpingography (HSG)** is most often used to evaluate the patency of the fallopian tubes in women who may be infertile. After a radio-opaque dye is injected transcervically, fluoroscopy (live x-ray) is used to determine whether dye spills into the peritoneal cavity (Fig. 32.4). HSG can also be used to define the size and shape of the uterine cavity and to detect developmental abnormalities, such as a unicornuate, septate, or didelphic uterus (see Chapter 4, Embryology and Anatomy). It also can demonstrate most endometrial polyps, submucous myomata, or intrauterine adhesions that are significant enough to have important reproductive consequences.

## PROCEDURES

Gynecologic procedures include diagnostic procedures such as biopsy and colposcopy, as well as procedures used as treatment modalities. Some procedures, such as laparoscopy and hysteroscopy, can be performed for both diagnosis and treatment and are chosen specifically for this reason.

## Genital Tract Biopsy

Biopsies of the vulva, vagina, cervix, and endometrium are frequently necessary in gynecology. These procedures are usually comfortably performed in the office; they require either no anesthesia or local anesthesia.

Vulvar biopsies are performed to evaluate visible lesions, persistent pruritus, burning, or pain. A circular, hollow metal instrument 3–5 mm in diameter, called a punch, is used to remove a small disk of tissue for evaluation (Fig. 32.5). For hemostasis, local pressure or anticoagulants (styptics) such as Monsel solution (ferric subsulfate) or silver nitrate sticks are often used. Sutures are rarely necessary. Local anesthesia is required for this type of biopsy.

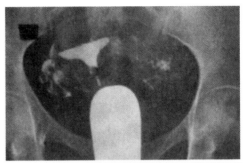
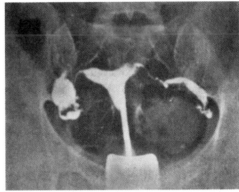
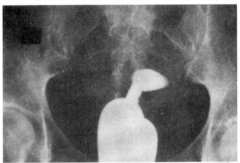

FIGURE 32.4.  Hysterosalpingography.

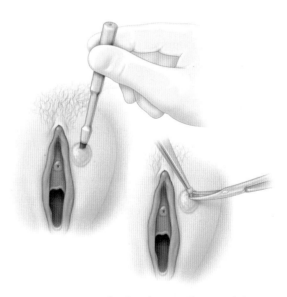

FIGURE 32.5.  Biopsy of vulvar lesion. The punch is rotated in place to incise tissue.

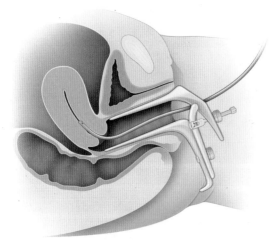

FIGURE 32.6. Endometrial biopsy. (Figure adapted from the American College of Obstetricians and Gynecologists, © 2008.)

Vaginal biopsy is performed to assess suspicious masses and to evaluate the vagina in the presence of cervical abnormalities. Women who have had a prior hysterectomy for cervical cancer should continue to have Pap tests performed on the vaginal cuff; if a result is abnormal, a vaginal biopsy may be required. Vaginal biopsy is performed with pinch biopsy forceps. Local anesthesia is rarely required.

**Cervical biopsy** is performed with biopsy forceps and, perhaps, a colposcope (see below). No anesthesia is necessary. Indications for cervical biopsy include chronic cervicitis, suspected neoplasm, or ulcer.

**Endometrial biopsy (EMB)** is generally used to evaluate abnormal uterine bleeding, such as menorrhagia, metrorrhagia, or menometrorrhagia. EMB is accomplished with a small-diameter catheter with a mild suction mechanism (Fig. 32.6). Various types are available. Anesthesia is not necessary, but many patients are more tolerant of EMB when given ibuprofen (400–800 mg) 1 hour prior to the procedure.

## Colposcopy

**Colposcopy** is performed to evaluate abnormal Pap results. It facilitates detailed evaluation of the surface of the cervix, vagina, and vulva when premalignancy or malignancy is suspected based on history, physical examination, or cytology. Cervical biopsy of suspicious lesions is frequently performed during colposcopy. Chapter 43, Cervical Neoplasia and Carcinoma, provides more detail about colposcopy.

## Cryotherapy

**Cryotherapy** is a technique that destroys tissue by freezing. A hollow metal probe (cryoprobe) is placed on the tis-

sue to be treated. The probe is then filled with a refrigerant gas (nitrous oxide or carbon dioxide) that causes it to cool to an extremely low temperature (between −65 and −85 degrees C), freezing the tissue with which the cryoprobe is in contact. Cryotherapy is most often used to treat cervical intraepithelial neoplasia and other benign lesions such as condyloma. The formation of ice crystals within the cells of the treated tissue leads to tissue destruction and subsequent sloughing. Patients who have had cryotherapy of the cervix can expect to have a watery discharge for several weeks as the tissues slough and healing occurs. Although cryotherapy is inexpensive, well-tolerated, and generally effective, it is less precise than other methods of tissue destruction, such as laser ablation or electrosurgery.

## Laser Vaporization

Highly energetic coherent light beams (light amplification by stimulated emission of radiation [LASER]) may be directed onto tissues, facilitating tissue destruction or incision, depending on the specific wavelength of light used and the power density of the beam. Infrared ($CO_2$) is the most common type of laser used in gynecologic procedures. Yttrium-aluminum-garnet (YAG), argon, or potassium-titanyl-phosphate (KTP) lasers, all of which have different effects on tissues, are also used. Some can be used in the presence of saline or water. The type of laser is selected according to the indication or desired effect of the surgery. Although expensive, the great precision that laser offers makes it a useful tool in specific clinical settings.

Laser therapy is used to treat vaginal and vulvar lesions, such as condyloma, vaginal intraepithelial neoplasia (VAIN), and vulvar intraepithelial neoplasia (VIN). Laser is also used to treat other dermatologic vulvar disorders, including molluscum contagiosum and lichen sclerosis atrophia. Prior to the development of LEEP (see below), laser ablation and conization were common treatment modalities for cervical epithelial neoplasia ablation and cervical conization.

## Dilation and Curettage

*Dilation and curettage (D&C) is a procedure in which the cervix is dilated using a series of graduated dilators, followed by curettage (scraping) of the endometrium, for both diagnostic (histologic) and therapeutic reasons.* D&C usually is performed under anesthesia in the operating room. Some common indications for D&C include abnormal uterine bleeding, incomplete or missed abortion, inability to perform EMB in the office, postmenopausal bleeding, and suspected endometrial polyp(s). With the availability of newer imaging procedures, D&C is now less commonly performed.

## Hysteroscopy

Hysteroscopy is the visualization of the endometrial cavity using a narrow telescope-like device (Fig. 32.7) attached to a light source, camera, and distension medium (often normal saline). It is used to view lesions such as polyps, intrauterine adhesions (synechiae), septa, and submucous myomas. Special instruments allow directed resection of such abnormalities. Hysteroscopy is commonly performed in the outpatient setting under general anesthesia; however, it can also be performed in the office as a diagnostic procedure or in conjunction with either endometrial ablation or sonohysterography.

A procedure for nonreversible sterilization has been designed to be used in conjunction with the hysteroscope. In this procedure, metal coils are inserted into the ostium of each fallopian tube under direct visualization. Scarring of the tubal ostia then occurs. To confirm that the tubes are occluded, an HSG must be performed three months later.

## Endometrial Ablation

**Endometrial ablation** is used to burn away the uterine lining. The procedure is used to treat abnormal uterine bleeding in women who do not wish to become pregnant. It is not a method of sterilization; therefore, women who undergo ablation must use some other form of birth control. Various ablation devices are available; some use heat, and others use cryotherapy. Some, but not all, of the available techniques involve direct visualization of the endometrium with a hysteroscope. Many women opt for endometrial ablation because it is a minor procedure, thus avoiding major surgery in the form of a hysterectomy. The procedure can be performed in either the surgical suite or office. In the office, a combination of nonsteroidal anti-inflammatory drugs, a local anesthetic, and an anxiolytic is used to provide pain relief.

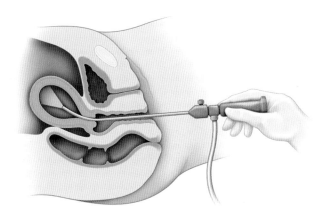

FIGURE 32.7. Hysteroscopy. (Figure adapted from the American College of Obstetricians and Gynecologists, © 2006.)

## Pregnancy Termination

Pregnancy termination refers to the planned interruption of pregnancy before viability and is often referred to as induced abortion. It is generally accomplished surgically through dilation of the cervix and evacuation of the uterine contents, accomplished under local anesthesia. In the first and early second trimester, removal of the products of conception uses either a suction or a sharp curette. Suction curettes are often preferred, because they are less likely to cause uterine damage such as endometrial scarring or perforation. In the second trimester, destructive grasping forceps may be used to remove the pregnancy through a dilated cervix (dilation and evacuation [D&E]).

Alternatively, in the first trimester (within 9 weeks of the first day of the last menstrual period), pregnancy can be terminated using medical rather than surgical techniques. Medical abortion may be carried out using one of the following methods:

- Mifepristone and misoprostol pills
- Mifepristone pills and vaginal misoprostol
- Methotrexate and vaginal misoprostol
- Vaginal misoprostol alone

A woman who is still pregnant after an attempted medical abortion needs to have a surgical abortion.

## Cervical Conization

Conization is a surgical procedure in which a cone-shaped sample of tissue, encompassing the entire cervical transformation zone and extending up the endocervical canal, is removed from the cervix (Fig. 32.8). It may be required as the definitive diagnostic procedure in the evaluation of an abnormal Pap test when the colposcopic examination is inadequate, or when colposcopic biopsy findings are inconsistent with Pap test results. Colposcopy-guided conization may also be used therapeutically in cases of cervical intraepithelial neoplasia (CIN). Various techniques for conization are available, including cold knife (scalpel), laser excision, or electrosurgery (loop electrosurgical excision procedure [LEEP], also called large loop excision of the transformation zone [LLETZ]). Laser excision and LEEP are often performed in the office. Long-term complications may include cervical insufficiency and stenosis.

## Laparoscopy

Laparoscopy is the visualization of the pelvis and abdominal cavity using an endoscopic telescope, which is most often placed via an incision in the periumbilical region (Fig. 32.9). The procedure may be diagnostic or therapeutic. Laparoscopic evaluation and treatment may be performed for conditions such as chronic pelvic pain, endometriosis, infertility, pelvic masses, ectopic pregnancies, and congenital abnormalities. Sterilization (bilateral

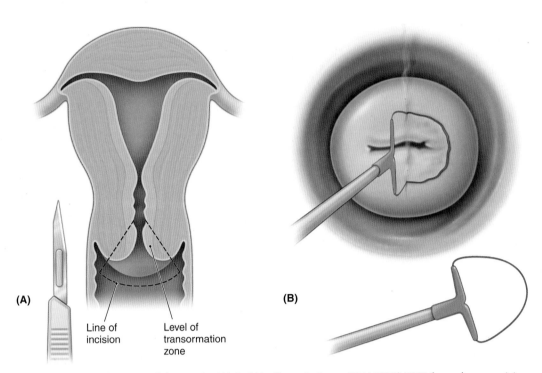

**(A)**

Line of
incision

Level of
transormation
zone

**(B)**

FIGURE 32.8. Conization of the cervix. (A) Cold knife technique. (B) LLETZ/LEEP (large loop excision of the transformation zone/loop electrosurgical excision procedure) technique.

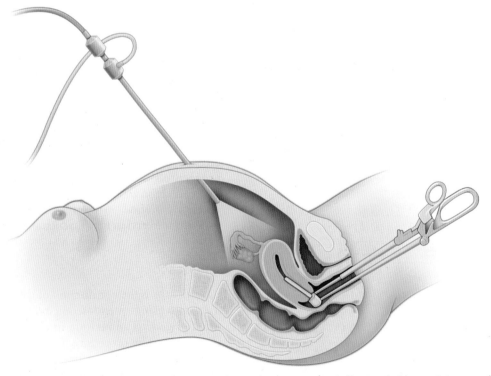

FIGURE 32.9. Laparoscopy. (Figure adapted from the American College of Obstetricians and Gynecologists, © 2008.)

tubal ligation) using techniques such as bipolar cautery, clips, or bands can be accomplished easily via laparoscopy (see Chapter 25, Sterilization). During the procedure, carbon dioxide is insufflated to distend the peritoneal cavity to provide visualization. Additional instruments with diameters of 5–15 mm may be inserted via other laparoscopic incisions. The number, length, and location of incisions depend on the instruments needed and the size of any tissue specimens that are to be removed. Transvaginal insertion of a uterine manipulator facilitates these maneuvers.

After laparoscopy, the most common complaints include incisional pain and shoulder pain due to referred pain of diaphragmatic irritation from the gas used to provide visualization. Rare, but serious complications include damage to major blood vessels, the bowel, and other intra-abdominal or retroperitoneal structures. However, when compared with laparotomy, laparoscopy has several advantages, including avoidance of long hospital stays, smaller incisions, quicker recovery, and decreased pain.

## Hysterectomy

Hysterectomy, removal of the uterus, is still one of the most commonly performed surgical procedures. In the United States, more than 500,000 hysterectomies are completed annually. The indications for hysterectomy are numerous; they include abnormal uterine bleeding that has not responded to conservative management, pelvic pain, postpartum hemorrhage, symptomatic leiomyomas, symptomatic uterine prolapse, cervical or uterine cancer, and severe anemia from uterine hemorrhage.

Patients are often confused by inaccurate terms used to describe types of hysterectomy. To many patients, a "complete" hysterectomy means removal of the uterus, fallopian tubes, and ovaries, and a "partial" hysterectomy means removal of the uterus but not the tubes and ovaries. However, the correct term for the removal of both tubes and both ovaries is a bilateral salpingo-oophorectomy, and this procedure is generally not part of a hysterectomy. Thus, it is important to determine exactly what procedure a patient may have had. Equally important is what a patient is expecting when a surgical procedure is planned. A total hysterectomy is the removal of the entire uterus, whereas a supracervical (or subtotal) hysterectomy removes the uterine corpus while leaving the cervix. The uterus may be removed by several different routes.

### ABDOMINAL HYSTERECTOMY

Abdominal hysterectomy is performed via a laparotomy incision. The laparotomy incision can be either transverse, usually Pfannenstiel, or vertical. The decision to perform a laparotomy involves many factors—the skill of the surgeon, the size of the uterus, concern for extensive pathology (e.g., endometriosis or cancer), the need to perform adjunct surgery during the surgery (e.g., lymph node dissection, appendectomy, omentectomy), and previous intra-abdominal scarring or surgeries.

### VAGINAL HYSTERECTOMY

Vaginal hysterectomy is preferred if there is adequate uterine mobility (descent of the cervix and uterus toward the introitus), the bony pelvis is of an appropriate configuration, the uterus is not too large, and there is no suspected adnexal pathology. In general, vaginal hysterectomy is performed for benign disease. The advantage of vaginal surgery is less pain than with abdominal surgery, quicker return of normal bowel function, and a shorter hospital stay. If indicated, a unilateral or bilateral salpingo-oophorectomy can be performed in conjunction with a vaginal hysterectomy.

### LAPAROSCOPIC-ASSISTED VAGINAL HYSTERECTOMY

Laparoscopic-assisted vaginal hysterectomy (LAVH), with or without a bilateral salpingo-oophorectomy, is often performed for patients who desire minimally invasive surgery and may not have adequate descensus of their uterus to undergo a vaginal hysterectomy. LAVH can be accomplished by performing most or all of the procedure laparoscopically; then the uterus is removed through the vagina. The vaginal cuff can then be sutured transvaginally or laparoscopically.

### TOTAL LAPAROSCOPIC HYSTERECTOMY

Many skilled laparoscopic surgeons are now performing a hysterectomy totally via the laparoscopic approach. This is usually accomplished with the assistance of a morcellator, which divides the uterus into multiple smaller specimens that can be removed through the ports. Even large uteri can be safely removed through small incisions.

## UROGYNECOLOGY PROCEDURES

Many gynecologists perform urogynecology procedures in the office and operating room. These procedures include the Q-tip test, urodynamic tests, cystoscopy, transvaginal tape (sling), and the Burch procedure. A description of these procedures can be found in Chapter 28.

## PREOPERATIVE, INTRAOPERATIVE, AND POSTOPERATIVE CONSIDERATIONS

Any surgical procedure carries risks. Naturally, more invasive procedures carry higher risks. Before patients sign preoperative surgical consent forms, they should be counseled on the risks of infection, hemorrhage, damage to surrounding structures (bowel, bladder, blood vessels, and other anatomic structures). Many hospitals require that patients also sign a consent form for a blood transfusion in case of an emergency. Some patients refuse to sign such consents for blood transfusion for personal or religious reasons, and this should be clearly documented in the chart. A discussion with the patient regarding the safety of the blood used for transfusion should address the risk of acquiring human immunodeficiency virus (HIV), hepatitis B and C viruses, and other blood-borne pathogens.

Preoperative testing, which could include blood work, urinalysis, other laboratory tests (glucose, creatinine, hemoglobin, coagulation parameters), pregnancy testing, electrocardiogram, and imaging studies (e.g., CT, MRI) should be individualized based on the patient's age (especially in pediatric patients), concurrent medical problems, route of anesthesia, and surgical procedure planned.

*Minor procedures are now more commonly performed in the office setting for patient convenience, avoidance of general anesthesia, and improved reimbursement.* In addition, not all patients are surgical candidates, and nonsurgical therapeutic options should always be considered. Patients may have such significant medical problems (e.g., poorly controlled diabetes, heart disease, pulmonary disease) that they might not tolerate anesthesia or surgery.

Several intraoperative and perioperative issues should be considered. Prophylactic antibiotics are indicated for some gynecologic surgeries and should be administered within 30 minutes of surgery. Often, a Foley catheter is inserted prior to surgery to prevent the bladder from becoming distended during the procedure. A preoperative pelvic examination of the anesthetized patient can sometimes prove useful.

Postoperatively, a nurse and a member of the anesthesia team assess the patient in the postanesthesia care unit. The patient is either discharged to home or admitted to the hospital, depending on the type of procedure performed and the condition of the patient. An operative note will have been written in the chart immediately postoperatively, outlining the preoperative diagnosis, postoperative diagnosis, procedure, surgeon(s), type of anesthesia, amount and type of intravenous fluid administered, any other fluids given (transfusions or other products), urine output (if indicated), findings, pathology specimens sent, complications, and a statement of patient's condition upon completion of the procedure. Postoperative orders for inpatient stays should include a notation of the procedure performed, the name of the attending physician and service, frequency of vital signs, parameters for calling the physician, diet, activity, intravenous fluids, pain medications, resumption of any home medications (antihypertensives, diabetic drugs, antidepressants, etc.), antiemetic medications, deep venous thrombosis (DVT) prophylaxis, Foley catheter, incentive spirometer, and any necessary laboratory studies.

During a postoperative hospitalization, the patient should be seen at least daily. Careful assessment and monitoring of pain, bladder and bowel function, nausea and vomiting, and vital signs are routine. Early ambulation can reduce the risk of thromboembolism. The most common surgical complications are fever, urinary tract infections, surgical site drainage and bleeding, minor separation of skin incisions, hemorrhage, pneumonia, ileus, and minor surgical site infection(s). Less common postoperative complications include skin and subcutaneous wound separation, fascial dehiscence or evisceration, bowel perforation, urinary tract injury, severe hemorrhage requiring reoperation, DVT, pulmonary embolism (PE), abscess, sepsis, fistulas, and anesthetic reactions.

Fever is defined as two oral temperatures of greater than or equal to 38°C at 4-hour intervals. Primary sources of fever include the respiratory and urinary tracts, the incision(s), thrombophlebitis, and any medications or transfusions. **Atelectasis** occurs when patients do not take large inspiratory breaths due to abdominal discomfort. Use of an incentive spirometer can minimize the risk of atelectasis and pneumonia. Use of an indwelling urinary catheter should be minimized, because placement for more than 24 hours increases the risk of urinary tract infection (cystitis or pyelonephritis). Ambulatory status affects breathing (hypoventilation) and possible thrombosis (DVT or PE). The wound should be assessed for any signs of infection. If there are no easily visible incisions as with vaginal surgery, a pelvic examination and/or imaging of the pelvis may be needed. If the fever resolves after withdrawal of a medication, then a presumptive diagnosis of drug reaction can be made. If the patient has received blood products, the possibility of a reaction to antigens in the transfusion should be investigated as a cause of the fever. Antibiotics should be ordered only when infection is suspected.

## SUGGESTED READINGS

American College of Obstetricians and Gynecologists. Antibiotic prophylaxis for gynecologic procedures. ACOG Practice Bulletin No. 74. *Obstet Gynecol.* 2006:108(1):225–234.

American College of Obstetricians and Gynecologists. Diagnosis and management of vulvar skin disorders. ACOG Practice Bulletin No. 93. *Obstet Gynecol.* 2008;111(_):1243–1253.

American College of Obstetricians and Gynecologists. Endometrial ablation. ACOG Practice Bulletin No. 81. *Obstet Gynecol.* 2007; 109(_):1233–1248.

American College of Obstetricians and Gynecologists. Management of abnormal cervical cytology and histology. ACOG Practice Bulletin No. 66. *Obstet Gynecol.* 2005;106(_):645–664.

American College of Obstetricians and Gynecologists. Patient safety in obstetrics and gynecology. ACOG Committee Opinion No. 286. *Obstet Gynecol.* 2003;102(_):883–885.

Breitkopf DM. Gynecologic imaging. In: American College of Obstetricians and Gynecologists. *Precis, An Update in Obstetrics and Gynecology: Gynecology.* 3rd ed. American College of Obstetricians and Gynecologists; 2006:15–25.

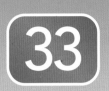

# Reproductive Cycles

**Topic 45:** Normal and Abnormal Uterine Bleeding

The student should understand the normal reproductive cycle in order to diagnose and treat common menstrual abnormalities.

I n the female reproductive cycle, ovulation is followed by menstrual bleeding in a cyclic, predictable sequence. This recurring process is established during puberty (average age of menarche is 12.43 years) and continues until the years prior to menopause (average age 51.4 years). Regular ovulatory cycles are usually established by the third year after menarche, and continue until the perimenopause. Therefore, between 15 and 45 years of age, a woman has approximately 30 years of ovulatory reproductive cycles. The reproductive cycles may be interrupted by conditions including pregnancy, lactation, illness, gynecologic disorders and endocrine disorders, and exogenous factors such as hormone-based contraceptives and various other medications.

*The duration of an adult reproductive cycle, from the beginning of one menses to the beginning of the next menses, averages approximately 28 days, with a range of 23 to 35 days, and comprises three distinct phases.* The **follicular phase** begins with the onset of menses (the first day of the menstrual cycle) and ends on the day of the **luteinizing hormone (LH)** surge. **Ovulation** occurs within 30–36 hours of the LH surge. The **luteal phase** begins on the day of the LH surge and ends with the onset of menses. The follicular and luteal phases each last approximately 14 days in reproductive-age women; however, variability in cycle length is more frequent at the extremes of the reproductive age. The duration of the luteal phase remains relatively constant, while the duration of the follicular phase can vary.

## HYPOTHALAMIC-PITUITARY-OVARIAN AXIS

*Hypothalamic-pituitary-ovarian axis refers to the complex interactions between the hypothalamus, pituitary, and ovaries that regulate the reproductive cycle.* These interactions are based on the interplay of the hormones released by these structures: gonadotropin-releasing hormone (GnRH), the gonadotropins **follicle-stimulating hormone (FSH)** and

LH, and the ovarian sex steroid hormones, estrogen and progesterone. Through stimulatory and inhibitory actions, these hormones directly and indirectly stimulate oocyte development and ovulation, endometrial development to facilitate embryo implantation, and menstruation. Feedback loops between the hypothalamus, pituitary, and ovaries are presented in Figure 33.1.

*Disruption of any of these communication and feedback loops results in alterations of hormone levels, which can lead to disorders of the reproductive cycle; ultimately, ovulation, reproduction, and menstruation can be affected.*

## Hypothalamic GnRH Secretion

The **gonadotropin-releasing hormone** is secreted in a pulsatile fashion from the arcuate nucleus of the hypothalamus. GnRH reaches the anterior pituitary through the hypothalamic–pituitary portal vascular system. The pulsatile secretion of GnRH stimulates and modulates pituitary gonadotropin secretion. Due to its remote location and a half-life of 2 to 4 minutes, GnRH cannot be directly measured, thus measurements of LH pulses are used to indicate GnRH pulsatile secretion. Ovarian function requires the pulsatile secretion of GnRH in a specific pattern that ranges from 60-minute to 4-hour intervals. *Therefore, the hypothalamus serves as the pulse generator of the reproductive cycle.* Coordinated GnRH release is stimulated by various neurotransmitters and catecholamines as well as by the inherent pulsatility of the GnRH neurons.

## Pituitary Gonadotropin Secretion

The pituitary gonadotropins FSH and LH are glycoprotein hormones secreted by the anterior pituitary gland. FSH and LH are also secreted in pulsatile fashion in response to the

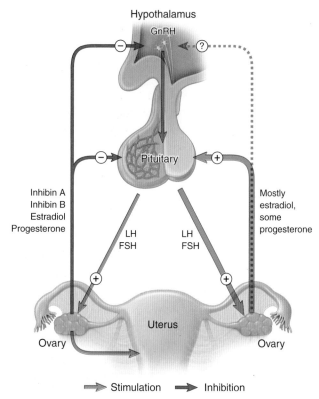

FIGURE 33.1. The reproductive cycle requires complex interactions and feedback between the hypothalamus, pituitary, and ovaries which are simplified in this diagram. CNS = central nervous system; GnRH = gonadotropin-releasing hormone; FSH = follicle stimulating hormone; LH = luteinizing hormone.

during childhood; thus, at menarche, 300,000 to 500,000 oocytes remain.

The immature oocyte is encircled by a single layer of **granulosa cells,** followed by a thin basement membrane that separates the follicle from the surrounding ovarian stroma. Early follicular maturation occurs independent of gonadotropins; the granulosa cells proliferate into multiple layers, and the surrounding stromal cells differentiate into **theca cells.** Granulosa cells produce estrogens, including estrone and **estradiol,** the latter being the more potent of the two. Theca cells produce androgens which serve as the precursors required for granulosa cell estrogen production. Androgens (androstenedione and testosterone) enter the granulosa cells by diffusion and are converted to estrogen. The two-cell theory of estrogen synthesis is diagrammed in Figure 33.2.

During follicular development, FSH binds to FSH-receptors on the granulosa cells, causing cellular proliferation and increased binding of FSH and, hence, increased production of estradiol. Estradiol stimulates the proliferation of LH-receptors on theca and granulosa cells, and LH stimulates the theca cells to produce androgens. Greater androgen production leads to increased estradiol production. Rising estrogen levels influence the pituitary gland through negative feedback and results in suppression of

pulsatile release of GnRH; the magnitude of secretion and the rates of secretion of FSH and/or LH are determined largely by the levels of ovarian steroid hormones, **estrogen** and **progesterone,** and other ovarian factors (such as inhibin, activin, and follistatin).

When a woman is in a state of relative estrogen deficiency, as in the early follicular phase, the principal gonadotropin secreted is FSH. The ovary responds to FSH secretion with estradiol production, with subsequent negative feedback on the pituitary inhibiting FSH secretion and positive feedback facilitating LH secretion.

## Ovarian Steroid Hormone Secretion

*At midcycle, there is a marked increase in LH secretion (the LH surge), which triggers ovulation.* With ovulation, the ovarian follicle is converted into a corpus luteum and begins secreting progesterone.

At birth, the human ovary contains approximately one to two million primordial follicles. Each follicle contains an oocyte that is arrested in prophase of the first meiotic division. A large number of these inactive primordial follicles undergo a degenerative process known as atresia

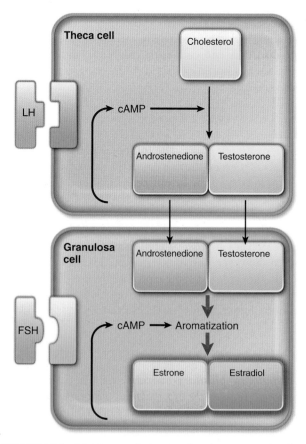

FIGURE 33.2. The two-cell theory of estrogen production.

FSH and LH secretion. In the late follicular phase, peak estradiol concentrations from the dominant follicle have positive feedback on the pituitary, which stimulates the midcycle surge of LH secretion that is necessary for ovulation. *With ovulation, the dominant ovarian follicle releases its oocyte and transitions to a progesterone-secreting ovarian cyst, the* **corpus luteum.** The process of follicular maturation is presented in Figure 33.3.

## REPRODUCTIVE CYCLE

As discussed, the reproductive cycle is divided into three phases: menstruation and the follicular phase, ovulation, and the luteal phase. These three phases refer to the status of the ovary during the reproductive cycle. In contrast, *when referring to the endometrium, the phases of the menstrual cycle are termed the* **proliferative** *and* **secretory phases.**

### Phase I: Menstruation and the Follicular Phase

*The first day of menstrual bleeding is considered day 1 of the menstrual cycle.* When conception does not occur, the involution of the corpus luteum and, hence, the decline of progesterone and estrogen levels cause menstruation. Normal menstruation lasts 3 to 7 days, during which women lose 20 to 60 mL of dark, nonclotting blood. Menstruation consists of blood and desquamated superficial endometrial tissues. Prostaglandins in the secretory endometrium and menstrual blood produce contractions of the uterine vasculature and musculature, which in turn cause endometrial ischemia and uterine cramping. These prostaglandin-associated uterine contractions also aid expulsion of the menstrual

blood and tissue. Rising estrogen levels in the early follicular phase induce endometrial healing which leads to cessation of menstruation.

At the end of the luteal phase, serum concentrations of estradiol, progesterone, and LH reach their lowest levels. In response to low hormone levels, FSH begins to rise in the late luteal phase before the onset of menstruation to recruit the next cohort of follicles. *Thus, during menstruation, follicular growth has already been initiated for the new reproductive cycle.* Estradiol levels rise during the follicular phase, causing a decline in FSH. LH remains low in the early follicular phase, but increasing estrogen levels have positive feedback on LH release, and LH starts to rise by the midfollicular phase. Although several follicles begin the maturation process, only the follicle with the greatest number of granulosa cells and FSH receptors and the highest estradiol production becomes the dominant follicle; the nondominant follicles undergo atresia.

### Phase II: Ovulation

As the dominant follicle secretes an increasing amount of estradiol, there is marked positive feedback to the pituitary gland to secrete LH. By days 11 to 13 of the cycle, the LH surge occurs, which triggers ovulation. The LH surge begins 34 to 36 hours prior to ovulation, and peak LH secretion occurs 10 to 12 hours prior to ovulation. With the LH surge, the granulosa and theca cells undergo distinct changes and begin production of progesterone. Meiosis of the primary follicle resumes after the LH surge and the first polar body is released; the oocyte then arrests in metaphase of the second meiotic division until fertilization occurs.

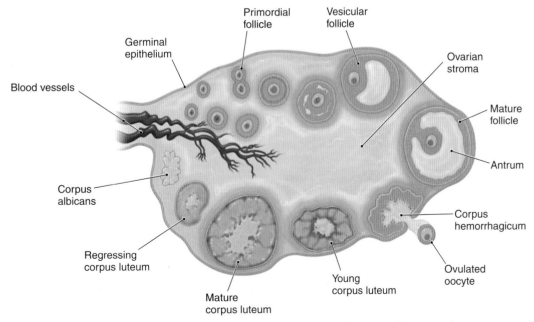

**FIGURE 33.3.  Ovarian follicle development during the reproductive cycle.**

During ovulation, the oocyte is expelled from the follicle, and the follicle is converted into the corpus luteum.

Some women experience a twinge of pain ("**mittel-schmerz**") at the time of ovulation and can precisely identify the time of ovulation. Other women do not experience this brief discomfort, but can recognize characteristic symptoms that occur due to progesterone production after ovulation.

## Phase III: Luteal Phase

*The luteal phase of the menstrual cycle is characterized by an alteration in the balance of sex steroid secretion from predominance of estrogen to predominance of progesterone.* The process of follicular development has led to increased numbers of LH receptors on the granulosa and theca cells. The mid-cycle LH surge stimulates these LH receptors and converts the enzymatic machinery of these cells to produce and secrete progesterone; this process is called **luteinization.** Progesterone has negative feedback on pituitary secretion of FSH and LH, thus both hormones are suppressed during the luteal phase. The corpus luteum also produces estradiol in a pattern that parallels progesterone secretion.

The production of progesterone begins approximately 24 hours before ovulation and rises rapidly thereafter. Maximal progesterone production occurs 3 to 4 days after ovulation. The lifespan of the corpus luteum ends approximately 9 to 11 days after ovulation; if conception does not occur, the corpus luteum undergoes involution (a progressive decrease in size) and progesterone production sharply declines. This withdrawal of progesterone releases FSH from negative feedback, thus FSH levels begin to rise prior to menstruation and the initiation of a new cycle.

The carefully orchestrated sequence of estrogen production and then progesterone production is essential for proper endometrial development to allow implantation of an embryo. If the oocyte becomes fertilized and implantation occurs, the resulting zygote begins secreting human chorionic gonadotropin (hCG), which sustains the corpus luteum for another 6 to 7 weeks. Adequate progesterone production by the corpus luteum is necessary to sustain the early pregnancy. By 9 to 10 weeks of pregnancy, placental steroidogenesis is well-established and the placenta assumes progesterone production.

The corpus luteum measures approximately 2.5 cm in diameter, has a characteristic deep yellow color, and can be seen on gross inspection of the ovary if surgery is performed during the luteal phase of the cycle. As the function of the corpus luteum declines, it decreases in volume and loses its yellow color. After a few months, the corpus luteum becomes a white fibrous streak within the ovary, called the **corpus albicans.**

Reproductive cycle changes in gonadotropins, steroid hormones, ovarian follicles, and the endometrium are summarized in Figure 33.4.

## CLINICAL MANIFESTATIONS OF HORMONAL CHANGES

Hormonal changes induced by the hypothalamic-pituitary-ovarian axis and the adrenal gland trigger puberty, and hormones continue to exert a cyclic influence until a woman reaches menopause. At that time, the lack of cyclic ovarian function results in the permanent cessation of menstruation.

*Various female structures undergo changes in response to the reproductive cycle hormones: the endometrium and endocervix, breasts, vagina, and the hypothalamus.* Changes in the endocervix and breasts can be directly observed. Daily assessment of basal body temperature can identify changes in the hypothalamic thermoregulation center. Other changes can be assessed by cytologic examination of a sample from the vaginal epithelium or histologic evaluation of an endometrial biopsy. A careful history may identify symptoms associated with hormone effects, such as abdominal bloating, fluid retention, mood and appetite changes, and uterine cramps at the onset of menstruation.

### Endometrium

Within the uterus, the endometrium undergoes dramatic histologic changes during the reproductive cycle. During menstruation, the entire endometrium is expelled and only the basal layer remains. During the follicular phase, the rise in estrogen levels stimulates endometrial cell growth: the endometrial stroma thickens and the endometrial glands become elongated to form the proliferative endometrium. In an ovulatory cycle, the endometrium reaches maximal thickness at the time of ovulation.

When ovulation occurs, the predominant hormone shifts from estrogen to progesterone and distinct changes occur within the endometrium at almost daily intervals. Progesterone causes differentiation of the endometrial components and converts the proliferative endometrium into a secretory endometrium. The endometrial stroma becomes loose and edematous, while blood vessels entering the endometrium become thickened and twisted. The endometrial glands, which were straight and tubular during the proliferative phase, become tortuous and contain secretory material within the lumen. With the withdrawal of progesterone at the end of the luteal phase, the endometrium breaks down and is sloughed during menses.

If ovulation does not occur and estrogen continues to be produced, the endometrial stroma continues to thicken and the endometrial glands continue to elongate. Only an endometrial biopsy will identify proliferative endometrium. The endometrium eventually outgrows its blood supply and sections of the endometrium slough intermittently. Without progesterone withdrawal to initiate desquamation of the entire endometrium, bleeding is acyclic and occurs outside of hormonal control irregularly and for prolonged periods of time. When women present with abnormal

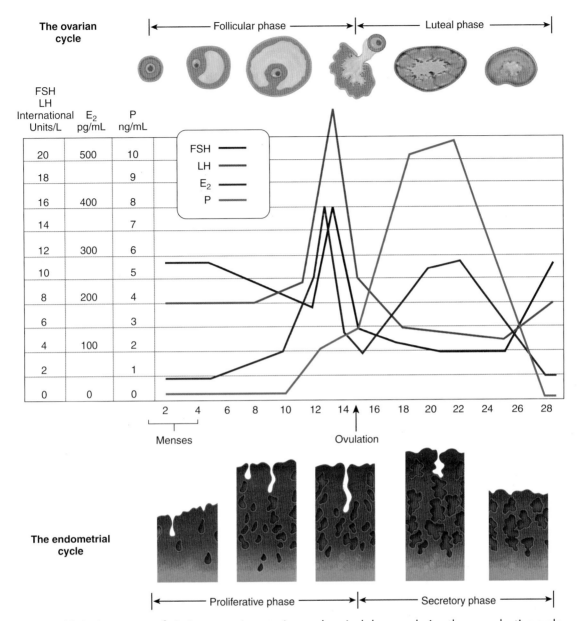

FIGURE 33.4. A summary of pituitary, ovarian, uterine, and vaginal changes during the reproductive cycle.

uterine bleeding, anovulatory bleeding is a common diagnosis (see Chapter 35, Amenorrhea and Abnormal Uterine Bleeding).

## Endocervix

The endocervix contains glands that secrete mucus in response to hormonal stimulation. Under the influence of estrogens, the endocervical glands secrete large quantities of thin, clear, watery mucus. Endocervical mucus production is maximal at the time of ovulation. This mucus facilitates sperm capture, storage, and transport. With ovulation, progesterone reverses the effect of estrogen on the endocervical mucus, and mucus production diminishes.

Some women monitor their cervical mucus to optimize the timing of intercourse when trying to conceive or in order to avoid conception. However, the timing of these changes is nonspecific and is an unreliable method of contraception.

## Breasts

Estrogen exposure is necessary for pubertal breast development; however, reproductive cycle changes in the breast occur primarily due to progesterone effect. The ductal elements of the breast, nipple, and areola respond to progesterone secretion. Some women will notice more breast tenderness and fullness in the luteal phase due to progesterone-mediated changes.

## Vagina

Estrogen promotes growth of the vaginal epithelium and maturation of the superficial epithelial cells of the mucosa. During sexual stimulation, the presence of estrogen aids vaginal transudation and lubrication, which facilitates intercourse. During the luteal phase of the reproductive cycle, the vaginal epithelium retains its thickness, but the secretions are markedly diminished.

## Hypothalamic Thermoregulation Center

Progesterone is a hormone with thermogenic effects; under the influence of progesterone, the hypothalamus shifts the basal body temperature upward by $0.5°F$ to $1.0°F$ over the average preovulatory temperature. This shift occurs abruptly with the beginning of progesterone secretion and quickly returns to baseline with the decline in progesterone secretion. Therefore, these changes in basal body temperature reflect changes in plasma progesterone concentration.

*Since the basal body temperature assumes basal conditions at rest, it should be performed immediately in the morning upon awakening, prior to any activity.*

Special thermometers with an expanded scale are available for this purpose. Identification of this characteristic biphasic curve provides retrospective, indirect evidence of ovulation; however, some ovulatory women do not demonstrate these changes (see Fig. 33.2).

## SUGGESTED READING

Bradshaw KD. The ovary and the menstrual cycle. In: American College of Obstetricians and Gynecologists. *Precis: An Update in Obstetrics and Gynecology: Reproductive Endocrinology.* 3rd ed. Washington, DC: American College of Obstetricians and Gynecologists; 2007:56–68.

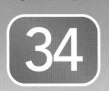

# 34 Puberty

P uberty is an endocrine process that involves the physical, emotional, and sexual transition from childhood to adulthood. It occurs gradually in a series of well-defined events and milestones. When puberty is early or delayed, an understanding of the hormonal events of puberty and the sequence of physical changes is essential to diagnosis of a potential problem. Knowledge of the events of puberty is also key to understanding the process of reproduction.

## NORMAL PUBERTAL DEVELOPMENT

A series of endocrine events initiate the onset of secondary sexual maturation. The hypothalamic–pituitary–gonadal axis begins to function during fetal life and remains active during the first few weeks following birth, after which time the axis becomes quiescent secondary to enhanced negative feedback of estrogen. The hypothalamic–pituitary–gonadal axis again becomes active during puberty, triggering the production of gonadotropin-releasing hormone (GnRH). The gonadotropins control production of sex steroids from the ovary, and higher levels cause the physical changes of puberty. At approximately 6 to 8 years of age, adrenarche, the increase in production of androgens, occurs in the adrenal glands. Adrenarche involves the increased production of dehydroepiandrosterone (DHEA), which can be converted to more potent androgens (testosterone and dihydrotestosterone).

*The process of secondary sexual maturation requires approximately 4 years.* It takes place in an orderly, predictable sequence that includes growth acceleration, breast development (thelarche), pubic hair development (pubarche) [maximum growth rate], menarche, and ovulation. The initial event is accelerated growth; however, this may be subtle, and breast budding is easier to detect as the first event. The sequence of breast development and pubic hair growth is referred to as Tanner's classification of sexual maturity (Fig. 34.1).

The ages at which some of these events occur are presented in Table 34.1. There is a strong relationship between body fat content and the onset of puberty. Mild to moderate obesity results in earlier puberty, whereas thinness results in later puberty. The onset of puberty is also marked by significant ethnic differences. Puberty usually begins earlier in African-American and Mexican-American girls than in white girls, and much of this difference may result from differences in body mass index (see Table 34.1). In contrast, puberty tends to begin in Asian-American girls later than in white girls. Body mass index may account for most of this difference, although as yet undefined genetic or environmental factors may also be important.

## ABNORMALITIES OF PUBERTAL DEVELOPMENT

The abnormalities of puberty include precocious puberty, primary amenorrhea, delayed sexual maturation, and incomplete sexual maturation.

*The presence of any of these disorders requires investigation of both the hypothalamic–pituitary–gonadal axis as well as the reproductive outflow tract.*

The initial evaluation should begin with measurement of pituitary gonadotropin (follicle-stimulating hormone [FSH] and luteinizing hormone [LH]) levels, which helps distinguish a hypothalamic–pituitary etiology from a gonadal etiology.

### Precocious Puberty

Precocious puberty is the onset of secondary sexual characteristics prior to the age 6 in black girls and age 7 in white

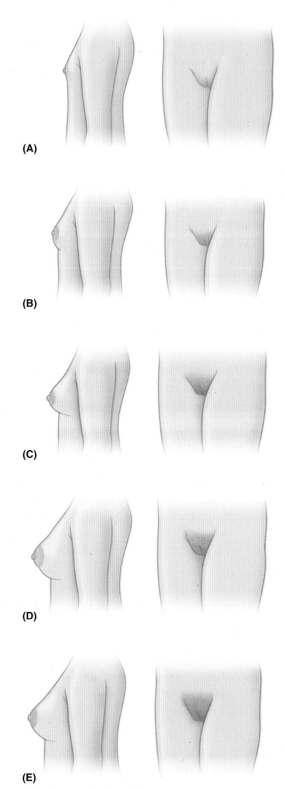

(A)

(B)

(C)

(D)

(E)

FIGURE 34.1. Tanner staging of breast and pubic hair development, which includes five stages. (From American College of Obstetricians and Gynecologists. *Precis, An Update in Obstetrics and Gynecology: Reproductive Endocrinology.* 3rd ed. Washington, DC: American College of Obstetricians and Gynecologists; 2007; modified from Speroff L, Glass RH, Kase NG. *Clinical Gynecologic Endocrinology and Infertility* 7th ed. Baltimore, MD: Lippincott Williams & Wilkins; 2005.)

| TABLE 34.1 | Ethnicity and Onset of Puberty | | |
|---|---|---|---|
| | Mean Age (years) | | |
| Event | African Americans | Mexican Americans | Whites |
| Thelarche | 9.5 | 9.8 | 10.3 |
| Pubarche | 9.5 | 10.3 | 10.5 |
| Menarche | 12.3 | 12.5 | 12.7 |

From American College of Obstetricians and Gynecologists. *Precis, An Update in Obstetrics and Gynecology: Reproductive Endocrinology.* 3rd ed. Washington, DC: American College of Obstetricians and Gynecologists; 2007; after Wu T, Mendola P, Buck GM. Ethnic differences in the presence of secondary sex characteristics and menarche among US girls: The Third National Health And Nutrition Examination Survey, 1988–1994. *Pediatrics.* 2002;110(4):752–757. Reproduced with permission.

girls. *Precocious puberty is caused by either GnRH-dependent or GnRH-independent sex hormone production* (Box 34.1). GnRH-dependent, or true (central) precocious puberty, develops secondary to early activation of the hypothalamic–pituitary–gonadal axis. The most common causes are idiopathic; other causes include infection, inflammation, or injury of the central nervous system. In idiopathic precocious puberty, the arcuate nucleus in the hypothalamus is prematurely activated. This causes early sexual maturation with early reproductive capability. The elevated estrogen levels affect the skeleton, resulting in short stature in adulthood secondary to premature closure of the epiphyseal plates. These individuals are at risk for sexual abuse and have psychosocial problems related to their early sexual development. Occasionally, GnRH-dependent precocious puberty results from neoplasms of the hypothalamic–pituitary stalk. In this situation, although sexual development begins early, the rate of sexual development is slower than usual. Transient inflammatory conditions of the hypothalamus may also result in GnRH-dependent precocious puberty; however, sexual development may begin and end abruptly. Laboratory studies show either an appropriate rise in gonadotropins or a steady gonadotropin level in the prepubertal range.

*GnRH-independent sex hormone production, or precocious pseudopuberty (peripheral), results from sex hormone production (androgens or estrogens) independent of hypothalamic–pituitary stimulation.* This condition can be caused by ovarian cysts or tumors, McCune–Albright syndrome, adrenal tumors, or iatrogenic causes. Some tumors, such as granulosa cell tumors, teratoma, or dysgerminomata, directly secrete androgen. Physical examination usually reveals a palpable pelvic mass and leads to further evaluation/imaging studies.

*McCune–Albright syndrome (polyostotic fibrous dysplasia) is characterized by multiple bone fractures, café-au-lait spots, and precocious puberty.* Premature menarche can be the first sign

---

**BOX 34.1**
## Causes of Precocious Sexual Development

**Gonadotropin-Releasing Hormone–Dependent (Central) Causes**

**Idiopathic Origin**
- Central nervous system tumors
- Hypothalamic hamartoma
- Craniopharyngiomata
- Gliomata
- Metastatic
- Arachnoid or suprasellar cysts

**Central Nervous System Infection/Inflammation**
- Encephalitis
- Meningitis
- Granulomata

**Central Nervous System Injury**
- Irradiation
- Trauma
- Hydrocephalus

**Gonadotropin-Releasing Hormone–Independent (Peripheral) Causes**

**Exogenous Sex Steroid Administration**

**Primary Hypothyroidism**

**Ovarian Tumors**
- Granulosa–theca cell
- Lipoid cell
- Gonadoblastoma
- Cystadenoma
- Germ cell

**Simple Ovarian Cyst**

**McCune–Albright Syndrome**

**Incomplete Precocious Sexual Development**

**Premature Thelarche**
- Nonprogressive, idiopathic
- Progresses to precocious puberty

**Premature Adrenarche**
- Idiopathic
- Congenital adrenal hyperplasia
- Precursor to polycystic ovary syndrome
- Adrenal or ovarian tumor (rare)

---

of the syndrome. The syndrome is thought to result from a defect in cellular regulation with a mutation in the alpha subunit of the G protein that stimulates cAMP formation, which causes affected tissues to function autonomously. This mutation causes the ovary to produce estrogen without the need for FSH, resulting in sexual precocity.

*Adrenal causes of precocious puberty include adrenal tumors or enzyme-secreting defects, such as congenital adrenal hyperplasia (CAH).* Tumors are very rare and must secrete estrogen to cause early sexual maturation. The most common form of CAH, 21-hydroxylase deficiency, presents at birth with the finding of ambiguous genitalia. However, the nonclassical form, previously known as late-onset CAH, tends to present at adolescence. In this disorder, the adrenal glands are unable to produce adequate amounts of cortisol as a result of a partial block in the conversion of 17-hydroxyprogesterone to deoxycortisol. Deficiency of the 21-hydroxylase enzyme leads to a shunting away from aldosterone and cortisol production in cholesterol biosynthesis toward the production of androgens (testosterone and estradiol), which results in precocious adrenarche. *A pathognomonic finding for 21-hydroxylase deficiency is an elevated 17-hydroxyprogesterone level.* Plasma renin is also measured to determine the amount of mineralocorticoid deficiency. Medical therapy is instituted as early as possible and is aimed at steroid/mineralocorticoid replacement, depending on the

severity of the deficiency. In the nonclassical form of CAH, patients present with premature adrenarche, anovulation, and hyperandrogenism, appearing somewhat like patients with polycystic ovarian syndrome.

*Iatrogenic causes such as drug ingestion must be considered in all children who present with precocious puberty.*

These children may exhibit increased pigmentation of the nipples and areola of the breast secondary to ingestion of oral contraceptives, anabolic steroids, and hair or facial creams. *The main goals of treatment of precocious puberty are to arrest and diminish sexual maturation until a normal pubertal age, as well as to maximize adult height.* Therapy for GnRH-independent precocious puberty involves administration of a GnRH agonist. Results occur rapidly and continue during the first year of treatment. Treatment for GnRH-independent precocious puberty attempts to suppress gonadal steroidogenesis.

## Delayed Puberty

There is wide variation in normal pubertal development. *However, puberty is considered delayed when secondary sex characteristics have not appeared by age 13, there is no evidence of menarche by age 15 to 16, or when menses have not began 5 years after the onset of thelarche.* These findings should prompt the physician to initiate a workup to determine the cause of the delay. The most common causes of delayed puberty are shown in Box 34.2.

### HYPERGONADOTROPIC HYPOGONADISM

*The most common cause of delayed puberty with an elevated FSH is gonadal dysgenesis, or Turner syndrome.* In this condition, there is an abnormality in or absence of one of the X chromosomes in all cell lines. Patients have streak gonads, with an absence of ovarian follicles; therefore, gonadal sex hormone production does not occur at puberty. These patients typically have primary amenorrhea, short stature, webbed neck (pterygium coli), shield chest with widely spaced nipples, high arched palate, and an increased carrying angle of the elbow (cubitus valgus) [see Fig. 34.2].

> *Estrogen administration should be initiated at the normal time of initiation of puberty, and growth hormone should be initiated very early (often prior to estrogen therapy) and aggressively to normalize adult height.*

Estrogen is necessary to stimulate breast development, genital tract maturation, and the beginning of menstruation. Low-dose estrogen is used to initiate secondary sexual maturation, and the dose is increased once breast budding and menarche occur. If an excessive amount of

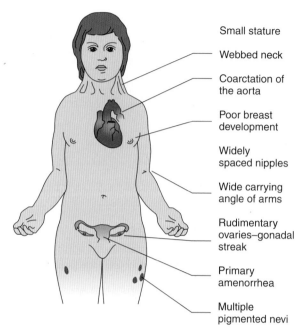

FIGURE 34.2. Clinical features of Turner syndrome. In Turner syndrome there is an abnormality or absence of one of the X chromosomes in all cell lines. Patients have streak gonads with an absence of ovarian follicles and, therefore, no gonadal sex hormone production at puberty. These patients typically present with primary amenorrhea, short stature, webbed neck (pterygium coli), shield chest with widely spaced nipples, high-arched palate, and an increased carrying angle of the elbow (cubitus valgus). (Modified from Rubin R, Strayer DS. *Rubin's Pathology*. 5th ed. Baltimore, MD: Lippincott Williams & Wilkins; 2008:195.)

Labels on figure:
- Small stature
- Webbed neck
- Coarctation of the aorta
- Poor breast development
- Widely spaced nipples
- Wide carrying angle of arms
- Rudimentary ovaries–gonadal streak
- Primary amenorrhea
- Multiple pigmented nevi

estrogen is administered initially, epiphyseal closure may begin, and long bone growth is truncated and adult height compromised. A delay in estrogen administration can lead to the development of osteoporosis in the teenage years. Progestins should not be given until the patient has reached Tanner stage IV, because premature progestin therapy may prevent the breast from developing completely, thus resulting in an abnormal contour (a more tubular breast).

### HYPOGONADOTROPIC HYPOGONADISM

The arcuate nucleus of the hypothalamus secretes GnRH in cyclic bursts (or a pulsatile fashion), which stimulates release of gonadotropins from the anterior pituitary gland. Dysfunction of the arcuate nucleus disrupts the short hormonal loop between the hypothalamus and pituitary. As a result, FSH and LH secretion does not occur. Consequently, the ovaries are not stimulated to secrete estradiol, and secondary sexual maturation is delayed. *The most common cause of this type of delayed puberty is constitutional (physiologic) delay.* Other causes include Kallmann syndrome; anorexia, exercise, or stress; pituitary tumors/pituitary disorders; hyperprolactinemia; and drug use.

---

**BOX 34.2**
## Causes of Delayed Puberty

**Hypergonadotropic Hypogonadism (FSH >30 mIU/mL)**
- Gonadal dysgenesis (Turner syndrome)

**Hypogonadotropic Hypogonadism (FSH + LH <10 mIU/mL)**
- Constitutional (physiologic) delay
- Kallmann syndrome
- Anorexia/Extreme exercise
- Pituitary tumors/pituitary disorders
- Hyperprolactinemia
- Drug use

**Anatomic Causes**
- Müllerian agenesis
- Imperforate hymen
- Transverse vaginal septum

Constitutional delay of puberty represents approximately 20% of all cases of delayed puberty. *It is thought to be a normal variant of the development process and trends can be seen within families.* Children with constitutional delay usually have not only delay of secondary sexual maturation, but also short stature with an appropriate delay of bone maturation.

*In the Kallmann syndrome, the olfactory tracts are hypoplastic, and the arcuate nucleus does not secrete GnRH.* Young women with Kallmann syndrome have little or no sense of smell and do not have breast development. This condition can be diagnosed on initial physical examination by challenging the olfactory function with known odors such as coffee or rubbing alcohol. Once the condition is recognized and treated, the prognosis for successful secondary sexual maturation and reproduction is excellent. Secondary sexual maturation can be stimulated by the administration of exogenous hormones or by the administration of pulsatile GnRH. Patients typically can have normal reproductive function. Ovulation is induced by the administration of exogenous gonadotropin, and progesterone is given in the luteal phase to allow implantation of the embryo.

*Other causes of hypothalamic amenorrhea include weight loss, strenuous exercise (such as ballet dancing or long-distance running), anorexia nervosa, or bulimia.* These conditions all result in suppressed gonadotropin levels with low estrogen levels. The correction of the underlying abnormality (such as weight gain in patients with weight loss) restores normal gonadotropin levels, stimulating ovarian steroidogenesis and the resumption of pubertal development.

*Craniopharyngioma is the most common tumor associated with delayed puberty.* This tumor develops in the pituitary stalk with suprasellar extension from nests of epithelium derived from the Rathke pouch. The radiologic hallmark is the appearance of a (supra)sellar calcified cyst. Calcifications are present in approximately 70% of craniopharyngiomas.

## ANATOMIC CAUSES

During fetal life, müllerian ducts develop and fuse in the female fetus to form the upper reproductive tract (i.e., the fallopian tubes, uterus, and upper vagina). The lower and midportion of the vagina develop from the canalization of the genital plate.

*Müllerian agenesis, or Mayer-Rokitansky–Küster–Hauser syndrome, is the most common cause of primary amenorrhea in women with normal breast development.* In this syndrome, there is congenital absence of the vagina and usually an absence of the uterus and fallopian tubes. Ovarian function is normal, because the ovaries are not derived from müllerian structures; therefore, all the secondary sexual characteristics of puberty occur at the appropriate time. Physical examination leads to the diagnosis of müllerian agenesis. Renal anomalies (e.g., reduplication of the ureters, horseshoe kidney, or unilateral renal agenesis) occur in 40% to 50% of cases. Skeletal anomalies such as scoliosis occur in 10% to 15% of cases. Mayer-Rokitansky–Küster–Hauser syndrome is generally sporadic in expression, although occasional occurrences in families can be seen.

There are several therapeutic approaches to this condition. Nonsurgical approaches should be tried first, using dilators and pressure on the dimple between the urethra and the rectum, twice a day. This tissue is quite pliable and, with increasing dilator size, a normal-length vagina can be achieved. An artificial vagina may be created by repetitive pressure by vaginal dilators on the perineum or by surgical construction followed by a split-thickness skin graft. After creation of a vagina, these women are able to have sexual intercourse. With the advances in assisted reproductive technologies, including in vitro fertilization (IVF) and use of a surrogate mother (gestational carrier), it is possible for a woman with this condition to have a genetic child by using her oocytes.

*The simplest genital tract anomaly is imperforate hymen.* In this condition, the genital plate canalization is incomplete, and the hymen is, therefore, closed. Menarche occurs at the appropriate time, but because there is obstruction to the passage of menstrual blood, it is not apparent. This condition presents with pain in the area of the uterus and a bulging, bluish-appearing vaginal introitus. Hymenotomy is the definitive therapy. This condition may be confused with a transverse vaginal septum. Transverse vaginal septa can occur along the vagina at any level and result in obstruction to outflow of menses. A vaginal septum can be resected and primarily repaired via a procedure called a Z-vaginoplasty. Prolonged obstruction to menstruation can be associated with an increased incidence of endometriosis.

## SUGGESTED READINGS

American College of Obstetricians and Gynecologists. *Precis, An Update in Obstetrics and Gynecology: Reproductive Endocrinology.* 3rd ed. Washington, DC: American College of Obstetricians and Gynecologists; 2007:31–55.

American College of Obstetricians and Gynecologists. *Guidelines for Women's Health Care: A Resource Manual.* 3rd ed. Washington, DC: American College of Obstetricians and Gynecologists; 2007.

# Amenorrhea and Abnormal Uterine Bleeding

Topic 43:  Amenorrhea

Topic 45:  Normal and Abnormal Uterine Bleeding

Students should be able to discuss the endocrine and anatomic causes of the absence of menstruation (amenorrhea) and irregular menstruation (oligomenorrhea) and their evaluation and management. Students should also be able to discuss the normal menstrual cycle and the evaluation and management of the causes of menses at times other than expected (abnormal uterine bleeding).

menorrhea (the absence of menstruation) and abnormal uterine bleeding are the most common gynecologic disorders of reproductive-age women. Amenorrhea and abnormal uterine bleeding are discussed as separate topics in this chapter. However, the pathophysiology underlying amenorrhea and abnormal uterine bleeding is often the same.

**Abnormal uterine bleeding** is a difference in frequency, duration, and amount of menstrual bleeding (Box 35.1). A logical approach to terminology is to separate abnormal bleeding into two broad categories: abnormal bleeding associated with ovulatory cycles, which usually have organic causes; and bleeding due to anovulatory causes, which is usually diagnosed through exclusion based on history.

## AMENORRHEA

If a young woman has never menstruated by age 13 without secondary sexual development or by age 15 with secondary sexual development, she is classified as having **primary amenorrhea.** If a menstruating woman has not menstruated for 3 to 6 months or for the duration of three typical menstrual cycles for the patient with oligomenorrhea, she is classified as having **secondary amenorrhea.** The designation of primary or secondary amenorrhea has no bearing on the severity of the underlying disorder or on the prognosis for restoring cyclic ovulation. Terms often confused with these include **oligomenorrhea,** defined as a reduction of the frequency of menses, with cycle lengths of greater than 35 days but less than 6 months, and **hypomenorrhea,** defined as a reduction in the number of days or the amount of menstrual flow.

Amenorrhea not caused by pregnancy occurs in 5% or less of all women during their menstrual lives.

## Causes of Amenorrhea

When endocrine function along the hypothalamic–pituitary–ovarian axis is disrupted or an abnormality develops in the genital outflow tract (obstruction of the uterus, cervix, or vagina or scarring of the endometrium), menstruation ceases. Causes of amenorrhea are divided into those arising from (1) pregnancy, (2) hypothalamic–pituitary dysfunction, (3) ovarian dysfunction, and (4) alteration of the genital outflow tract.

### PREGNANCY

*Because pregnancy is the most common cause of amenorrhea, it is essential to exclude pregnancy in the evaluation of amenorrhea.*

A history of breast fullness, weight gain, and nausea suggest the diagnosis of pregnancy, which is confirmed by a positive human chorionic gonadotropin (hCG) assay. It is important to rule out pregnancy to allay the patient's anxiety and to avoid unnecessary testing. Also, some treatments for other causes of amenorrhea can be harmful to an ongoing pregnancy. Lastly, the diagnosis of ectopic pregnancy should be entertained in the presence of abnormal menses and a positive pregnancy test, as this would necessitate medical or surgical intervention.

### BOX 35.1
### Types of Abnormal Uterine Bleeding

Polymenorrhea—frequent menstrual bleeding
  (frequency, 21 days or less)
Menorrhagia—prolonged or excessive uterine
  bleeding that occurs at regular intervals (the
  loss of 80 mL or more of blood that lasts for
  more than 7 days)
Metrorrhagia—irregular menstrual bleeding or
  bleeding between periods
Menometrorrhagia—frequent menstrual bleeding
  that is excessive and irregular in amount and
  duration

American College of Obstetricians and Gynecologists. Management of anovulatory bleeding. ACOG Practice Bulletin 14. Washington, DC: American College of Obstetricians and Gynecologists; 2000.

### BOX 35.2
### Causes of Hypothalamic–Pituitary Amenorrhea

**Functional Causes**
Weight loss
Excessive exercise
Obesity

**Drug-Induced Causes**
Marijuana
Psychoactive drugs, including antidepressants

**Neoplastic Causes**
Prolactin-secreting pituitary adenomas
Craniopharyngioma
Hypothalamic hamartoma

**Psychogenic Causes**
Chronic anxiety
Pseudocyesis
Anorexia nervosa

**Other Causes**
Head injury
Chronic medical illness

## HYPOTHALAMIC–PITUITARY DYSFUNCTION

Release of hypothalamic gonadotropin-releasing hormone (GnRH) occurs in a pulsatile fashion, modulated by catecholamine secretion from the central nervous system and by feedback of sex steroids from the ovaries. When this pulsatile secretion of GnRH is disrupted or altered, the anterior pituitary gland is not stimulated to secrete follicle-stimulating hormone (FSH) and luteinizing hormone (LH). The result is an absence of folliculogenesis despite estrogen production, no ovulation, and lack of corpus luteum with its usual production of estrogen and progesterone. Because of the lack of sex hormone production with no stimulation of the endometrium, there is no menstruation.

Alterations in catecholamine secretion and metabolism in sex steroid hormone feedback or an alteration of blood flow through the hypothalamic–pituitary portal plexus can disrupt the signaling process that leads to ovulation. This latter disruption can be caused by tumors or infiltrative processes that impinge on the pituitary stalk and alter blood flow.

The most common causes of hypothalamic–pituitary dysfunction are presented in Box 35.2. Most hypothalamic–pituitary amenorrhea is of functional origin and can be corrected by modifying causal behavior, by stimulating gonadotropin secretion, or by giving exogenous human menopausal gonadotropins.

The physician cannot differentiate hypothalamic–pituitary causes of amenorrhea from ovarian or genital outflow causes by medical history or even physical examination alone. However, there are some clues in the medical history and physical examination that would suggest a hypothalamic–pituitary etiology for amenorrhea. A his-

tory of any condition listed in Box 35.2 should cause the physician to consider hypothalamic–pituitary dysfunction.

*The definitive method to identify hypothalamic–pituitary dysfunction is to measure FSH, LH, and prolactin levels in the blood. In these conditions, FSH and LH levels are in the low range. The prolactin level is normal in most conditions, but is elevated in prolactin-secreting pituitary adenomas.*

## OVARIAN DYSFUNCTION

In ovarian failure, the ovarian follicles are either exhausted or are resistant to stimulation by pituitary FSH and LH. *As the ovaries cease functioning, blood concentrations of FSH and LH increase.* Women with ovarian failure experience the symptoms and signs of estrogen deficiency. A summary of causes is presented in Box 35.3.

## ALTERATION OF THE GENITAL OUTFLOW TRACT

Obstruction of the genital outflow tract prevents overt menstrual bleeding even if ovulation occurs. *Most cases of outflow obstruction result from congenital abnormalities in the*

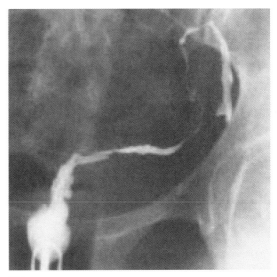

**(A)**

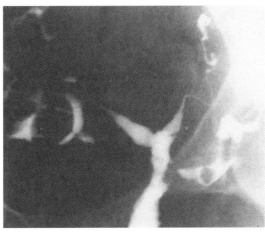

**(B)**

FIGURE 35.1. Asherman syndrome. A. Hysterosalpingogram of a patient with Asherman syndrome. Note the thin sliver of endometrial cavity. B. The same patient after hysteroscopic resection of intrauterine adhesions. Both fallopian tubes are now visualized. (Knockenhauer ES, Blackwell RE. Operative hysteroscopic procedures. In: Azziz R, Murphy AA, eds. *Practical Manual of Operative Laparoscopy and Hysteroscopy.* 2nd ed. New York: Spring-Verlag; 1997:290.)

*development and canalization of the müllerian ducts.* Imperforate hymen and no uterus or vagina are the most common anomalies that result in primary amenorrhea. Surgical correction of an imperforate hymen allows for menstruation and fertility. Less-commonly encountered anomalies, such as a transverse vaginal septum, are more difficult to correct, and even with attempted surgical correction, menstruation and fertility are often not restored.

*Scarring of the uterine cavity (Asherman syndrome) is the most frequent anatomic cause of secondary amenorrhea* (Fig. 35.1). Women who undergo dilation and curettage (D&C) for retained products of pregnancy (especially when infection is present) are at risk for developing scarring of the endometrium. Cases of mild scarring can be corrected by surgical lysis of the adhesions performed by hysteroscopy and D&C. However, severe cases are often refractory to therapy. Estrogen therapy should be added to the surgical treatment postoperatively to stimulate endometrial regeneration of the denuded areas. In some cases, a balloon or intrauterine (contraceptive) device may be placed in the uterine cavity to help keep the uterine walls apart during healing.

## Treatment of Amenorrhea

The first step is to establish a cause for the amenorrhea. The progesterone "challenge test" is commonly used to determine whether or not the patient has adequate estrogen, a competent endometrium, and a patent outflow tract. An injection of 100 mg of progesterone in oil or a 5-day to 14-day course of oral medroxyprogesterone acetate or micronized progesterone is expected to induce progesterone withdrawal bleeding within a few days after completing the oral course. If bleeding does occur, the patient is likely to be anovulatory or oligo-ovulatory. If withdrawal bleeding does not occur, the patient may be hypoestrogenic or have an anatomic condition such as Asherman syndrome or outflow tract obstruction.

*Hyperprolactinemia associated with some pituitary adenomas (or other medical conditions) results in amenorrhea and galactorrhea (a milky discharge from the breast).* Approximately 80% of all pituitary tumors secrete prolactin, causing galactorrhea, and these patients are treated with either cabergoline (Dostinex) or the dopamine agonist bromocriptine (Parlodel). In approximately 5% of patients with hyperprolactinemia and galactorrhea, the underlying etiology is hypothyroidism. A low serum thyroxine (T4) level eliminates negative feedback signaling to the hypothalamic–pituitary axis. As a result, TRH (thyrotropin-releasing hormone) levels increase. Positive feedback signaling that stimulates dopamine secretion is also absent, causing a decrease in dopamine levels. Elevated TRH stimulates release of prolactin from the pituitary gland. The reduced dopamine secretion results in elevated levels of TSH (thyroid-stimulating hormone) and prolactin.

In patients who desire pregnancy, ovulation can be induced through the use of clomiphene citrate, human menopausal gonadotropins, pulsatile GnRH, or aromatase inhibitors. In patients who are oligo-ovulatory or anovulatory (polycystic ovary syndrome), ovulation can usually be induced with clomiphene citrate. In patients with hypogonadotropic hypogonadism, ovulation can be induced with pulsatile GnRH or human menopausal gonadotropins. Women with genital tract obstruction require surgery to create a vagina or to restore genital tract integrity. Menstruation will never be established if the uterus is absent. Women with premature menopause may require exogenous estrogen therapy.

## ABNORMAL UTERINE BLEEDING

Failure to ovulate results in either amenorrhea or irregular uterine bleeding. Irregular bleeding that is unrelated to anatomic lesions of the uterus is referred to as **anovulatory uterine bleeding.** It is most likely to occur in association with anovulation as found in polycystic ovarian disease, exogenous obesity, or adrenal hyperplasia.

*Women with hypothalamic amenorrhea (hypothalamic–pituitary dysfunction) and no genital tract obstruction are in a state of estrogen deficiency.* Estrogen is inadequate to stimulate growth and development of the endometrium. Therefore, there is inadequate endometrium for uterine bleeding to occur. *In contrast, women with oligo-ovulation and anovulation with abnormal uterine bleeding have constant, noncyclic blood estrogen concentrations that stimulate growth and development of the endometrium.* Without the predictable effect of ovulation, progesterone-induced changes do not occur. Initially, these patients have amenorrhea because of the chronic, constant estrogen levels but, eventually, the endometrium outgrows its blood supply and sloughs from the uterus at irregular times and in unpredictable amounts (see Box 35.1).

When there is chronic stimulation of the endometrium from low plasma concentrations of estrogens, the episodes of uterine bleeding are infrequent and light. Alternatively, with chronic stimulation of the endometrium from increased plasma concentrations of estrogens, the episodes of uterine bleeding can be frequent and heavy. Because amenorrhea and abnormal uterine bleeding both result from anovulation, it is not surprising that they can occur at different times in the same patient.

Subtle alterations in the mechanisms of ovulation can produce abnormal cycles, even when ovulation occurs (e.g., the luteal phase defect). In the **luteal phase defect,** ovulation does occur; however, the corpus luteum of the ovary is not fully developed to secrete adequate quantities of progesterone to support the endometrium for the usual

13 to 14 days and is not adequate to support a pregnancy if conception does occur. The menstrual cycle is shortened, and menstruation occurs earlier than expected. Although this is not classical anovulatory uterine bleeding, it is considered to be in the same category. Another example is midcycle spotting, in which patients report bleeding at the time of ovulation. In the absence of demonstrable pathology, this self-limited bleeding can be attributed to the sudden drop in estrogen level that occurs at this time of the cycle.

## Diagnosis of Abnormal Uterine Bleeding

Diagnosis of abnormal uterine bleeding should be suspected when vaginal bleeding is not regular, not predictable, and not associated with premenstrual signs and symptoms that usually accompany ovulatory cycles. These signs and symptoms include breast fullness, abdominal bloating, mood changes, edema, weight gain, and uterine cramps.

> *Before anovulatory uterine bleeding can be diagnosed, anatomic causes including neoplasia should be excluded.*

In a reproductive-aged woman, complications of pregnancy as a cause of irregular vaginal bleeding should be excluded. Other anatomic causes of irregular vaginal bleeding include uterine leiomyomata, inflammation or infection of the genital tract, hyperplasia or carcinoma of the cervix or endometrium, cervical and endometrial polyps, and lesions of the vagina (Box 35.4). Pelvic ultrasonography or sonohysterography may assist in diagnosing these lesions. Women with organic causes for bleeding may have regular ovulatory cycles with superimposed irregular bleeding.

If the diagnosis is uncertain based on history and physical examination alone, a woman may keep a basal body temperature chart for 6 to 8 weeks to look for the shift in the basal temperature that occurs with ovulation. An ovulation predictor kit may also be used. Luteal phase progestin may also be measured. In cases of anovulation and abnormal bleeding, an endometrial biopsy may reveal endometrial hyperplasia. Because abnormal uterine bleeding results from chronic, unopposed estrogenic stimulation of the endometrium, the endometrium appears proliferative or, with prolonged estrogenic stimulation, hyperplastic. Without treatment, these women are at increased risk for endometrial cancer.

## Treatment of Abnormal Uterine Bleeding

The risks to a woman with anovulatory uterine bleeding include anemia, incapacitating blood loss, endometrial hyperplasia, and carcinoma. Uterine bleeding can be severe enough to require hospitalization. Both hemor-

---

> ### BOX 35.4
> ### Anatomic Causes of Abnormal Uterine Bleeding
>
> Uterine Lesions
>   Myomas
>   Polyps
>   Endometrial carcinoma
>
> Cervical Lesions
>   Neoplasia
>   Polyps
>   Cervicitis
>   Cervical condyloma
>
> Vaginal Lesions
>   Carcinoma, sarcoma, or adenosis
>   Laceration or trauma
>   Infections
>   Inflammation or ulceration secondary to foreign
>     bodies
>
> Bleeding from Other Sites
>   Urethral caruncle
>   Infected urethral diverticulum
>   Gastrointestinal bleeding
>   Labial lesion (neoplasm, trauma, infection)

rhage and endometrial hyperplasia can be prevented by appropriate management.

*The primary goal of treatment of anovulatory uterine bleeding is to ensure regular shedding of the endometrium and consequent regulation of uterine bleeding.* If ovulation is achieved, conversion of the proliferative endometrium into secretory endometrium will result in predictable uterine withdrawal bleeding.

A progestational agent may be administered for a minimum of 10 days. The most commonly used agent is medroxyprogesterone acetate. When the progestational agent is discontinued, uterine withdrawal bleeding ensues, thereby mimicking physiologic withdrawal of progesterone.

As an alternative, administration of oral contraceptives suppresses the endometrium and establishes regular, predictable withdrawal cycles. No particular oral contraceptive preparation is better than any of the others for this purpose. Women who take oral contraceptives as treatment of abnormal uterine bleeding often resume abnormal uterine bleeding after therapy is discontinued.

If a patient is being treated for a particularly heavy bleeding episode, once organic pathology has been ruled out, treatment should focus on two issues: (1) control of the acute episode, and (2) prevention of future recurrences. Both high-dose estrogen and progestin therapy as well as combination treatment (oral contraceptive pills, four per day) have been advocated for management of heavy abnormal bleeding in the acute phase. Long-term preventive management may include either intermittent progestin treatment or oral contraceptives. Uterine bleeding that does not respond to medical therapy often is managed surgically with endometrial ablation or hysterectomy. Before proceeding with endometrial ablation, one must rule out endometrial carcinoma.

## SUGGESTED READINGS

ACOG Committee on Adolescent Health Care. Menstruation in girls and adolescents: using the menstrual cycle as a vital sign. ACOG Committee Opinion No. 349. *Obstet Gynecol.* 2006;108(5): 1323–1328.

American College of Obstetricians and Gynecologists. *Abnormal Uterine Bleeding.* ACOG Patient Education Pamphlet AP095. Washington, DC: American College of Obstetricians and Gynecologists; 2008. http://www.acog.org/publications/patient_ education/bp095.cfm. Accessed October 27, 2008.

American College of Obstetricians and Gynecologists. *Guidelines for Women's Health Care: A Resource Manual.* 3rd ed. Washington, DC: American College of Obstetricians and Gynecologists; 2007.

American College of Obstetricians and Gynecologists. *Management of Anovulatory Bleeding.* ACOG Practice Bulletin 14. Washington, DC: American College of Obstetricians and Gynecologists; 2000.

American College of Obstetricians and Gynecologists. *Quality Improvement in Women's Health Care.* Washington, DC: American College of Obstetricians and Gynecologists; 2000:55.

Bruce CR. Abnormal uterine bleeding. In: *Precis, An Update in Obstetrics and Gynecology: Reproductive Endocrinology.* 3rd ed. Washington, DC: American College of Obstetricians and Gynecologists; 2007: 69–80.

Guzick DS. Polycystic ovary syndrome. *Obstet Gynecol.* 2004;103(1): 181–193.

# 36 Hirsutism and Virilization

This chapter deals primarily with APGO Educational Topic:

Topic 44: Hirsutism and Virilization

Students should be able to describe variations in hirsutism and virilization; discuss the relationship of ovarian, adrenal, pituitary, and pharmacologic causes of hirsutism and virilization; and discuss the evaluation and management of hirsutism and virilization.

**H**irsutism *is excess terminal hair in a male pattern of distribution.* It is manifested initially by the appearance of midline terminal hair. Terminal hair is darker, coarser, and kinkier than vellus hair, which is soft, downy, and fine. Care must be taken to evaluate the possibility that excess terminal hair is familial, not pathological, in origin. A scale used for the evaluation of hirsutism is shown in Figure 36.1. When a woman is exposed to excess androgens, terminal hair first appears on the lower abdomen and around the nipples, next around the chin and upper lip, and finally between the breasts and on the lower back. Usually, a woman with hirsutism also has acne. For women in Western cultures, terminal hair on the abdomen, breasts, and face is considered unsightly and presents a cosmetic problem. As a result, at the first sign of hirsutism, women often consult their physician to seek a cause for the excess hair growth and seek treatment to eliminate it.

*Virilization is defined as masculinization of a woman and is associated with a marked increase in circulating* **testosterone.** As a woman becomes virilized, she first notices enlargement of the clitoris, followed by temporal balding, deepening of the voice, involution of the breasts, and a remodeling of the limb–shoulder girdle as well as hirsutism. Over time, she takes on a more masculine appearance.

Hirsutism and virilization may be clinical clues to an underlying androgen excess disorder.

> *When evaluating and treating hirsutism and virilization, the sites of androgen production and the mechanisms of androgen action should be considered.*

Idiopathic (constitutional or familial) hirsutism (a diagnosis of exclusion) is the most common nonpathologic etiology, representing about one-half of all cases. The most common pathologic causes of hirsutism are polycystic ovarian syndrome, followed by congenital adrenal hyperplasia. These conditions must be diagnosed by laboratory evaluations. Treatment of androgen excess should be directed at suppressing the source of androgen excess or blocking androgen action at the receptor site.

## ANDROGEN PRODUCTION AND ANDROGEN ACTION

In women, **androgens** are produced in the adrenal glands, the ovaries, and adipose tissue, where there is extraglandular production of testosterone from androstenedione. The following three androgens may be measured when evaluating a woman with hirsutism and virilization.

1. **Dehydroepiandrosterone** (DHEA): a weak androgen secreted principally by the adrenal glands. (This is generally measured as dehydroepiandrosterone sulfate [DHEA-S] because of its longer half-life, making it a more reliable measure.)
2. **Androstenedione:** a weak androgen secreted in equal amounts by the adrenal glands and ovaries.
3. **Testosterone:** a potent androgen secreted by the adrenal glands and ovaries and produced in adipose tissue from the conversion of androstenedione.

The sites of androgen production and proportions produced are presented in Table 36.1. In addition, testosterone is also converted within hair follicles and within genital skin to **dihydrotestosterone** (DHT), which is an androgen even more potent than testosterone. This metabolic conversion is the result of the local action of $5\alpha$-reductase on testosterone at these sites. This is the basis for constitutional hirsutism, which is discussed later.

Adrenal androgen production is controlled by reciprocal feedback regulation through pituitary secretion of adrenocorticotropic hormone (ACTH). ACTH stimulates the adrenal cortical production of cortisol. In the metabolic

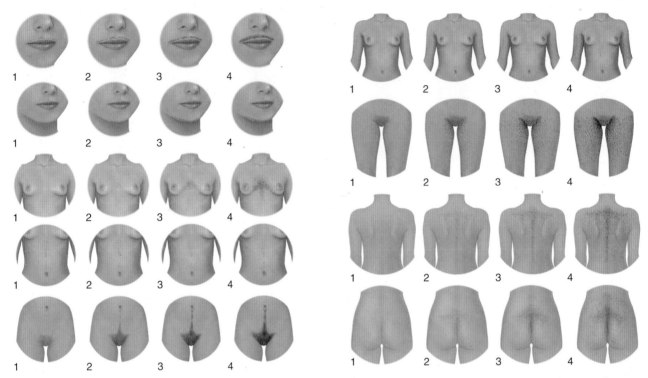

FIGURE 36.1. Modified Ferriman-Gallwey scale, a clinical tool for assessing the extent and distribution of hirsutism.

sequence of cortisol production, DHEA is one precursor hormone. In enzymatic deficiencies of adrenal steroidogenesis (21-hydroxylase deficiency and 11β-hydroxylase deficiency), DHEA accumulates and is further metabolized to androstenedione and testosterone. The flow of adrenal hormone production is shown in Figure 36.2.

Ovarian androgen production is regulated by luteinizing hormone (LH) secretion from the pituitary gland. LH stimulates theca-lutein cells surrounding the ovarian follicles to secrete androstenedione and, to a lesser extent, testosterone. These androgens are precursors for estrogen production by granulosa cells of the ovarian follicles. In conditions of sustained or increased LH secretion, androstenedione and testosterone increase.

Extraglandular testosterone production occurs in adipocytes (fat cells) and depends on the magnitude of adrenal and ovarian androstenedione production. When androstenedione production increases, there is a dependent increase in extraglandular testosterone production. When a woman becomes obese, the conversion of androstenedione to testosterone is increased.

*Testosterone is the primary androgen that causes increased hair growth, acne, and the physical changes associated with virilization.* After testosterone is secreted, it is bound to a carrier protein—**sex hormone-binding globulin** (SHBG)—and primarily circulates in plasma as a bound steroid hormone. Bound testosterone is unable to attach to testosterone receptors and is, therefore, metabolically inactive. Only a small fraction (1% to 3%) of testosterone is unbound (free). This small fraction of free hormones exerts the effects. The liver produces SHBG. Estrogens stimulate hepatic production of SHBG. Greater estrogen production is associated

**TABLE 36.1  Sites of Androgen Production**

| Site | DHEA-S(%) | Androstenedione (%) | Testosterone (%) |
|---|---|---|---|
| Adrenal glands | 90 | 50 | 25 |
| Ovaries | 10 | 50 | 25 |
| Extraglandular | 0 | 0 | 50 |

DHEA-S = dehydroepiandrosterone sulfate.

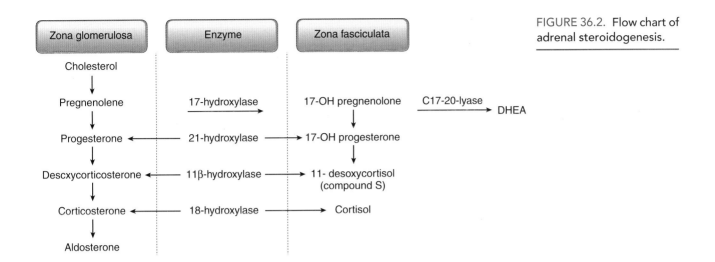

FIGURE 36.2. Flow chart of adrenal steroidogenesis.

with less free testosterone, whereas decreased estrogen production is associated with increased free testosterone. Therefore, measurement of total testosterone alone may not reflect the amount of biologically active testosterone.

**Testosterone receptors** are scattered throughout the body. For the purpose of this discussion, testosterone receptors are considered only in hair follicles, sebaceous glands, and genital skin. Free testosterone enters the cytosol of testosterone-dependent cells. There it is bound to a testosterone receptor and carried into the nucleus of the cell to initiate its metabolic action. *When testosterone is excessive, increased hair growth, acne, and rugation of the genital skin is seen.* Some individuals have increased 5α-reductase within hair follicles, resulting in excessive local production of DHT.

Excess androgen production has several causes, including polycystic ovarian syndrome, testosterone-secreting tumors, adrenal disorders, and iatrogenic and idiopathic causes. Figure 36.3 presents a scheme for the evaluation of hirsutism that encompasses the various conditions that lead to this condition.

## POLYCYSTIC OVARY SYNDROME

*Polycystic ovary syndrome (PCOS) is the most common cause of androgen excess and hirsutism.*

The etiology of this disorder is unknown. Some cases appear to result from a genetic predisposition, whereas others seem to result from obesity or other causes of LH excess.

*Symptoms of PCOS include oligomenorrhea or amenorrhea, acne, hirsutism, and infertility.* The disorder is characterized by chronic anovulation or extended periods of infrequent ovulation (oligo-ovulation). It is a syndrome primarily defined by excess androgen. The definition of PCOS has varied in the past, resulting in the National Institutes of Health (NIH)-convening consensus conferences in 1990 and 2000. In 2003 the Rotterdam consensus workshop

developed a more encompassing definition of PCOS. To establish the diagnosis, the patient should have two of the following criteria:

- Oligo-ovulation or anovulation usually marked by irregular menstrual cycles
- Biochemical or clinical evidence of hyperandrogenism
- Polycystic appearing ovaries on ultrasound (Fig. 36.4)

It is also important to rule out other endocrine disorders that can mimic PCOS, such as congenital adrenal hyperplasia, Cushing syndrome, and hyperprolactinemia.

*In many women with PCOS, obesity seems to be the common factor (seen in 50% of patients), and the acquisition of body fat coincides with the onset of PCOS.* In fact, Stein and Leventhal first described PCOS as women with hirsutism, irregular cycles, and obesity. (PCOS was originally called Stein-Leventhal syndrome.) PCOS is related to obesity by the following mechanism: LH stimulates the theca-lutein cells to increase androstenedione production. Androstenedione undergoes aromatization to estrone within adipocytes. Although estrone is a weak estrogen, it has a positive-feedback action or stimulating effect on the pituitary secretion of LH. LH secretion is, therefore, stimulated by increased estrogen. With increasing obesity comes increased conversion of androstenedione to estrone. With the increased rise in androstenedione, there is coincident increased testosterone production, which causes acne and hirsutism (Fig. 36.5).

*Hormonal studies in women with PCOS show the following: (1) increased LH:FSH (follicle-stimulating hormone) ratio, (2) estrone in greater concentration than estradiol, (3) androstenedione at the upper limits of normal or increased, and (4) testosterone at the upper limits of normal or slightly increased.*

Therefore, PCOS can be viewed as one of excess androgen and excess estrogen. The unopposed long-term elevated

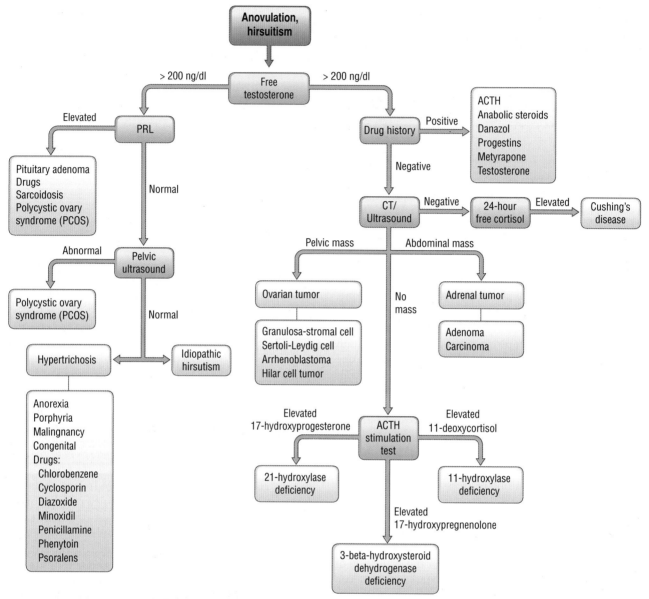

FIGURE 36.3. Scheme for the evaluation of hirsutism. ACTH = adrenocorticotropic hormone; CT = computed tomography; PRL = prolactin.

estrogen levels that characterize PCOS increases the risk of abnormal uterine bleeding, endometrial hyperplasia, and, in some cases, the development of endometrial carcinoma.

The typical woman with PCOS has many of the signs of **metabolic syndrome** (Syndrome X). Approximately 40% of patients with PCOS have impaired glucose tolerance, and 8% have overt type 2 diabetes mellitus. These patients should be screened for diabetes. Classic lipid abnormalities include elevated triglyceride levels, low high-density lipoprotein (HDL) levels, and elevated low-density lipoprotein (LDL) levels. Hypertension is also common in individuals with this condition. The combination of the preceding abnormalities potentially increases the risk of cardiovascular disease.

**Acanthosis nigricans** has also been found in a significant percentage of these patients. The HAIR-AN syndrome (*h*yperandrogenism, *i*nsulin resistance, *a*canthosis *n*igricans) constitutes a defined subgroup of patients with PCOS. Administration of the insulin-sensitizing agent metformin in these patients also reduces androgen and insulin levels.

*PCOS is a functional disorder whose treatment should be targeted to interrupt the disorder's positive-feedback cycle.*

The most common therapy for PCOS is the administration of oral contraceptives, which suppresses pituitary LH

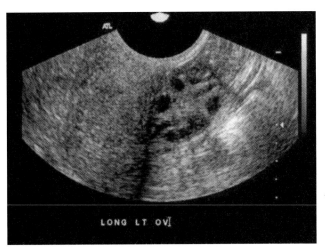

FIGURE 36.4. Ultrasound of polycystic ovary showing the characteristic "string-of-pearls" appearance of the cysts. (From Guzick DS. Polycystic ovary syndrome. *Obstet Gynecol.* 2004;103(1):187.)

production. Suppressing LH causes decreased production of androstenedione and testosterone. The ovarian contribution to the total androgen pool is thereby decreased. Acne clears, new hair growth is prevented, and there is decreased androgenic stimulation of existing hair follicles. By preventing estrogen excess, oral contraceptives also prevent endometrial hyperplasia, and women have cyclic, predictable, withdrawal bleeding episodes.

*If a woman with PCOS wishes to conceive, oral contraceptive therapy is not a suitable choice.* If the patient is obese, a weight-reduction diet designed to restore the patient to a normal weight should be encouraged. *With body weight reduction alone, many women resume regular ovulatory cycles and conceive spontaneously.* In some women, ovulation induction with clomiphene citrate is needed and is facilitated by weight reduction. Insulin sensitizers (metformin) alone or with clomiphene citrate may be used to reduce insulin resistance, control weight, and facilitate ovulation.

*Hyperthecosis is a more severe form of PCOS.* In cases of hyperthecosis, androstenedione production may be so great that testosterone reaches concentrations that cause virilization. Women with this condition may exhibit temporal balding, clitoral enlargement, deepening of the voice, and remodeling at the limb–shoulder girdle. Hyperthecosis is often refractory to oral contraceptive suppression. It is also more difficult to successfully induce ovulation in women with this condition.

## OVARIAN NEOPLASMS

Several androgen-secreting ovarian tumors can cause hirsutism and virilization, including Sertoli-Leydig cell tumors and three rare neoplasms.

### Sertoli–Leydig Cell Tumors

*Sertoli–Leydig cell tumors (also called androblastoma and arrhenoblastoma) are ovarian neoplasms that secrete testosterone.* These tumors constitute <0.4% of ovarian tumors and usually occur in women between the ages of 20 and 40. *The tumor is most often unilateral (95% of cases) and may reach a size of 7 to 10 cm in diameter.*

The history and physical examination give critical clues in diagnosing subjects who present with hirsutism and testosterone-secreting ovarian tumors. Testosterone-

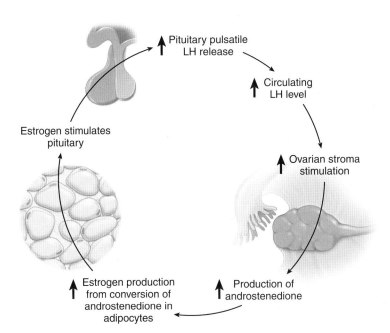

FIGURE 36.5. Proposed mechanism that demonstrates how obesity leads to polycystic ovary syndrome. LH = luteinizing hormone.

secreting tumors usually have a more rapid onset and more severe hirsutism with virilizing signs. *Women with a Sertoli–Leydig cell tumor have a rapid onset of acne, hirsutism (75% of patients), amenorrhea (30% of patients), and virilization.* A characteristic clinical course of two overlapping stages is described: first, the stage of defeminization, characterized by amenorrhea, breast atrophy, and loss of the subcutaneous fatty deposits responsible for the rounding of the feminine figure; and second, the stage of masculinization, characterized by clitoral hypertrophy, hirsutism, and deepening of the voice. These changes may occur over 6 months or less.

Laboratory studies of this disorder show suppression of FSH and LH, low plasma androstenedione, and marked elevation of testosterone. An ovarian mass may be palpable on pelvic examination. Once the diagnosis is suspected, there should be no delay in surgical removal of the involved ovary. The contralateral ovary should be inspected, and if it is found to be enlarged, it should be bisected for gross inspection.

Following surgical removal of a Sertoli–Leydig cell tumor, ovulatory cycles return spontaneously, and further progression of hirsutism is arrested. If the clitoris has become enlarged, it does not revert to its pretreatment size. However, temporal hair is restored, and the body habitus becomes feminine once again. Terminal hair in a sexual distribution will not revert to vellus hair, but the growth and pigmentation will slow. Most patients will require mechanical removal of excess hair following removal of the ovarian tumor. *The 10-year survival rates for this low-grade malignant ovarian tumor approximate 90% to 95%.*

## Uncommon Virilizing Ovarian Tumors

**Gynandroblastoma** is a rare ovarian tumor, having both granulosa cell and arrhenoblastoma components. The predominant clinical feature is masculinization, although estrogen production may simultaneously produce endometrial hyperplasia and irregular uterine bleeding.

**Lipid (lipoid) cell tumors** are usually small ovarian tumors containing sheets of round, clear, pale-staining cells with a differential histologic diagnosis of hilar cell tumors, stromal luteoma of pregnancy, and Sertoli–Leydig cell tumors. The clinical presentation is masculinization or defeminization associated with elevated 17-ketosteroids in many cases.

**Hilar cell tumors** arise from an overgrowth of mature hilar cells or from ovarian mesenchyme and are typically found in postmenopausal women. They are characterized clinically by masculinization, which supports the idea that hilar cells are the homologs of the interstitial or Leydig cells of the testis. Histologically, the tumors contain pathognomonic Reinke albuminoid crystals in most cases, and grossly, they are always small, unilateral, and benign. Treatment is surgical removal for these three rare tumors.

## ADRENAL ANDROGEN EXCESS DISORDERS

Adrenal disorders that cause an increase in androgen production can lead to hirsutism and virilization; the most common are congenital adrenal hyperplasia, Cushing syndrome, and adrenal neoplasms.

## Congenital Adrenal Hyperplasia

**Congenital adrenal hyperplasia** (CAH) is caused by enzyme deficiencies that result in precursor (substrate) excess, thus resulting in androgen excess. DHEA is a precursor for androstenedione and testosterone.

*The most common cause of increased adrenal androgen production is adrenal hyperplasia as a result of 21-hydroxylase deficiency; 21-hydroxylase catalyzes the conversion of progesterone and 17α-hydroxyprogesterone to desoxycorticosterone and compound S.*

When 21-hydroxylase is deficient, there is an accumulation of progesterone and 17α-hydroxyprogesterone, which are metabolized subsequently to DHEA. This disorder affects approximately 2% of the population and is caused by an alteration in the genes for 21-hydroxylase, which are carried on chromosome 6. The genetic defect is autosomal recessive and has variable penetrance.

*In the most severe form of 21-hydroxylase deficiency, the newly born female infant is simply virilized (ambiguous genitalia) or is virilized and suffers from life-threatening salt wasting (Box 36.1).* However, milder forms are more common and can appear at puberty or even later in adult life. A mild deficiency of 21-hydroxylase is frequently associated with

---

**BOX 36.1**

**Manifestations of 21-Hydrolase Deficiency**

- **Severe:**
  - Newborn female infant
  - Virilized (ambiguous genitalia), or virilized and has life-threatening salt wasting
- **Mild:**
  - Frequently associated with terminal body hair, acne, subtle alterations in menstrual cycles and infertility
  - Patients can also have sonographic evidence of polycystic-appearing ovaries.
- **Manifested at puberty**
  - Adrenarche may precede thelarche.
  - History of pubic hair growth occurring before the onset of breast development may be a clinical clue.

terminal body hair, acne, subtle alterations in menstrual cycles, and infertility. These patients can also have sonographic evidence of polycystic-appearing ovaries. *When 21-hydroxylase deficiency is manifested at puberty, adrenarche may precede thelarche.* The history of pubic hair growth occurring before the onset of breast development may be a clinical clue to this disorder. The diagnosis of 21-hydroxylase deficiency is made by measuring increased 17-OH progesterone in plasma during the follicular phase (preferably measured while fasting). Patients with classic 21-hydroxylase deficiency will have significantly elevated plasma 17-OH progesterone levels, usually over 2000 ng/dL. Those with less severe 21-hydroxylase deficiency may have mildly elevated basal levels, 200 ng/dL, and an increase to usually 1000 ng/dL in response to ACTH stimulation. Dehydroepiandrosterone sulfate (DHEA-S) and androstenedione will also be elevated and contribute to the hirsutism and virilizing signs.

*A less-common cause of adrenal hyperplasia is 11β-hydroxylase deficiency.* The enzyme 11β-hydroxylase catalyzes the conversion of desoxycorticosterone to cortisol. A deficiency in this enzyme also results in increased androgen production. The clinical features of 11β-hydroxylase deficiency are mild hypertension and mild hirsutism. The diagnosis of 11β-hydroxylase deficiency is made by demonstrating increased plasma desoxycorticosterone.

Treatment of CAH is aimed at restoring normal cortisol levels. In CAH, cortisol production is reduced secondary to enzymatic block. This decreased cortisol production results in a compensatory increase in ACTH secretion to attempt to stimulate cortisol production. This increased ACTH production results in the oversecretion of precursor molecules proximal to the enzymatic block, which results in oversecretion of androgens. In patients with a high-grade enzymatic block, inadequate amounts of glucocorticoids and mineralocorticoids are made, resulting in salt loss, which can be life-threatening. *Nonclassic CAH can be managed easily by supplementing glucocorticoids.* Usually, prednisone, 2.5 mg daily (or its equivalent), suppresses adrenal androgen production to within the normal range. When this therapy is instituted, facial acne usually clears promptly, ovulation is restored, and there is no new terminal hair growth.

*Medical therapy for adrenal and ovarian disorders cannot resolve hirsutism.* It can only suppress new hair growth. Hair that is present must be controlled by shaving, bleaching, using depilatory agents, by electrolysis or laser hair ablation.

## Cushing Syndrome

**Cushing syndrome** *is an adrenal disease resulting in adrenal excess.* As a result of an adrenal neoplasm or an ACTH-producing tumor, the patient demonstrates signs of corticosteroid excess that include truncal obesity, moonlike facies, glucose intolerance, skin thinning with striae, osteo-

porosis, proximal muscle weakness in addition to evidence of hyperandrogenism, and menstrual irregularities.

## Adrenal Neoplasms

Androgen-secreting adrenal adenomas cause a rapid increase in hair growth associated with severe acne, amenorrhea, and sometimes virilization. In androgen-secreting adenomas, DHEA-S is usually elevated above 6 mg/mL. The diagnosis of this rare tumor is established by computed axial tomography (CAT) or magnetic resonance imaging (MRI) of the adrenal glands. Adrenal adenomas must be removed surgically.

## CONSTITUTIONAL HIRSUTISM

Occasionally after a diagnostic evaluation for hirsutism, there is no explanation for the cause of the disorder. By exclusion, this condition is often called **constitutional hirsutism.** Data support the hypothesis that women with constitutional hirsutism have greater activity of 5α-reductase than do unaffected women.

Treatment of constitutional hirsutism is primarily androgen blockade and mechanical removal of the excess hair. Spironolactone 100 mg/day is the most commonly used androgen blocker. Spironolactone also inhibits testosterone production by the ovary and reduces 5α-reductase activity. Other androgen blockers include flutamide and cyproterone acetate. The activity of 5α-reductase can also be inhibited directly through the use of drugs such as finasteride (5 mg orally daily). Eflornithine hydrochloride 13.9% is an irreversible inhibitor of L-ornithine decarboxylase, which slows and shrinks hair. This cream has been approved for facial use with satisfactory local effects. Patients taking an androgen receptor or 5α-reductase blocker should be placed on concomitant oral contraceptives because of the teratogenic and demasculinizing effects on a fetus should pregnancy occur. Oral contraceptives may also improve the efficacy of these treatments through the decreased androgen and increased SHBG production effects associated with their use.

## IATROGENIC ANDROGEN EXCESS

Some drugs with androgen activity have been implicated in hirsutism and virilization, including danazol and progestin-containing oral contraceptives.

## Danazol

*Danazol is an attenuated androgen used for the suppression of pelvic endometriosis.* It has androgenic properties, and some women develop hirsutism, acne, and deepening of the voice while taking the drug. If these symptoms occur, the value of the danazol should be weighed against the side effects before continuing therapy. Symptoms of voice changes may be irreversible upon discontinuation of treatment. Pregnancy should be ruled out before initiating a course of danazol therapy, because it can produce virilization of the female fetus.

## Oral Contraceptives

The progestins in oral contraceptives are impeded androgens. Rarely, a woman taking oral contraceptives develops acne and even hirsutism. If this occurs, another product with a less-androgenic progestin should be selected, or the pill should be discontinued. Moreover, evaluation for the coincidental development of late-onset adrenal hyperplasia should be done.

## SUGGESTED READINGS

American College of Obstetricians and Gynecologists. *Guidelines for Women's Health Care: A Resource Manual.* 3rd ed. Washington, DC: ACOG; 2007.

American College of Obstetrics and Gynecology. *Management of Anovulatory Bleeding. ACOG Practice Bulletin No. 14.* Washington, DC: ACOG;2000.

American College of Obstetricians and Gynecologists. Management of infertility caused by ovulatory dysfunction. ACOG Practice Bulletin No. 34. *Obstet Gynecol.* 2002;99(2):347–358.

American College of Obstetricians and Gynecologists. Polycystic ovary syndrome. ACOG Practice Bulletin No. 41. *Obstet Gynecol.* 2002;100(6):1389–1402. [Reaffirmed 2006]

*Precis, An Update in Obstetrics and Gynecology: Reproductive Endocrinology.* 3rd ed. Washington, DC: American College of Obstetricians and Gynecologists; 2007: 84–96.

# 37 Menopause

Topic 47: Menopause

Students should be able to define perimenopause and menopause and describe the neuroendocrine changes associated with each and the results of these changes, as well as the evaluation and management of each of these life stages, including counseling and hormonal and nonhormonal management regimens.

**M**enopause *is the permanent cessation of menses after cessation of estrogen production.* **Perimenopause** *is the period before menopause, i.e., the transition from the reproductive to the nonreproductive years. The time period during which the changes of menopause occur is called the* **climacteric.** An increasing proportion of American women are included in these groups, because the female life expectancy has lengthened and the number of women in this age group is expanding (Fig. 37.1). Many women are expected to live 30 to 35 years—one third of their life expectancy—after menopause.

## MENSTRUATION AND MENOPAUSE

Whereas male gametes are renewed on a daily basis, female gametes are of a fixed number that is progressively reduced throughout a woman's reproductive life. At the time of birth, the female infant has approximately 1 to 2 million oocytes; by puberty, she has approximately 400,000 oocytes remaining. By age 30 to 35, the number of oocytes will have decreased to approximately 100,000. For the remaining reproductive years, the process of oocyte maturation and ovulation becomes increasingly inefficient.

A woman ovulates approximately 400 oocytes during her reproductive years. The process of **oocyte selection** is complex and new information is making the process clearer. During the reproductive cycle, a cohort of oocytes is stimulated to begin maturation, but only 1 or 2 dominant follicles complete the process and are eventually ovulated.

**Follicular maturation** is induced and stimulated by the pituitary release of the follicle-stimulating hormone (FSH) and luteinizing hormone (LH). FSH binds to its receptors in the follicular membrane of the oocyte and stimulates follicular maturation, providing estradiol ($E_2$), which is the major estrogen of the reproductive years. LH stimulates the theca luteal cells surrounding the oocyte to produce androgens as well as estrogens and serves as the triggering mechanism to induce ovulation. With advanc-

ing reproductive age, the remaining oocytes become increasingly resistant to FSH. Thus, plasma concentrations of FSH begin to increase several years in advance of actual menopause, when the FSH is generally found to be >30 mIU/mL (Table 37.1).

Menopause marks the end of a woman's natural reproductive life. *The average age for menopause in the United States is between 50 and 52 years of age (median 51.5),* with 95% of women experiencing this event between the ages of 44 and 55. The age of menopause is not influenced by the age of menarche, number of ovulations or pregnancies, lactation, or the use of oral contraceptives. Race, socioeconomic status, education, and height also have no effect on the age of menopause. Genetics and lifestyle can affect the age of menopause. Undernourished women and smokers do tend to have an earlier menopause, although the effect is slight. Approximately 1% of women undergo menopause before the age of 40, which is generally referred to as **premature ovarian failure.**

Contrary to popular belief, the ovaries of postmenopausal women are not quiescent. Under the stimulation of LH, theca cell islands in the ovarian stroma produce hormones, primarily the androgens testosterone and androstenedione. Testosterone appears to be the major product of the postmenopausal ovary. Testosterone concentrations decline after menopause, but remain two times higher in menopausal women with intact ovaries than in those whose ovaries have been removed. **Estrone** is the predominant endogenous estrogen in postmenopausal women. It is termed **extragonadal estrogen,** because the concentration is directly related to body weight. Androstenedione is converted to estrone in fatty tissue (Table 37.2).

*Because estrogen promotes endometrial proliferation, obese women have a higher risk of endometrial hyperplasia and carcinoma. Conversely, slender women are at a higher risk for menopausal symptoms.*

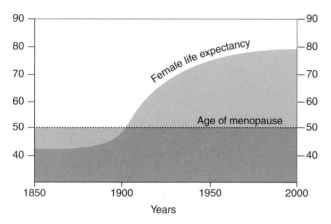

FIGURE 37.1. **Age of menopause and female life expectancy.**

| TABLE 37.1 | Relative Changes in Follicle-stimulating Hormone (FSH) as a Function of Life Stages | |
|---|---|---|
| **Life Stages** | **FSH (mIU/mL)** | |
| Childhood | <4 | |
| Prime reproductive years | 6–10 | |
| Perimenopause | 14–24 | |
| Menopause | >30 | |

## SYMPTOMS AND SIGNS OF MENOPAUSE

Menopause is a physiologic process that can be associated with symptoms that may affect a woman's quality of life.

*Decreased estrogen production can result in multiple systemic effects (Fig. 37.2). Many of these symptoms can be ameliorated with hormone therapy. The need for hormone therapy should be individualized based on a woman's specific risk factors.*

### Menstrual Cycle Alterations

Beginning at approximately 40 years of age, the number of a woman's ovarian follicles diminishes, and subtle changes occur in the frequency and length of menstrual cycles. A woman may note shortening or lengthening of her cycles. The luteal phase of the cycle remains constant at 13 to 14 days, whereas the variation of cycle length is related to a change in the follicular phase. As a woman approaches menopause, the frequency of ovulation decreases from 13 to 14 times per year to 11 to 12 times per year. With advancing reproductive age, ovulation frequency may decrease to 3 to 4 times per year.

With the change in reproductive cycle length and frequency, there are concomitant changes in the plasma concentration of FSH and LH. More FSH is required to

stimulate follicular maturation. Beginning in the late 30s and early 40s, the concentration of FSH begins to increase from normal cyclic ranges (6–10 IU/L) to perimenopausal levels (14–24 IU/L). During this period, women begin to experience symptoms and signs of decreasing estrogen levels. Levels of FSH are 30 IU/L or more at menopause.

### Hot Flushes and Vasomotor Instability

*Coincident with the change in reproductive cycle length and frequency, the **hot flush** is the first physical manifestation of decreasing ovarian function and is a symptom of vasomotor instability.*

Hot flushes are recurrent, transient episodes of flushing, perspiration, and a sensation ranging from warmth to intense heat on the upper body and face, sometimes followed by chills. When they occur during sleep and are associated with perspiration, they are termed **night sweats.** Occasional hot flushes begin several years before actual menopause. Other conditions that can cause hot flushes include thyroid disease, epilepsy, infection, and use of certain drugs.

*The hot flush is the most common symptom of decreased estrogen production and is considered one of the hallmark signs of perimenopause.* However, its incidence varies widely. Some U.S. studies have found that about 75% of women experienced hot flushes during the transition from the perimenopause to postmenopause. Outside the United States, rates vary even more widely, from about 10% in Hong

| TABLE 37.2 | Steroid Hormone Serum Concentrations in Premenopausal Women, Postmenopausal Women, and Women After Oophorectomy | | |
|---|---|---|---|
| **Hormone** | **Premenopausal (Normal Ranges)** | **Postmenopausal** | **Postoophorectomy** |
| Testosterone (ng/dL) | 325 (200–600) | 230 | 110 |
| Androstenedione (ng/dL) | 1500 (500–3000) | 800–900 | 800–900 |
| Estrone (pg/mL) | 30–200 | 25–30 | 30 |
| Estradiol (pg/mL) | 35–500 | 10–15 | 15–20 |

**Vulva and vagina**
Dyspareunia (atrophic vaginitis)
Blood-stained discharge (atrophic vaginitis)
Pruritus vulvae

**Bladder and urethra**
Frequency, urgency
Stress incontinence

**Uterus and pelvic floor**
Uterovaginal prolapse

**Skin and mucous membranes**
Dryness or pruritus
Easily traumatized
Loss of resilience and pliability
Dry hair or loss of hair
Minor hirsutism of face
Dry mouth
Voice changes: reduction in
    upper registry

**Cardiovascular system**
Angina and coronary heart disease

**Skeletal**
Fracture of hip or wrist
Backache

**Breasts**
Reduced size
Softer consistency
Reduced support

**Emotional symptoms**
Fatigue or diminished drive
Irritability
Apprehension
Altered libido
Insomnia
Feelings of inadequacy or nonfulfillment
Headache, tension

**Metabolic**
Vasomotor symptoms: hot flashes
Diaphoresis

FIGURE 37.2. Effects of menopause.

Kong to 62% in Australia. Reasons for these differences are unknown. In the United States, prevalence rates also differ among racial and ethnic groups, with African-Americans most frequently reporting symptoms (45.6%), followed by Hispanics (35.4%), whites (31.2%), Chinese (20.5%), and Japanese (17.6%). More recent studies seem to indicate that differences in body mass index (BMI) would be a more reliable indicator of the incidence of hot flushes.

Hot flushes have a rapid onset and resolution. When a hot flush occurs, a woman experiences a sudden sensation of warmth. The skin of the face and the anterior chest wall become flushed for approximately 90 seconds. With resolution of the hot flush, a woman feels cold and breaks out

into a "cold sweat." The entire phenomenon lasts less than 3 minutes. The exact cause of hot flushes has not been determined, although it seems that declining estradiol-17$\beta$ secretion by the ovarian follicles plays a significant role. As a woman approaches menopause, the frequency and intensity of hot flushes increase. Hot flushes may be disabling, especially at night. When perimenopausal and post-menopausal women receive hormone therapy, hot flushes usually resolve in 3 to 6 weeks. If a menopausal woman does not receive hormone therapy, hot flushes usually resolve spontaneously within 2 to 3 years, although some women experience them for 10 years or longer.

## Sleep Disturbances

Declining estradiol levels induce a change in a woman's sleep cycle so that restful sleep becomes difficult and for some, impossible. The latent phase of sleep (i.e., the time required to fall asleep) is lengthened; the actual period of sleep is shortened. Therefore, perimenopausal and post-menopausal women complain of having difficulty falling asleep and of waking up soon after going to sleep.

*Sleep disturbances are one of the most common and disabling effects of menopause.*

Women with marked sleep aberration are often tense and irritable and have difficulty with concentration and interpersonal relationships. With hormone therapy, the sleep cycle is restored to the premenopausal state.

## Vaginal Dryness and Genital Tract Atrophy

*The vaginal epithelium, cervix, endocervix, endometrium, myometrium, and uroepithelium are estrogen-dependent tissues. With decreasing estrogen production, these tissues become atrophic, resulting in various symptoms.* The vaginal epithelium becomes thin and cervical secretions diminish. Women experience vaginal dryness while attempting or having sexual intercourse, leading to diminished sexual enjoyment and dyspareunia. **Atrophic vaginitis** also may present with itching and burning. The thinned epithelium is also more susceptible to becoming infected by local flora. This discomfort can be relieved with systemic or topical hormone therapy or the topical use of estrogen.

The endometrium also becomes atrophic, sometimes resulting in postmenopausal spotting. The paravaginal tissues that support the bladder and rectum become atrophic. When this is combined with the effects of child bearing, it can result in loss of support for the bladder (cystocele) and rectum (rectocele). In addition, uterine prolapse is more common in the hypoestrogenic patient. Because of atrophy of the lining of the urinary tract, there may be symptoms of dysuria and urinary frequency, a condition called **atrophic**

**urethritis.** Hormone therapy can relieve the symptoms of urgency, frequency, and dysuria. Loss of support to the urethrovesical junction may result in stress urinary incontinence; in some cases, hormone therapy plus pelvic muscle (Kegel) exercises may relieve some of these symptoms.

## Mood Changes

Perimenopausal and postmenopausal women often complain of volatility of affect. Some women experience depression, apathy, and "crying spells." These feelings may be related to menopause, to sleep disturbances, or both. The physician should provide counseling and emotional support as well as medical therapy, if indicated. *Although sex steroid hormone receptors are present in the central nervous system, there is insufficient evidence about the role of estrogens in central nervous system function.*

## Skin, Hair, and Nail Changes

*Some women notice changes in their hair and nails with the hormonal changes of menopause.* Estrogen influences skin thickness. With declining estrogen production, the skin tends to become thin, less elastic, and eventually more susceptible to abrasion and trauma. Estrogen stimulates the production of the sex hormone-binding globulin, which binds androgens and estrogens. With declining estrogen production, less sex hormone-binding globulin is available, thus increasing the level of free testosterone. Increased testosterone levels may result in increased facial hair. Moreover, changes in estrogen production affect the rate of hair shedding. Hair from the scalp is normally lost and replaced in an asynchronous way. With changes in estrogen production, hair is shed and replaced in a synchronous way, resulting in the appearance of increased scalp hair loss. This is a self-limiting condition and requires no therapy, but patients do require reassurance. Nails become thin and brittle with estrogen deprivation, but are restored to normal with estrogen therapy.

## Osteoporosis

**Bone demineralization** is a natural consequence of aging. Diminishing bone density occurs in both men and women. However, the onset of bone demineralization occurs 15 to 20 years earlier in women than in men by virtue of acceleration after ovarian function ceases. Bone demineralization not only occurs with natural menopause, but also has been reported in association with decreased estrogen production in certain groups of young women (such as those with eating disorders or elite athletes). Other factors contribute to the risk of osteoporosis (Box 37.1).

Estrogen receptors are present in osteoblasts, which suggests a permissive and perhaps even an essential role for estrogen in bone formation. *Estrogen affects the development of cortical and trabecular bone, although the effect on the latter*

---

### BOX 37.1
### Risk Factors for Osteoporotic Fractures

Adult Fracture
Fracture in first-degree relative
White race
Advanced age
Dementia
Poor health/frailty
Cigarette use
Low body weight
Estrogen deficiency
Early menopause or bilateral oophorectomy (<45 yr old)
Prolonged premenopausal amenorrhea (> 1yr)
Alcoholism
Inadequate physical activity

yr = year.

---

*is more pronounced. Bone density diminishes at the rate of approximately 1% to 2% per year in postmenopausal women, compared with approximately 0.5% per year in perimenopausal women* (Fig. 37.3). Hormone therapy, especially when combined with appropriate calcium supplementation and weight-bearing exercise, can help slow bone loss in menopausal women. Weight-bearing activity such as walking for as little as 30 minutes a day increases the mineral content of older women.

*Calcium supplementation is beneficial to prevent bone loss; 1500 mg of daily calcium intake for menopausal women is recommended.* Calcium therapy combined with estrogen

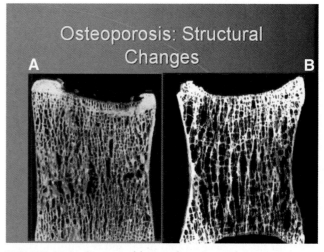

FIGURE 37.3. Structural bone changes with osteoporosis. (A) Normal bone. (B) Osteoporotic trabecular bone. (From Randolph JF, Lobo RA. Menopause. In: *Precis: Reproductive Endocrinology.* 3rd ed. Washington, DC: ACOG;2007:185.)

therapy is more effective. In addition, for those with limited sun exposure or those lacking other dietary sources, supplementation with vitamin D should be considered: 10 μg from ages of 51 to 70; 15 μg, older than 71.

Progressive, linear decrease in bone mineral mass is noted in women who do not receive hormone therapy in the first 5 to 10 years following menopause. When hormone therapy is initiated before or at the time of menopause, bone density loss is greatly reduced. Hormone therapy begun in a woman 5 or more years after menopause may still have a positive effect on bone density loss. *However, osteoporosis is not the primary indication for hormone therapy.* Several bisphosphonates such as alendronate, ibandronate, or risedronate can be used for the management of menopause-associated bone loss. These agents reduce bone resorption through the inhibition of osteoclastic activity (Table 37.3).

*Selective estrogen receptor modulators (SERMs) provide another nonhormonal management option.* Most estrogenic responses are mediated in the body by one of two receptors, either ER (alpha) or ER (beta). SERMs are ER ligands, which act like estrogens in some tissues but block estrogen action in others. Examples include tamoxifen and raloxifene, which exhibit ER antagonist activity in the breast but agonist activity in the bone. As with the bisphosphonates, they also lack the capabilities of mitigating many of the other estrogen deprivation symptoms, such as hot flushes and sleeplessness, and may even exacerbate these symptoms.

## Cardiovascular Lipid Changes

*With perimenopause, changes occur in the cardiovascular lipid profile.* Total cholesterol increases, high-density lipoprotein (HDL) cholesterol decreases, and low-density lipoprotein (LDL) cholesterol increases. Hormone therapy may promote changes in the lipid profile that are favorable to the cardiovascular system. Retrospective case control studies suggest that estrogens have a cardioprotective effect. However, recent data from the Women's Health Initiative (WHI) suggest that no such protection exists in placebo control clinical trials, though these trials have been criticized because of the late onset of treatment following menopause. *At this time, hormone therapy should not be offered to patients with the primary goal of protection against heart disease.*

## PREMATURE OVARIAN FAILURE

The diagnosis of premature ovarian failure applies to the approximately 1% of women who experience menopause before the age of 40 years. *The diagnosis should be suspected in a young woman with hot flushes and other symptoms of hypoestrogenism and secondary amenorrhea (e.g., a woman seeking treatment for infertility).* The diagnosis is confirmed by laboratory findings of menopausal FSH levels. Interestingly, hot flushes are not as common as might be expected in this group of patients. The diagnosis has profound emotional implications for most patients, especially if their desires for childbearing have not been fulfilled, as well as metabolic and constitutional implications. There are many causes of premature loss of oocytes and premature menopause; some of the more common causes are discussed below. Given its potential dramatic impact, premature ovarian failure demands a careful workup in order to identify the underlying cause and permit appropriate management.

## Genetic Factors

Several factors influence a woman's reproductive life span. Genetic information that determines the length of a woman's reproductive life is carried on the distal long arm of the X chromosome. Partial deletion of the long arm of one X chromosome results in premature ovarian failure. Total loss of the long arm of the X chromosome, as seen in Turner syndrome, results in ovarian failure at birth or in early childhood. When suspected, these diagnoses can be established by careful mapping of the X chromosome.

## Gonadotropin-Resistant Ovary Syndrome (Savage Syndrome)

Some women with premature ovarian failure have an adequate number of ovarian follicles, yet these follicles are resistant to FSH and LH. A number of pregnancies have been reported in women with the gonadotropin-resistant ovary syndrome during the administration of exogenous estrogen. This fact supports a role for estrogens in stimulating FSH receptors in the ovarian follicles.

| TABLE 37.3 | Nonhormonal Regimens for Osteoporosis | |
|---|---|---|
| **Drug** | **Drug Class** | **Mechanism of Action** |
| Risedronate | Bisphosphonate | Inhibits osteoclast bone resorption |
| Ibandronate | Bisphosphonate | Inhibits osteoclast bone resorption |
| Alendronate | Bisphosphonate | Inhibits osteoclast bone resorption |
| Calcium carbonate | Natural | Inhibits osteoclast bone resorption (bisphosphonate) |
| Raloxifene | Selective estrogen receptor modulator (SERM), selectively binds estrogen receptors, inhibiting bone resorption and turnover | Inhibits bone resorption & turnover |

## Autoimmune Disorders

Some women develop autoantibodies against thyroid, adrenal, and ovarian endocrine tissues. These autoantibodies may cause ovarian failure. Occasionally these women respond to hormone therapy with subsequent resumption of ovulation.

## Smoking

*Women who smoke tobacco can undergo ovarian failure some 3 to 5 years earlier than the expected time of menopause.* It is established that women who smoke metabolize estradiol primarily to 2-hydroxyestradiol. The 2-hydroxylated estrogens are termed **catecholestrogens** because of their structural similarity to catecholamines. The catecholestrogens act as antiestrogens and block estrogen action. The mechanism for premature ovarian failure in smokers is unknown. However, the effects of smoking should be considered in smokers who are experiencing symptoms of estrogen deficiency.

## Alkylating Cancer Chemotherapy

Alkylating cancer chemotherapeutic agents affect the membrane of ovarian follicles and hasten follicular atresia. One of the consequences of cancer chemotherapy in reproductive-age women is loss of ovarian function. Young women being treated for malignant neoplasms should be counseled of this possibility and advised that they may be candidates for follicular retrieval and cryopreservation as a means for attempting future pregnancy.

## Hysterectomy

Surgical removal of the uterus (hysterectomy) in reproductive-age women is associated with menopause some 3 to 5 years earlier than the expected age. The mechanism for this occurrence is unknown. It is likely to be associated with alteration of ovarian blood flow resulting from the surgery.

## MANAGEMENT OF MENOPAUSE

The changes of menopause result from declining 17-β estradiol production by the ovarian follicles. 17-β estradiol and its metabolic by-products, estrone and estriol, are used in hormone therapy, the objective of which is to diminish the signs and symptoms of menopause. *Several different estrogen preparations are available through various routes of administration, including oral medications, transdermal preparations, and topical preparations.* When administered orally, 17-β estradiol is oxidized in the enterohepatic circulation to estrone. 17-β estradiol remains unaltered when it is administered transdermally, transbucally, transvaginally, intravenously, or intramuscularly. Unfortunately, intramuscular estradiol administration results in unpredictable fluctuations in plasma concentration. When estradiol is administered across the vaginal epithelium, absorption is poorly controlled, and pharmacologic plasma concentrations of estradiol can result. Transdermal administration of estradiol results in steady, sustained estrogen blood levels and may be a preferable alternative to oral dosing for many patients.

*The administration of continuous unopposed estrogens can result in endometrial hyperplasia and an increased risk of endometrial adenocarcinoma. Therefore, it is essential to administer a progestin in conjunction with estrogens in women who have not undergone hysterectomy.* Progestins may include any variety of synthetics, such as medroxyprogesterone acetate and norethindrone or micronized progesterone. To achieve this protective effect, the progestin chosen may be given continuously in low doses or sequentially in higher doses. Sequential dosing is usually for 10 or 12 days each calendar month. Progestins may be associated with unacceptable side effects, such as affective symptoms and weight gain. If estrogen is administered alone because of unacceptable side effects of progestins, then it is imperative to counsel the patient about the need for yearly endometrial biopsy.

*There are two principal regimens for hormone therapy.* Continuous estrogen replacement with cyclic progestin administration results in excellent resolution of symptoms and cyclic withdrawal bleeding from the endometrium. One of the difficulties of this method of therapy is that many postmenopausal women do not want to continue having menstrual cycles. As a result, many physicians and patients choose to avoid the problem of cyclic withdrawal bleeding by the daily administration of both an estrogen and a low-dose progestin.

There are a variety of estrogen preparations available. Most perimenopausal and menopausal women respond to one of these preparations, all of which ameliorate acute menopause symptoms and relieve vaginal atrophy. The administration of progestins for 10 to 12 days each month converts the proliferative endometrium into a secretory endometrium, brings about endometrial sloughing, and prevents endometrial hyperplasia or cellular atypia. Continuous progestin therapy may be used to produce endometrial atrophy.

Numerous preparations combining estrogen and progestins are available in both oral and transdermal formulation. The most widely used contain a combination of conjugated equine estrogens and medroxyprogesterone acetate in one tablet. Newer preparations include a combination of micronized estradiol and norethynodrel acetate or ethinyl estradiol and norethindrone acetate. Transdermal preparations include a combination of micronized estradiol and norethindrone acetate. *Low-dose oral contraceptives may also be used to relieve the vasomotor symptoms of menopause.*

## CAUTIONS IN HORMONE THERAPY

The results of the WHI in 2002 revealed epidemiologic findings that have modified the contemporary use of hormone therapy. This large, multicenter, randomized clinical trial (approximately 17,000 women) studied the effects of hormone therapy, dietary modification, and calcium and vitamin D supplementation as related to heart disease, fractures, breast cancer, and colorectal cancer. *Although there are features of this study that are not applicable to many younger menopause patients, the overall results suggested that when compared to placebo, a combination of conjugated equine estrogens and continuous low-dose medroxyprogesterone acetate resulted in an increased risk of heart attack, stroke, thromboembolic disease, and breast cancer, with a reduced risk of colorectal cancer and hip fractures.* Some of the data contradicted prior large-scale observational studies, and thus many physicians have changed their practice regarding hormone therapy to center more on the relief of short-term symptoms of estrogen deprivation, including hot flushes, sleeplessness, and vaginal atrophy. Although reappraisals of the study have focused on its flaws, current opinion suggests that initiation early in menopause is associated with a good risk-benefit ratio, with preference for the transdermal route. Nonetheless, the current recommendations from numerous organizations, including ACOG, is that hormone therapy should only be used for the short-term relief of menopausal symptoms and should be individually tailored to a woman's need for treatment (Box 37.2).

Hormone therapy in women with prior history of breast and endometrial cancer is controversial. Currently, prospective studies are underway using low-dose hormone therapy in women with a prior history of limited-lesion, successfully treated breast cancer. Similar studies in women with prior treated limited-lesion endometrial cancer have been completed and show no increased risk of recurrence for estrogen users.

---

### BOX 37.2
### Contraindications to Hormone Therapy

- Undiagnosed abnormal genital bleeding
- Known or suspected estrogen-dependent neoplasia except in appropriately selected patients
- Active deep vein thrombosis, pulmonary embolism, or a history of these conditions
- Active or recent arterial thromboembolic disease (stroke, myocardial infarction)
- Liver dysfunction or liver disease
- Known or suspected pregnancy
- Hypersensitivity to hormone therapy preparations

---

## ALTERNATIVES TO HORMONE THERAPY

Because of the controversy surrounding hormone therapy, many women are seeking alternative therapies. When counseling patients, one must take a holistic approach. Most women seek relief of the most common symptom of menopause—hot flushes—but as noted above, the menopause affects women in different ways. *As women age, their risk for heart disease begins to rise and, thus, it is important to advocate heart-healthy lifestyle changes.* Likewise, preventive counseling about osteoporosis, as previously discussed, should also be included. Alternative therapies for the short-term treatment of common symptoms of menopause include the following:

- Soy and isoflavones may be helpful in the short-term (≤2 years) treatment of vasomotor symptoms. Given the possibility that these compounds may interact with estrogen, these agents should not be considered free of potential harm in women with estrogen-dependent cancers.
- St. John's wort may be helpful in the short-term (≤2 years) treatment of mild to moderate depression in women.
- Black cohosh may be helpful in the short-term (≤6 months) treatment of women with vasomotor symptoms.
- Soy and isoflavone intake over prolonged periods may improve lipoprotein profiles and protect against osteoporosis. Soy in foodstuffs may differ in biological activity from soy and isoflavones in supplements.

Most well-controlled studies of the common over-the-counter remedies have not shown dramatic improvements. In addition, many of these over-the-counter botanical supplements are not U.S. Food and Drug Administration (FDA)-regulated. Consequently, there is little quality control. Patients need to be informed that "natural" does not necessarily mean safe. Moreover, many of these products have undesired side effects. Many soy products interact with thyroid medications, while Dong quai and red clover potentiate warfarin and other anticoagulants.

One of the most commonly utilized off-label medications is progesterone. Numerous randomized, placebo controlled studies have demonstrated its efficacy, usually in the form of medroxyprogesterone acetate, in the treatment of hot flushes. Selective serotonin reuptake inhibitors (SSRIs) have also been used with some success. In randomized, double blind studies, venlafaxine, paroxetine, and fluoxetine were all shown to significantly decrease hot flushes. In addition, both gabapentin and cetirizine were found to provide moderate relief of vasomotor symptoms.

*Lastly, patients should be advised of the potential relief achieved by lifestyle changes, such as eating a healthy diet that is less than 30% fat and rich in calcium, regular exercise, maintaining a healthy weight, avoidance of smoking, limiting alcohol intake, and getting regular health care.* These practices may not only help relieve some menopausal symptoms, but may help prevent other health problems.

## SUGGESTED READINGS

American College of Obstetricians and Gynecologists. Compounded bioidentical hormones. ACOG Committee Opinion No. 322. *Obstet Gynecol.* 2005;106(5):1139–1140.

American College of Obstetricians and Gynecologists. *Guidelines for Women's Health Care: A Resource Manual.* 3rd ed. Washington, D.C.: ACOG; 2007.

American College of Obstetricians and Gynecologists. *Management of Anovulatory Bleeding. ACOG Practice Bulletin No. 14.* Washington, DC: ACOG;2000.

American College of Obstetricians and Gynecologists. Non-contraceptive uses of the levonorgestrel intrauterine system. ACOG Committee Opinion No. 337. *Obstet Gynecol.* 2006;107(6):1479–1482.

American College of Obstetricians and Gynecologists. Osteoporosis: Clinical management guidelines for obstetrician-gynecologists. ACOG Practice Bulletin No. 50. *Obstet Gynecol.* 2004;103(1):203–216.

American College of Obstetricians and Gynecologists. Use of botanicals for management of menopausal symptoms. ACOG Practice Bulletin No. 28. *Obstet Gynecol.* 2001;97(6, Suppl):1–11.

American College of Obstetricians and Gynecologists. *Precis, An Update in Obstetrics and Gynecology: Reproductive Endocrinology.* 3rd ed. Washington, D.C.: American College of Obstetricians and Gynecologists; 2007:181–197.

# 38 | Infertility

Topic 48: Infertility

Students should be able to define infertility and discuss the causes, evaluation, and management of female and male infertility. Students should also be aware of the psychosocial issues associated with infertility.

---

*nfertility affects approximately 15% of reproductive-age couples in the United States.* **Reproductive age** generally encompasses ages 15 to 44 years, although pregnancy can occur outside of this age range. *Infertility is the failure of a couple to conceive after 12 months of frequent, unprotected intercourse.* The probability of achieving a pregnancy in one menstrual cycle is termed **fecundability,** and is estimated to be 20% to 25% in healthy young couples. Similarly, **fecundity** is the probability of achieving a live birth in one menstrual cycle. Fecundability and fecundity both decrease over time; in other words, the probability of conceiving in a given menstrual cycle decreases as the duration of time to achieve conception increases (Fig. 38.1). After 12 months without using contraception, approximately 50% of couples will conceive spontaneously within the following 36 months. If a couple does not conceive by this point, then infertility will likely persist without medical intervention.

Infertility is a condition that encompasses a wide spectrum of reversible and irreversible disorders, and many successful treatments are available. Today, greater numbers of men and women are seeking infertility treatment due to increased public awareness of infertility and available treatments, improvements in the availability and range of fertility treatments, improvements in physicians' ability to evaluate and diagnose infertility, and changes in social acceptance of infertility. Furthermore, many individuals and same-sex couples as well seek fertility treatments to conceive. Although this chapter discusses infertility from the standpoint of a heterosexual couple, it is recognized that fertility treatments offer the opportunity of parenthood to many other individuals and couples.

*Today, 85% of infertile couples who undergo appropriate treatment can expect to have a child.* However, fertility treatment can be a difficult experience for an individual or a couple. The inability to conceive or carry a pregnancy can be emotionally stressful, and fertility treatment can be a significant financial burden. *The psychologic stress associated*

*with infertility must be recognized and patients should be counseled accordingly.*

## ETIOLOGY OF INFERTILITY

*Successful conception requires a specific series of complex events: (1) ovulation of a competent oocyte, (2) production of competent sperm, (3) juxtaposition of sperm and oocyte in a patent reproductive tract and subsequent fertilization, (4) generation of a viable embryo, (5) transport of the embryo into the uterine cavity, and (6) successful implantation of the embryo into the endometrium (Fig. 38.2).*

> *Any defect in one or more of the essential steps in reproduction can result in diminished fertility or infertility.*

Furthermore, some degree of male infertility is implicated in up to 40% of couples. Conditions that affect fertility are divided into four main categories:

1. Female factors (65%)
2. Male factors (20%)
3. Unexplained or other conditions (15%)

## EVALUATION OF INFERTILITY

The most common causes of male and female infertility are investigated during the initial evaluation of infertility. It is important to recognize that more than one factor may be involved in a couple's infertility (Table 38.1). As with any medical condition, a careful history and evaluation should reveal factors that may be involved in a couple's infertility, such as medical disorders, medications, prior surgeries, pelvic infections or pelvic pain, sexual dysfunction, and environmental and lifestyle factors (e.g., diet, exercise, tobacco use, drug use).

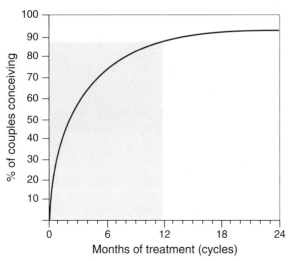

FIGURE 38.1.  Conception rates for fertile couples.

## Ovulation

A history of regular, predictable menses strongly suggests ovulatory cycles. Furthermore, many women experience characteristic symptoms associated with ovulation and the production of progesterone: unilateral pelvic discomfort (mittelschmerz), fullness and tenderness of the breasts, decreased vaginal secretions, abdominal bloating, slight increase in body weight, and occasional episodes of depression. These changes rarely occur in anovulatory women. Therefore, a history of regular menses with associated cyclic changes may be considered presumptive evidence of ovulation.

*Secretion of progesterone by the corpus luteum dominates the luteal phase of the menstrual cycle, and persists if conception occurs.*

The timing of the initial evaluation depends primarily on the age of the female partner and a couple's risk factors for infertility. *Because there is a decline in fecundity with advancing maternal age, women over age 35 may benefit from a preliminary evaluation before 12 months of attempted conception.* The initial assessment and treatment of infertility is commonly provided by an obstetrician-gynecologist. More specialized evaluation and treatment may be performed by a reproductive endocrinologist.

Progesterone acts on the endocervix to convert the thin, clear endocervical mucus into a sticky mucoid material. Progesterone also changes the brain's thermoregulatory center setpoint, resulting in a basal body temperature rise of approximately 0.6°F. In the absence of pregnancy, involution of the corpus luteum is associated with an abrupt decrease in progesterone production, normalization of the basal body temperature, and the commencement of menstruation.

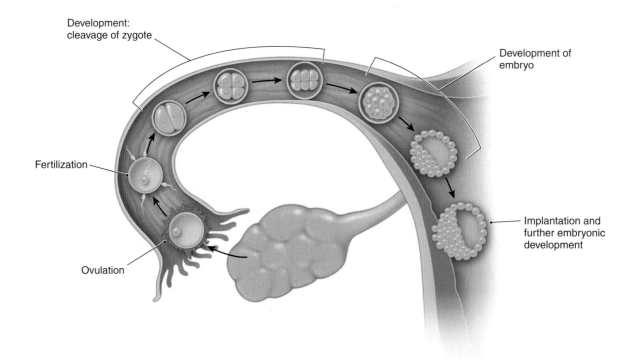

FIGURE 38.2.  Steps in successful conception: ovulation, production of viable sperm and fertilization, development of the zygote, early embryonic development, and implantation of the embryo into the endometrium.

TABLE
**38.1**     Tests Performed During the Evaluation of the Infertile Couple

| Evaluation of | Initial Evaluation | Further Evaluation |
|---|---|---|
| **Female** | | |
| Ovulation | History and physical examination<br>Basal body temperature charting<br>Ovulation predictor kits | Mid-luteal phase progesterone level<br>Ultrasonography<br>Endometrial biopsy (not routine)<br>Endocrine testing |
| Uterus | Ultrasonography | Saline-infusion sonography<br>Hysterosalpingography<br>MRI<br>Hysteroscopy |
| Fallopian tubes and peritoneum | Hysterosalpingography | Laparoscopy with chromotubation |
| **Male** | Semen analysis<br>Repeat semen analysis if indicated<br>Postcoital test (not routine) | Genetic evaluation<br>FSH, LH, testosterone level evaluation<br>Prolactin level evaluation<br>Epididymal sperm aspiration<br>Testicular biopsy |

FSH = follicle-stimulating hormone; LH = luteinizing hormone; MRI = magnetic resonance imaging.

*Two tests provide indirect evidence of ovulation and can help predict the timing of ovulation.* **Basal body temperature** measurement reveals a characteristic biphasic temperature curve during most ovulatory cycles (Fig. 38.3). Special thermometers are available for this use. Upon awakening in the morning, the temperature must be obtained immediately before any physical activity. The temperature drops at the time of menses, and then rises 2 days after the peak of the luteinizing hormone (LH) surge, coinciding with a rise in peripheral levels of progesterone. Oocyte release occurs 1 day before the first temperature elevation, and the temperature remains elevated for up to 14 days. This test for ovulation is readily available, although cumbersome to use; it can retrospectively identify ovulation and the optimal time for intercourse, but can be difficult to interpret. **Urine LH kits** are also used to prospectively assess the presence and timing of ovulation based on increased excretion of LH in the urine. Ovulation occurs approximately 24 hours after urinary evidence of the LH surge. However, due to the pulsatile nature of LH release, an LH surge can be missed if the test is only performed once daily.

Other diagnostic tests assess ovulation using **serum progesterone** levels and the **endometrial response** to progesterone. A mid-luteal phase serum progesterone level can be used to retrospectively assess ovulation. A value above 3 ng/mL implies ovulation; however, values between 6 to 25 ng/mL may occur in a normal ovulatory cycle. Due to the pulsatile nature of hormone secretion, a single low progesterone assessment should be repeated. Another diagnostic procedure is the **luteal phase endometrial biopsy.** The identification of secretory endometrium consistent with the day of the menstrual cycle confirms the presence of progesterone; hence ovulation is implied. However, this procedure is invasive, and histologic assessment of the endometrium does not reliably differentiate infertile and fertile women. Therefore, the endometrial biopsy is not routinely performed to assess ovulation or the endometrium.

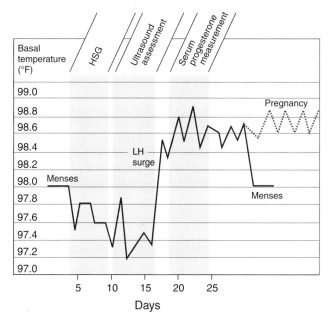

FIGURE 38.3. Biphasic basal body temperature pattern that occurs with an ovulatory cycle.

LH=luteinizing hormone.

If **oligo-ovulation** (sporadic and unpredictable ovulation) or **anovulation** (absence of ovulation) is established, usually based on a menstrual cycle history of irregular cycles, further testing is indicated to determine the underlying cause. A common cause of ovulatory dysfunction in reproductive-age women is **polycystic ovary syndrome** (PCOS); other causes include thyroid disorders and hyperprolactinemia. Women with PCOS often present with oligomenorrhea and signs of hyperandrogenism such as hirsutism, acne, and weight gain (see Chapter 36, Hirsutism and Virilization). Furthermore, some infertile women present with **amenorrhea,** and this usually signifies anovulation. Important causes of amenorrhea include pregnancy (a pregnancy test should always be given), hypothalamic dysfunction (usually stress-related), ovarian failure, or obstruction of the reproductive tract. Depending on the individual case, laboratory testing for ovulatory dysfunction may include assessment of serum levels of human chorionic gonadotropin (hCG), thyroid-stimulating hormone (TSH), prolactin, total testosterone, dehydroepiandrosterone sulfate (DHEA-S), follicle-stimulating hormone (FSH), LH, and estradiol.

*Treatment of the etiology of ovulatory dysfunction may lead to resumption of ovulation and improved fertility.*

## Anatomic Factors

The pelvic anatomy should be assessed as a part of the infertility evaluation. Abnormalities of the uterus, fallopian tubes, and peritoneum can all play a role in infertility.

### UTERUS

Uterine abnormalities are commonly not sufficient to cause infertility; these disorders are usually associated with pregnancy loss. *However, assessment of the uterus is particularly important if there is a history that causes concern, such as abnormal bleeding, pregnancy loss, preterm delivery, or previous uterine surgery.* Potential uterine abnormalities include leiomyomas, endometrial polyps, intrauterine adhesions, or congenital anomalies (such as a septate, bicornuate, unicornuate, or didelphyic uterus) (Fig. 38.4). Assessment of the uterus and endometrial cavity can be accomplished with several imaging techniques; sometimes, a combination of modalities is necessary to best assess pelvic anatomy (Box 38.1).

### FALLOPIAN TUBES AND PERITONEUM

*The fallopian tubes are dynamic structures that are essential for ovum, sperm, and embryo transport and fertilization.*

At ovulation, the fimbriated end of the fallopian tube picks up the oocyte from the site of ovulation or from the pelvic cul-de-sac. The oocyte is transported to the ampullary portion of the fallopian tube where fertilization occurs

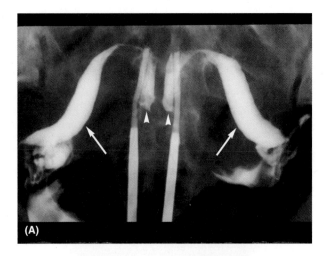

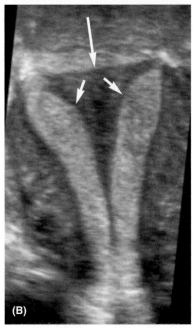

FIGURE 38.4. Uterine abnormalities. A. X-ray hysterosalpingogram confirms a didelphic uterus, with paired contrast-filled cervical canals (arrowheads) and uterine cavities (arrows). B. Three-dimensional sonogram indicating a septate uterus. The endometrium is separated into two components (short arrows) and the uterine fundus (long arrow) has a smooth external contour. Courtesy of Dr. Beryl Benacerraf. (From Doubilet PM, Benson CB. *Atlas of Ultrasound in Obstetrics and Gynecology.* Philadelphia: Lippincott Williams & Wilkins; 2003:291.)

(see Fig. 38.2). Subsequently, a zygote and then an embryo are formed. At 5 days following fertilization, the embryo enters the endometrial cavity, where implantation into the secretory endometrium occurs, followed by further embryo growth and development.

The fallopian tubes and pelvis can be evaluated with hysterosalpingography (HSG) or laparoscopy. There

## Procedures Used in the Evaluation of Female Infertility

**Transvaginal ultrasonography:** Used to visualize the vagina, cervix, uterus, and ovaries.

**Saline-infusion sonography:** Assesses the myometrium, endometrium, and adnexa; sometimes used in conjunction with magnetic resonance imaging.

**Hysterosalpingography** (HSG): Provides information about the uterus and fallopian tubes' structure and function.

**Hysteroscopy:** Used for evaluation and treatment of abnormalities identified by imaging studies, such as removal of small leiomyomata, polyps, and adhesions

**Laparoscopy:** Used to visualize the pelvic organs as well as treat certain conditions, including endometriosis. Saline-infusion of the fallopian tubes can also be performed to test their patency.

are several important characteristics of a normal HSG (Fig. 38.5). The uterine cavity should be smooth and symmetrical; indentations or irregularities of the cavity suggest the presence of leiomyomas, endometrial polyps, or intrauterine adhesions. The proximal two-thirds of the fallopian tube should be thin, approximating the diameter of a pencil lead. The distal one-third comprises the ampulla, and should appear dilated in comparison to the proximal portion of the tube. Free spill of dye from the fimbria into the pelvis is appreciated as the cul-de-sac and other structures such as bowel are outlined by the accumulating dye. Failure to observe dispersion of dye through a fallopian tube or throughout the pelvis suggests the possibility of pelvic adhesions that restrict normal fallopian tube mobility. Examples of abnormal hysterosalpingograms are shown in Figure 38.6.

**Pelvic adhesions** that affect the fallopian tubes or peritoneum may occur because of pelvic infection (e.g., pelvic inflammatory disease, appendicitis), endometriosis, or abdominal or pelvic surgery. The sequelae of any of these processes or events can include fallopian tube scarring and obstruction. Pelvic infections are usually associated with sexually transmitted infections that cause acute salpingitis; commonly implicated organisms are *Chlamydia*

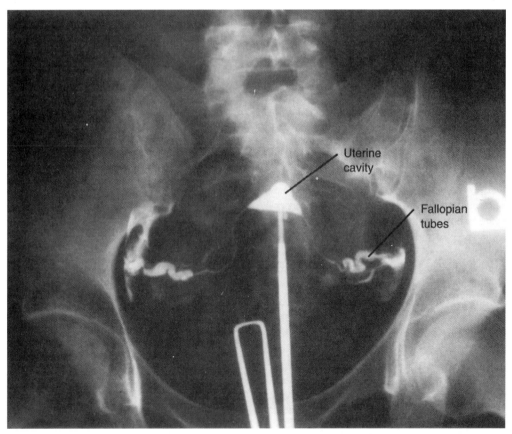

FIGURE 38.5. A hysterosalpingogram demonstrating a patent female reproductive tract with normal anatomy.

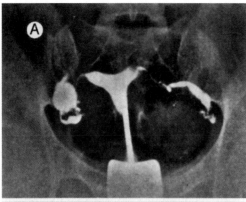

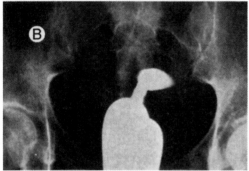

FIGURE 38.6. Abnormal hysterosalpingograms. (A) Bilateral hydrosalpinges (dilated fallopian tubes) with distal obstruction at the fimbriated ends, no free spill of dye seen. (B) Bilateral proximal tubal occlusion; uterus overdistended with radiopaque dye.

*trachomatis* and *Neisseria gonorrhea* (see Chapter 27, Sexually Transmitted Diseases). Endometriosis occurs with higher frequency in infertile women compared to fertile women, and can cause scarring and distortion of the fallopian tubes and other pelvic organs (see Chapter 29, Endometriosis).

The HSG detects approximately 70% of anatomic abnormalities of the genital tract. When there are abnormalities, further diagnostic evaluation and treatment can be performed with hysteroscopy and laparoscopy. Hysteroscopy evaluates the endometrium and the architecture of the uterine cavity. Laparoscopy assesses pelvic structures including the uterus, ovaries, and fallopian tubes as well as the pelvic peritoneum. During laparoscopy, **chromotubation** should be performed: similar to the HSG, a catheter is placed in the uterus and colored dye is injected into the uterus while tubal patency and function is directly assessed by laparoscopy. Laparoscopy also allows the diagnosis and treatment of any pelvic abnormalities, such as adhesions and endometriosis.

## MALE INFERTILITY

Because male infertility is common, it is important to also perform a **semen analysis** when initiating evaluation of the female partner. The semen specimen is usually obtained by masturbation after 2 to 3 days of abstinence; frequent ejaculation may lower the sperm concentration. It is important to collect the entire ejaculate, because the first part contains the greatest density of sperm. Analysis of the specimen should be performed within 1 hour of ejaculation (see Table 38.1). The standard semen analysis evaluates the quantity and quality of seminal fluid, sperm concentration, and sperm motility and morphology. Normal semen measurements have been established by the World Health Organization (Table 38.2). A normal semen analysis excludes a male cause for infertility in more than 90% of heterosexual couples. Certain abnormalities identified by the semen analysis are associated with specific etiologies of male infertility (Table 38.3). Sperm function can be further evaluated with specialized diagnostic tests, but these tests are not routinely used.

Besides the semen analysis, the **postcoital test** has historically been used to evaluate sperm concentration and their interaction with the cervical mucus. To perform this test, a sample of cervical mucus must be obtained 2 to 12 hours after intercourse that occurs 1 to 3 days prior to ovulation. The sample is placed on a glass slide and examined under a microscope. Standard criteria include the presence of at least 5 motile sperm per high-powered field. However, the diagnostic utility and validity of this test is limited; thus, its routine use is not indicated. Furthermore, conventional fertility treatments such as intrauterine insemination and in vitro fertilization (IVF) bypass any abnormalities of the cervix or cervical mucus.

If the results of the semen analysis are abnormal, it should be repeated in 1 to 2 weeks. Persistent abnormalities in the semen necessitate further investigation. The male partner should be evaluated by a urologist or reproductive endocrinologist who specializes in male infertility. Occasionally, male infertility may be the presenting sign of a serious medical condition, such as testicular cancer or a pituitary tumor. Etiologies of male infertility include congenital, acquired, or systemic disorders that can be grouped into the following categories: hypothalamic-pituitary disease that causes gonadal dysfunction (1% to 2%), testicular disease (30% to 40%), post-testicular defects that cause

| TABLE 38.2 | Reference Values for Semen Analysis |
|---|---|
| **Element** | **Reference Value** |
| Ejaculate volume | 1.5–5.0 mL |
| pH | >7.2 |
| Sperm concentration | >20 million/mL |
| Motility | >50%<br>≥25% with rapid progressive motility |
| Normal morphology | >30% normal forms |

| TABLE 38.3 | Causes of Abnormal Semen |
|---|---|
| **Finding** | **Cause** |
| Low semen volume | Ejaculatory dysfunction<br>Retrograde ejaculation<br>Hypogonadism<br>Poor collection technique |
| Acidic semen | Ejaculatory duct obstruction<br>Congenital absence of the vas deferens and/or seminal vesicles |
| Azoospermia or oligospermia | Genetic disorders<br>Endocrine disorders<br>Varicocele<br>Cryptorchidism<br>Infections<br>Exposure to toxins, radiation, medications<br>Genital tract obstruction<br>Idiopathic |
| Decreased motility (asthenospermia) | Prolonged abstinence<br>Immunologic factors: antisperm antibodies<br>Partial genital tract obstruction<br>Infection<br>Sperm structural defects<br>Idiopathic |
| Abnormal morphology (teratospermia) | Varicocele<br>Genetic disorder<br>Cryptorchidism<br>Infections<br>Exposure to toxins, radiation, medications<br>Idiopathic |

disorders of sperm transport or ejaculation (10% to 20%), and unexplained infertility (40% to 50%).

*Abnormalities in spermatogenesis are a major cause of male infertility.* Unlike oocytes, which undergo development in a cyclic fashion, sperm are being produced constantly by the testes. As sperm develop within the germinal epithelium of the testis, they are released into the epididymis where maturation occurs before ejaculation.

*Sperm production and development takes approximately 70 days. Therefore, abnormal results of the semen analysis reflect events that occurred more than 2 months before the specimen collection.*

Alternatively, a minimum of 70 days is required to observe changes in sperm production following initiation of any therapy.

Further evaluation of the infertile male includes endocrine and genetic testing. Endocrine evaluation is appropriate for individuals with abnormal sperm concentrations or signs of androgen deficiency. Serum testosterone, FSH, and LH levels will identify primary hypogonadism (low testosterone, or elevated FSH and LH) or secondary hypogonadism (low testosterone, FSH, and LH). A low LH level in the presence of **oligospermia** (sperm concentration less than 5 million/mL) and a normal testosterone level may indicate exogenous steroid use. A serum **prolactin** level should be assessed in men with low testosterone levels.

*Genetic abnormalities may affect sperm production or transport.* **Genetic testing** is indicated in men with **azoospermia** (no sperm) and severe oligospermia. The most common abnormalities identified include gene mutations in the cystic fibrosis transmembrane conductase regulator (CFTR), somatic and sex chromosome abnormalities, and microdeletions of the Y chromosome. Men with mutations in one or both copies of the CFTR gene often exhibit congenital bilateral absence of the vas deferens or other obstructive defects, and many have no pulmonary symptoms. A karyotype may reveal abnormalities, such as Klinefelter syndrome (47 XXY) or chromosome inversions and translocations. Special testing must be performed to search for Y chromosome microdeletions, because they are not detected by routine karyotype analysis; these microdeletions are associated with altered testicular development and spermatogenesis. If a genetic condition is identified, genetic counseling is strongly recommended.

Men with azoospermia can be further evaluated by two diagnostic procedures. If an obstructive process is suspected (obstructive azoospermia), then sperm should accumulate just before the obstruction. For example, men with congenital absence of the vas deferens or those who underwent a vasectomy have a swollen epididymis where constant production of sperm results in a small collection. **Percutaneous epididymal sperm aspiration (PESA)** or **microsurgical epididymal sperm aspiration (MESA)** procedures can retrieve motile, healthy sperm. If no obstruction is present (nonobstructive azoospermia) and a testicular abnormality is suspected, a testicular biopsy may identify a few sperm present in the seminiferous tubules. With either procedure, small numbers of sperm are obtained compared to a normal ejaculated specimen. These retrieved sperm can be used to try to achieve pregnancy; however, the female partner must undergo IVF, and a single sperm is used to fertilize a singe oocyte (intracytoplasmic sperm injection).

## UNEXPLAINED INFERTILITY

*For some couples, comprehensive evaluation of both partners does not identify an etiology for their infertility. Specifically, test results identify a normal semen analysis, evidence of ovulation, a normal uterine cavity, and patent fallopian tubes.* Approximately 15% of couples are considered to have unexplained infertility. This diagnosis usually signifies the presence of one or more mild abnormalities in the highly orchestrated sequence of events that results in successful conception. These abnormalities may lie below the level of detection of current tests or may not be detected by current tests. These couples have a low rate of spontaneous conception, approximately 1% to 3% each month; this rate is influenced by the age of the female partner and the duration of infertility. If laparoscopy is performed on the female partner, subtle abnormalities such as pelvic adhesions and mild endometriosis may be identified and treated. However, it is reasonable to proceed with medical treatment of infertility without performing laparoscopy.

## TREATMENT

A couple's infertility may be related to one or several abnormalities in one or both partners. *Numerous medical, surgical, and assisted reproductive technology (ART) therapies are available for treating the infertile couple.* For couples with unexplained infertility, empiric treatment may overcome the negative effects of one or more mild abnormalities. These couples, as well as the majority of infertile couples, tend to proceed through fertility treatment in a stepwise fashion, starting with conservative and then with more aggressive ovarian stimulation, inseminations, and eventually proceeding to IVF (explained below).

Surgical procedures are indicated in certain circumstances. If a woman presents with pelvic pain and infertility, laparoscopy may be used to identify and treat the cause of her pelvic pain as well as evaluate pelvic anatomy from a fertility standpoint. If an obstructed fallopian tube is identified with HSG, it may be possible to correct the obstruction surgically. For these operations to be successful, the endosalpinx must be healthy. If the tubal damage is significant enough to impair gamete transport, then an ART such as IVF may be necessary. When indicated, abnormalities of the uterine cavity such as submucosal leiomyomas, endometrial polyps, intrauterine adhesions, and a septum can be surgically corrected with a hysteroscopic procedure.

### Ovarian Stimulation

**Ovulation induction** is indicated in women with anovulation or oligo-ovulation. *However, any identified condition associated with ovulatory disorders should be treated before initiating ovulation-induction therapy. Such conditions include thyroid disorders, hyperprolactinemia, PCOS, and high levels of stress (including psychologic stress, intense exercise, or eating disorders).*

*The most commonly used medication for ovulation induction is clomiphene citrate.* Clomiphene is a selective estrogen receptor modulator (SERM) that competitively inhibits estrogen binding to the estrogen receptors at the hypothalamus and pituitary. The anti-estrogen effects of clomiphene induce gonadotropin release from the pituitary, which stimulates follicle development in the ovaries. Clomiphene is administered daily for 5 days in the follicular phase of the menstrual cycle, starting between cycle days 3 to 5. If ovulation does not occur, the dose is increased for the subsequent month. Women with ovulatory disorders associated with oligomenorrhea may not have regular menses and may require a progesterone-induced menses to start their clomiphene cycle. When used in women who are already ovulatory, clomiphene may stimulate development of several mature follicles.

With clomiphene, ovulation can occur between 5 to 12 days after the last pill, and it can be monitored in several ways. Urine LH kits can be used each day starting on cycle day 10; when ovulation occurs, exposure to sperm through intercourse or **intrauterine insemination (IUI)** should occur. Transvaginal ultrasound performed on cycle day 11 or 12 may identify a developing follicle. When ultrasound is used and a mature follicle is identified (average diameter >18 mm), ovulation can be triggered by administering a subcutaneous injection of hCG. The exogenous hCG effectively simulates the LH surge and ovulation occurs; this practice enables the proper timing of intercourse or insemination. Some couples prefer to not monitor ovulation, and have regular midcycle intercourse. In this situation, a serum progesterone level on cycle day 21 can identify if ovulation has occurred. *The use of clomiphene is associated with a 10% risk of multiple gestations, the majority of which are twin gestations, and a small risk of ovarian hyperstimulation and cyst formation.*

Alternatively, exogenous gonadotropins can be given to stimulate follicular development. The use of gonadotropins is commonly referred to as **controlled ovarian hyperstimulation** (COH). This therapy aims to achieve monofollicular ovulation in anovulatory women (particularly those who do not respond to clomiphene), and ovulation of several mature follicles in other infertile women. Available preparations include purified human menopausal gonadotropins (FSH and LH are extracted from the urine of postmenopausal women), and recombinant human FSH. The dose of medication is tailored to a woman's age, body weight, infertility diagnosis, and response to previous fertility treatments. These medications are more potent than clomiphene and require frequent monitoring of follicle growth that usually includes transvaginal ultrasonography and serum estradiol measurements. When at least one mature follicle is identified (average follicle diameter of 18 mm and serum estradiol concentration >200 pg/mL), hCG is administered to trigger ovulation. Timed inseminations are commonly performed within 12 to 36 hours from hCG administration. The risks of this therapy include ovarian **hyperstimulation syndrome (OHSS),** which can require intensive therapy; a 25% incidence of multiple gestations; and an increased risk of ectopic pregnancy.

### Intrauterine Insemination

Before performing IUI, an ejaculated semen specimen is washed to remove prostaglandins, bacteria, and proteins. The sperm is then suspended in a small amount of medium.

To perform IUI, a speculum is inserted into the vagina, the specimen is placed in a thin flexible catheter, and the catheter is advanced through the cervix into the uterine cavity where the specimen is deposited (Fig. 38.7). A total motile sperm count (concentration multiplied by motility) of at least one million must be present, as pregnancy is rarely achieved with lower counts. *In couples with infertility, and particularly in those with mild male infertility, pregnancy rates are increased with IUI.* However, more severe male infertility may necessitate the use of ART to achieve pregnancy. If the male partner is azoospermic and no sperm are identified during testicular biopsy, or if a woman does not have a male partner, IUI with anonymous donor sperm is an available alternative.

## Assisted Reproductive Technologies

All fertility procedures that involve manipulation of gametes, zygotes, or embryos to achieve conception comprise the assisted reproductive technologies (ART). In the United States, IVF accounts for more than 99% of all ART procedures. *The process of IVF involves ovarian stimulation to produce multiple follicles, retrieval of the oocytes from the ovaries, oocyte fertilization in vitro in the laboratory, embryo incubation in the laboratory, and transfer of embryos into a woman's uterus through the cervix.* The required medications for IVF include gonadotropins to stimulate follicle development, a gonadotropin-releasing hormone analogue (agonist or antagonist) to prevent premature ovulation during follicle development, and hCG to initiate the final maturation of oocytes prior to their retrieval. As with COH, the IVF process necessitates careful monitoring of ovarian response with transvaginal ultrasonography and serum estradiol measurements.

Depending on the etiology of infertility, fertilization can be achieved "naturally" by placing tens of thousands of sperm together with a single oocyte, or with **intracytoplasmic sperm injection** (ICSI) by which a single sperm is injected directly into the oocyte (Fig. 38.8). Therefore,

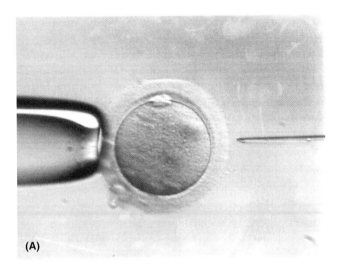

(A)

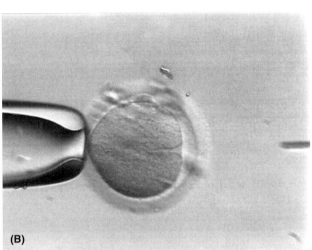

(B)

FIGURE 38.8. Intracytoplasmic sperm injection. A. An oocyte is being held by a holding pipette. The injection pipette contains a single sperm. B. The injection pipette has penetrated the zona pellucida and plasma membrane of the oocyte, and the sperm has been microinjected into the oocyte. (Courtesy of James H. Liu, MD. From Fritz MA, Dodson WC, Meldrum D, Johnson JV. Infertility. In: *Precis, An Update in Obstetrics and Gynecology: Reproductive Endocrinology.* 3rd ed. Washington, DC: American College of Obstetricians and Gynecologists; 2007:161.)

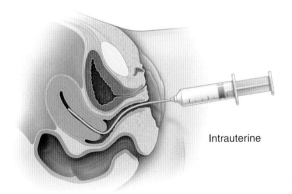

Intrauterine

FIGURE 38.7. Intrauterine insemination technique.

IVF provides the tools necessary to bypass the normal mechanisms of gamete transport, fertilization, and embryo transport. *After oocyte retrieval, daily progesterone supplementation is necessary to insure the appropriate secretory changes in the endometrium and to support the potential pregnancy; if conception occurs, supplementation is continued until at least 10 weeks of gestation.*

Indications for IVF include the following: absent or blocked fallopian tubes, tubal sterilization, failed surgery to achieve tubal patency, severe pelvic adhesions, severe endometriosis, poor ovarian response to stimulation, oligo-ovulation, severe male factor infertility, unexplained infertility, or failed treatment with less aggressive therapies. *Success rates with IVF depend on the etiology of infertility and the age of the female partner.* The chance of conception with one IVF cycle depends on the number and quality of embryos transferred, and can be as high as 40% to 50%, with a 30% rate of multiple gestations and at least a 15% rate of spontaneous abortion.

## COUNSELING

A team approach is frequently helpful in ensuring that patients receive an adequate workup and appropriate counseling. Counseling of patients who are treated with ART should include information regarding the risk of multiple gestation, ethical issues surrounding multifetal pregnancy reduction, and adoption. Clinicians should also be familiar with any state laws regarding infertility services and treatment or insurance coverage.

## SUGGESTED READINGS

American College of Obstetricians and Gynecologists. *Guidelines for Women's Health Care: A Resource Manual.* 3rd ed. Washington, DC: American College of Obstetricians and Gynecologists; 2007.

American College of Obstetricians and Gynecologists. Management of infertility caused by ovulatory dysfunction. ACOG Practice Bulletin No. 34. *Obstet Gynecol.* 2002;99(1):347–358.

Meldrum D. Assisted reproductive technologies. In: American College of Obstetricians and Gynecologists. *Precis, An Update in Obstetrics and Gynecology: Reproductive Endocrinology.* 3rd ed. Washington, DC: American College of Obstetricians and Gynecologists; 2007:140–172.

# Premenstrual Syndrome and Premenstrual Dysphoric Disorder

This chapter deals primarily with APGO Educational Topic:

Topic 49: Premenstrual Syndrome and Premenstrual Dysphoric Disorder

The student should be able to diagnose, distinguish, and plan effective management for PMS and PMDD.

P *remenstrual syndrome (PMS) is a group of physical, mood-related, and behavioral changes that occur in a regular, cyclic relationship to the luteal phase of the menstrual cycle and that interfere with some aspect of the patient's life.* These symptoms occur in most cycles, resolving usually with onset of menses, but certainly by cessation of menses. This cyclic symptom complex varies both in severity and in the degree of disruption of the patient's work, home, or leisure life. The Diagnostic and Statistical Manual of Mental Disorders, 4th edition (DSM-IV), *lists the diagnostic criteria for premenstrual dysphoric disorder (PMDD) as a specific set of at least 5 of 11 possible symptoms, with at least 1 core symptom—specifically depressed mood, anxiety or tension, irritability, or decreased interest in activities (anhedonia).* These symptoms occur regularly during the luteal phase of the menstrual cycle.

*PMDD identifies women with PMS who have more severe emotional symptoms that may require more intensive therapy.*

The pathophysiology of both entities is not well-elucidated. Neither condition should be confused with normal cyclic symptoms associated with ovulation.

## INCIDENCE

Premenstrual symptoms occur in approximately 75% to 85% of women. *PMS that causes significant disruption of daily life occurs in approximately 5% to 10% of women. PMDD, rigorously diagnosed as outlined in the DSM-IV, affects only 3% to 5% of women.* PMS and PMDD can begin with menarche, but can also present later in life, even in a woman's 40s, though this is often a reflection of the hesitancy of women to seek medical help for their symptoms. The expression or symptom dominance of these disorders dif-

fers depending on ethnicity and culture. There is some evidence that the incidence of PMDD varies across cultures as well, with high rates in Mediterranean cultures and the Middle East and low rates in Asia. Twin studies also demonstrate concordance, implying a genetic contribution to the development of these disorders.

## SYMPTOMS

Over 200 symptoms have been attributed to PMS. Each patient presents with her own constellation of symptoms, thus making specific symptoms less important than the cyclic occurrence of the symptoms. Somatic symptoms that are most common include abdominal bloating and fatigue. Other symptoms include breast swelling and pain (**mastodynia**), headache, acne, digestive upset, dizziness, sensitivity to external stimuli, and hot flushes. The most common behavioral symptom is emotional lability. Other behavioral symptoms include irritability, depressed mood, anxiety, hostility, lachrymosity, increased appetite, difficulty concentrating, and changes in libido. Box 39.1 presents the diagnostic criteria for PMDD as described in the DSM-IV. Box 39.2 lists the diagnostic criteria for PMS. The criteria for the diagnosis of PMDD are more rigorous than those of PMS and emphasize the existence of mood-related symptoms. PMS can be diagnosed on the basis of either mood or physical symptoms.

### Etiology

*Many theories have been proposed to explain PMS, including altered levels of estrogen, progesterone, endorphins, catecholamines, vitamins, and minerals, but none provides a single, unified explanation that accounts for all the variations that are seen.*

---

**BOX 39.1**
**Diagnostic Criteria for Premenstrual Dysphoric Disorder**

A. In most menstrual cycles during the past year, ≥5 of the following were present most of the time during the last week of the luteal phase, began to remit within a few days of menses onset, and were absent in the week post-menses, with at least one of the symptoms being items 1, 2, 3, or 4 ("core symptoms") listed below:

  1. Markedly depressed mood, feelings of hopelessness, self-deprecation
  2. Marked anxiety, tension, feelings of being "keyed up" or "on edge"
  3. Suddenly feeling sad or tearful, with increased sensitivity to personal rejection
  4. Persistent and marked irritability, anger, or increased interpersonal conflicts
  5. Decreased interest in usual activities
  6. Subjective sense of having difficulty in concentrating

  7. Lethargy, fatigue, or marked lack of energy
  8. Marked change in appetite and cravings for certain foods
  9. Hypersomnia or insomnia
  10. Feeling overwhelmed or out of control
  11. Other physical symptoms, such as breast tenderness or swelling, headaches, joint or muscle pain, a sensation of "bloating," or weight gain, pain, etc.

B. The disturbance markedly interferes with work or school, or with usual social activities and relationships with others

C. The disturbance is not merely an exacerbation of the symptoms of another disorder, although it may be superimposed on one

D. Criteria A, B, and C must be confirmed by prospective daily ratings during at least 2 consecutive symptomatic cycles (the diagnosis may be made provisionally prior to this confirmation)

Reprinted with permission from American Psychiatric Association. *The Diagnostic and Statistical Manual of Mental Disorders.* 4th ed. Text Revision. (DSM-IV-TR). Arlington, VA. American Psychiatric Association, 2000.

---

No compelling variations in any of these substances have been found in women who have symptoms, compared to women without symptoms, with the exception of some preliminary studies on serotonin. Although it has been proposed that a low luteal-phase progesterone level is the cause of what is now recognized as PMS or PMDD, measurement of serum progesterone values and clinical results of progesterone supplementation have not supported this theory.

*Currently the data support a theory of* **serotoninergic dysregulation** *as the basis for PMS/PMDD.* Normal cyclic hormonal fluctuations can trigger an abnormal serotonin response. Monoamine oxidase reduces serotonin availability, progesterone potentiates monoamine oxidase, and estrogen potentiates monoamine oxidase inhibitors. Thus, the availability of serotonin is decreased in the progesterone-dominant luteal phase. However, the interaction must be more complex, because replacement of progesterone alone does not ameliorate PMS symptoms. Absolute levels of progesterone have not been found to be different in women with PMS and those without, and monoamine oxidase inhibitors do not improve symptoms in these patients. More recent data implicates γ-aminobutyric acid (GABA) as an important factor in decreasing levels of allopregnanolone, a progesterone metabolite.

## Diagnosis

Virtually any condition that results in mood or physical changes in any cyclic fashion may be included in the dif-ferential diagnosis of PMS (Box 39.3). Studies have shown that a patient's recall of symptoms and timing of symptoms is often biased and thus inaccurate, because of widespread societal expectations and cultural prominence of "the premenstrual syndrome." *The majority of patients who present for treatment of PMS do not actually demonstrate symptoms restricted to the luteal phase.*

*The diagnosis of PMS and PMDD can be very subjective and thus should be rigorously established using the criteria outlined.*

The physician must remain open-minded at the outset, and not prematurely exclude the primary problem. In the differential diagnosis, the physician should consider medical problems, psychiatric disorders, and premenstrual exacerbations of medical and/or psychiatric conditions: Perimenopause can also present with similar symptoms (see Chapter 37, Menopause).

Because the etiology of PMS and PMDD is not clear, no definitive historical, physical examination, or laboratory markers are available to aid in diagnosis. *At present, the diagnosis of PMS and PMDD is based on documentation of the relationship of the patient's symptoms to the luteal phase.* Prospective documentation of symptoms can be accom-

---

BOX 39.2
## Diagnostic Criteria for Premenstrual Syndrome

1. Premenstrual syndrome can be diagnosed if the patient reports at least 1 of the following affective and somatic symptoms during the 5 days before menses in each of 3 menstrual cycles:

   **Affective Symptoms**
   Depression
   Angry outbursts
   Irritability
   Anxiety
   Confusion
   Social Withdrawal

   **Somatic Symptoms**
   Breast tenderness
   Abdominal bloating
   Headache
   Swelling of extremities

2. These symptoms are relieved within 4 days of the onset of menses, without recurrence until at least cycle day 13. The symptoms are present in the absence of any pharmacologic therapy, hormone ingestion, or drug or alcohol use. The symptoms occur reproducibly during 2 cycles of prospective recording. The patient suffers from identifiable dysfunction in social or economic performance.

Adapted with permission from Mortola JF, Girton L, Yen SS. Depressive episodes in premenstrual syndrome. *Am J Obstet Gynecol.* 1989;161(1 Pt 1):1682–1687.

---

plished using a **menstrual diary** in two or more consecutive menstrual cycles. The patient is asked to monitor her symptoms and the pattern of menstrual bleeding for 2 or more cycles. For PMS, she needs only to have one of the listed symptoms, but must have a symptom-free period. For PMDD, the patient is asked to also monitor the severity of symptoms. She must demonstrate 5 of the listed 11 symptoms (see Box 39.2), one of which must be a core symptom. She also must demonstrate a symptom-free follicular phase. If her symptoms persist during the follicular phase but are less severe, one must consider luteal phase worsening of a different disorder (sometimes called **entrainment**).

*Many physical and psychiatric disorders are known to worsen in the luteal phase, including irritable bowel syndrome and major depressive disorder.*

It is important to distinguish these disorders from PMDD. A variety of diagnostic tools exist to assist patients with keeping their menstrual diaries. Figure 39.1 shows one such tool called "Daily Record of Severity of Problems."

*Patients with PMS should be evaluated to rule out specific pathology, although it is also important to understand that no specific physical findings are diagnostic of PMS.*

It is reasonable to perform a complete blood count and evaluate the thyroid-stimulating hormone (TSH) level, because thyroid disease and anemia are quite common in young menstruating women; however, there is no evidence that anemia or thyroid disease occur more frequently in patients who present for treatment of PMS or PMDD.

## TREATMENT

The prospective charting of symptoms not only documents the cyclic or noncyclical nature of the patient's symptoms, but also allows her to play a key role in the diagnostic and management team. This will allow her to regain some control of her symptoms. For some women, providing a diagnostic label helps relieve the fear that they are "going crazy." Often a patient's symptoms become more bearable as she gains insight. The symptom calendar is usually continued during the treatment phase to monitor the effectiveness of treatment and to suggest the need for further focused therapy.

### Nonpharmacologic Treatment

Diet recommendations emphasize eating fresh rather than processed foods. The patient is encouraged to eat more fruits and vegetables and minimize refined sugars and fats. Minimizing salt intake may help with bloating, and eliminating caffeine and alcohol from the diet can reduce nervousness and anxiety. None of these therapies have shown statistically significant improvements in PMS and PMDD, but they are reasonable, benign, a good part of general health improvement, and in some studies have demonstrated trends towards improvement. Clearly these interventions yield low risks and are generally healthful behaviors.

*Lifestyle interventions that have demonstrated significant improvement in symptoms include aerobic exercise and calcium carbonate and magnesium supplementation.* Aerobic exercise, as opposed to static (e.g., weightlifting) exercise, has been found to be helpful in some patients, possibly by increasing endogenous production of endorphins. Calcium decreases water retention, food cravings, pain, and negative affect, compared with placebo.

Other interventions have been studied, but demonstrate conflicting results. These include vitamins E and D or chaste-tree berry extract, as well as relaxation therapy,

---

**BOX 39.3**
**Differential Diagnosis of Premenstrual Syndrome**

Allergy
Breast disorders (fibrocystic change)
Chronic fatigue states
   Anemia
   Chronic cytomegalovirus infection
   Lyme disease
Connective tissue disease (lupus erythematosus)
Drug and substance abuse
Endocrinologic disorders
   Adrenal disorders (Cushing syndrome,
    hypoadrenalism)
   Adrenocorticotropic hormone-mediated
    disorders
   Hyperandrogenism
   Hyperprolactinemia
   Panhypopituitarism
   Pheochromocytoma
   Thyroid disorders (hypothyroidism,
    hyperthyroidism)
Family, marital, and social stress (physical or
   sexual abuse)

Gastrointestinal conditions
   Inflammatory bowel disease (Crohn disease,
    ulcerative colitis)
   Irritable bowel syndrome
Gynecologic disorders
   Dysmenorrhea
   Endometriosis
   Pelvic inflammatory disease
   Perimenopause
   Uterine leiomyomata
Idiopathic edema
Neurologic disorders
   Migraine
   Seizure disorders
Psychiatric and psychological disorders
   Anxiety neurosis
   Bulimia
   Personality disorders
   Psychosis
   Somatoform disorders
   Unipolar and bipolar affective disorders

From Smith RP. *Gynecology in Primary Care*. Baltimore, MD: Lippincott Williams & Wilkins; 1996:434.

---

cognitive therapy, and light therapy. Many of these therapies have no untoward side effects, and can be considered for certain patients. Studies have shown that B6 supplementation has limited clinical benefit. Patients should be cautioned that dosages in excess of 100 mg/d may cause medical harm, including peripheral neuropathy. Studies of evening primrose oil demonstrate no benefit. Alternative therapies include meditation, aromatherapy, reflexology, acupuncture, acupressure, and yoga. Further research is warranted in these areas.

## Pharmacologic Treatment

*In addition to lifestyle changes, behavioral therapies, and dietary supplementation, some pharmacologic agents have been shown to provide symptomatic relief.* **Nonsteroidal anti-inflammatory agents (NSAIDs)** have been found in controlled trials to be useful in PMS patients with dysmenorrhea, breast pain, and leg edema, but not useful in treating other aspects of PMS. This effect is possibly related to prostaglandin production in various sites in the body. Spironolactone decreases bloating, but does not relieve other symptoms.

Because the underlying mechanism appears to be normal hormone fluctuations triggering an abnormal serotonin response, it would seem that medications to induce anovulation should be beneficial in the treatment of PMS/PMDD. *The research on PMS/PMDD has been fraught with multiple challenges because the strict criteria for diagnosis of PMS/PMDD have only recently been established and standardized, many previous studies suffered from poor methodology, and the placebo effect (30% to 70%) in patients with PMS/PMDD is significant.* Because symptoms are associated with ovulatory cycles, suppressing ovulation is beneficial for some patients with PMS and can be accomplished by using oral contraceptives, **danazol**, or **gonadotropin-releasing hormone (GnRH)** agonists. Oral contraceptives are a logical first choice for patients who also require contraception. Some patients, however, find that their symptoms worsen when taking oral contraceptives.

*As an overall clinical approach, treatments should be employed in increasing orders of complexity.*

Using this principle, in most cases, the therapies should be used in the following order:

**Step 1.** Supportive therapy, complex carbohydrate diet, nutritional supplements (calcium, magnesium, vitamin E), spironolactone

**Step 2.** Selective serotonin reuptake inhibitors (SSRIs), with fluoxetine or sertraline as the initial choice; for women

## DAILY RECORD OF SEVERITY OF PROBLEMS

**Please print and use as many sheets as you need for at least two FULL months of ratings.**

Name or Initials _____

Month/Year _____

Each evening note the degree to which you experienced each of the problems listed below. Put an "x" in the box which corresponds to the severity: 1 - not at all, 2 - minimal, 3 - mild, 4 - moderate, 5 - severe, 6 - extreme.

| | | |
|---|---|---|
| Enter day (Monday="M", Thursday="R", etc) > | | |
| Note spotting by entering "S" > | | |
| Note menses by entering "M" > | | |
| Begin rating on correct calendar day > | | 1 2 3 4 5 6 7 8 9 10 11 12 13 14 15 16 17 18 19 20 21 22 23 24 25 26 27 28 29 30 31 |

1. Felt depressed, sad, "down,", or "blue" or felt hopeless; or felt worthless or guilty — 6 5 4 3 2 1

2. Felt anxious, tense, "keyed up" or "on edge" — 6 5 4 3 2 1

3. Had mood swings (i.e., suddenly feeling sad or tearful) or was sensitive to rejection or feelings were easily hurt — 6 5 4 3 2 1

4. Felt angry, or irritable — 6 5 4 3 2 1

5. Had less interest in usual activities (work, school, friends, hobbies) — 6 5 4 3 2 1

6. Had difficulty concentrating — 6 5 4 3 2 1

7. Felt lethargic, tired, or fatigued; or had lack of energy — 6 5 4 3 2 1

8. Had increased appetite or overate; or had cravings for specific foods — 6 5 4 3 2 1

9. Slept more, took naps, found it hard to get up when intended; or had trouble getting to sleep or staying asleep — 6 5 4 3 2 1

10. Felt overwhelmed or unable to cope; or felt out of control — 6 5 4 3 2 1

11. Had breast tenderness, breast swelling, bloated sensation, weight gain, headache, joint or muscle pain, or other physical symptoms — 6 5 4 3 2 1

At work, school, home, or in daily routine, at least one of the problems noted above caused reduction of productivity or inefficiency — 6 5 4 3 2 1

At least one of the problems noted above caused avoidance of or less participation in hobbies or social activities — 6 5 4 3 2 1

At least one of the problems noted above interfered with relationships with others — 6 5 4 3 2 1

© pending, Jean Endicott, Ph.D. and Wilma Harrison, M.D.

**FIGURE 39.1.** Daily Record of Severity of Problems. © Jean Endicott, PhD and Wilma Harrison, MD.

who do not respond, consider an anxiolytic for specific symptoms

**Step 3.** Hormonal ovulation suppression (oral contraceptives or GnRH agonists)

*The medical treatment of PMDD differs from that of PMS. Ovulation suppression does not seem to help patients with PMDD.* Though many medications have been studied, only four are U.S. Food and Drug Administration (FDA)-approved for the treatment of PMDD: fluoxetine, sertraline, paroxetine controlled-release, and drospirenone/ethinyl estradiol.

*In patients who have been diagnosed with PMDD using the strict criteria, the gold standard of treatment is the **SSRIs**.*

In a Cochrane Data Base Review, 15 randomized placebo-controlled trials demonstrated benefit with SSRIs. The combination of drospirenone and ethinyl estradiol is the only oral contraceptive regimen that has demonstrated benefit and is the newest therapeutic choice for the treatment of PMDD. SSRIs are effective when dosed continuously (daily dosage); or dosed intermittently (taken only during the luteal phase [the 14 days prior to onset of menses]). Patients often report improvement with their first cycle of use, lending credence to the idea that the pathophysiology of PMDD is different from that of major depressive disorder, in which treatment can take weeks to demonstrate improvement. Side effects of SSRIs include gastrointestinal upset, insomnia, sexual dysfunction, weight gain, anxiety, hot flushes, and nervousness.

*The use of danazol and GnRH agonists has been demonstrated to be beneficial in short-term studies, but long-term effects of such drugs for PMS/PMDD have not been fully evaluated, and these medications are associated with significant, often prohibitive, side effects.* The use of either constitutes a "medical oophorectomy" and may be used as a trial before surgical oophorectomy is undertaken. Oophorectomy should be reserved for those severely affected patients who meet strict diagnostic criteria and who do not respond to any potentially effective therapy other than GnRH agonists.

## SUGGESTED READINGS

American College of Obstetricians and Gynecologists. *Guidelines for Women's Health Care: A Resource Manual.* 3rd ed. Washington, D.C.: ACOG; 2007.

American College of Obstetricians and Gynecologists. Premenstrual Syndrome. ACOG Practice Bulletin 15. *Obstet Gynecol.* 2000; 95(4):1–9.

*Precis, An Update in Obstetrics and Gynecology: Reproductive Endocrinology.* 3rd ed. Washington, D.C.: American College of Obstetricians and Gynecologists; 2007:102–112, 203–205.

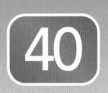

# Cell Biology and Principles of Cancer Therapy

Understanding the fundamentals of cell biology is important in the recognition of the behavior of malignant tumors and their response to therapy.

Treatment of cancers involving the breast and genital organs may involve surgery, chemotherapy, radiation therapy, or hormone therapy, used alone or in combination. The specific treatment plan depends on the type of cancer, the stage of the cancer, and the characteristics of the individual patient. *Individualizing treatment is an important aspect of cancer therapy.*

## CELL CYCLE AND CANCER THERAPY

Knowledge of the cell cycle is important in understanding cancer therapies. The ideal cancer treatment would be a drug that targets only cancer cells with no effect on healthy tissues.

*In order to optimally target only cancerous tissue, it is imperative to understand not only how normal cells function, but also how cancer cells differ from normal cells.*

Many treatments are based on the fact that cancer cells are constantly dividing, making them more vulnerable to agents that interfere with cell division.

*The cell cycle consists of four phases* (Fig. 40.1). During the $G_1$ phase (postmitotic phase), RNA and protein synthesis, cell growth, and DNA repair take place. Once these processes are complete, the cell enters the S phase (synthesis phase), during which the DNA is completely replicated. The $G_2$ phase is a period of additional synthesis of RNA, protein, and specialized DNA. Cell division occurs during the M phase (mitosis). After mitosis, cells can again enter the $G_1$ phase, or can "drop out" of the cell cycle and enter a resting phase ($G_0$). Cells in $G_0$ do not engage in the synthetic activities characteristic of the cell cycle and are not vulnerable to therapies aimed at actively growing and dividing cells. The **growth fraction** is the proportion of cells in a tumor that are actively involved in cell division

(i.e., not in the $G_0$ phase). The growth fraction of tumors decreases as they enlarge, because vascular supply and oxygen levels are decreased. *Surgical removal of tumor tissue (cytoreductive debulking surgery) can result in $G_0$ cells reentering the cell cycle, thus making them more vulnerable to chemotherapy and radiation therapy.*

The **generation time** is the length of the cell cycle, from one M phase to the next M phase. For a given cell type, the lengths of the S and M phases are relatively constant, whereas $G_2$ and especially $G_1$ vary. The variable length of $G_1$ can be explained by cells entering the resting phase ($G_0$) for a period and then reentering the cycle. The length of $G_1$ has a profound effect on the cell's susceptibility to treatment.

Chemotherapeutic agents and radiation kill cancer cells by first-order kinetics. This means that each dose kills a constant fraction of tumor cells, instead of a constant number. The resulting clinical implication is that several intermittent doses are more likely to be curative than a single large dose.

## CHEMOTHERAPY

**Chemotherapeutic agents** can be (1) **cell cycle (phase)-nonspecific,** which means that they can kill in all phases of the cell cycle and are useful in tumors with a low growth index, or (2) **cell cycle (phase)-specific,** which means that they kill in a specific phase of the cell cycle and are most useful in tumors that have a large proportion of actively dividing cells. Figure 40.1 illustrates common drugs and their sites of action within the cell cycle.

Several classes of **antineoplastic drugs** are available (Table 40.1). **Alkylating agents** and **alkylating-like agents** bind and cross-link DNA, interfering with DNA replication and, ultimately, with RNA transcription. Dividing cells, especially those in the late $G_1$ and S phases, are most sensitive to the effects of these drugs; however, these drugs are considered phase-nonspecific (i.e., they are effective in all phases of the cell cycle). The major side effect of the

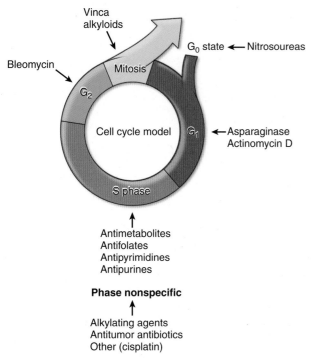

FIGURE 40.1. Actions of antineoplastic agents within the cell cycle.

alkylating agents is myelosuppression. The alkylating-like agents behave similarly, and include the platinum-based agents cisplatin and carboplatin.

**Antitumor antibiotics** inhibit DNA-directed RNA synthesis and also are involved in the formation of free radicals, causing strand breakage. They are phase-nonspecific. Their general side effects are similar to those of the alkylating agents; however, each individual drug has its own individual toxicity.

**Antimetabolites** are structural analogs of normal molecules necessary for cell function. They competitively interfere with the enzymes involved with normal synthesis of nucleic acids and, therefore, are most active during the S phase of cell division. They may cause bone marrow suppression or gastrointestinal mucositis when given in a bolus.

**Plant (vinca) alkaloids** interfere with the M phase of cell division by preventing the assembly of microtubules. They may cause bone marrow suppression or an anaphylactoid reaction.

**Topoisomerase inhibitors** result in cell death by inhibiting topoisomerase I (TOPO-I), an enzyme required for DNA replication. In a normally replicating cell, TOPO-I induces reversible single-strand breaks in the DNA. TOPO-I inhibitors complex with the DNA and TOPO-I and prevent repair of the breaks in the single strand of DNA, thus resulting in cellular death.

| TABLE 40.1 | Classes of Chemotherapeutic Drugs | | |
|---|---|---|---|
| **Class** | **Mechanism of Action** | **Primary Toxicities** | **Representative Drugs** |
| Alkylating agents | Bind and cross-link DNA either inter-strand, intrastrand, or to proteins; prevents replication and transcription | Hemorrhagic cystitis, alopecia, nephrotoxicity | Cyclophosphamide, ifosfamide, melphalan |
| Alkylating-like agents | Cross-link DNA strands (interstrand) | Nephrotoxicity, neurotoxicity, myelosuppression | Cisplatin, carboplatin |
| Antibiotics | Interfere with DNA replication through free radical formation and intercalation between bases | Variable | Bleomycin, actinomycin D |
| Antimetabolites | Block enzymes required for DNA synthesis | Gastrointestinal, myelosuppression, dermatologic, hepatotoxicity | Methotrexate, 5-fluorouracil |
| Plant (vinca) alkaloids | Inhibit microtubule assembly | Myelosuppression | Vincristine, vinblastine, paclitaxel |
| Topoisomerase inhibitors | Inhibit topoisomerase, resulting in DNA strand breaks | Myelosuppression, alopecia, gastrointestinal | Etoposide, Topotecan |

Endocrine therapy with **selective estrogen receptor modulators** (SERMs) acts in estrogen-sensitive breast tumors to block the interaction of estrogen with estrogen receptors (ERs). The therapeutic importance of cellular ERs has been well established in breast cancers. ER-positive tumors are responsive to endocrine therapy. Normally, estrogen enters cells and binds to ERs in the cytoplasm. The complex is translocated to the nucleus, where it binds to acceptor sites on chromosomes, resulting in activation of RNA and protein synthesis. SERMs act as competitive inhibitors of estrogen binding; the SERM–ER complex binds to chromosomes, but does not activate cell metabolism. The subsequent decrease in cellular activity and cell division results in reduced tumor growth. The two SERMs most frequently prescribed in the United States are tamoxifen and raloxifene. Although relatively nontoxic, this class of drugs is related to an increased risk of endometrial cancer and uterine sarcomas and an increase in benign endometrial pathology.

**Aromatase inhibitors** (AIs), which suppress intra-tumor and plasma estrogen levels, are being used in post-menopausal patients for treatment of advanced breast cancer that has progressed beyond tamoxifen therapy.

**Progestational agents** have been found to be useful in the treatment of early-stage endometrial cancer when surgery is either not feasible, unsafe, or not desired. Progestational therapy is also useful for some patients with recurrent disease. The most common progestational agents used are medroxyprogesterone and megestrol. Other hormonal agents that have demonstrated efficacy in cases of recurrent disease include tamoxifen (SERM), goserelin (synthetic hormone), anastrozole (AI), and arzoxifene (SERM).

*Antineoplastic drugs are toxic because they act on normal as well as cancer cells.* Table 40.2 describes the major applications and side effects of antineoplastic agents. Rapidly dividing cell types of the erythroid, myeloid, and megakaryocytic lineages are most sensitive to damage by common neoplastic drugs. Anemia, granulocytopenia (neutropenia), and thrombocytopenia are predictable side effects. Patients with anemia will often experience incapacitating lethargy. Patients with neutropenia are at high risk for fatal sepsis, and those with sustained thrombocytopenia are at risk for spontaneous gastrointestinal or acute intracranial hemorrhage. Prophylactic antibiotics are administered to patients with febrile neutropenia or in neutropenic patients to prevent serious infection. Platelet transfusions can be used to decrease the risk of hemorrhage.

The use of single agents is limited by development of drug resistance and toxicity. **Combination chemotherapy** is used to counteract these limitations. Several strategies can be used to select drugs for combination chemotherapy. In **sequential blockade,** the drugs block sequential enzymes in a single biochemical pathway. In **concurrent blockade,** the drugs attack parallel biochemical pathways leading to the same end product. Complementary inhibition inter-feres with different steps in the synthesis of DNA, RNA, or protein.

The interactions between drugs used in combination are defined as **synergistic** (result in improved antitumor activity or decreased toxicity, compared with when each agent is used alone), **additive** (result in enhanced antitumor activity equal to the sum of the antitumor activities resulting from using the individual agents separately), or **antagonistic** (result in less antitumor activity than if each individual agent is used alone). Drugs used in combinations should (1) be effective when used singly, (2) have different mechanisms of action, and (3) be additive or, preferably, synergistic in action.

*Chemotherapy is administered in various regimens.* **Adjuvant** chemotherapy is usually a set course of combination chemotherapy that is given in a high dose to patients who have no evidence of residual cancer after radiotherapy or surgery. The purpose is to eliminate any residual cancer cells, typically with the intent to cure disease. **Neoadjuvant** chemotherapy aims to eradicate micrometastases or reduce inoperable disease in order to prepare patients for surgery and/or radiotherapy. **Induction** chemotherapy is usually a combination chemotherapy given in a high dose to cause a remission. **Maintenance** chemotherapy (consolidation chemotherapy) is a long-term and low-dose regimen that is given to a patient in remission to maintain the remission by inhibiting the growth of remaining cancer cells.

## RADIATION THERAPY

**Ionizing radiation** causes the production of free hydrogen ions and hydroxyl ($\cdot$OH) radicals. With sufficient oxygen, hydrogen peroxide ($H_2O_2$) is formed, which disrupts the structure of DNA and, eventually, the cell's ability to divide. As with chemotherapy, killing is by first-order kinetics. *Because dividing cells are more sensitive to radiation damage and because not all cells in a given tumor are dividing at any one time, fractionated doses of radiation are more likely to be effective than a single dose.* Providing multiple lower doses of radiation also reduces the deleterious effects on normal tissues.

The basis of fractionated dosage comes from the **"four Rs"** of radiobiology:

1. **Repair of sublethal injury.** When a dose is divided, the number of normal cells that survive is greater than if the dose were given at one time (higher total amounts of radiation can be tolerated in fractionated as opposed to single doses).
2. **Repopulation.** Reactivation of stem cells occurs when radiation is stopped; thus regenerative capacity depends on the number of available stem cells.
3. **Reoxygenation.** Cells are more vulnerable to radiation damage with oxygen present; as tumor cells are killed, surviving tumor cells are brought into contact with capillaries, making them radiosensitive.

| TABLE 40.2 | Major Application and Side Effects of Chemotherapeutic Agents | | |
|---|---|---|---|
| **Drug** | **Application** | **Dose-Limiting Toxicity** | **Other Toxicities** |
| Paclitaxel (mitotic inhibitor) | Ovarian cancer, endometrial cancer (advanced), granulosa cell tumors | Myelosuppression (neutropenia), peripheral neuropathy | Alopecia, myalgias/arthralgias, GI toxicity, hypersensitivity reaction |
| Carboplatin (alkylating-like agent) | Ovarian cancer, endometrial cancer (advanced), granulose cell tumors | Myelosuppression (thrombocytopenia) | Nephrotoxicity, ototoxicity, GI toxicity, alopecia, hypersensitivity reaction |
| Cisplatin (alkylating-like agent) | Cervical cancer, germ cell tumors | Nephrotoxicity | Neurotoxicity, GI toxicity, hypersensitivity reaction |
| Bleomycin (antibiotic) | Germ cell tumors | Pulmonary fibrosis | Dermatologic (mucositis, hyperpigmentation) |
| Topotecan (topoisomerase inhibitor) | Ovarian cancer | Myelosuppression (neutropenia) | Alopecia, GI toxicity |
| Liposomal doxorubicin | Ovarian cancer | Myelosuppression | Palmar-plantar erythrodysesthesia, GI toxicity (stomatitis, N&V), cardiac (minimal) |
| Gemcitabine hydrochloride (antimetabolite) | Ovarian cancer | Neutropenia | Hepatotoxicity, nephrotoxicity, hemolytic uremic syndrome |
| Etoposide (topoisomerase inhibitor) | Germ cell tumors, gestational trophoblastic neoplasia | Myelosuppression (neutropenia) | Alopecia, GI toxicity, acute MI, acute leukemia |
| Ifosfamide (alkylating agent) | Uterine sarcoma | Hemorrhagic cystitis | Nephrotoxicity, GI toxicity, alopecia, mild leukopenia |
| Methotrexate (antimetabolite) | Gestational trophoblastic neoplasia, molar pregnancies | Myelosuppression (all cell lines) | Hepatotoxicity, nephrotoxicity, dermatologic (photosensitivity, rashes, vasculitis) |
| Dactinomycin/ Actinomycin D (antibiotic) | Endometrial cancer, gestational trophoblastic neoplasia | Myelosuppression (all cell lines) | GI toxicity (N&V, mucositis), alopecia, extravasation necrosis |
| Cyclophosphamide (alkylating agent) | Gestational trophoblastic neoplasia | Myelosuppression | Hemorrhagic cystitis, alopecia, SIADH |
| Vincristine (plant alkaloid) | Gestational trophoblastic neoplasia | Myelosuppression | Alopecia, GI toxicity, myalgias, peripheral neuropathy |

GI = gastrointestinal; MI = myocardial infarction; N&V = nausea and vomiting; SIADH = syndrome of inappropriate secretion of antidiuretic hormone.

4. **Redistribution in the cell cycle.** Because tumor cells are in various phases of the cell cycle, fractionated doses make it more likely that a given cell is irradiated when it is most vulnerable.

The *rad* has been used as a measure of the amount of energy absorbed per unit mass of tissue. A standard measure of absorbed dose is the *Gray*, which is defined as 1 joule per kilogram; *1 Gray is equal to 100 rad.* Radiation is delivered in two general ways: external irradiation (teletherapy) and local irradiation (brachytherapy). **Teletherapy** depends on the use of high-energy (>1 million eV) beams, because

this spares the skin and delivers less toxic radiation to the bone. Tolerance for external radiation depends on the vulnerability of surrounding normal tissues. Teletherapy usually is used to shrink tumors before localized radiation. **Brachytherapy** depends on the inverse square law: the dose of radiation at a given point is inversely proportional to the square of the distance from the radiation source. To put the radioactive material at the closest possible distance, brachytherapy uses encapsulated sources of ionizing radiation implanted directly into tissues (interstitial) or placed in natural body cavities (intracavitary). **Intracavitary devices** can be placed within the uterus, cervix, or vagina, and then (after) loaded with radioactive sources as either low-dose radiotherapy (cesium-137), high-dose radiotherapy (iridium-192, cobalt-60), or as interstitial implants. This method protects health personnel from radiation exposure. A new method of treating early breast cancer involves high–dose-rate brachytherapy inserted by balloon catheter into the cavity created by lumpectomy. **Interstitial implants** use isotopes (iridium-192, iodine-125) formulated as wires or seeds. These implants are usually temporary, but permanent seed implants are being investigated.

New strategies are being developed for radiation therapy. For example, **intraoperative** therapy is being used for previously irradiated patients with recurrent disease who would require unacceptably high dosages of external radiation.

*Complications associated with radiation therapy can be acute or late (chronic).* **Acute reactions** affect rapidly dividing tissues, such as epithelia (skin, gastrointestinal mucosa, bone marrow, and reproductive cells). Manifestations are cessation of mitotic activity, cellular swelling, tissue edema, and tissue necrosis. Early problems associated with irradiation of gynecologic cancers include enteritis, acute cystitis, vulvitis, proctosigmoiditis, topical skin desquamation, and, occasionally, bone marrow depression. **Chronic complications** occur months to years after completion of radiation therapy. These include obliteration of small blood vessels or thickening of the vessel wall, fibrosis, and reductions in epithelial and parenchymal cell populations. Chronic proctitis, hemorrhagic cystitis, formation of ureterovaginal or vesicovaginal fistula, rectal or sigmoid stenosis, and bowel obstructions, as well as gastrointestinal fistulae may result.

## NOVEL CHEMOTHERAPEUTIC AGENTS

The next horizon for cancer treatment is molecularly targeted agents, cancer vaccines, and gene therapy. Several drugs are currently available that target specific molecules or proteins in cancer cells. For example, trastuzumab is a DNA-derived monoclonal antibody to the human epidermal growth factor receptor 2 protein (HER-2). Treatment with trastuzumab is currently indicated in patients with metastatic breast cancer whose tumors overexpress HER-2. Some ovarian, cervical, and endometrial tumors express the HER-2/*neu* receptor; therefore, investigation is currently ongoing regarding the usefulness of this

agent in gynecologic tumors. Additionally, bevacizumab is a monoclonal antibody designed to target the VEGF protein and inhibit angiogenesis in tumors. It is currently under investigation for possible treatment of a variety of tumors, including epithelial ovarian cancer.

**Tumor vaccines** are also currently being investigated for the treatment of ovarian cancer. The underlying principle behind these therapeutic vaccines is to inoculate the patient with a modified cancer cell line in an attempt to stimulate the patient's immune system to recognize and eliminate the tumor. Inactivated virus strains have also been studied as a vector for the vaccines in hopes of creating higher immunogenicity. Currently the response to this type of therapy has been modest, but studies are ongoing.

Because a large proportion of gynecologic cancers result from loss of genetic function through DNA mutations, investigational therapies have also focused on genetic manipulation of the tumors, or **gene therapy.** For instance, because half of ovarian cancers exhibit deleterious mutations in the *p53* gene, research has focused on delivering a normal *p53* gene product to the tumor using a variety of viral vectors. The hope is that the wild-type gene product would then be expressed by the tumor and the growth would then be inhibited. So far, response has been minimal, but investigation continues.

The potential benefits of these novel therapeutic concepts are manifold, whether considered as primary or adjunct therapy. *Work in this area is in the experimental stage, but the goal of eliminating cancer cells with minimal toxicity remains the goal of cancer therapeutics.*

## SUGGESTED READINGS

American College of Obstetricians and Gynecologists. Breast cancer screening. ACOG Practice Bulletin No. 42. *Obstet Gynecol.* 2003;101(5):821–832.

American College of Obstetricians and Gynecologists. Diagnosis and treatment of cervical carcinomas. ACOG Practice Bulletin No. 35. *Obstet Gynecol.* 2002;99(5):855–867.

American College of Obstetricians and Gynecologists (ACOG). *Guidelines for Women's Health Care: A Resource Manual.* 3rd ed. Washington, D.C.: ACOG; 2007.

American College of Obstetricians and Gynecologists. Selective estrogen receptor modulators. ACOG Practice Bulletin No. 39. *Obstet Gynecol.* 2002;100(5):835–844.

Genetics and gynecologic cancer. In: *Precis, An Update in Obstetrics and Gynecology: Oncology,* 3rd ed. Washington, DC: American College of Obstetricians and Gynecologists; 2008:10–20.

# 41 Gestational Trophoblastic Neoplasia

This chapter deals primarily with APGO Educational Topic:

Topic 50: Gestational Trophoblastic Neoplasia

The student should be familiar with the morbidity and mortality associated with this unique neoplasm.

G *estational trophoblastic neoplasia (GTN) is a rare variation of pregnancy of unknown etiology and usually presents as a benign disease called* **hydatidiform mole** (molar pregnancy). *GTN is a clinical spectrum that includes all neoplasms that derive from abnormal placental (trophoblastic)* proliferation. There are two varieties of molar pregnancies, complete mole (no fetus), and incomplete mole (fetal parts in addition to molar degeneration.) *Persistent or* **malignant disease** *will develop in approximately 20% of patients with molar pregnancy. Persistent or malignant GTN is responsive to chemotherapy.*

Key clinical features of GTN include: (1) clinical presentation as pregnancy, (2) reliable means of diagnosis by pathognomonic ultrasound findings, and (3) a specific tumor marker (quantitative serum **human chorionic gonadotropin [hCG]**). *Persistent GTN may occur with any pregnancy, although it most commonly follows molar pregnancy.*

## EPIDEMIOLOGY

The incidence of molar pregnancy varies among different national and ethnic groups. The highest incidence occurs among Asian women living in Asia (1 in 200 pregnancies). The incidence in the United States is approximately 1 in 1500 pregnancies, with a recurrence rate of 1% to 2%. It is more common in older women. It is associated with low dietary carotene consumption and vitamin A deficiency. Partial moles are associated with history of infertility and spontaneous abortion.

## HYDATIDIFORM MOLE

A hydatidiform mole includes abnormal proliferation of the syncytiotrophoblast and replacement of normal placental trophoblastic tissue by **hydropic placental villi**. **Complete moles** do not have identifiable embryonic or fetal structures. **Partial moles** are characterized by focal trophoblastic proliferation, degeneration of the placenta, and identifiable fetal or embryonic structures.

*The genetic constitutions of the two types of molar pregnancy are different* (Table 41.1). Complete moles have chromosomes entirely of paternal origin as the result of the fertilization of a blighted ovum by a haploid sperm that reduplicates, or rarely, fertilization of a blighted ovum with two sperm. *The karyotype of a complete mole is usually 46XX. The fetus of a partial mole is usually a triploid.* This consists of one haploid set of maternal chromosomes and two haploid sets of paternal chromosomes, the consequence of dispermic fertilization of a normal ovum. *Complete moles are more common than partial moles and are more likely to undergo malignant transformation.*

## Clinical Presentation

Patients with molar pregnancy have findings consistent with a confirmed pregnancy as well as uterine size and date discrepancy, exaggerated subjective symptoms of pregnancy, and painless second-trimester bleeding. *With the increased early prevalence of first-trimester ultrasound, moles are now frequently diagnosed in the first trimester of pregnancy before symptoms are present.* Abnormal bleeding is the most characteristic presenting symptom which prompts evaluation for threatened abortion. Lack of fetal heart tones detected at the first obstetric appointment can also prompt evaluation (depending on the estimated gestational age). Ultrasound imaging confirms the diagnosis of molar pregnancy by its characteristic "**snowstorm**" appearance and absence of fetal parts (complete mole) [Fig. 41.1]. In cases of partial mole, ultrasonography reveals an abnormally formed fetus. Quantitative hCG levels are excessively elevated for gestational age, and the uterus is usually larger than expected.

Molar pregnancies may present with other signs and symptoms, including severe nausea and vomiting, marked crepancy of the uterine fundus and absent fetal heart tones, but also changes associated with developing severe hypertension, such as hyperreflexia. Bimanual pelvic examination may reveal large adnexal masses (**theca lutein cysts**), which represent marked enlargement of the ovaries secondary to hCG stimulation.

With earlier diagnosis, the medical complications of molar pregnancy are becoming less common.

*In any woman who presents with findings suggestive of severe hypertension prior to 20 weeks in pregnancy, a molar pregnancy should be immediately suspected.*

Twin pregnancies with a normal fetus coexisting with a complete or partial mole are exceedingly rare. Women with these pregnancies should be treated in a tertiary hospital center with specialized care. Medical complications in molar twin gestations rarely allow these pregnancies to reach term. These pregnancies also have a higher risk of persistent metastatic or nonmetastatic gestational trophoblastic disease (GTD).

An **invasive mole** is histologically identical to a complete mole. It invades the myometrium without any intervening endometrial stroma seen on histological sample. It is often diagnosed months after evacuation of a complete

gestational hypertension, proteinuria, and, rarely, clinical hyperthyroidism. *Most of these findings can be attributed to the high levels of hCG produced by the abnormal pregnancy.* Some patients experience tachycardia and shortness of breath, arising from intense hemodynamic changes associated with acute hypertensive crisis. In these patients physical examination reveals not only date and size dis-

TABLE 41.1    **Features of Partial and Complete Hydatidiform Moles**

| Feature | Partial Mole | Complete Mole |
|---|---|---|
| Karyotype | Triploid | 46XX, rarely 46XY |
| Pathology | | |
| Fetus | Often present | Absent |
| Amnion, fetal RBCs | Usually present | Absent |
| Villous edema | Variable, focal | Diffuse |
| Trophoblastic proliferation | Focal, slight to moderate | Diffuse |
| Clinical Presentation | | |
| Diagnosis | Missed abortion | Molar gestation |
| Uterine size | Small or appropriate for gestational age | 50% large for gestational age |
| Theca lutein cysts | Rare | >25% depending on diagnostic modality |
| Medical complications | Rare | Becoming rare with early diagnosis |
| Postmolar invasion and malignancy | <5% | 15% and 4% respectively |

RBC = red blood cells.
Table modified from *ACOG Practice Bulletin #53* June 2004. Updated information from Berkowitz RS, and Goldstein DP. Gestational trophoblastic disease. In: Hoskins WJ, Perez CA, Young RC, eds. *Principles and Practice of Gynecologic Oncology.* 4th ed. Philadelphia, PA: Lippincott Williams & Wilkins; 2005:1057–1061.

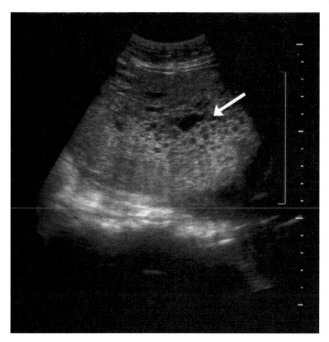

FIGURE 41.1. "Snowstorm" appearance of complete mole on ultrasound examination. The arrow points to intrauterine tissue. (From Soper JT. Gestational trophoblastic disease. Obstet Gynecol. 2006;108(1):178.)

mole, when hCG levels do not fall appropriately as **persistent metastatic** or **nonmetastatic GTD.** Occasionally, it may be diagnosed on curettage at the time of initial molar evacuation.

*Whereas both partial and complete molar pregnancies present as abnormal pregnancies, partial mole most often presents as a missed abortion.* Vaginal bleeding is less common in partial molar pregnancy than in complete molar pregnancy. Uterine growth is less than expected for the gestational age in partial molar pregnancy. Ultrasound reveals molar degeneration of the placenta and a grossly abnormal fetus or embryo. Medical complications, theca lutein cysts, and subsequent malignancies are rare (see Table 41-1).

---

**B O X   4 1 . 2**
**Preoperative Evaluation of Molar Pregnancy**

1. Baseline quantitative hCG level
2. Baseline chest x-ray to check for metastatic disease
3. Complete blood count
4. Blood type with type and screen
5. Clotting function studies
6. Other appropriate tests if clinical evidence of hyperthyroidism and/or gestational hypertension

---

## Treatment

*In most cases of molar pregnancy the definitive treatment is prompt evacuation of the uterine contents.* Uterine evacuation is done most often by dilation of the cervix, and suction curettage followed by gentle sharp curettage. Because the evacuation of larger moles is sometimes associated with uterine atony and excessive blood loss, appropriate preparations should be made for uterotonic administration and blood transfusion, if needed. In rare cases of a late presenting partial molar pregnancy, there may be an additional need for larger grasping instruments to remove the abnormal fetus.

> *In general, the larger the uterus, the greater the risk of pulmonary complications associated with trophoblastic emboli, fluid overload, and anemia.*

This is particularly true in patients with severe associated gestational hypertension, who may experience concomitant hemoconcentration and alteration in vascular hemodynamics (see the section on preeclampsia in Chapter 16, Hypertension in Pregnancy). Hysterectomy or induction of labor with prostaglandins is not usually recommended, because of the increased risk of blood loss and other sequelae. The bilaterally enlarged multicystic ovaries (**theca lutein cysts**) resulting from follicular stimulation by high levels of circulating hCG, do not represent malignant changes. *The theca lutein cysts invariably regress within a few months of evacuation, and therefore do not require surgical removal.*

Patients who have no interest in further childbearing or have other indications for hysterectomy may be treated by hysterectomy with ovarian preservation. Despite removal of the entire primary neoplasm, the risk of persistent GTD is 3% to 5%.

## Postevacuation Management

*Because of the predisposition for recurrence, patients should be monitored closely for 6 to 12 months after the evacuation of a molar pregnancy.* Rh-negative patients should be given Rh-immune globulin. Follow-up consists of periodic physical examination to check for vaginal metastasis and appropriate involution of pelvic structures. Quantitative *hCG* levels should be checked within 48 hours following evacuation, every 1 to 2 weeks while elevated, and at 1 to 2 months thereafter. Quantitative hCG levels that rise or reach a plateau are an indication of persistent disease and the need for further treatment after a new pregnancy has been ruled out. *During the first year, the patient should be treated with oral contraceptive pills (OCPs) or other reliable contraceptive method to prevent an intercurrent pregnancy.* (Multiple studies have proven the safety of OCP use after a molar pregnancy.) The risk of recurrence after 1 year of remission is

<1%. The risk of recurrence with subsequent pregnancies is 1% to 2%. There is no increase in congenital anomalies or complications in future pregnancies.

## MALIGNANT GESTATIONAL TROPHOBLASTIC NEOPLASIA

Postmolar or **persistent GTD** is only one of the many forms of malignant GTD. Although invasive moles are histologically identical to antecedent molar pregnancies while invading the myometrium, **choriocarcinomas** are a malignant transformation of trophoblastic tissue. Instead of hydropic chorionic villi, the tumor has a red granular appearance on cut suction and consists of intermingled syncytiotrophoblastic and cytotrophoblastic elements with many abnormal cellular forms. Clinically, choriocarcinomas are characterized by rapid myometrial and uterine-vessel invasion and systemic metastases resulting from hematogenous embolization. Lung, vagina, central nervous system, kidney, and liver are common metastatic locations. Choriocarcinoma may follow a molar pregnancy, normal-term pregnancy, abortion, or ectopic pregnancy. In the United States, choriocarcinoma is associated with approximately 1 in 150,000 pregnancies, 1 in 15,000 abortions, 1 in 5000 ectopic pregnancies, and 1 in 40 molar pregnancies.

Early identification and treatment are important. *Abnormal bleeding for more than 6 weeks after any pregnancy should be evaluated with hCG testing to exclude a new pregnancy or GTD.* Failure of quantitative hCG levels to regress after treatment of a molar pregnancy suggests that further treatment is needed. Identified metastatic sites should not be biopsied to avoid bleeding complications. *Most GTN, including malignant forms, are highly sensitive to chemotherapy and often results in a cure, allowing for future reproduction.*

*Nonmetastatic persistent GTN is completely treated by single-agent chemotherapy.* Single-agent chemotherapy is either **methotrexate** or **actinomycin D.** The prognosis for metastatic GTN is more complex, divided into good and poor prognostic categories (Table 41-2). The World Health Organization (WHO) has developed a prognostic scoring system for GTN that includes a number of epidemiologic and laboratory findings; this system was later combined into the International Federation of Gynecology and Obstetrics (FIGO) staging system (Table 41-3). *A FIGO score of 7 or above classifies metastatic GTN as high-risk, requiring multi-agent chemotherapy.* The combination chemotherapeutic regimen with the highest success rates is: **etoposide, methotrexate, actinomycin D, cyclophosphamide, and Oncovin (vincristine)) [EMACO].** Adjunctive radiotherapy is sometimes performed with patients who have brain or liver metastasis. Surgery may be necessary to control hemorrhage, remove chemotherapy-resistant disease, and treat other complications to stabilize high-risk patients during intensive chemotherapy. Cure rates for non-metastatic and good-prognosis metastatic disease approach 100%. Cute rates for poor-prognosis metastatic disease are 80% to 90%.

| TABLE 41.2 | Clinical Classification of Malignant Gestational Trophoblastic Disease |
|---|---|
| **Category** | **Criteria** |
| Nonmetastatic gestational trophoblastic disease | No evidence of metastases; not assigned to prognostic category |
| Metastatic gestational trophoblastic disease | Any extra uterine metastasis |
|   Good prognosis | No Risk Factors:<br>1. Short interval from antecedent pregnancy <4 mo.<br>2. Pretherapy hCG level <40,000 mIU/mL<br>3. No brain or liver metastases<br>4. No antecedent term pregnancy<br>5. No prior chemotherapy |
|   Poor prognosis | Any Risk Factor:<br>1. >4 mo. since last pregnancy<br>2. Pretherapy hCG level >40,000 mIU/mL<br>3. Brain or liver metastases<br>4. Antecedent term pregnancy<br>5. Prior chemotherapy |

From American College of Obstetricians and Gynecologists. Diagnosis and treatment of gestational trophoblastic disease. ACOG Practice Bulletin No. 53. *Obstet Gynecol.* 2004;103:1365–1377.

| TABLE 41.3 | Revised FIGO Scoring System |

| Finding | FIGO* Score | | | |
|---|---|---|---|---|
| | 0 | 1 | 2 | 4 |
| Age (years) | ≤39 | ≥39 | – | – |
| Antecedent pregnancy | Hydatidiform mole | Abortion | Term pregnancy | – |
| Interval from last pregnancy | <4 mo | 4–6 mo | 7–12 mo | >12 mo |
| Pretreatment hCG level | <1000 | 1000–10,000 | >10,000–100,000 | >100,000 |
| Largest tumor size including uterus | 3–4 cm | 5 cm | – | – |
| Site of metastases | Lung, vagina | Spleen, kidney | Gastrointestinal tract | Brain, liver |
| Number of metastases | 0 | 1–4 | 4–8 | >8 |
| Previous failed chemotherapy | – | – | Single drug | 2 or more drugs |

*FIGO = International Federation of Gynecology and Obstetrics.
**The total score for a patient is obtained by adding the individual scores for each prognostic factor. Total Score: 0–6 = low risk, ≥7 high risk.**

## PLACENTAL SITE TUMORS

Placental site tumor is a rare form of trophoblastic disease. The tumor is comprised of monomorphic populations of intermediate cytotrophoblastic cells that are locally invasive at the site of placental implantation. The tumor only secretes small amounts of hCG, and can be better followed by human placental lactogen levels. This tumor is rarely metastatic and is much more resistant to standard chemotherapy. Hysterectomy as initial therapy is often curative.

## SUGGESTED READING

American College of Obstetricians and Gynecologists. Diagnosis and treatment of gestational trophoblastic disease. ACOG Practice Bulletin No. 53. *Obstet Gynecol.* 2004;103(#): 1365–1377.

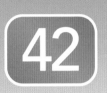

# 42 Vulvar and Vaginal Disease and Neoplasia

**Topic 51:** Vulvar Neoplasms

Students should be able to describe the risk factors associated with vulvar neoplasms and common vulvar diseases, as well as their appropriate evaluation and management. They should also be able to explain the indications for vulvar biopsy and describe the standard techniques.

E valuation of vulvar symptoms and examination of patients for vulvar disease and neoplasia constitute a significant part of healthcare for women. *The major symptoms of vulvar disease are pruritus, burning, non-specific irritation, and/or appreciation of a mass.* The vulvar region is particularly sensitive to irritants, more so than other regions of the body. It has been suggested that the layer overlying the vulva—the stratum corneum—may be less of a barrier to irritants, thereby making the vulva more susceptible to irritations and contributing to the "itch-scratch" cycle. Noninflammatory vulvar pathology is found in women of all ages, but is especially significant in perimenopausal and postmenopausal women because of concern regarding the possibility of vulvar neoplasia.

Diagnostic aids for the assessment of noninflammatory conditions are relatively limited in number and include careful history, inspection, and biopsy. *Because vulvar lesions are often difficult to diagnose, use of vulvar biopsy is central to good care.* **Punch biopsies** of vulvar abnormalities are most helpful to determine if cancer is present or to histologically determine the specific cause of a perceived abnormality of the vulva. Cytologic evaluation of the vulva is of limited value, as the vulvar skin is keratinized and epithelium shedding does not occur as readily as that of the cervix. **Colposcopy** is useful for evaluating known vulvar atypia and intraepithelial neoplasia.

This chapter provides discussions of a range of vulvar pathologic conditions, including non-neoplastic dermatoses, vestibulitis, benign vulvar mass lesions, vulvar intraepithelial neoplasia, and vulvar cancer. Benign vaginal masses and vaginal neoplasia are also discussed. Inflammatory conditions of the vulva are discussed in Chapter 28, Vulvovaginitis.

## BENIGN VULVAR DISEASE

In the past, the classification of benign, noninfectious vulvar disease used descriptive terminology based on gross clinical morphologic appearance such as leukoplakia, kraurosis vulvae, and hyperplastic vulvitis. Currently, these diseases are classified into three categories: squamous cell hyperplasia, lichen sclerosus, and other dermatoses.

In 2006, the International Society for the Study of Vulvar Disease (ISSVD) constructed a new classification using **histologic morphology** based on consensus among gynecologists, dermatologists, and pathologists involved in the care of women with vulvar disease. Common ISSVD classifications are outlined in Table 42.1.

## Lichen Sclerosus

**Lichen sclerosus** has confused clinicians and pathologists because of inconsistent terminology and its frequent association with other types of vulvar pathology, including those of the acanthotic variety. As with the other disorders, chronic vulvar pruritus occurs in most patients. *Typically, the vulva is diffusely involved, with very thin, whitish epithelial areas, termed "onion skin" epithelium* (Fig. 42.1B). The epithelium has been termed "cigarette paper" skin and described as "parchment-like." Most patients have involvement on both sides of the vulva, with the most common sites being the labia majora, labia minora, the clitoral and periclitoral epithelium, and the perineal body. The lesion may extend to include a perianal "halo" of atrophic, whitish epithelium, forming a figure-8 configuration with the vulvar changes. *In severe cases, many normal anatomic landmarks are lost, including obliteration of the labial and periclitoral architecture as well as severe stenosis of the vaginal introitus.* Some patients have areas of cracked skin, which are prone to bleeding with minimal trauma. Patients with these severe anatomic changes complain of difficulty in having normal coital function.

*The etiology of lichen sclerosus is unknown, but a familial association has been noted, as well as disorders of the immune*

| TABLE 42.1 | 2006 ISSVD Classification of Vulvar Dermatoses: Most Common Pathologic Subsets and Their Clinical Correlates | |
|---|---|---|
| **Histologic Pattern** | **Characteristic** | **Clinical Correlate** |
| Lichenoid | Bandlike lymphocytic infiltration of the upper dermis and epidermal basal layer damage | Lichen sclerosus<br>Lichen planus |
| Dermal homogenization/ sclerosis | Partial or complete obliteration of collagen bundle boundaries with "hyalinized/glassy" dermis | Lichen sclerosus |
| Acanthotic (formerly squamous cell hyperplasia) | Hyperkeratosis-increased number of epithelial cells leading to epidermal thickening or hyperplasia | Lichen simplex chronicus<br>    Primary (idiopathic)<br>    Secondary (superimposed on lichen<br>    sclerosis/planus)<br>Psoriasis |
| Spongiotic | Intercellular edema within the epidermis with widening of the intercellular space | Irritant dermatitis<br>Allergic contact dermatitis |

IVSSD = International Society for the Study of Vulvar Disease.

*system, including thyroid disorders and Class II human leukocyte antigens.* However, the response to topical steroids further indicates the underlying inflammatory process and the role of prostaglandins and leukotrienes in the hallmark symptom of pruritus. *Histologic evaluation and confirmation of lichen sclerosis is often necessary and useful, because they allow specific therapy.* The histologic features of the lichenoid pattern include a band of chronic inflammatory cells, consisting mostly of lymphocytes, in the upper dermis with a zone of homogeneous, pink-staining, collagenous-like material beneath the epidermis due to cell death. The obliteration of boundaries between collagen bundles gives the dermis a "hyalinized" or "glassy" appearance. This dermal homogenization/ sclerosis pattern is virtually pathognomonic.

In 27% to 35% of patients, there are associated areas of acanthosis characterized by **hyperkeratosis**—an increase in the number of epithelial cells (keratinocytes) with flattening of the rete pegs. These areas may be mixed through-out or adjacent to the typically lichenoid areas. In patients with this mixed pattern, both components need to be treated to effect resolution of symptoms. Patients in whom a large acanthotic component has been histologically confirmed should be treated initially with well-penetrating corticosteroid creams. With improvement of these areas (usually 2 to 3 weeks), therapy can then be directed to the lichenoid component.

*Treatment for lichen sclerosis includes the use of topical steroid (clobetasol) preparations in an effort to ameliorate symptoms.* The lesion is unlikely to resolve totally. Intermittent treatment may be needed indefinitely, which is in marked contrast to acanthotic lesions, which usually totally resolve within 6 months.

*Lichen sclerosus does not significantly increase the patient's risk of developing cancer.*

FIGURE 42.1. The three "lichens." (A) Lichen simplex chronicus; sclerosus; (B) Lichen simplex chronicus; (C) Lichen planus. (Used with permission from Foster DC. Vulvar disease. *Obstet Gynecol.* 2002;100(1): 149.)

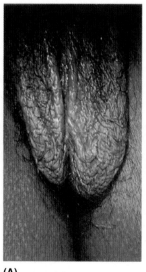
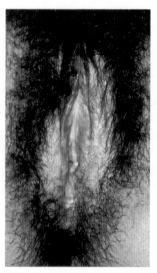
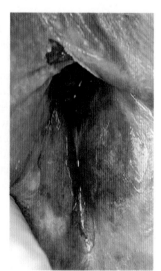

(A)                    (B)                    (C)

It has been estimated that this risk is in the 4% range. However, due to the frequent coexistence with acanthosis, the condition needs to be followed carefully and a rebiopsy performed, because therapeutically resistant acanthosis can be a harbinger of squamous cell carcinoma (SCC).

## Lichen Simplex Chronicus

In contrast to many dermatologic conditions that may be described as "rashes that itch," lichen simplex chronicus can be described as *"an itch that rashes."* Most patients develop this disorder secondary to an irritant dermatitis, which progresses to lichen simplex chronicus as a result of the effects of chronic mechanical irritation from scratching and rubbing an already irritated area. *The mechanical irritation contributes to epidermal thickening or hyperplasia and inflammatory cell infiltrate, which, in turn, leads to heightened sensitivity that triggers more mechanical irritation.*

*Accordingly, the history of these patients is one of progressive vulvar pruritus and/or burning,* which is temporarily relieved by scratching or rubbing with a washcloth or some similar material. Etiologic factors for the original pruritic symptoms often are unknown, but may include sources of skin irritation such as laundry detergents, fabric softeners, scented hygienic preparations, and the use of colored or scented toilet tissue. These potential sources of symptoms must be investigated. Any domestic or hygienic irritants must be removed, in combination with treatment, to break the cycle described.

*On clinical inspection, the skin of the labia majora, labia minora, and perineal body often shows diffusely reddened areas with occasional hyperplastic or hyperpigmented plaques of red to reddish brown* (see Fig. 42.1A). One may also find occasional areas of linear hyperplasia, which show the effect of grossly hyperkeratotic ridges of epidermis. Biopsy of patients who have these characteristic findings is usually not warranted.

Empiric treatment to include antipruritic medications such as diphenhydramine hydrochloride (Benadryl) or hydroxyzine hydrochloride (Atarax) that inhibit nighttime, unconscious scratching, combined with a mild to moderate topical steroid cream applied to the vulva, usually provides relief. A steroid cream, such as hydrocortisone (1% or 2%) or, for patients with significant areas of obvious hyperkeratosis, triamcinolone acetonide or betamethasone valerate may be used. *If significant relief is not obtained within 3 months, diagnostic vulvar biopsy is warranted.*

*The prognosis for this disorder is excellent when the offending irritating agents are removed and a topical steroid preparation is used appropriately.* In most patients, these measures cure the problem and eliminate future recurrences.

## Lichen Planus

Although **lichen planus** is usually a desquamative lesion of the vagina, occasional patients develop lesions on the vulva near the inner aspects of the labia minora and vulvar vestibule. Patients may have areas of whitish, lacy bands (Wickham striae) of keratosis near the reddish ulcerated-like lesions characteristic of the disease (see Figure 42.1C). *Typically, complaints include chronic vulvar burning and/or pruritus and insertional (i.e., entrance) dyspareunia and a profuse vaginal discharge.* Because of the patchiness of this lesion and the concern raised by atypical appearance of the lesions, biopsy may be warranted to confirm the diagnosis in some patients. In lichen planus, biopsy shows no atypia. Examination of the vaginal discharge in these patients frequently reveals large numbers of acute inflammatory cells without significant numbers of bacteria. Accordingly, the diagnosis most often can be made by the typical history of vaginal/vulvar burning and/or insertional dyspareunia, coupled with a physical examination that shows the bright red patchy distribution; and a wet prep that shows large numbers of white cells. Histologically the epithelium is thinned, and there is a loss of the rete ridges with a lymphocytic infiltrate just beneath, associated with basal cell liquefaction necrosis.

Treatment for lichen planus is topical steroid preparations similar to those used for lichen simplex chronicus. This may include the use of intravaginal 1% hydrocortisone douches. Length of treatment for these patients is often shorter than that required to treat lichen simplex chronicus, although lichen planus is more likely to recur.

## Psoriasis

**Psoriasis** *is an autosomal dominant inherited disorder that can involve the vulvar skin as part of a generalized dermatologic process.* With approximately 2% of the general population suffering from psoriasis, the physician should be alert to its prevalence and the likelihood of vulvar manifestation, because it may appear during menarche, pregnancy, and menopause.

The lesions are typically slightly raised round or ovoid patches with a silver scale appearance atop an erythematous base. These lesions most often measure approximately $1 \times 1$ to $1 \times 2$ cm. Though pruritus is usually minimal, these silvery lesions will reveal punctate bleeding areas if removed (Auspitz sign). *The diagnosis is generally known because of psoriasis found elsewhere on the body, obviating the need for vulvar biopsy to confirm the diagnosis.* Histologically, a prominent **acanthotic pattern** is seen, with distinct dermal papillae that are clubbed and chronic inflammatory cells between them.

Treatment often occurs in conjunction with consultation by a dermatologist. Like lesions elsewhere, vulvar lesions usually respond to topical coal tar preparations, followed by exposure to ultraviolet light as well as corticosteroid medications, either topically or by intralesional injection. Coal tar preparations are extremely irritating to the vagina and labial mucous membranes and should not be used in these areas. *Because vulvar application of some of the photoactivated preparations can be somewhat awkward, topical steroids are most effective, using compounds such as betamethasone valerate 0.1%.*

## Dermatitis

**Vulvar dermatitis** falls into two main categories: **eczema** and **seborrheic dermatitis.** Eczema can be further subdivided into **exogenous** and **endogenous forms. Irritant** and **allergic contact dermatitis** are forms of exogenous eczema. They are usually reactions to potential irritants or allergens found in soaps, laundry detergents, textiles, and feminine hygiene products. Careful history can be helpful in identifying the offending agent and in preventing recurrences. **Atopic dermatitis** is a form of endogenous eczema that often affects multiple sites, including the flexural surfaces of the elbows and knees, retroauricular area, and scalp. The lesions associated with these three forms of dermatitis can appear similar: symmetric eczematous lesions, with underlying erythema. Histology alone will not distinguish these three types of dermatitis. They all exhibit a **spongiotic pattern** characterized by intercellular edema within the epidermis, causing widening of the space between the cells. Therefore, these entities must often be distinguished clinically.

*Although **seborrheic dermatitis** is a common problem, isolated vulvar seborrheic dermatitis is rare.* It involves a chronic inflammation of the sebaceous glands, but the exact cause is unknown. The diagnosis is usually made in patients complaining of vulvar pruritus who are known to have seborrheic dermatitis in the scalp or other hair-bearing areas of the body. The lesion may mimic other entities such as psoriasis or lichen simplex chronicus. *The lesions are pale red to a yellowish pink and may be covered by an oily appearing, scaly crust.* Because this area of the body remains continually moist, occasional exudative lesions include raw "weeping" patches, caused by skin maceration, which are exacerbated by the patient's scratching. *As with psoriasis, vulvar biopsy is usually not needed when the diagnosis is made in conjunction with known seborrheic dermatitis in other hair-bearing areas.* The histologic features of seborrheic dermatitis are a combination of those seen in the acanthotic and spongiotic patterns.

Treatment for vulvar dermatitis involves removing the offending agent, if applicable, initial perineal hygiene and the use of a 5% solution of aluminum acetate several times a day, followed by drying. Topical corticosteroid lotions or creams containing a mixture of an agent that penetrates well, such as betamethasone valerate, in conjunction with crotamiton, can be used for symptom control. As with LSC, the use of antipruritic agents as a bedtime dose in the first 10 days to 2 weeks of treatment frequently helps break the sleep/scratch cycle and allows the lesions to heal. Table 42.2 summarizes the clinical characteristics of the common vulvar dermatoses.

## Vestibulitis

**Vulvar vestibulitis** is a condition of unknown etiology. It involves the acute and chronic inflammation of the vestibular glands, which lie just inside the vaginal introitus near the hymeneal ring. The involved glands may be circumferential to include areas near the urethra, but this condition most commonly involves posterolateral vestibular glands between the 4 and 8 o'clock positions (Fig. 42.2). *The diagnosis should be suspected in all patients who present with new onset insertional dyspareunia.* Patients with this condition frequently complain of progressive insertional dyspareunia to the point where they are unable to have intercourse. The history may go on for a few weeks, but most typically involves progres-

| TABLE 42.2 | Clinical Characteristics of the Common Vulvar Dermatoses | |
|---|---|---|
| **Disorder** | **Lesion** | **Hallmarks** |
| Lichen sclerosis | Atrophic, thin, whitish epithelium with frequent perianal halo or "keyhole" distribution | "Cigarette paper," parchment-like skin, halo or loss of elasticity |
| Lichen planus | White lacy network (Wickham striae) with flat-topped lilac papules and plaques | Erosive vaginitis with demarcated edges |
| Lichen simplex chronicus | Lichenified, hyperplastic plaques of red to reddish brown | Symmetric with variable pigmentation |
| Psoriasis | Annular pink plaques with silvery scale that bleed if removed (Auspitz sign) | Elbows, knees, scalp also often affected |
| Dermatitis Irritant, allergic, or atopic | Eczematous lesions with underlying erythema | Symmetric with extension into areas of irritant or allergen contact |
| Seborrheic | Pale red to yellowish pink plaques, often oily appearing, scaly crust | Other hair-bearing areas often affected–scalp and chest; also back and face |

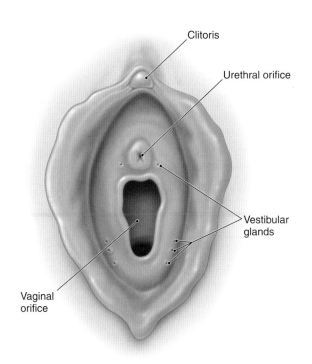

FIGURE 42.2. **Vestibular glands.**

sive worsening over the course of 3 or 4 months. Patients also complain of pain on tampon insertion and at times during washing or bathing the perineal area.

Physical examination is the key to diagnosis. Because the vestibular glands lie between the folds of the hymenal ring and the medial aspect of the vulvar vestibule, diagnosis is frequently missed when inspection of the perineum does not include these areas: *Once the speculum has been placed in the vagina, the vestibular gland area becomes impossible to identify.* After carefully inspecting the proper anatomic area, a light touch with a moistened cotton applicator recreates the pain exactly and allows for quantification of the pain. In addition, the regions affected are most often evident as small, reddened, patchy areas.

Because the cause of vestibulitis is unknown, treatments vary and range from changing or eliminating environmental factors, temporary sexual abstinence, and application of cortisone ointments and topical lidocaine (jelly); to more radical treatments such as surgical excision of the vestibular glands. A combination of treatment modalities may be necessary. Treatment must be individualized, based on the severity of patient symptoms and the sexual disability.

Some patients may benefit from low-dose tricyclic medication (amitriptyline and desipramine) or fluoxetine to help break the cycle of pain. Other limited reports suggest the use of calcium citrate to change the urine composition by removing oxalic acid crystals. Those advocating changing the urine chemistry cite evidence to suggest that oxalic acid crystals are particularly irritating when precipitated in the urine of patients with high urinary oxalic acid composi-

tion. Other modalities include biofeedback, physical therapy with electrical stimulation, or intralesional injections with triamcinolone and bupivacaine.

## Vulvar Lesions

**Sebaceous** or **inclusion cysts** are caused by inflammatory blockage of the sebaceous gland ducts and are small, smooth, nodular masses, usually arising from the inner surfaces of the labia minora and majora, that contain cheesy, sebaceous material. They may be easily excised if their size or position is troublesome.

The round ligament inserts into the labium majus, carrying an investment of peritoneum. On occasion, peritoneal fluid may accumulate therein, causing a **cyst of the canal of Nuck or hydrocele.** If such cysts reach symptomatic size, excision is usually required.

**Fibromas** (fibromyomas) arise from the connective tissue and smooth muscle elements of vulva and vagina and are usually small and asymptomatic. Sarcomatous change is extremely uncommon, although edema and degenerative changes may make such lesions suspicious for malignancy. Treatment is surgical excision when the lesions are symptomatic or with concerns about malignancy. **Lipomas** appear much like fibromas, are rare, and are also treated by excision if symptomatic.

**Hidradenoma** is a rare lesion arising from the sweat glands of the vulva. It is almost always benign, is usually found on the inner surface of the labia majora, and is treated with excision.

**Nevi** are benign, usually asymptomatic, pigmented lesions whose importance is that they must be distinguished from malignant melanoma, 3% to 4% of which occur on the external genitalia in females. Biopsy of pigmented vulvar lesions may be warranted, depending on clinical suspicion.

## VULVAR INTRAEPITHELIAL NEOPLASIA

Much like the vulvar dermatoses, the classification and terminology of VIN is still evolving and has undergone multiple revisions and reclassifications over the years. There are currently three grading systems: (1) the World Health Organization (WHO) three-grade system of VIN 1, 2, and 3; (2) the clinical, Bethesda-like, two-grade system of low- and high-grade vulvar intraepithelial lesions; and (3) the revised 2004 International Society for the Study of Vulvar Disease (ISSVD) classification, which divides VIN into two types: usual and differentiated. VIN, usual type is further divided into 3 subtypes: warty, basaloid, and mixed. These grading systems are summarized in Table 42.3.

### VIN 1

**VIN 1,** or mild dysplasia, is a low-grade lesion that demonstrates minimal to mild squamous atypia limited to the

| TABLE 42.3 | Grading Systems for Vulvar Intraepithelial Neoplasia (VIN) | |
|---|---|---|
| **2003 WHO** | **Clinical, "Bethesda-like"** | **2004 ISSVD** |
| VIN 1 (mild dysplasia) | Low-grade VIN | Term abolished |
| VIN 2 (moderate dysplasia) | High-grade VIN | VIN, usual type |
| VIN 3 (severe dysplasia, CIS) | | a. VIN, warty<br>b. VIN, basaloid<br>c. VIN, mixed |
| VIN 3, simplex type (CIS) | | VIN, differentiated type |

CIS = carcinoma in situ; ISSVD = International Society for the Study of Vulvar Disease; WHO = World Health Organization.

lower epidermis. VIN 1 is either a non-neoplastic, reactive atypia or is an effect of a human papillomavirus (HPV) infection. VIN 1 occurs most often in condylomata acuminata. Lesions that are condylomatous in origin do not have the features of attenuated maturation, pleomorphism, and atypical mitotic figures that are other forms of VIN.

Because the features of VIN 1 are an uncommon histologic finding and there is little evidence that VIN 1 is a cancer precursor, it may be misleading to classify these lesions as true intraepithelial neoplasia. In 2004, the ISSVD abolished the term *VIN 1* from their classification system. *The diagnosis of VIN 1 must be made by biopsy, and treatment is the same as for condyloma.*

## VIN, Usual Type

The ISSVD combined VIN 2 and 3 into **VIN, usual type.** These are high-grade, HPV-related lesions distinguished only by degree of abnormality. They represent true neoplasia with a high predilection for progression to severe intraepithelial lesions and, eventually, carcinoma, if left untreated. Almost 60% of women with VIN 3 or vaginal intraepithelial neoplasia (VAIN) 3 will also have cervical intraepithelial neoplasia (CIN) lesions. Furthermore, 10% of women with CIN 3 will have either VIN or VAIN.

Smoking or secondhand smoke is a common social-history finding in patients with VIN. *Presenting complaints include vulvar pruritus, chronic irritation, and a development of raised mass lesions.* Normally, the lesions are localized, fairly well-isolated, and raised above the normal epithelial surface to include a slightly rough texture. They are usually found along the posterior, hairless area of vulva and in the perineal body, but can occur anywhere on the vulva. The color changes in these lesions range from white, hyperplastic areas to reddened or dusky, patch-like involvement, depending on whether associated hyperkeratosis is present. Figure 42.3 illustrates the variation in appearance of VIN.

In patients without obvious raised or isolated lesions, careful inspection of the vulva is warranted, using a colposcope. Applying a 3%- to 5%-solution of acetic acid to the

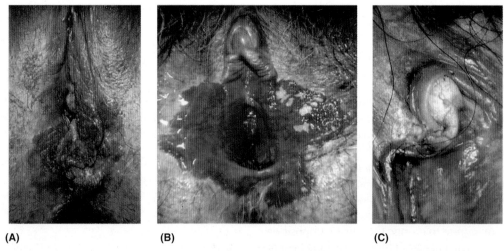

(A)                    (B)                    (C)

FIGURE 42.3. Variation in appearance of vulvar intraepithelial neoplasia. (A) Large, hypertrophic, pigmented lesion; (B) Associated with erosive lichen planus; (C) Isolated to the clitoris. (Used with permission from Foster DC. Vulvar disease. *Obstet Gynecol.* 2002;100(1):157.)

vulva for 2 to 5 minutes often accentuates the white lesions and may also help in revealing abnormal vascular patterns. *These areas must be selectively biopsied in multiple sites to thoroughly investigate the type of VIN and reliably exclude invasive carcinoma.*

VIN, usual type is subdivided into three histologic subtypes–warty, basaloid, or mixed–depending on the features present. They all have atypical mitotic figures and nuclear pleomorphism, with loss of normal differentiation in the lower one third to one half of the epithelial layer. Full-thickness loss of maturation indicates lesions that are at least severely dysplastic, including areas that may represent true carcinoma in situ (CIS).

*The goal in treating VIN, usual type is to quickly and completely remove all involved areas of skin.* These lesions can be removed after appropriate biopsies confirm the absence of invasive cancer. Removal options include wide local excision or laser ablation. A variety of nonsurgical treatments for patients with VIN, usual type have been reported, including corticosteroids, 5-fluorouracil, and imidazoquinolones (particularly imiquimod). Results to date are inconclusive. *Careful evaluation to exclude invasive disease is of paramount importance, as VIN, usual type is seen adjacent to 30% of SCCs of the vulva.*

## VIN, Differentiated Type

The less common simplex type of VIN (CIS) in the WHO system is now called **VIN, differentiated type** by the ISSVD (see Table 42.3). The lesion is either a hyperkeratotic plaque, warty papule, or an ulcer, seen primarily in older women. It is often associated with keratinizing SCCs or lichen sclerosus, and is not HPV-related. It is thought that VIN, differentiated type is underdiagnosed due to a relatively short intraepithelial phase before progression to invasive carcinoma. Clinical awareness of this entity and its features as different from VIN, usual type would help to improve diagnosis before cancer has supervened. Biopsy is mandatory and the mainstay of treatment is excision.

## PAGET DISEASE

**Paget disease** is characterized by extensive intraepithelial disease whose gross appearance is described as a fiery red background mottled with whitish hyperkeratotic areas. The histology of these lesions is similar to that of the breast lesions, with large, pale cells of apocrine origin below the surface epithelium (Fig. 42.4). Although not common, Paget disease of the vulva may be associated with carcinoma of the skin. Similarly, patients with Paget disease of the vulva have a higher incidence of underlying internal carcinoma, particularly of the colon and breast.

*The treatment for vulvar Paget disease is wide local excision or simple vulvectomy*, depending on the amount of involve-

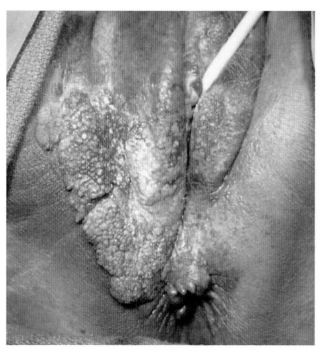

FIGURE 42.4. Paget disease. Large, pale cells of apocrine origin involving the surface epithelium. (Used with permission from Berek, JS. *Berek and Novak's Gynecology.* 14th ed. Philadelphia, (PA): Lippincott Williams & Wilkins; 2007: Figure 17.20.)

ment. Recurrences are more common with this disorder than with VIN, necessitating wider margins when local excision or vulvectomy is performed.

## VULVAR CANCER

*Vulvar carcinoma accounts for approximately 5% of all gynecologic malignancies.* Approximately 90% of these carcinomas are squamous **cell carcinomas.** The second most common variety is melanoma, which accounts for 2% of all vulvar carcinomas, followed by sarcoma. Less-common types include basal cell carcinoma and adenocarcinoma.

The typical clinical profile of vulvar carcinoma includes women in their postmenopausal years, most commonly between the ages of 70 and 80. However, about 20% of these cancers are discovered in women younger than 50 years of age. *Vulvar pruritus is the most common presenting complaint.* In addition, patients may notice a red or white ulcerative or exophytic lesion arising most commonly on the posterior two-thirds of either labium majus. An exophytic ulcerative lesion need not be present, further underscoring the need for thorough biopsy in patients of the age group who complain of vulvar symptoms. *Patients in this older age group may be reluctant to consult their physicians about these signs and symptoms, and physicians are further reluctant to investigate the symptoms and findings thoroughly via vulvar biopsy, which can result in a delay in treatment.*

Although a specific cause for vulvar cancer is not known, progression has been shown from prior intraepithelial lesions, including those that are associated with certain types of HPV. Smokers have a high preponderance in this population of patients.

## Natural History

Squamous cell carcinoma of the vulva generally remains localized for long periods of time and then spreads in a predictable fashion to the regional lymph nodes, including those of the inguinal and femoral chain. Lesions 2 cm wide and 0.5 cm deep have an increased chance of nodal metastases. The overall incidence of lymph node metastasis is approximately 30%. Lesions arising in the anterior one-third of the vulva may spread to the deep pelvic nodes, bypassing regional inguinal and femoral lymphatics.

## Evaluation

The staging classification for vulvar cancer was revised by the Federation of Gynecology and Obstetrics (FIGO) in 1995 (Table 42.4). Prior to 1988, vulvar cancers were staged clinically. However, noted discrepancies in regard to predicting nodal metastasis led to a change from clinical to surgical staging. This staging convention uses the analysis of

| TABLE 42.4 | International Federation of Gynecology and Obstetrics 1995 Staging of Vulvar Cancer |
|---|---|
| **Stage** | **Definition** |
| 0 | Carcinoma in situ; intraepithelial carcinoma |
| I | Tumor confined to the vulva and/or perineum, 2 cm or less in greatest dimension; no nodal metastasis |
| IA | Stromal invasion no greater than 1.0 mm* |
| IB | Stromal invasion greater than 1.0 mm* |
| II | Tumor confined to the vulva and/or perineum, more than 2 cm in greatest dimension; no nodal metastasis |
| III | Tumor of any size which invades any of the following: lower urethra, vagina, anus, and/or unilateral regional node metastasis |
| IV |  |
| IVA | Tumor invades any of the following: upper urethra, bladder mucosa, rectal mucosa, or is fixed to bone and/or bilateral regional node metastasis |
| IVB | Any distant metastasis including pelvic lymph nodes |

*The depth of invasion is defined as the measurement of the tumor from the epithelial-stromal junction of the adjacent most superficial dermal papilla to the deepest point of invasion.

the removed vulvar tumor and microscopic assessment of the regional lymph nodes as its basis.

## Treatment

Although the mainstay for the treatment of invasive vulvar cancer is **surgical,** many advances have been made to help individualize patients into treatment categories in an effort to reduce the amount of radical surgery, while not compromising survival. Accordingly, not all patients undergo radical vulvectomy with bilateral nodal dissections. Individualized approaches include the following:

- Conservative vulvar operations for unifocal lesions
- Elimination of routine pelvic lymphadenectomy
- Avoidance of groin dissection in unilateral lesions 1 mm deep
- Elimination of contralateral groin dissection in unilateral lesions 1 cm from the midline with negative ipsilateral nodes
- Separate groin incisions for patients with indicated bilateral groin dissection
- Postoperative radiation therapy to decrease groin recurrence in patients with two or more positive groin nodes

Concomitant use of radiation and chemotherapy (5-fluorouracil plus cisplatin or mitomycin or cisplatin alone) is gaining favor for treatment of vulvar cancers that require radiation therapy. Treatment with chemotherapy in cases of recurrent vulvar cancer has only limited value.

## Prognosis

The corrected 5-year survival rate for all vulvar carcinoma is approximately 70%. Five-year survival rates for squamous cell cancer are 60% to 80% for stage I and II disease. Survival rates for patients with stage III disease are 45%, and those with stage IV have rates of 15%.

## Other Types of Vulvar Cancer

### MELANOMA

*Melanoma is the most common nonsquamous cell cancer of the vulva.* Vulvar melanoma usually presents with a raised, irritated, pruritic, pigmented lesion. Most commonly, melanotic lesions are located on the labia minora or the clitoris. Melanoma accounts for approximately 6% of all vulvar malignancies, and when suspected, wide local excision is necessary for diagnosis and staging. Survival approaches 100% when the lesions are confined to the intrapapillary ridges, decreasing rapidly as involvement includes the papillary dermis, reticular dermis, and finally subcutaneous tissues. In the latter instance, survival is generally 20% because of substantial incidence of nodal involvement. Because early diagnosis and treatment by wide excision are so crucial, it is important to recognize that irritated, pigmented, vulvar lesions mandate excisional biopsy for definitive treatment.

### CARCINOMA OF THE BARTHOLIN GLAND

**Carcinoma of the Bartholin gland** is uncommon (1% to 2% of all vulvar carcinomas). Malignancies that arise from the Bartholin gland include adenocarcinomas, squamous cell carcinomas, adenosquamous carcinomas, and adenoid cystic and transitional-cell carcinomas. These arise mainly as a result of changes occurring within the different histologic areas of the gland and ducts leading from it. Bartholin carcinoma on average occurs in women over the age of 50; however, any new Bartholin mass in a woman over the age of 40 should be excised. Treatment of diagnosed Bartholin cancers is radical vulvectomy and bilateral lymphadenectomy. Recurrence is disappointingly common, and a 5-year overall survival rate of 65% is noted.

## VAGINAL DISEASE

Vaginal disease can be classified into three broad categories: benign, precancerous, and cancerous. There are important differences in the management and prognosis of these conditions.

> *Vaginal neoplasias are rare and usually occur secondary to cervical or vulvar cancers that have spread to the vagina from the primary site.*

### Benign Vaginal Masses

**Gartner duct cysts** arise from vestigial remnants of the wolffian or mesonephric system that course along the outer anterior aspect of the vaginal canal. These cystic structures are usually small and asymptomatic, but on occasion they may be larger and symptomatic so that excision is required.

**Inclusion cysts** are usually seen on the posterior lower vaginal surface, resulting from imperfect approximation of childbirth lacerations or episiotomy. They are lined with stratified squamous epithelium, their content is usually cheesy, and they may be excised if symptomatic.

### Vaginal Intraepithelial Neoplasia (VAIN)

**Vaginal intraepithelial neoplasia (VAIN)** can be classified into three types:

- VAIN I involves the basal epithelial layers
- VAIN 2 involves up to two-thirds of the vaginal epithelium
- VAIN 3 involves most of the vaginal epithelium (carcinoma in situ)

VAIN is most commonly located in the upper third of the vagina, a finding that may be partially related to its association with the more common cervical neoplasias. It is estimated that one-half to two-thirds of all patients with VAIN have had cervical or vulvar neoplasia.

Patients with VAIN I and II can be monitored and typically will not require therapy. Many of these patients have human papillomavirus infection and atrophic change of the vagina. Topical estrogen therapy may be useful in some women.

**VAIN III** appears to occur more commonly in the third decade of life onward, although its exact incidence is unknown. One-half to two-thirds of patients with VAIN III have a previous or coexistent neoplasm of the lower genital tract. Approximately 1% to 2% of patients who undergo hysterectomy for CIN III and many patients who undergo radiation therapy for other gynecologic malignancy ultimately develop VAIN III. This is one of the arguments for yearly Pap smears after hysterectomy. The importance of VAIN III is its potential for progression to invasive vaginal carcinoma, as the lesions themselves are usually asymptomatic and have no intrinsic morbidity.

VAIN III must be differentiated from other causes of red, ulcerated, or white hyperplastic lesions of the vagina such as herpes, traumatic lesions, hyperkeratosis associated with chronic irritation (e.g., from a poorly fitting diaphragm), or adenosis. Inspection and palpation of the vagina are the mainstays of diagnosis, but, unfortunately, this is often done in a cursory fashion during the routine pelvic examination. *Pap smears of the vaginal epithelium can disclose findings that are useful in the diagnosis, although colposcopy with directed biopsy is the definitive method of diagnosis, just as it is with CIN.*

The goals of treatment of VAIN III are ablation of the intraepithelial lesion while preserving vaginal depth, caliber, and sexual function. Laser ablation, local excision, and chemical treatment with 5-fluorouracil cream are all used for limited lesions; total or partial vaginectomy with application of a split thickness skin graft is usually reserved for failure of the previously described treatments. Cure rates of 80% to 95% may be expected.

### Vaginal Cancer

Invasive vaginal cancer accounts for approximately 1% to 3% of gynecologic malignancies. Squamous cell carcinoma makes up approximately 80% to 90% of these malignancies, which occur primarily in women 55 years of age or older. *The remainder of vaginal carcinomas consists of adenocarcinoma of the vagina and vaginal melanoma.*

The staging of vaginal carcinoma is nonsurgical (Table 42.5). Radiation therapy is the mainstay of treatment for SCC of the vagina. Radical hysterectomy combined with upper vaginectomy and pelvic lymphadenectomy are used for selected patients. Upper vaginal lesions and pelvic

| TABLE 42.5 | International Federation of Gynecology and Obstetrics (FIGO) Staging of Carcinoma of the Vagina |
|---|---|
| **Stage** | **Definition** |
| 0 | Carcinoma *in situ;* intraepithelial neoplasia grade 3 |
| I | Carcinoma limited to the vaginal wall |
| II | Carcinoma involving subvaginal tissue but not extending to the pelvic wall |
| III | Carcinoma extending to the pelvic wall |
| IV | Carcinoma extending beyond the true pelvis or has involved the mucosa of the bladder or rectum; bullous edema as such does not permit a case to be allotted to Stage IV |
| IVA | Tumor invades bladder and/or rectal mucosa and/or direct extension beyond the true pelvis |
| IVB | Spread to distant organs |

exenteration and radical vulvectomy are used for selected patients with lower vaginal lesions involving the vulva. Most young women with clear cell carcinoma have lesions located in the upper one-half of the vagina, and wish to maintain ovarian and vaginal function. Radical hysterectomy with upper vaginectomy combined with pelvic lymphadenectomy is often the primary treatment for these patients, with radiation therapy following. The overall 5-year survival rate for squamous cell carcinoma of the vagina is approximately 42%, and for clear cell adenocarcinoma of the vagina, 78%, with stage I and II patients having the best prognosis. Melanoma is treated with radical surgery; radiation and chemotherapy have little efficacy.

**Sarcoma botryoides** (or embryonal rhabdomyosarcoma) is a rare tumor that presents as a mass of grapelike polyps protruding from the introitus of pediatric-age patients. It arises from the undifferentiated mesenchyme of the lamina propria of the anterior vaginal wall. Bloody discharge is an associated symptom in these tumors. The tumor spreads locally, although it may have distant hematogenous metastases. Combination chemotherapy appears to be effective, resulting in a marked reduction in tumor size. This permits more conservative surgery than was performed in the past, preserving as much bowel and bladder function as possible.

## SUGGESTED READINGS

American College of Obstetricians and Gynecologists. Cervical cytology screening. ACOG Practice Bulletin No. 45. *Obstet Gynecol.* 2003;102(2):417–427.

American College of Obstetricians and Gynecologists. Evaluation and management of abnormal cervical cytology and histology in the adolescent. ACOG Committee Opinion No. 330. *Obstet Gynecol.* 2006;107(4):963–968.

American College of Obstetricians and Gynecologists (ACOG). *Guidelines for Women's Health Care: A Resource Manual.* 3rd ed. Washington, D.C.: ACOG; 2007.

Patient Education pamphlet, "Disorders of the Vulva"

Sideri M, Jones RW, Wilkinson EJ, Preti M, Heller DS, Scurry J, Haefner H, Neill S. Squamous vulvar intraepithelial neoplasia: 2004 modified terminology, ISSVD Vulvar Oncology Subcommittee. *J Reprod Med.* 2005;50(11):807–810.

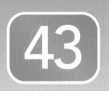

# 43

# Cervical Neoplasia and Carcinoma

Topic 52:  Cervical Disease and Neoplasia

The student should understand how detection and treatment of preinvasive lesions reduces medical and social costs of, as well as mortality from, carcinoma of the cervix.

A lthough the incidence and mortality from cervical cancer have decreased substantially in the past several decades among women in the United States, cervical cancer remains the third most common gynecologic cancer. In countries where cytologic screening is not widely available, cervical cancer remains common. Worldwide, it is the second most common cancer among women, the third most common cause of cancer-related death, and the most common cause of mortality from gynecologic malignancy.

Cervical cancer can be thought of as a "controllable" cancer. It is preceded by an identifiable precursor lesion (**cervical intraepithelial neoplasia, CIN**) that may (but not always) progress to invasive cancer. CIN can be easily detected by an inexpensive and noninvasive screening test (Pap test) that may be augmented with adjunctive tests such as HPV DNA typing and a follow-up diagnostic procedure (colposcopy). CIN is treatable with simple and effective therapies, including cryotherapy, laser ablation, loop electrosurgical excision procedure (LEEP), and cold knife cone biopsy, all of which have high cure rates. It is also one of only a few cancers for which a vaccine exists that may have a significant impact in reducing an individual's risk.

## CERVICAL INTRAEPITHELIAL NEOPLASIA

### Etiology

Cervical cancer and CIN are caused by human papillomavirus (HPV). Of the approximately 80 types of HPV, about 30 infect the anogenital tract. Approximately 15 of these types (16, 18, 31, 33, 35, 39, 45, 51, 52, 56, 58, 59, 68, 73, and 82) are associated with cancer and are known as **high-risk HPV types.** The majority of cervical cancers are caused by just four of these high-risk HPV types: 16, 18, 31, and 45. Low-risk HPV types are not associated with cancer. However, low-risk types 6 and 11 are associ-

ated with **genital warts** (**condylomata acuminata**) and with low-grade squamous intraepithelial lesions.

HPV infects the cells of the cervix. The size and shape of the cervix change depending on age, hormonal status, and number of children (parity). In reproductive-age women, the cervix measures 7–8 mm at its widest point. The upper part of the cervix that opens into the endometrial cavity is called the **internal os;** the lower part that opens into the vagina is called the **external os.** The exterior portion of the cervical canal is called the **exocervix,** and the interior cervical canal is called the **endocervical canal.** The walls of the endocervical canal contain numerous folds and plicae.

The histology of the cervix is complex (Fig. 43.1, A and B). Overlying the fibrous stroma of the cervix is the cervical epithelium, a meshwork of cells. The epithelium is of two types: columnar (glandular) and stratified non-keratinizing squamous epithelia. The columnar epithelium consists of a single layer of mucus-secreting cells that are arranged into deep folds or crypts. The area where the two types of epithelia meet is called the **squamocolumnar junction (SCJ).** The SCJ is clinically important, as it is the site where over 90% of lower genital tract neoplasias arise. During childhood, the SCJ is located just inside the external os. Under the influence of hormones and the acidification of the vaginal environment during puberty, subcolumnar cells undergo metaplasia, a process of transformation. The metaplasia of these cells causes the SCJ to "roll out," or evert, from its original position inside the external os to a position on the enlarged cervical surface. Columnar epithelium is also rolled onto the cervical surface, where it is exposed to vaginal secretions, irritants, and a changing hormonal milieu. The area between the original SCJ and the active SCJ is called the **transformation zone (TZ).** As metaplasia continues, the metaplastic epithelium covers and eventually becomes indistinguishable from the original squamous epithelium. Glands

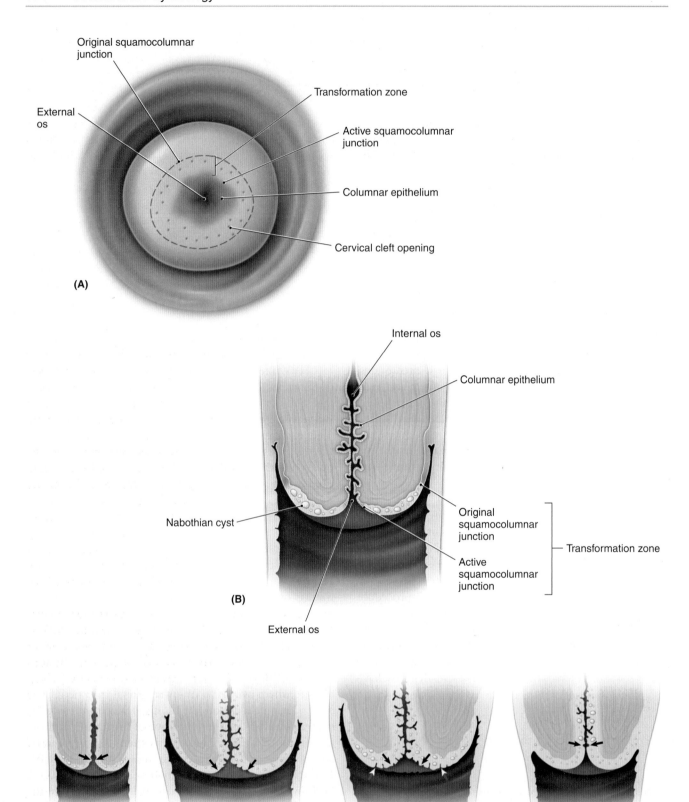

FIGURE 43.1. Anatomy of the cervix. (A) The cervix and the transformation zone. (B) Anterior view of the cervix and excocervix. (C) Different locations of the transformation zone and the squamocolumnar junction during a woman's lifetime. The arrows mark the active transformation zone. (Based on Berek JS. *Berek and Novak's Gynecology*. 14th ed. Philadelphia, PA: Lippincott Williams & Wilkins; 2007:563–565.)

within the columnar epithelium may become trapped during this metaplastic activity by squamous epithelium, causing **Nabothian cysts.** These cysts are not considered pathologic, but a normal consequence of the dynamic histology of the cervix.

The metaplastic cells within the TZ represent the newest and least mature cells in the cervix, and it is thought that they are the most vulnerable to oncogenic change. The rate of metaplasia is highest during adolescence and early pregnancy. During perimenopause, the new SCJ recedes upward into the endocervical canal, often out of direct visual contact (Figure 43.1C).

HPV infection of cervical cells may or may not result in neoplastic change. Most HPV infections are transient, indicating that the host's immune system is able to eradicate the virus before it can cause neoplastic changes in cervical cells. It is likely that several as-yet unidentified host or environmental factors act as cofactors. If the HPV DNA is not integrated into the host genome, encapsulated virions are produced that are expressed morphologically as "koilocytes." If HPV DNA is integrated into the host DNA, the expression of the cell's regulatory genes may be altered, leading to the transformation of the cells into intraepithelial lesions or cancer.

## Risk Factors

Several factors have been identified that may increase the risk of cervical neoplasia (Box 43.1). A higher incidence of HPV infection and progression of intraepithelial neoplasia is seen in immunosuppressed patients, including those infected with HIV as well as those who are organ transplant recipients, who have chronic renal failure or a history of Hodgkin lymphoma, or have undergone

> ### BOX 43.1
> ### Risk Factors for Cervical Neoplasia
>
> - More than 1 sexual partner or have a male sexual partner who has had sex with more than 1 person
> - First intercourse at an early age (younger than 18 years)
> - Male sexual partner who has had a sexual partner with cervical cancer
> - Smoking
> - Human immunodeficiency virus (HIV) infection
> - Organ (especially kidney) transplant
> - STD infection
> - Diethylstilbestrol (DES) exposure
> - History of cervical cancer or high-grade squamous intraepithelial lesions
> - Infrequent or absent Pap screening tests

immunosuppressive therapy for other reasons. Another factor is cigarette smoking. The risk of cervical cancer is 3.5 times greater among smokers than among nonsmokers. Carcinogens from cigarette smoke have been found in high concentrations in the cervical mucus of smokers, suggesting a plausible biologic explanation for this association. First intercourse at a young age may increase a woman's risk for cervical neoplasia because of the high rate of metaplasia that occurs in the transformation zone during adolescence and a higher proportion of new or immature cervical cells in this region.

Persistent HPV infection increases the risk of persistent or progressive cervical dysplasia. HPV 16 infection is more likely to be persistent than infections caused by other oncogenic HPV types. Individuals may possess a genetic susceptibility to cervical cancer, but the relative risks are small.

## Classification

The goal of all cervical cancer classification systems is to establish management guidelines that decrease the likelihood of progression of precursor lesions to more advanced lesions. The 2001 Bethesda System is the most widely used system in the United States for reporting and classifying cervical cytologic studies. Established in 1988 and updated in 1991 and 2001, The Bethesda Classification outlines the various possible results of the Pap test, specifies accepted methodologies of reporting the Pap results, and provides for interpretation of findings. This categorization allows for defined management options regarding the initial results of the Pap test (Box 43.2). Details about how the Pap test is performed are found in Chapter 1, The Woman's Health Examination. Guidelines for cervical cancer screening are found in Chapter 2, The Obstetrician–Gynecologist's Role in Screening and Preventive Care.

The classification used by the Bethesda system divides epithelial lesions into two categories: squamous lesions and glandular lesions. In both categories, lesions are either precancerous or cancerous. Squamous precursor lesions are described as either **atypical squamous cells (ASC), low-grade squamous intraepithelial lesions (LSIL)** or **high-grade squamous intraepithelial lesions (HSIL),** while cancerous lesions are termed **invasive squamous carcinoma.** ASC is further divided into **ASC of undetermined significance (ASC-US),** and **ASC–cannot exclude HSIL (ASC-H).** Precancerous glandular lesions are classified as **atypical (AGC); atypical, favor neoplastic;** and **endocervical adenocarcinoma in situ (AIS).** Cancerous glandular lesions are classified as **adenocarcinoma.** AGC is also classified as endocervical, endometrial, or not otherwise specified (NOS).

Before the intraepithelial lesion terminology was created, the term **cervical intraepithelial neoplasia (CIN)** was used, and lesions were graded as **CIN 1, CIN 2,** or **CIN 3.** The CIN classification system replaced an even

---

**BOX 43.2**
**The 2001 Bethesda System**

**Specimen Type:**  *Indicate conventional smear (Pap smear) vs. liquid-based vs. other*

**Specimen Adequacy**
- Satisfactory for evaluation (*describe presence or absence of endocervical/transformation zone component and any other quality indicators, e.g., partially obscuring blood, inflammation, etc.*)
- Unsatisfactory for evaluation . . . (*specify reason*)
  - Specimen rejected/not processed (*specify reason*)
  - Specimen processed and examined, but unsatisfactory for evaluation of epithelial abnormality because of (*specify reason*)

**General Categorization (*optional*)**
- Negative for Intraepithelial Lesion or Malignancy
- Epithelial Cell Abnormality: See Interpretation/Result (*specify 'squamous' or 'glandular' as appropriate*)
- Other: See Interpretation/Result (*e.g., endometrial cells in a woman[3] 40 years of age*)

**Interpretation/Result**

*Negative for Intraepithelial Lesion or Malignancy*
**Organisms:**
- *Trichomonas vaginalis*
- Fungal organisms morphologically consistent with *Candida* spp
- Shift in flora suggestive of bacterial vaginosis
- Bacteria morphologically consistent with *Actinomyces* spp.
- Cellular changes consistent with Herpes simplex virus

**Other Non Neoplastic Findings (*Optional to report; list not inclusive*):**
- Reactive cellular changes associated with
  - inflammation (includes typical repair)
  - radiation
  - intrauterine contraceptive device (IUD)

- Glandular cells status post hysterectomy
- Atrophy

*Other*
- Endometrial cells (*in a woman[3] 40 years of age*) (*Specify if 'negative for squamous intraepithelial lesion'*)

*Epithelial Cell Abnormalities*
**Squamous Cell**
- Atypical squamous cells
  - of undetermined significance (ASC-US)
  - cannot exclude HSIL (ASC-H)
- Low grade squamous intraepithelial lesion (LSIL) encompassing: HPV/mild dysplasia/CIN 1
- High grade squamous intraepithelial lesion (HSIL) encompassing: moderate and severe dysplasia, CIS/CIN 2 and CIN 3
  - with features suspicious for invasion (*if invasion is suspected*)
- Squamous cell carcinoma

**Glandular Cell**
- Atypical
  - endocervical cells
  - endometrial cells
  - glandular cells
- Atypical
  - endocervical cells, favor neoplastic
  - glandular cells, favor neoplastic
- Endocervical adenocarcinoma in situ
- Adenocarcinoma
  - endocervical
  - endometrial
  - extrauterine
  - not otherwise specified (NOS)

*Other Malignant Neoplasms:* (*specify*)

**Educational Notes and Suggestions (*optional*)**
*Suggestions should be concise and consistent with clinical follow-up guidelines published by professional organizations (references to relevant publications may be included).*

---

earlier classification scheme that used the term **dysplasia** and classified precancerous lesions as mild, moderate, or severe. With each revision, the terminology for cervical cancer results has become more precise and reflects the current scientific understanding of the progression of cervical cancer. The CIN terminology, however, is still used with the current Bethesda terminology. LSIL encompasses HPV infection, mild dysplasia, or CIN 1. HSIL encompasses CIN 2 and CIN 3. CIN 3 is also designated carcinoma in situ (Table 43.1).

Despite decades of study, the natural history of cervical intraepithelial lesions is still not completely understood.

TABLE 43.1  Comparison of Pap Test Descriptive Conventions

| CIN system | Normal | Inflammatory | | CIN I or CIN II | | CIN III | Suggestive of cancer |
|---|---|---|---|---|---|---|---|
| Bethesda 2001 | Negative for intraepithelial lesion or malignancy | ASC-US | ASC-H | LSIL | HSIL | | Squamous cell carcinoma |
| Histology | Basal cells | WBCs | | Basement membrane | | | Invasive cervical cancer |

The once widely held concept that low-grade lesions are necessary precursors to the high-grade lesions that, in turn, may progress to invasive cancer has been questioned as the sole pathogenesis. It has been observed, for example, that many women present with CIN 2 or CIN 3 without prior CIN 1 lesions. Although multiple longitudinal studies have attempted to document rates of "progression" and "regression" of CIN, results of these studies must be interpreted with caution due to varying methods of diagnostic criteria, populations, and duration of follow-up.

## Evaluation of Abnormal Pap Test Results

An abnormal cervical cytologic finding from a Pap test should be followed by visual inspection of the vagina and a bimanual examination. The first objective is to exclude the presence of invasive carcinoma. Once this has been accomplished, the objectives are to determine the grade and distribution of the intraepithelial lesion. Options for evaluation include repeat cytology, HPV DNA testing, colposcopy with directed biopsies (see Chapter 32, Gynecologic Procedures), and endocervical assessment.

### COLPOSCOPY AND ENDOCERVICAL CURETTAGE

**Colposcopy with directed biopsy** has been the criterion of disease detection and remains the technique of choice for treatment decisions. A **colposcope** is a binocular stereomicroscope with variable magnification (usually 7× to 15×) and a light source with a green filter to aid in the identification of abnormal appearing blood vessels that may be associated with intraepithelial neoplasia. With colposcopy, areas with changes consistent with dysplasia are identified, allowing directed biopsy (i.e., biopsy of the area where dysplasia is

most likely). Colposcopic criteria such as white epithelium, abnormal vascular patterns, and punctate lesions help identify such areas (Fig. 43.2). To facilitate the examination, the cervix is washed with a 3% to 4% acetic acid solution, which acts as an epithelial desiccant of intracellular protein, enhancing visualization of dysplastic lesions. Lesions usually appear with relatively discrete borders near the SCJ within 10–90 seconds of acetic acid application. Tissue samples for biopsy can be collected; the number of samples obtained will vary depending on the number and severity of abnormal areas found.

Visualization of the entire SCJ is required for a colposcopy to be considered satisfactory. If the SCJ is not visualized in its entirety, or if the margins of abnormal areas are not seen in their entirety, the colposcopic assessment is termed unsatisfactory, and other evaluations such as cervical conization or **endocervical curettage (ECC)** is indicated. In this procedure, a small curette is used to collect cells from the endocervical canal. An endocervical brush can be used to retrieve additional cells dislodged in the curette specimen. This endocervical sample is obtained so that potential disease farther inside the cervical canal, which is not visualized by the colposcope, may be detected. The cervical biopsies and ECC are then submitted separately for pathologic assessment.

### HUMAN PAPILLOMAVIRUS DNA TESTING

Testing for the presence of high-risk HPV DNA is now being used as an adjunct screening tool for cervical neoplasia in women older than 30 years of age. It is also used as a triage tool for women with Pap test results reported as ASC-US and in the management of non-adolescent women with LSIL. HPV DNA can identify women whose Pap test

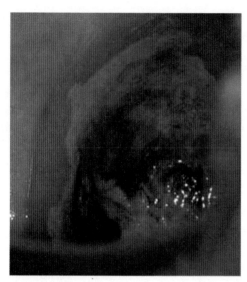

FIGURE 43.2. Colposcopic image of the cervix. The white epithelium and course mosaic pattern of the underlying capillaries in this colpophotograph are suggestive of cervical intraepithelial neoplasia. (CASE STUDIES IN COLPOSCOPY Case #53—March 2007. Kevin J. Mitchell, MD, Chair, with pathology courtesy of Mary Chacho MD, Department of Pathology, Danbury Hospital, Danbury, CT, 2006-08 Section on the Cervix. Downloaded on 7-21-08 from http://www.asccp.org/edu/case_studies.shtml#)

results are caused by other, non-HPV-associated phenomena, such as infection, thus preventing unnecessary colposcopic evaluations. Because HPV is more prevalent in younger women and the rate of CIN 2 and CIN 3 increases with age, HPV DNA testing is more useful as a triage tool in older women. HPV DNA testing is also used in the initial workup of women with AGC.

## Management Guidelines for Cervical Epithelial Cell Abnormalities

The American Society for Colposcopy and Cervical Pathology (ASCCP) issues guidelines and protocols for the appropriate management of women with cervical cytologic or histologic abnormalities. The most recent updates to these recommendations occurred in 2006 and were published in 2007. These guidelines, including practice algorithms, are available at www.asccp.org/concensus/cytological/shtml. The following sections summarize these guidelines.

### LOW-GRADE SQUAMOUS INTRAEPITHELIAL LESIONS AND ATYPICAL SQUAMOUS CELLS OF UNDETERMINED SIGNIFICANCE

A patient with an ASC-US result should either undergo HPV DNA testing or repeat cytology at 6 and 12 months

following the abnormal Pap test result. The rationale for HPV DNA testing is that a negative result obviates the need for colposcopy; patients with ASC-US who are negative for high-risk HPV DNA may be followed routinely. Women who screen positive for HPV DNA with ASC-US results on two repeated tests should be managed in the same way as women with LSIL—both groups should be referred for a colposcopic evaluation. Patients with ASC-US results at either the 6th- or 12th-month repeat cytology screening should also be referred for colposcopy; if both repeat tests are negative, then the patient may resume routine screening. Patients with LSIL are not referred for HPV DNA testing, because 83% of LSIL patients are positive for HPV, and the test is of little prognostic significance.

About 3% of Pap test results are reproducibly classified as LSIL. Management and follow-up are the same following colposcopy for women with LSIL and women with HPV DNA-positive ASC-US. If no CIN is found, cytologic testing is repeated at 6 and 12 months or HPV DNA testing is repeated at 12 months. A positive result for either ASC or HPV DNA warrants a repeat colposcopy; women with negative results for ASC or HPV DNA may resume routine screening (Figs. 43.3 and 43.4).

Management protocols differ for adolescents and pregnant women. ASC and LSIL are more common in adolescents and the likelihood of spontaneous regression is higher. Because HPV DNA positivity is also higher in this population, using HPV DNA screening as a triage method is not useful. Adolescents with LSIL or ASC-US may be managed with repeat cytologic testing at 12 months. Those whose repeat test results show HSIL are referred for colposcopy. Pregnant women with LSIL should not undergo ECC and should not have more than one colposcopy during pregnancy. Colposcopic examination for evaluation of ASC-US can be deferred until at least 6 weeks following delivery.

Earlier guidelines for postmenopausal women with LSIL Pap test results offered repeat cytologic screening after treatment with vaginal estrogen cream as a triage option, as atrophy of the vaginal mucosa may contribute to the abnormal test result. However, current guidelines recommend that postmenopausal women with LSIL and ASC-US test results be managed in the same way as the general population.

### HIGH-GRADE SQUAMOUS INTRAEPITHELIAL LESION (HSIL) AND ATYPICAL SQUAMOUS CELLS—CANNOT EXCLUDE HIGH-GRADE SQUAMOUS INTRAEPITHELIAL LESION (ASC-H)

In the United States, approximately 0.5% of all Pap test results are reported as HSIL. The rate of HSIL decreases with age. CIN 2 or CIN 3 is identified in 84% to 97% of women with HSIL Pap test results, and invasive cancer is

## Management of Women with Atypical Squamous Cells of Undetermined Significance (ASC-US)

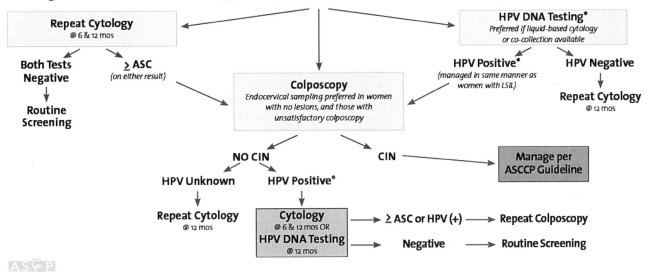

*Test only for high-risk (oncogenic) types of HPV

FIGURE 43.3. Management of Women with Atypical Squamous Cells of Undetermined Significance (ASCCP). (Reprinted from *The Journal of Lower Genital Tract Disease* Vol. 11 Issue 4, with permission of ASCCP ©American Society for Colposcopy and Cervical Pathology 2007. No copies of the algorithms may be made without prior consent of ASCCP.)

## Management of Women with Low-grade Squamous Intraepithelial Lesion (LSIL) *

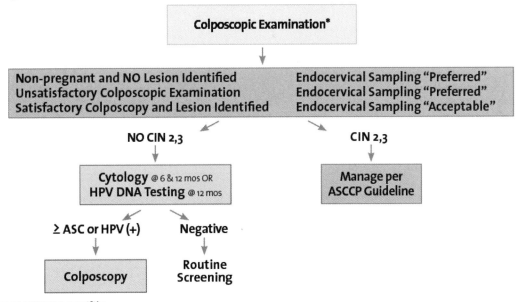

*Management options may vary if the woman is pregnant, postmenopausal, or an adolescent - (see text)

FIGURE 43.4. Management of Women with LSIL (ASCCP) (Reprinted from *The Journal of Lower Genital Tract Disease* Vol. 11 Issue 4, with permission of ASCCP ©American Society for Colposcopy and Cervical Pathology 2007. No copies of the algorithms may be made without prior consent of ASCCP.)

identified in 2%. Because the rate of CIN 2 or CIN 3 is so high in adults with HSIL cytologic findings, immediate treatment with the loop electrosurgical excision procedure (LEEP; see below) is an acceptable management approach. In women planning a future pregnancy, the risks of a LEEP procedure—which include preterm delivery, premature rupture of membranes, and low-birth-weight infants—should be taken into consideration. The other management approach is colposcopic examination, followed by appropriate treatment and follow-up (see Fig. 43.4).

ASC-H is evaluated by colposcopy because, like HSIL, it carries a higher risk of underlying CIN 2–3 lesions. If no CIN 2 or CIN 3 is found, the patient may be followed up by repeat screening at 6 and 12 months or an HPV-DNA test at 12 months. A positive CIN 2, 3, or HPV DNA result on any of these follow-up tests warrants a colposcopic examination; if results of all follow-up tests are negative, the patient may return to routine screening (Fig. 43.5).

## ATYPICAL GLANDULAR CELLS AND OTHER GLANDULAR ABNORMALITIES

Glandular cell abnormalities comprise 0.4% of epithelial cell abnormalities. The risk associated with AGC is dramatically higher than that seen with ASC. The risk associated with glandular abnormalities increases as the description in the Bethesda classification system advances from AGC—Not Otherwise Specified (AGC-NOS) to AGC, Favor Neoplasia (AGC-FN) and, finally, to adenocarcinoma in situ (AIS). Women with AGC of any type except for atypical endometrial cells should undergo colposcopic evaluation, HPV DNA testing, and ECC. If a woman is older than 35 years of age or is at risk for endometrial neoplasia (she has unexplained vaginal bleeding or conditions suggesting chronic anovulation), endometrial sampling should also be performed. Women with atypical endometrial cells should have an endometrial biopsy and ECC.

Knowledge of HPV status in women with AGC who do not have CIN 2 or CIN 3 or glandular neoplasia allows expedited triage. Women who test positive for HPV at the time of their Pap screening test should have a repeat Pap test and HPV DNA test at 6 months; those who test negative for HPV, at 12 months. Women with a positive HPV test and an abnormal Pap test result should be referred to colposcopy; women who have negative results on both tests can resume routine screening. In contrast, if HPV status is not known, the Pap test should be repeated every 6 months until there are four consecutive negative results, before a woman can resume routine screening (Fig. 43.6).

## Treatment

Both excisional and ablative techniques are used to treat CIN. The underlying concept in the treatment of CIN is that excision or ablation of the precursor lesion prevents progression to carcinoma. **Ablative methods** destroy the

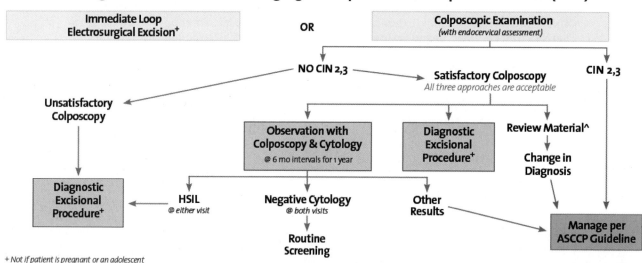

FIGURE 43.5. Management of Women with HSIL (ASCCP). (Reprinted from *The Journal of Lower Genital Tract Disease* Vol. 11 Issue 4, with permission of ASCCP ©American Society for Colposcopy and Cervical Pathology 2007. No copies of the algorithms may be made without prior consent of ASCCP.)

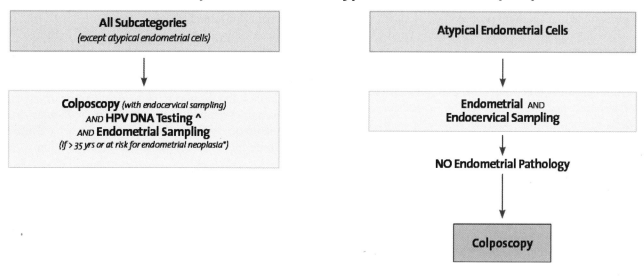

## Initial Workup of Women with Atypical Glandular Cells (AGC)

**All Subcategories**
*(except atypical endometrial cells)*

↓

**Colposcopy** *(with endocervical sampling)*
AND **HPV DNA Testing** ^
AND **Endometrial Sampling**
*(if > 35 yrs or at risk for endometrial neoplasia\*)*

**Atypical Endometrial Cells**

↓

**Endometrial** AND
**Endocervical Sampling**

↓

**NO Endometrial Pathology**

↓

**Colposcopy**

^ *If not already obtained. Test only for high-risk (oncogenic) types.*
\* *Includes unexplained vaginal bleeding or conditions suggesting chronic anovulation.*

FIGURE 43.6. Initial Workup of Women with AGC (ASCCP). (Reprinted from *The Journal of Lower Genital Tract Disease* Vol. 11 Issue 4, with permission of ASCCP ©American Society for Colposcopy and Cervical Pathology 2007. No copies of the algorithms may be made without prior consent of ASCCP.)

affected cervical tissue and include cryotherapy, laser ablation, electrofulguration, and cold coagulation, all of which are outpatient procedures that can be performed with regional anesthesia. Ablative methods should be used only with an adequate colposcopy and appropriate correlation between Pap test results and colposcopically directed biopsy.

Laser therapy is now only rarely performed in the United States. **Cryotherapy** is a commonly used outpatient method used to treat persistent CIN 1. The procedure involves covering the SCJ and all identified lesions with a stainless steel probe, which is then supercooled with liquid nitrogen or compressed gas (carbon dioxide or nitrous oxide). The size and shape of the probe depends on the size and shape of the cervix and the lesion to be treated. The most common technique involves a 3-minute freeze followed by a 5-minute thaw, with a repeat 3-minute freeze. The thaw period between the two freezing episodes allows the damaged tissue from the first freeze to become edematous and swell with intracellular fluid. With the second freeze, the edematous cellular architecture is refrozen and extends the damaged area slightly deeper into the tissue. Healing after cryotherapy may take up to 4 or 5 weeks, because the damaged tissue slowly sloughs and is replaced by new cervical epithelium. This process is associated with profuse watery discharge often mixed with necrotic cellular debris. The healing process is complete within 2 months. A follow-up Pap test is usually preformed

12 weeks following the freezing to ascertain the effectiveness of the procedure. The cure rate for CIN 1 using this technique approaches 90%.

**Excisional methods** remove the affected tissue and provide a specimen for pathologic evaluation. These methods include cold-knife conization (CKC), loop electrosurgical excision procedures (LEEP or large loop excision of the transformation zone [LLETZ]), laser conization, and electrosurgical needle conization. These procedures are performed under regional or general anesthesia. A cone-shaped specimen is removed from the cervix, which encompasses the SCJ, all identified lesions on the ectocervix, and a portion of the endocervical canal, the extent of which depends on whether the ECC was positive or negative. Because LEEP uses electrosurgical energy, thermal damage may occur at the margins of the specimen, obscuring the histology. Thermal damage is usually not considered a problem in the evaluation of squamous epithelial abnormalities, but it may be a substantial issue in the evaluation of glandular epithelial lesions, where abnormal cells in the bottom of glandular crypts may be altered. In cases of glandular abnormalities, CKC may be more appropriate.

If the margins of the biopsy are not free of disease, the patient should have either repeat conization or close follow-up because of the possibility that disease remains. If the margins are positive for a high-grade epithelial lesion or carcinoma in situ, the most appropriate treatment may be hysterectomy, if the patient has no desire for future childbearing. If the patient wants to preserve her fertility, colposcopy with ECC and HPV-DNA testing is an acceptable management protocol.

Excisional procedures are also indicated in the following situations:

- When an ECC is positive
- Unsatisfactory colposcopy: If the SCJ is not visualized in its entirety or if the margins of abnormal areas are not seen in their entirety during colposcopy, the colposcopic assessment is termed unsatisfactory and other evaluation such as cervical conization or endocervical curettage (ECC) is indicated.
- If a substantial discrepancy is seen between the screening Pap test and the histologic data from biopsy and ECC (i.e., the biopsy does not explain the source of the abnormal Pap test).: In this situation, which occurs in approximately 10% of colposcopies with directed biopsies and ECC, more tissue needs to be obtained by an excisional procedure for further testing.

CKC is associated with an increased risk of preterm labor, low–birth-weight infants, and cesarean delivery. LEEP and LLETZ are also associated with an increased risk of preterm labor, low–birth-weight infants, and premature rupture of membranes. Both types of excisional procedures are also associated with the usual risks of any surgery (bleeding, infection, and anesthetic risks).

## Follow-up

After treatment for noninvasive epithelial cell abnormalities, either by ablation or excision, a period of follow-up Pap tests every 6 months for 2 years is generally recommended, with variations depending on the severity of the lesion treated. Most patients may return to a routine screening thereafter. If a subsequent Pap test is abnormal, it is evaluated in the same manner as a new abnormal Pap test. The importance of follow-up should be stressed to the patient, because of the greater risk of recurrent abnormalities.

## CERVICAL CARCINOMA

Between 1950 and 1992, the death rate from cervical cancer declined by 74%. The main reason for this steep decrease is the increasing use of the Pap test for cervical cancer screening. The death rate continues to decline by approximately 4% per year. Despite the progress made in early detection and treatment, approximately 11,000 new cases of invasive cervical carcinoma are diagnosed annually with 3870 deaths.

The average age at diagnosis for invasive cervical cancer is approximately 50 years, although the disease may occur in the very young as well as the very old patient. In studies following patients with advanced CIN, this precursor lesion precedes invasive carcinoma by approximately 10 years. In some patients, however, this time of progression may be considerably less.

The etiology of cervical cancer is HPV in more than 90% of the cases. The two major histologic types of invasive cervical carcinomas are squamous cell carcinomas and adenocarcinomas. Squamous cell carcinomas comprise 80% of cases, and adenocarcinoma or adenosquamous carcinoma comprise approximately 15%. The remaining cases are made up of various rare histologies that behave differently from squamous cell cancer and adenocarcinoma.

### Clinical Evaluation

The signs and symptoms of early cervical carcinoma are variable and nonspecific, including watery vaginal discharge, intermittent spotting, and postcoital bleeding. Often the symptoms go unrecognized by the patient. Because of the accessibility of the cervix, accurate diagnosis often can be made with cytologic screening, colposcopically directed biopsy, or biopsy of a gross or palpable lesion. In cases of suspected microinvasion and early-stage cervical carcinoma, conization of the cervix is indicated to evaluate the possibility of invasion or to define the depth and extent of microinvasion. CKC provides the most accurate evaluation of the margins.

Staging is based on the International Federation of Gynecology and Obstetrics (FIGO) Staging Classification (Box 43.3). This classification is based both on the histologic assessment of the tumor sample and on physical and laboratory examination to ascertain the extent of disease. It is useful because of the predictable manner in which cervical carcinoma spreads by direct invasion and by lymphatic metastasis (Fig. 43.7). Careful clinical examination should be performed on all patients. Examinations should be conducted by experienced examiners, and may be performed under anesthesia. Pretreatment evaluation of women with cervical carcinoma often can be helpful if provided by an obstetrician–gynecologist with advanced surgical training, experience, and demonstrated competence, such as a gynecologic oncologist. Various optional examinations, such as ultrasonography, computed tomography (CT), magnetic resonance imaging (MRI), lymphangiography, laparoscopy, and fine-needle aspiration, are valuable for treatment planning and to help define the extent of tumor growth, especially in patients with locally advanced disease (i.e., stage IIb or more advanced). Surgical findings provide extremely accurate information about the extent of disease and will guide treatment plans, but will not change the results of clinical staging.

### Management

The clinician should be familiar with the options for treating women with both early and advanced cervical cancer

---

**BOX 43.3**
**FIGO Staging of Cervical Cancer**

**Stage I**
Stage I is carcinoma strictly confined to the cervix; extension to the uterine corpus should be disregarded.
- Stage IA: Invasive cancer identified only microscopically. All gross lesions even with superficial invasion are stage IB cancers. Invasion is limited to measured stromal invasion with a maximum depth of 5 mm* and no wider than 7 mm. [Note: *The depth of invasion should be 5 mm or less taken from the base of the epithelium, either surface or glandular, from which it originates. Vascular space involvement, either venous or lymphatic, should not alter the staging.]
  - Stage IA1: Measured invasion of the stroma 3 mm or less in depth and 7 mm or less in diameter.
  - Stage IA2: Measured invasion of stroma more than 3 mm but 5 mm or less in depth and 7 mm or less in diameter
- Stage IB: Clinical lesions confined to the cervix or preclinical lesions greater than stage IA.
  - Stage IB1: Clinical lesions 4 cm or less in size
  - Stage IB2: Clinical lesions 4 cm or more in size

**Stage II**
Stage II is carcinoma that extends beyond the cervix but has not extended onto the pelvic wall. The carcinoma involves the vagina but not as far as the lower third section.

- Stage IIA: No obvious parametrial involvement. Involvement of as much as the upper two thirds of the vagina
- Stage IIB: Obvious parametrial involvement, but not onto the pelvic sidewall

**Stage III**
Stage III is carcinoma that has extended onto the pelvic sidewall and/or involves the lower third of the vagina. On rectal examination, there is no cancer-free space between the tumor and the pelvic sidewall. All cases with a hydronephrosis or nonfunctioning kidney should be included, unless they are known to be due to other causes.
- Stage IIIA: No extension onto the pelvic sidewall, but involvement of the lower third of the vagina
- Stage IIIB: Extension onto the pelvic sidewall or hydronephrosis or nonfunctioning kidney

**Stage IV**
Stage IV is carcinoma that has extended beyond the true pelvis or has clinically involved the mucosa of the bladder and/or rectum.
- Stage IVA: Spread of the tumor onto adjacent pelvic organs
- Stage IVB: Spread to distant organs

From Quinn MA, Benedet JL, Odicino F, Maisonneuve P, Beller U, Creasman WT, et al. Carcinoma of the cervix uteri. International Federation of Gynecology and Obstetrics. FIGO annual report on the results of treatment in gynecological cancer, S43, copyright Elsevier 2006. Originally published in *International Journal of Gynecology and Obstetrics*, volume 95, supplement.

---

and should facilitate referrals for this treatment. Surgery or radiation therapy may be options for treatment, depending on the stage and size of the lesion:

- Patients with squamous cell cancers and those with adenocarcinomas should be managed similarly, except for those with microinvasive disease. Criteria for microinvasive adenocarcinomas have not been established.
- For stage Ia1, microinvasive squamous carcinoma of the cervix, treatment with conization of the cervix or simple extrafascial hysterectomy may be considered.
- Stage Ia2, invasive squamous carcinoma of the cervix, should be treated with radical hysterectomy with lymph node dissection or radiation therapy, depending on clinical circumstances.
- Stage Ib1 should be distinguished from stage Ib2 carcinoma of the cervix, because the distinction predicts

nodal involvement and overall survival and may therefore affect treatment and outcome.
- For stage Ib and selected IIa carcinomas of the cervix, either radical hysterectomy and lymph node dissection or radiation therapy with cisplatin-based chemotherapy should be considered. Adjuvant radiation therapy may be required in those treated surgically, based on pathologic risk factors, especially in those with stage Ib2 carcinoma.
- Stage IIb and greater should be treated with external-beam and brachytherapy radiation and concurrent cisplatin-based chemotherapy.

Brachytherapy delivers radiation close to the affected organ or structure. Both high- and low-dose brachytherapy are used to treat cervical cancer. The brachytherapy radiation is delivered using special apparatuses known as tandem and ovoid devices placed through the cervix into the uterus and

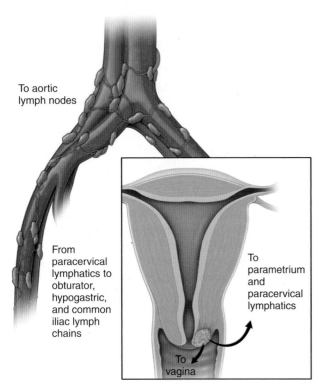

To aortic
lymph nodes

From
paracervical
lymphatics to
obturator,
hypogastric,
and common
iliac lymph
chains

To
parametrium
and
paracervical
lymphatics

To
vagina

FIGURE 43.7. Spread patterns of cervical carcinoma.

| TABLE 43.2 | Five-Year Survival Rates for Cervical Cancer |
|---|---|
| Stage | 5-Year Survival Rate |
| IA | >95% |
| IB1 | Approximately 90% |
| IB2 | 80%–85% |
| IIA/B | 75%–78% |
| IIIA/B | 47%–50% |
| IV | 20%–30% |

American Cancer Society, 2008.

at the apices of the vagina. The external beam radiation is applied primarily along the paths of lymphatic extension of cervical carcinoma in the pelvis.

The structures close to the cervix, such as the bladder and distal colon, tolerate radiation relatively well. Radiation therapy doses are calculated by individual-patient needs to maximize radiation to the tumor sites and potential spread areas, while minimizing the amount of radiation to adjacent uninvolved tissues. Complications of radiation therapy include radiation cystitis and proctitis, which are usually relatively easy to manage. Other more unusual complications include intestinal or vaginal fistulae, small bowel obstruction, or difficult-to-manage hemorrhagic proctitis or cystitis. Tissue damage and fibrosis incurred by radiation therapy progresses over many years, and these effects may complicate long-term management.

Following treatment for cervical carcinoma, patients should be monitored regularly, for example, with thrice-yearly follow-up examinations for the first 2 years and twice-yearly visits subsequently to year 5, with Pap tests annually and chest x-rays annually for up to 5 years. The five-year survival rates for cervical cancer are listed in Table 43.2.

Treatment for recurrent disease is associated with poor cure rates. Most chemotherapeutic protocols have only limited usefulness and are reserved for palliative efforts. Likewise, specific "spot" radiation to areas of recurrence also provides only limited benefit. Occasional patients with

central recurrence (i.e., recurrence of disease in the upper vagina or the residual cervix and uterus in radiation patients) may benefit from ultraradical surgery with partial or total pelvic exenteration. These candidates are few, but when properly selected, may benefit from this aggressive therapy.

## PREVENTION

Preventive approaches to cervical cancer include sexual abstinence, the use of barrier protection with or without spermicides, regular gynecologic examination and cytologic screening with treatment of precancerous lesions according to established protocols, and vaccination with the HPV vaccine. It is estimated that gynecologic examination and Pap tests administered according to current guidelines may reduce cancer incidence and mortality by 40%. Limiting the number of sexual partners also may decrease one's risk for STDs, including HPV.

The recently developed HPV vaccine prevents transmission and acquisition of type-specific HPV through sexual and nonsexual contact. Currently, the only approved vaccine on the market is active against oncogenic HPV types 16 and 18 as well as two types that cause genital warts, HPV types 6 and 11. Another vaccine currently being investigated is active against oncogenic HPV types 16 and 18. These two vaccines contain virus-like particles (VLPs) that consist of the main structural HPV-L1 protein but lack the viral genetic material and, hence, are noninfectious. These vaccines stimulate production of IgG-type specific antibodies to prevent acquisition of type specific HPV in the genital and vulvar areas. The quadrivalent vaccine has been shown to prevent 91% of new and 100% of persistent infections. Currently, HPV vaccines are only indicated for prophylaxis (Box 43-4). However, it is anticipated that the guidelines for their use will continue to change regarding age group, sex, and therapeutic indications. The development of new vaccines may also broaden the horizon for HPV treatment.

> ## BOX 43.4
> ### Current Guidelines for Administration of the Quadrivalent HPV Vaccine
>
> - The HPV vaccine is given in three doses over a 6-month period.
> - It is recommended as a routine vaccination for all girls aged 11–12 years. However, it can be given to girls as young as 9 years. Girls and young women aged 13–26 years who have either not yet received the vaccine or have not completed all doses also should be vaccinated.
> - Sexually active women can receive the quadrivalent HPV vaccine. Women with previous abnormal cervical cytology or genital warts also can receive the quadrivalent HPV vaccine. These patients should be counseled that the vaccine may be less effective in women who have been exposed to HPV before vaccination than in women who were HPV naive at the time of vaccination. Women with previous HPV infection will benefit from protection against disease caused by the HPV vaccine genotypes with which they have not been infected.
> - Testing for HPV is currently not recommended before vaccination.
> - The vaccine is not recommended for pregnant women, but is safe for women who are breastfeeding.
> - Current cervical cytology screening recommendations remain unchanged and should be followed regardless of vaccination status.
>
> From American College of Obstetricians and Gynecologists. Human papillomavirus vaccination. ACOG Committee Opinion No. 344. *Obstet Gynecol.* 2006;108(3):699–705.

## SUGGESTED READINGS

American College of Obstetricians and Gynecologists. Cervical cancer screening in adolescents. ACOG Committee Opinion No. 300. *Obstet Gynecol.* 2004;104(4):885–889.

American College of Obstetricians and Gynecologists. Cervical cytology screening. ACOG Practice Bulletin No. 45. *Obstet Gynecol.* 2003;102(2):417–427.

American College of Obstetricians and Gynecologists. Management of abnormal cervical cytology and histology. ACOG Practice Bulletin No. 66. *Obstet Gynecol.* 2005;106(3):645–664.

*Guidelines for Women's Health Care.* 3rd ed. Washington, DC: American College of Obstetricians and Gynecologists; 2007: 386–392,169–169.

Spitzer M, Moore DH. Cervical neoplasia. In: *Precis: Oncology.* 3rd ed. Washington, DC: American College of Obstetricians and Gynecologists; 2007:51–73.

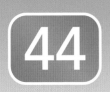
# Uterine Leiomyoma and Neoplasia

This chapter deals primarily with APGO Educational Topic:

Topic 53:  Uterine Leiomyomas

The student should understand how to diagnose and, if necessary, treat the most common gynecologic neoplasm.

*U*terine leiomyomata *(also called* **fibroids** *and* **myomas**) *represent localized proliferation of smooth muscle cells surrounded by a pseudocapsule of compressed muscle fibers.* The highest prevalence occurs during the fifth decade of a woman's life, when they may be present in 1 in 4 white women and 1 in 2 black women. *Uterine leiomyomata are clinically apparent in 25% to 50% of women, although studies in which careful pathologic examination of the uterus is carried out suggest that the prevalence may be as high as 80%.* Uterine fibroids vary in size, from microscopic to large multinodular tumors that literally fill the patient's abdomen. Leiomyomata are the most common indication for hysterectomy, accounting for approximately 30% of all such cases. Additionally, they account for a large number of more conservative operations, including myomectomy, uterine curettage, operative hysteroscopy, and uterine artery embolization (UAE).

Leiomyomata are classified into subgroups based on their anatomic relationship to the layers of the uterus. *The three most common types are* **intramural** *(centered in the muscular wall of the uterus),* **subserosal** *(just beneath the uterine serosa), and* **submucosal** *(just beneath the endometrium).* A subset of the subserosal category is the **pedunculated leiomyoma,** which appears on stump-like structures. Most leiomyomata initially develop from within the myometrium as intramural leiomyomata. Roughly 5% of uterine myomas originate from the cervix. Rarely, leiomyomata may occur without evidence of a uterine origin in places such as the broad ligament and peritoneal cavity. Leiomyomata are considered hormonally responsive, benign tumors, because estrogen may induce their rapid growth in high-estrogen states, such as pregnancy. In contrast, menopause generally causes cessation of tumor growth and even some atrophy. Estrogen may work by stimulating the production of progesterone receptors in the myometrium. In turn, progesterone binding to these sites stimulates the production of several growth factors, causing the growth of myomas. Although exact mechanisms are unknown, chromosomal translocations/deletions, peptide growth factor, and epidermal growth factor are implicated as potential pathogenic factors of leiomyomata. Sensitive DNA studies suggest that each myoma arises from a single smooth muscle cell and that, in many cases, the smooth muscle cell is vascular in origin.

The uterine smooth muscle may also develop a rare cancer, such as **leiomyosarcoma.** These are not thought to represent "degeneration" of a fibroid, but, rather, a new neoplasm. *Uterine malignancy is more typical in postmenopausal patients who present with rapidly enlarging uterine masses, postmenopausal bleeding, unusual vaginal discharge, and pelvic pain.* An enlarging uterine mass in a postmenopausal patient should be evaluated with considerably more concern for malignancy than one found in a younger woman. These heterologous, mixed tumors contain other sarcomatous tissue elements not necessarily found only in the uterus.

## SYMPTOMS

Bleeding is the most common presenting symptom in uterine fibroids. Although the kind of abnormal bleeding may vary, the most common presentation includes the development of progressively heavier menstrual flow that lasts longer than the normal duration (**menorrhagia,** defined as menstrual blood loss of >80 mL). This bleeding may result from significant distortion of the endometrial cavity by the underlying tumor. Three generally accepted but unproved mechanisms for increased bleeding include:

1. Alteration of normal myometrial contractile function in the small artery and arteriolar blood supply underlying the endometrium
2. Inability of the overlying endometrium to respond to the normal estrogen/progesterone menstrual phases, which contributes to efficient sloughing of the endometrium

**3.** Pressure necrosis of the overlying endometrial bed, which exposes vascular surfaces that bleed in excess of that normally found with endometrial sloughing

Characteristically, the best example of leiomyoma contributing to this bleeding pattern is by the so-called **submucous leiomyoma.** In this variant, most of the distortion created by the smooth muscle tumor projects toward the endometrial cavity, rather than toward the serosal surface of the uterus. Enlarging intramural fibroids likewise may contribute to excessive bleeding if they become large enough to significantly distort the endometrial cavity.

Blood loss from this type of menstrual bleeding may be heavy enough to contribute to chronic **iron-deficiency anemia** and, rarely, to profound acute blood loss. The occurrence of isolated submucous (subendometrial) leiomyomata is unusual. Commonly, these are found in association with other types of leiomyomata (Fig. 44.1).

*Another common symptom is a progressive increase in "pelvic pressure."* This may be a sense of progressive pelvic fullness, "something pressing down," and/or the sensation of a pelvic mass. Most commonly, this is caused by slowly enlarging myomas, which on occasion may attain a massive size. These leiomyomata are the most easily palpated on bimanual or abdominal examination and contributes to a characteristic "lumpy-bumpy," or cobblestone, sensation when multiple myomas are present. Occasionally, these large myomas present as a large asymptomatic pelvic or even abdominopelvic mass. Such large leiomyomata may cause an uncommon but significant clinical problem: pressure on the ureters as they traverse the pelvic brim leading to **hydroureter** (dilation of the ureter) and possibly **hydronephrosis** (dilation of the renal pelvis and calyces). These conditions can also occur if fibroids lower

within the pelvis grow laterally between the leaves of the broad ligament.

Another presentation is the onset of **secondary dysmenorrhea.** Other pain symptoms, although rare, may be the result of rapid enlargement of a leiomyoma. This can result in areas of tissue necrosis or areas of subnecrotic vascular ischemia, which contribute to alteration in myometrial response to prostaglandins similar to the mechanism described for primary dysmenorrhea. Occasionally, torsion of a pedunculated myoma can occur, resulting in acute pain. Dull, intermittent, low midline cramping (labor-like) pain is the clinical presentation when a submucous (subendometrial) myoma becomes pedunculated and progressively prolapses through the internal os of the cervix.

## DIAGNOSIS

The diagnosis of fibroids is usually based on physical examination or imaging studies. Occasionally, irregularities of the uterine cavity are detected during endometrial sampling. Often the diagnosis is incidental to pathologic assessment of a uterine specimen removed for other indications. *On abdominopelvic examination, uterine leiomyomata usually present as a large, midline, irregular-contoured mobile pelvic mass with a characteristic "hard feel" or solid quality.*

> *The degree of enlargement is usually stated in terms (weeks' size) that are used to estimate equivalent gestational size.*

The fibroid uterus is described separate from any adnexal disease, although on occasion a pedunculated myoma may be difficult to distinguish from a solid adnexal mass.

Pelvic ultrasound may be used for confirmation (when necessary) of uterine myomas, but the diagnosis remains a clinical one. There may be areas of acoustic "shadowing" amid otherwise normal myometrial patterns, and there may be a distorted endometrial stripe. Occasionally cystic components may be seen as hypoechogenic areas and are consistent in appearance with myomas undergoing degeneration. Adnexal structures, including the ovaries, are usually identifiable separate from these masses.

Computerized axial tomography (CAT) and magnetic resonance imaging (MRI) may be useful in evaluating extremely large myomas when ultrasonography may not image a large myoma well. Hysteroscopy, hysterosalpingography, and saline infusion ultrasonography are the best techniques for identifying intrauterine lesions such as submucosal myomata and polyps.

**Endometrial biopsy** should not be relied on to provide additional diagnostic information; however, an indirect appreciation for uterine enlargement may be gained by uterine sounding, which is part of this procedure. If a patient has irregular uterine bleeding and endometrial carcinoma is a consideration, endometrial sampling is useful to evaluate for this possibility, independent of the myomas.

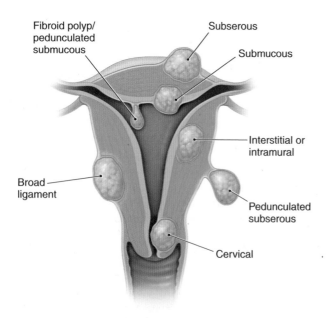

FIGURE 44.1. Common types of leiomyomata.

**Hysteroscopy** may be used to evaluate the enlarged uterus by directly visualizing the endometrial cavity. The increased size of the cavity can be documented, and submucous fibroids can be visualized and removed.

*Although the efficacy of hysteroscopic removal (resection) of submucous myomas has been documented, long-term follow-up suggests that up to 20% of patients require additional treatment during the subsequent 10 years.*

Surgical evaluation may be required when physical examination and ultrasound cannot differentiate whether the patient has a leiomyomata or other potentially more serious disease, such as adnexal neoplasia. Laparoscopic resection of subserosal or intramural myoma has gained in popularity, although the long-term benefit of this procedure has not been well-established.

## TREATMENT

*Most patients with uterine myomas do not require (surgical or medical) treatment.* Treatment is generally first directed toward the symptoms caused by the myomas. If this approach fails (or there are other indications present), surgical or other extirpative procedures may be considered.

For example, if a patient presents with menstrual aberrations that are attributable to the myomas, with bleeding that is not heavy enough to cause her significant hygiene or lifestyle problems—and the bleeding is also not contributing to iron-deficiency anemia—reassurance and observation may be all that are necessary. Further uterine growth may be assessed by repeat pelvic examinations or serial pelvic ultrasonography.

An attempt may be made to minimize uterine bleeding by using intermittent **progestin supplementation** and/or prostaglandin synthetase inhibitors, which decrease the amount of secondary dysmenorrhea and amount of menstrual flow. If significant endometrial cavity distortion is caused by intramural or submucous myomas, hormonal supplementation may be ineffective. If effective, this conservative approach can potentially be used until the time of menopause.

Of the surgical options available, **myomectomy** is warranted in patients who desire to retain childbearing potential or whose fertility is compromised by the myomas, creating significant intracavitary distortion. *Indications for a myomectomy include a rapidly enlarging pelvic mass, persistent bleeding, pain or pressure, or enlargement of an asymptomatic myoma to more than 8 cm in a woman who has not completed childbearing.* Contraindications to myomectomy include pregnancy, advanced adnexal disease, malignancy, and the situation where enucleation of the myomas would completely compromise the function of the uterus. Potential complications of myomectomy include excessive intraoperative blood loss; postoperative hemorrhage, infection, and pelvic adhesions; and even the need for emergent hys-

terectomy. Within 20 years of a myomectomy procedure, 1 in 4 women has a hysterectomy, the majority for recurrent leiomyomas.

Although **hysterectomy** is commonly performed for uterine myomas, it should be considered as definitive treatment only in symptomatic women who have completed childbearing. Indications should be specific and well-documented (Box 44.1). Depending on the size of

---

**BOX 44.1**
### Criteria for Hysterectomy for Leiomyomata*

**Indication**
**Leiomyomata**
*Confirmation of indication* (1, 2, or 3)
1. Asymptomatic leiomyomata of such size that they are palpable abdominally and are a concern to the patient
2. Excessive uterine bleeding evidenced by either of the following:
   a. Profuse bleeding with flooding or clots, or repetitive periods lasting >8 days
   b. Anemia caused by acute or chronic blood loss
3. Pelvic discomfort caused by myomata (a, b, or c):
   a. Acute and severe
   b. Chronic lower abdominal or low back pressure
   c. Bladder pressure with urinary frequency not caused by urinary tract infection

**Actions Before Procedure**
1. Confirm no cervical malignancy
2. Eliminate anovulation and other causes of abnormal bleeding
3. When abnormal bleeding is present, confirm no endometrial malignancy
4. Assess surgical risk from anemia and need for treatment
5. Consider patient's medical and psychological risks concerning hysterectomy

**Contraindications**
1. Desire to maintain fertility, in which case, myomectomy should be considered
2. Asymptomatic leiomyomata of 12 weeks' gestation determined by physical examination or ultrasound examination

Modified from the American College of Obstetricians and Gynecologists. Quality Assessment and Improvement in Obstetrics and Gynecology. Washington, DC: American College of Obstetricians and Gynecologists; 1994.

the fibroids and the skill of the surgeon, both myomectomy and hysterectomy can potentially be performed via laparoscopy. The ultimate decision whether to perform a hysterectomy should include an assessment of the patient's future reproductive plans as well as careful assessment of clinical factors, including the amount and timing of bleeding, the degree of enlargement of the tumors, and the associated disability for the individual patient. Uterine myomas alone do not necessarily warrant hysterectomy.

In addition to surgery, pharmacologic inhibition of estrogen secretion has been used to treat fibroids. This is particularly applicable in the perimenopausal years when women are more likely anovulatory, with relatively more endogenous estrogen. Pharmacologic removal of the ovarian estrogen source can be achieved by suppression of the hypothalamic-pituitary-ovarian axis through the use of **gonadotropin-releasing hormone agonists (GnRH analogs),** which can reduce fibroid size by as much as 40% to 60%. *This treatment is commonly used before a planned hysterectomy to reduce blood loss as well as the difficulty of the procedure. It can also be used as a temporizing medical therapy until natural menopause occurs.* Therapy is generally limited to 6 months of drug treatment.

In patients with an adequate endogenous estrogen source, this treatment does not permanently reduce the size of uterine myomas, as withdrawal of the medication predictably results in regrowth of the myomas. Although less successful, other pharmacologic agents such as **danazol** have also been used as medical treatment for myomas by reducing endogenous production of ovarian estrogen.

Other therapeutic modalities have been introduced, although their efficacy is yet to be demonstrated. Included in these are **myolysis** (via direct procedures or by the delivery of external radio or ultrasonic energy) and uterine artery embolization (UAE). The safety and efficacy of **UAE** have been studied to the point that it is now considered a viable alternative to hysterectomy and myomectomy for selected patients. The procedure involves selective uterine artery catheterization with embolization using polyvinyl alcohol particles, which creates acute infarction of the target myomas. For maximal efficacy, bilateral uterine artery cannulation and embolization is necessary. In assessing outcomes data, the three most common symptoms of myomas—bleeding, pressure, and pain—are ameliorated in over 85% of patients. Acute postembolization pain that requires hospitalization occurs in approximately 10% to 15% of patients. Other complications include delayed infection and/or passage of necrotic fibroids through the cervix up to 30 days after the procedure. *UAE is currently not recommended as a procedure to consider in patients who desire future childbearing.*

*MRI-guided focused ultrasound surgery is a new approach used to treat myomata.* A focused ultrasound unit delivers sufficient ultrasound energy to a targeted point to raise the temperature to approximately 70°C. This results in coagulative necrosis and a decrease in myoma size. Treatment is associated with minimal pain and appears to improve self-reported bleeding patterns and quality of life.

## EFFECT OF LEIOMYOMATA IN PREGNANCY

*Although leiomyomata are equivocally associated with infertility, patients with leiomyoma do become pregnant.* Pregnancy with small leiomyomata is usually unremarkable, with a normal antepartum course, labor, and delivery. However, women with myomas greater than 3 cm may have significantly increased rates of preterm labor, placental abruption, pelvic pain, and cesarean delivery. Myomas may sometimes cause pain, as they can outgrow their blood supply during pregnancy, resulting in **red or carneous degeneration.** Bed rest and strong analgesics are usually sufficient as treatment, although on occasion myomectomy may be needed. The risk of abortion or preterm labor following myomectomy during pregnancy is relatively high, so that prophylactic β-adrenergic tocolytics are frequently used. *Myomectomy during pregnancy should be limited to myomas with a discrete pedicle that can be clamped and easily ligated.* Myomas should otherwise not be removed during time of delivery, because bleeding may be profuse, resulting in hysterectomy. Vaginal birth after myomectomy is controversial and must be decided on a case-by-case basis. Removal of an intramural leiomyoma is especially hazardous for subsequent pregnancy. After myomectomy there is a significant risk of uterine rupture during a subsequent pregnancy, even at times remote from labor. When a myomectomy results in a defect through the myometrium, subsequent pregnancies should be delivered before active labor begins. Rarely, myomas are located below the fetus, in the lower uterine segment or cervix, causing a soft tissue dystocia, leading to a need for cesarean birth.

## SUGGESTED READINGS

American College of Obstetricians and Gynecologists. Alternatives to hysterectomy in the management of leiomyomas. ACOG Practice Bulletin No. 16. *Obstet Gynecol.* 2008;112(2 Pt 1):387–400.

American College of Obstetricians and Gynecologists. *Guidelines for Women's Health Care: A Resource Manual.* 3rd ed. Washington, D.C.: ACOG; 2007.

American College of Obstetricians and Gynecologists. Uterine artery embolization. ACOG Committee Opinion No. 293. *Obstet Gynecol.* 2004;103(2):403–404.

American College of Obstetricians and Gynecologists. *Precis: Gynecology.* 3rd ed. Washington, DC: American College of Obstetricians and Gynecologists; 2006:95–102.

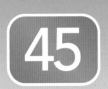

# Cancer of the Uterine Corpus

This chapter deals primarily with APGO Educational Topic:

Topic 54: Endometrial Carcinoma

The student should be familiar with the risk factors as well as the diagnosis and treatment of the most common gynecologic malignancy.

Approximately 2% to 3% of women will develop uterine cancer during their lifetime. Ninety-seven percent of all uterine cancers arise from the glands of the endometrium and are known as **endometrial carcinomas.** The remaining 3% of uterine cancers arise from mesenchymal uterine components and are classified as **sarcomas.**

*Endometrial carcinoma is the most common genital tract malignancy and the fourth most common cancer after breast, bowel, and lung carcinoma.* Approximately 39,000 new cases of endometrial carcinoma were diagnosed in 2007, resulting in over 7400 deaths. Fortunately, patients with this disease usually present early in the disease course with some form of abnormal uterine bleeding (AUB), particularly postmenopausal bleeding. With early diagnosis, survival rates are excellent.

## ENDOMETRIAL HYPERPLASIA

Endometrial hyperplasia is the most common precursor to endometrioid adenocarcinoma. In 1994, the World Health Organization defined a classification system of endometrial hyperplasia based on four types of simple and complex hyperplasia, with or without **atypia** (see Table 45.1).

## Types

### SIMPLE HYPERPLASIA

**Simple hyperplasia** is the least significant form of endometrial hyperplasia and is not commonly associated with progression to endometrial carcinoma. *In this type of hyperplasia, both glandular elements and stromal cell elements proliferate excessively.* Histologically, glands vary markedly in size, from small to cystically enlarged (the hallmark of this hyperplasia). Cystic glandular hyperplasia should not be confused with a normal postmenopausal variant—cystic involution of

the endometrium—which is histologically not a hyperplastic condition.

### COMPLEX HYPERPLASIA

*Complex hyperplasia represents an abnormal proliferation of primarily glandular elements without concomitant proliferation of stromal elements.* This increased gland-to-stroma ratio gives the endometrium a "crowded" picture, frequently with glands appearing almost back-to-back. As the severity of the hyperplasia increases, the glands become more crowded and more structurally bizarre. It is thought that complex hyperplasia represents a true intraepithelial neoplastic process, and it is occasionally found coexisting with areas of endometrial adenocarcinoma.

### HYPERPLASIA (SIMPLE OR COMPLEX) WITH CYTOLOGICAL ATYPIA

Hyperplasia characterized by significant numbers of glandular elements that exhibit **cytological atypia** and disordered maturation (loss of cellular polarity, nuclear enlargement with increased nucleus-to-cytoplasm ratio, dense chromatin, and prominent nucleoli), is considered a precursor lesion to endometrial carcinoma (Fig. 45.1).

## Pathophysiology and Risk Factors

*The primary process central to the development of endometrial hyperplasia (and most endometrial cancer) is overgrowth of the endometrium in response to excess unopposed estrogen.* Sources of estrogen may be **endogenous** (ovarian; peripheral conversion of androgenic precursors) or **exogenous** (Box 45.1). Endometrial proliferation represents a normal part of the menstrual cycle and occurs during the follicular, or estrogen-dominant, phase of the cycle. With continued estrogen stimulation through either endogenous mechanisms or by exogenous administration, simple endometrial

| TABLE 45.1 | World Health Organization's Classification of Endometrial Hyperplasia | |
|---|---|---|
| **Types** | | **Risk of progressing to cancer (%)** |
| Simple hyperplasia without atypia | | 1 |
| Complex hyperplasia without atypia | | 3 |
| Simple hyperplasia with atypia | | 8 |
| Complex hyperplasia with atypia | | 29 |

proliferation will become endometrial hyperplasia. Research suggests that this transformation may be time- and dose-dependent. When proliferation becomes hyperplasia is not clear, although studies showing sequential change suggest it requires 6 months or longer of stimulation without progesterone opposition. The risk factors for hyperplasia and endometrial cancer are identical (Table 45.2).

The risks of underlying endometrial cancer following biopsy-proven hyperplasia are as follows: 1% for simple, 3% for complex, and 8% for simple atypia. Complex atypical hyperplasia was reported to occur in 29% of cases. *In one study, more than 42% of women with endometrial atypia had invasive endometrial cancer demonstrated when hysterectomy was performed within 3 months.*

## PATIENT HISTORY

*AUB is the hallmark symptom of both endometrial hyperplasia and cancer.*

Further evaluation to rule out underlying carcinoma is warranted in two general scenarios: (1) a postmenopausal woman with any bleeding who is not on hormone replacement therapy, or (2) a premenopausal woman with AUB in the presence of additional risk factors (family history of breast, colon, or gynecologic cancer; obesity; prior endometrial hyperplasia; chronic anovulation; tamoxifen use; or estrogen therapy).

## EVALUATION

Histologic evaluation of a sample of the endometrium establishes the diagnosis of endometrial hyperplasia or carcinoma. **Endometrial biopsy** is most easily accomplished by any number of different atraumatic aspiration devices used in the office.

*The diagnostic accuracy of office endometrial biopsy is 90% to 98%, compared with dilation and curettage (D&C) or hysterectomy.*

The routine Pap smear is not reliable in diagnosing endometrial hyperplasia or cancer, as only 30% to 40% of patients with endometrial carcinoma have abnormal Pap test results. On the other hand, endometrial carcinoma must be considered, and endometrial sampling obtained, when atypical endometrial cells or atypical glandular cells of undetermined significance (AGUS) are found on the Pap smear.

*The most common indication for endometrial sampling is abnormal bleeding.* After ruling out pregnancy in premenopausal women, an adequate tissue sample can be obtained with relatively little discomfort. Further management is usually dictated by the results of the biopsy specimen. **Dilatation and curettage (D&C)** or **hysteroscopy** with directed endometrial biopsy may be undertaken when outpatient sampling is not possible (e.g., because of a stenotic cervical os or a patient who cannot tolerate the outpatient procedure) or when the outpatient sampling has been nondiagnostic.

Sometimes the office endometrial biopsy will be reported as having "insufficient tissue for diagnosis." In a postmenopausal woman who is not taking hormone therapy, this result is compatible with an atrophic condition of the endometrium. In other cases, the clinical suspicion of a possible hyperplastic endometrial process may be high enough to warrant hysteroscopic evaluation with directed sampling, which allows more complete evaluation of the endometrium as well as direct diagnosis of polyps, myomas, and structural abnormalities (Fig. 45.2).

**Transvaginal ultrasound** (with or without the installation of fluid for contrast, sonohysterography) may be used as an adjunct means of evaluation for endometrial hyperplasia as well as for polyps, myomas, and structural abnormalities of the uterus. An endometrial thickness of >5 mm in a postmenopausal patient, a polypoid mass, or fluid collection is often considered an indication for further evaluation and histologic samples. It is also useful in patients who have multiple medical problems, to help determine if the risks of endometrial sampling are less than the risk of not sampling. *Nevertheless, an endometrial stripe of less than 5 mm, although consistent with menopause and endometrial atrophy, does not exclude the possibility of a nonestrogen-dependent carcinoma of the atrophic endometrium* (Fig. 47.3). The value of transvaginal ultrasonography in a premenopausal woman is less significant, given day-to-day variations throughout menstrual cycle.

In women with breast cancer treated with tamoxifen, the optimal manner of monitoring the endometrium is unclear. *Tamoxifen acts as a weak estrogen and is associated with increased risk of endometrial hyperplasia and carcinoma.* Most agree that routine ultrasonography and endometrial biopsy in asymptomatic women are not necessary. Endometrial abnormalities should be excluded in the presence of new symptoms, such as bloody vaginal discharge, spotting, or AUB.

FIGURE 45.1. Complex hyperplasia with severe nuclear atypia of endometrium. (A) The proliferative endometrial glands reveal considerable crowding and papillary infoldings. The endometrial stroma, although markedly diminished, can still be recognized between the glands. (B) Higher magnification demonstrates disorderly nuclear arrangement and nuclear enlargement and irregularity. Some contain small nucleoli. (Provided by Gordana Stevanovic, MD, and Jianyu Rao, MD, Department of Pathology, UCLA; Berek JS, *Berek & Novak's Gynecology.* 14th ed. Philadelphia, PA: Lippincott Williams & Wilkins; 2007:1347, Figure 33.1.)

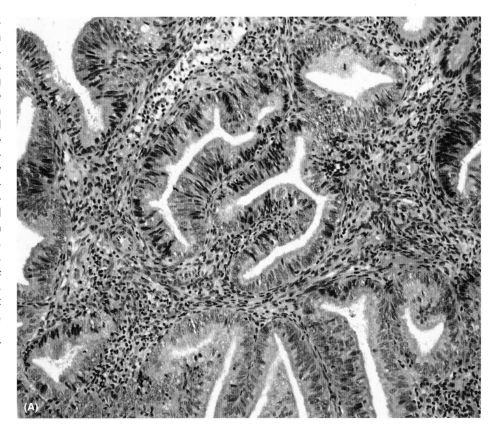

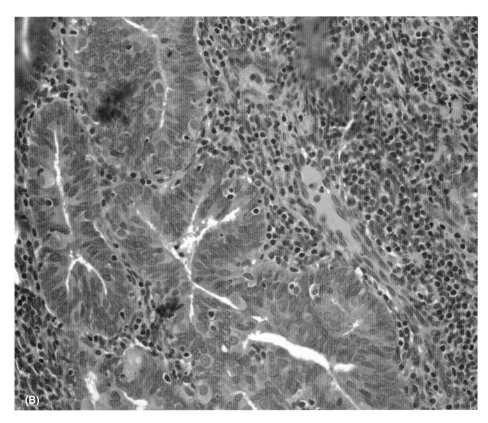

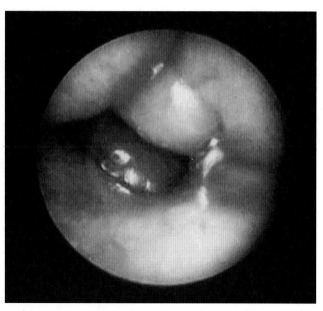

FIGURE 45.2. Diffuse hyperplasia as seen by hysteroscopy. The thickened walls of the uterus are closely opposed. (Baggish MS, Valle RF, Guedj H. *Hysteroscopy: Visual Perspectives of Uterine Anatomy, Physiology & Pathology.* 3rd ed. Philadelphia, PA: Lippincott Williams & Wilkins; 2007:233, Figure 18.19.)

## Management

The primary goals of treating endometrial hyperplasia are to reduce the risk of malignant transformation and to control the presenting symptoms. *Synthetic progesterones or other progestins are central in the medical treatment of endometrial hyperplasia.* They act through a number of pathways. First, they work to alter the enzymatic pathways, which eventually convert endogenous estradiol to weaker estrogens. Secondly, they decrease the number of estrogen receptors in the endometrial glandular cells, rendering them less susceptible to exogenous stimulation. Finally, the stimulation of progesterone receptors results in thinning of the endometrium and stromal decidualization. With time, this results in a decrease in endometrial glandular proliferation, which renders the endometrium atrophic.

In cases of hyperplasia without atypia, medical therapy is first utilized. The mean duration of progression from endometrial hyperplasia to carcinoma in those that do

| TABLE 45.2 | Risk Factors for Endometrial Hyperplasia and Cancer | |
|---|---|
| **Factors Influencing Risk** | **Estimated Relative Risk** |
| Long-term use of high dosages of menopausal estrogens | 10–20 |
| Residency in North America or Northern Europe | 3–18 |
| High cumulative doses of tamoxifen | 3–7 |
| Stein-Leventhal disease or estrogen-producing tumors | >5 |
| Obesity | 2–5 |
| Nulliparity | 3 |
| Older age | 2–3 |
| History of infertility | 2–3 |
| Late age of natural menopause | 2–3 |
| Early age of menarche | 1.5–2 |

Adapted from American College of Obstetricians and Gynecologists. *Management of Uterine Cancer.* ACOG Practice Bulletin # 65. Washington, DC: ACOG; 2005:2.

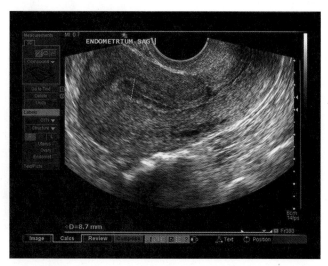

FIGURE 45.3. Endometrial stripe (calipers) as seen on ultrasound.

progress is relatively long: perhaps 10 years for those without atypia and 4 years for those with atypia. The most common treatment regimen is cyclic medroxyprogesterone acetate, or MPA, which is administered for 10 to 14 days each month for at least 3 to 6 months. Continuous administration is equally effective and may aid with compliance in patients who have an irregular cycle length.

Many view hyperplasia with atypia as a continuum with endometrial cancer. Hence, aggressive therapy for these patients is warranted, given the increased likelihood of progression to endometrial cancer. *After initial diagnosis, D&C is indicated to better sample the endometrium and exclude underlying endometrial cancer.* In young women who desire future fertility, long-term, high-dose progestin therapy may be used in an attempt to avoid a hysterectomy. As an alternative to oral therapy, the progesterone intrauterine contraceptive has been reported to have response rates ranging from 58% to 100%. Definitive therapy by hysterectomy is recommended after completing childbearing. Patients who are treated medically for atypical hyperplasia should also be followed with periodic endometrial sampling (every 3 months after therapy), so treatment response can be monitored.

## ENDOMETRIAL POLYPS

*Most endometrial polyps represent focal, accentuated, benign hyperplastic processes.* Their histologic architecture is characteristic and may commonly be found in association with other types of endometrial hyperplasia or even carcinoma.

Polyps occur most frequently in perimenopausal or immediately postmenopausal women, when ovarian function is characterized by persistent estrogen production due to chronic anovulation. The most common presenting symptom is abnormal bleeding. Small polyps may often be incidentally found as part of endometrial sampling or curettage done for evaluating AUB. Rarely, a large polyp may begin to protrude through the cervical canal. Such cases present with bleeding irregularities, and low, dull, midline pain, as the cervix is slowly dilated and effaced. In these cases, surgical removal is necessary to reduce the amount of bleeding and to prevent infection developing within the exposed endometrial surface. *Less than 5% of polyps show malignant change*, and when they do, they may represent any endometrial histologic variant. Polyps in postmenopausal women or women taking tamoxifen are more likely to be associated with endometrial carcinoma than those found in reproductive-age women.

## ENDOMETRIAL CANCER

Endometrial carcinoma is typically a disease of postmenopausal women. *Between 15% and 25% of postmenopausal women with bleeding have endometrial cancer.* A majority of cases are diagnosed while in stage I (72%). Despite recognition at early stages, endometrial cancer is the eighth leading site of cancer-related mortality among women in the United States.

Most primary endometrial carcinomas are **adenocarcinomas** (Fig. 45.4). Because squamous epithelium may

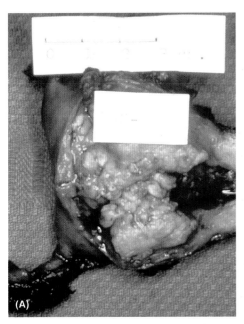
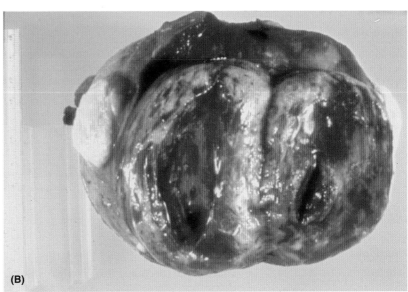

FIGURE 45.4. Types of endometrial tumors. (A) Endometrial adenocarcinoma. This polypoid exophytic tumor has invaded the outer third of the myometrium. (B) Serous carcinoma of the endometrium. The tumor is a polypoid mass arising in an atrophic uterus. Extensive myometrial lymphatic spread and involvement of the ovary are evident. (From Berek JS, Hacker NF. *Practical Gynecologic Oncology.* 4th ed. Philadelphia, PA: Lippincott Williams & Wilkins; 2005: Figures 6.42, 6.49.)

coexist with the glandular elements in an adenocarcinoma, descriptive terms that include the squamous element may be used. In cases where the squamous element is benign and makes up less than 10% of the histologic picture, the term **adenoacanthoma** is used. Uncommonly, the squamous element may appear malignant on histologic assessment and is then referred to as **adenosquamous carcinoma.** Other descriptions, such as **clear cell carcinoma** and **papillary serous adenocarcinoma,** may be applied, depending on the histologic architecture. All of these carcinomas are considered under the general category of adenocarcinoma of the endometrium and are treated in a similar manner.

## Pathogenesis and Risk Factors

Two kinds of endometrial carcinoma have been identified. Type I endometrial carcinoma is "**estrogen-dependent**" and accounts for approximately 90% of cases. It is most commonly caused by an excess of estrogen unopposed by progestins. These cancers tend to have low-grade nuclear atypia, endometrioid cell types, and an overall favorable prognosis. The second type, Type II or "**estrogen-independent**" endometrial carcinoma, occurs spontaneously, characteristically in thin, older postmenopausal women without unopposed estrogen excess, arising in an atrophic endometrium rather than a hyperplastic one. These cancers tend to be less well-differentiated, with a poorer prognosis. Estrogen-independent cancer is less common than estrogen-dependent cancer. Unusual histologic subtypes, including papillary serous adenocarcinoma and clear cell adenocarcinoma of the endometrium, tend to be more aggressive than the more common adenocarcinoma (Table 45.3).

*Endometrial carcinoma usually spreads throughout the endometrial cavity first and then begins to invade the myometrium, endocervical canal, and eventually the lymphatics.* Hematogenous spread occurs with endometrial carcinoma more readily than in cervical cancer or ovarian cancer. Invasion of adnexal structures may occur through lymphatics or direct implantation through the fallopian tubes. After extrauterine spread to the peritoneal cavity, cancer cells may spread widely in a fashion similar to that of ovarian cancer.

As mentioned earlier, the risk factors for developing endometrial cancer are identical to those for endometrial hyperplasia (see Table 45.2).

## Diagnosis

*Endometrial sampling, prompted by vaginal bleeding, most frequently establishes the diagnosis of endometrial cancer.* Vaginal bleeding or discharge is the only presenting complaint in 80% to 90% of women with endometrial carcinoma. In some, often older patients, cervical stenosis may sequester the blood in the uterus, with the

| TABLE 45.3 | Histologic Types of Endometrial Carcinoma | |
|---|---|---|
| **Histologic Type** | **Discussion** | **Percentage of Endometrial Carcinomas** |
| Endometrioid | Composed of glands that resemble normal endometrial glands but that contain more solid areas, less glandular formation, and more cytologic atypia as they become less well-differentiated | 80–85 |
| Endometrial carcinoma with squamous differentiation | Encompasses tumors with benign-appearing squamous areas (also called adenoacanthomas) and those with malignant-looking squamous elements (also called adenosquamous carcinomas) | 15–25 |
| Villoglandular | Endometrial cells with characteristics of endometrioid cells, arranged in papillary fibrovascular stalks, always well-differentiated | 2 |
| Secretory endometrial carcinoma | 50% of cells have intracytoplasmic mucin; most behave like well-differentiated endometrioid carcinoma; good prognosis | 5 |
| **Mucinous** | | |
| Papillary serous | Endometrial carcinoma that resembles serous carcinoma of the ovary and fallopian tube; very aggressive, poorer prognosis | 3–4 |
| Clear cell | Mixed histologic pattern; more common in older women; very aggressive, poor prognosis | <5 |
| Squamous | Generally pure cell type, some with glands; associated with older women and cervical stenosis; very poor prognosis | <1 |

presentation being hematometra or pyometra and a purulent vaginal discharge. In more advanced disease, pelvic discomfort or an associated sensation of pressure caused by uterine enlargement or extrauterine disease spread may accompany the complaint of vaginal bleeding or even be the presenting complaint. *Fewer than 5% of women found to have endometrial carcinoma are actually asymptomatic.*

*Special consideration should be given to the patient who presents with **postmenopausal bleeding** (i.e., bleeding that occurs after 6 months of amenorrhea in a patient who has been diagnosed as menopausal).*

In this group of patients, it is mandatory to assess the endometrium histologically because the risk of endometrial carcinoma is approximately 10% to 15%, although other causes are more common (Table 45.4). Other gynecologic assessments should also be made, including careful physical and pelvic examination, as well as a screening Pap smear. *Preoperative measurement of the CA 125 level may be appropriate, because it is frequently elevated in women with advanced-stage disease.* Elevated levels of CA 125 may assist in predicting treatment response or in posttreatment surveillance.

## Prognostic Factors

The current International Federation of Gynecology and Obstetrics (FIGO) staging of endometrial cancer (adopted in 1988) lists three grades of endometrial carcinoma:

- G1 is well-differentiated adenomatous carcinoma (less than 5% of the tumor shows a solid growth pattern).
- G2 is moderately differentiated adenomatous carcinoma with partly solid areas (6% to 50% of the tumor shows a solid growth pattern).
- G3 is poorly differentiated or undifferentiated (greater than 50% of the tumor shows a solid growth pattern).

Most patients with endometrial carcinoma have G1 or G2 lesions by this classification, with 15% to 20% having undifferentiated or poorly differentiated G3 lesions.

| TABLE 45.4 | Causes of Postmenopausal Uterine Bleeding | |
| --- | --- |
| Cause | Frequency (%) |
| Atrophy of the endometrium | 60–80 |
| Hormone therapy | 15–25 |
| Endometrial cancer | 10–15 |
| Endometrial polyps | 2–12 |
| Endometrial hyperplasia | 5–10 |

The FIGO staging system incorporates elements correlated with prognosis and risk of recurrent disease—histologic grade, nuclear grade, depth of myometrial invasion, cervical glandular or stromal invasion, vaginal and adnexal metastasis, cytology status, disease in the pelvic and/or paraaortic lymph nodes, and presence of distant metastases (Table 45.5). The single most important prognostic factor for endometrial carcinoma is **histologic grade.** Histologically, poorly differentiated or undifferentiated tumors are associated with a considerably poorer prognosis because of the likelihood of extrauterine spread through adjacent lymphatic and peritoneal fluid. **Depth of myometrial invasion** is the second most important prognostic factor.

*Survival rates vary widely, depending on the grade of tumor and depth of penetration into the myometrium.* A patient with a G1 tumor that does not invade the myometrium has a 95% 5-year survival rate, whereas a patient with a poorly differentiated (G3) tumor with deep myometrial invasion may have a 5-year survival rate of only 20%.

## Treatment

*Hysterectomy is the primary treatment of endometrial cancer. The addition of complete surgical staging with an assessment of retroperitoneal lymph nodes is not only therapeutic, but also is associated with improved survival.*

Complete surgical staging includes pelvic washings, bilateral pelvic and paraaortic lymphadenectomy, and complete resection of all disease. Sampling of the common iliac nodes, regardless of depth of penetration or histologic grade, may provide further information about the histologic grade and depth of invasion. Palpation of lymph nodes is equally inaccurate and should not substitute surgical resection of nodal tissue for histopathology.

Exceptions to the need for surgical staging include young or perimenopausal women with grade 1 endometrioid adenocarcinoma associated with atypical endometrial hyperplasia, and women at increased risk for mortality secondary to comorbidities. Women in the former group who desire to maintain their fertility may be treated with high-dose progestin monitored by serial endometrioid sampling. Women in the latter group may be treated with vaginal hysterectomy. In ultra-high-risk surgical patients, therapeutic radiation may be used as primary treatment, although results are suboptimal.

Postoperative radiation therapy should be tailored to known metastatic disease or used in cases of recurrence. In patients with surgical stage I disease, radiation therapy may reduce the risk of recurrence, but does not improve survival. *For women with positive lymph nodes (stage IIIc) disease, radiation therapy is critical in improving survival rates.* Women with intraperitoneal disease are treated with surgery, followed by systemic chemotherapy or radiation therapy or both.

| TABLE 45.5 | | International Federation of Gynecology and Obstetrics (FIGO) Surgical Staging System for Endometrial Cancer |
|---|---|---|
| **FIGO Stages*** | | **Surgical-Pathologic Findings** |
| 0 | | Carcinoma in situ |
| I | | Tumor confined to the uterus |
| | Ia | Tumor limited to endometrium |
| | Ib | Tumor invading less than 50% of myometrium |
| | Ic | Tumor invading 50% or more of myometrium |
| II | | Tumor invades cervix but confined to uterus |
| | IIa | Tumor limited to the glandular epithelium of the endocervix; there is no evidence of connective tissue stromal invasion |
| | IIb | Invasion of stromal connective tissue of the cervix |
| III | | Local and/or regional spread |
| | IIIa | Tumor involves serosa and/or adnexa (direct extension or metastasis) and/or cancer cells in ascites or peritoneal washings |
| | IIIb | Vaginal involvement (direct extension or metastasis) |
| | IIIc | Regional lymph node metastases to pelvic and/or periaortic nodes |
| IV | | |
| | IV a | Tumor invades bladder mucosa and/or bowel mucosa |
| | IV b | Distant metastases, including abdominal lymph nodes other than paraaortic, and/or inguinal lymph nodes; excludes metastasis to vagina, pelvic serosa, or adnexa |

*All cases of FIGO Stage I–IVA should be subclassified by histologic grade as follows: GX, grade cannot be assessed; G1, well-differentiated; G2, moderately differentiated; G3, poorly differentiated or undifferentiated.
Used with the permission of the American Joint Committee on Cancer (AJCC), Chicago, Illinois. The original source for this material is the *AJCC Cancer Staging Manual.* 6th ed. New York: Springer-Verlag; 2002. Available from: http://www.springeronline.com.

## Recurrent Endometrial Carcinoma

Postoperative surveillance for women who have not received radiation therapy involves speculum and recto-vaginal examinations every 3 to 4 months for 2 to 3 years, and then twice a year to detect pelvic recurrent disease, particularly in the vagina. *Women who have received radiation therapy have a decreased risk of vaginal recurrence as well as fewer therapeutic options to treat recurrence. Therefore, these women benefit less from frequent surveillance with cervical cytology screening and pelvic examinations for detection of recurrent disease.*

Recurrent endometrial carcinoma occurs in about 25% of patients treated for early disease, one-half within 2 years, and three-fourths within 3 to 4 years. In general, those with recurrent vaginal disease have a better prognosis than those with pelvic recurrence, who in turn fare better than those with distant metastatic disease (lung, abdomen, lymph nodes, liver, brain, and bone).

*Recurrent estrogen-dependent or progestin-dependent cancer may respond to high-dose* **progestin** *therapy.* A major advan-

tage of high-dose progestin therapy is its minimal complication rate. Chemotherapy with doxorubicin, cisplatin, and paclitaxel produces occasional favorable short-term results, but long-term remissions with these therapies are rare.

## Hormone Therapy after Treatment for Endometrial Carcinoma

The use of **estrogen therapy** in patients previously treated for endometrial carcinoma has long been considered contraindicated because of the concern that estrogen might activate occult metastatic disease.

*Hormone therapy can be used in the presence of the same indications as for any other woman, except that the selection of appropriate candidates for estrogen treatment should be based on prognostic indicators and the patient must be willing to assume the risk.*

Cautious individualized assessment of risks and benefits should therefore be made on a case-by-case basis.

## UTERINE SARCOMA

*Uterine sarcomas represent an unusual gynecologic malignancy accounting for approximately 3% of cancers involving the body of the uterus, and only about 0.1% of all myomas.* Progressive uterine enlargement occurring in the postmenopausal years should not be assumed to be the result of simple uterine leiomyomata, because appreciable endogenous ovarian estrogen secretion is absent, thereby minimizing the potential for growth of benign myomas. Even postmenopausal women on low-dose hormone therapy are not at risk for stimulation of uterine enlargement. When progressive growth is present in postmenopausal women, uterine sarcoma should be considered. Other symptoms of uterine sarcoma include postmenopausal bleeding, unusual pelvic pain coupled with uterine enlargement, and an increase in unusual vaginal discharge. Surgical removal is the method of most reliable diagnosis. Accordingly, hysterectomy is usually indicated in patients with documented, and especially progressive, uterine enlargement (Fig. 45-5).

The virulence of uterine sarcoma is directly related to the number of mitotic figures and degree of cellular atypia as defined histologically. These tumors are more likely to spread hematogenously than endometrial adenocarcinoma. When uterine sarcoma is suspected, patients should undergo a tumor survey to assess for distant metastatic disease. At the time of hysterectomy, it is necessary to thoroughly explore the abdomen and sample commonly affected node chains, including the iliac and periaortic areas. *The staging for uterine sarcoma is surgical and identical to that for endometrial adenocarcinoma.*

Unfortunately, the 5-year survival of patients with a uterine sarcoma is only 50%. Radiation and chemotherapy provide little benefit as adjuvant therapy to hysterectomy.

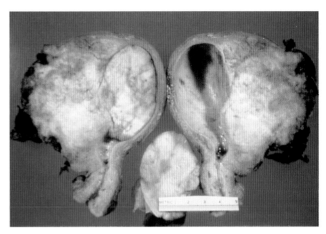

FIGURE 45.5. Uterine sarcoma. This hysterectomy specimen shows a large, partially necrotic polypoid mass filling the endometrial cavity and extensively invading the uterine wall. (From Berek JS, Hacker NF. *Practical Gynecologic Oncology.* 4th ed. Philadelphia, PA: Lippincott Williams & Wilkins; 2005:Figure 6.47.)

## SUGGESTED READINGS

American College of Obstetricians and Gynecologists, Committee on Gynecologic Practice. Tamoxifen and uterine cancer. ACOG Committee Opinion. No. 336. *Obstet Gynecol.* 2006;107(6): 1475–1478.

American College of Obstetricians and Gynecologists. *Guidelines for Women's Health Care: A Resource Manual.* 3rd ed. Washington, D.C.: ACOG; 2007.

American College of Obstetricians and Gynecologists. *Management of Endometrial Cancer.* ACOG Practice Bulletin No. 65. Washington, DC: American College of Obstetricians and Gynecologists; 2005.

American College of Obstetricians and Gynecologists. Cancer of the uterine corpus. In: *Precis, An Update in Obstetrics and Gynecology: Oncology.* 3rd ed. Washington, DC: American College of Obstetricians and Gynecologists; 2008: 74–87.

# 46 Ovarian and Adnexal Disease

Topic 55: Ovarian Neoplasms

The student should understand the physiologic and pathologic origins of both symptomatic and asymptomatic adnexal masses as well as the relevant diagnostic and therapeutic options.

T he area between the lateral pelvic wall and the cornu of the uterus is called the **adnexal space.** The structures in this space are called the adnexa and include the ovaries, fallopian tubes, upper portion of the broad ligament and mesosalpinx, and remnants of the embryonic müllerian duct. Of these, the organs most commonly affected by disease processes are the ovaries and fallopian tubes.

## DIFFERENTIAL DIAGNOSIS

Because the adnexal space is located near urinary and gastrointestinal organs, disorders of these organs may cause symptoms in the pelvic area that need to be distinguished from gynecologic disorders. The most common urologic disorders are upper and lower **urinary tract infection,** and the less common **renal and ureteral calculi.** Even rarer are anatomic abnormalities such as a **ptotic kidney,** which may present as a solid pelvic mass. An isolated pelvic kidney may likewise present as an asymptomatic, solid, cul-de-sac mass. Right adnexal signs and symptoms are associated with acute **appendicitis,** which should be considered in the differential diagnosis of acute right-lower-quadrant pain. Less commonly, symptoms in the right adnexa may be related to intrinsic **inflammatory bowel disease** involving the ileocecal junction. Left-sided bowel disease involving the rectosigmoid is seen more often in older patients, as in acute or chronic diverticular disease. Because of the age of these patients and the proximity of the left ovary to the sigmoid, **sigmoid diverticular disease** is included in the differential diagnosis of a left-sided adnexal mass. Finally, left-sided pelvic pain or a mass may be related to **rectosigmoid carcinoma.** Midline disease can sometimes be related to a process involving a Meckel diverticulum, or a sacral tumor.

## EVALUATION OF OVARIAN DISEASE

A thorough pelvic examination is essential for evaluation of the ovary. Symptoms that may arise from physiologic and pathologic processes of the ovary must be correlated with physical examination findings. Also, because some ovarian conditions are asymptomatic, incidental physical examination findings may be the only information available when an evaluation begins. Interpretation of examination findings requires knowledge of the physical characteristics of the ovary during the stages of the life cycle.

> In the **premenarchal age group,** the ovary should not be palpable.

If it is, a pathologic condition is presumed, and further evaluation is necessary.

*In the **reproductive-age group,** the normal ovary is palpable about half the time.* Important considerations include ovarian size, shape, consistency (firm or cystic), and mobility. In reproductive-age women taking oral contraceptives, the ovaries are palpable less frequently and are smaller and more symmetric than in women who are not using contraceptives.

In postmenopausal women, the ovaries are less responsive to gonadotropin secretion; therefore, their surface follicular activity diminishes over time, disappearing in most women within 3 years of the onset of natural menopause. Perimenopausal women are more likely to have residual functional cysts. In general, palpable ovarian enlargement in postmenopausal women should be assessed more critically than in a younger woman, because the incidence of ovarian malignant neoplasm is increased in this group.

*One-quarter of all ovarian tumors in postmenopausal women are malignant, whereas in reproductive-age women only about*

*10% of ovarian tumors are malignant.* This risk was considered so great in the past that any ovarian enlargement in a postmenopausal woman was an indication for surgical investigation, the so-called palpable postmenopausal ovary (PPO) syndrome. With the advent of more sensitive pelvic imaging techniques to assist in diagnosis, routine removal of minimally enlarged postmenopausal ovaries is no longer recommended.

CA-125 is a serum marker used to distinguish benign from malignant pelvic masses. Tumors can be evaluated by CA-125 assessments and ultrasound as well as consideration of family history. Simple, unilocular cysts less than 10 cm wide confirmed by transvaginal ultrasonography, are almost universally benign and may safely be followed without intervention regardless of age. Any CA-125 elevation in a postmenopausal woman with a pelvic mass is highly suspicious for cancer.

## FUNCTIONAL OVARIAN CYSTS

*Functional ovarian cysts are not neoplasms, but, rather, anatomic variations that arise as a result of normal ovarian function.* They may present as an asymptomatic adnexal mass or become symptomatic, requiring evaluation and possibly treatment.

When an ovarian follicle fails to rupture during follicular maturation, ovulation does not occur, and a **follicular cyst** may develop. This process, by definition, involves a lengthening of the follicular phase of the cycle, with resultant transient secondary amenorrhea. Follicular cysts are lined by normal granulosa cells, and the fluid contained in them is rich in estrogen.

A follicular cyst becomes clinically significant if it is large enough to cause pain or if it persists beyond one menstrual interval. For poorly understood reasons, the granulosa cells lining the follicular cyst persist through the time when ovulation should have occurred and continue to enlarge through the second half of the cycle. A cyst may enlarge beyond 5 cm and continue to fill with follicular fluid from the thickened granulosa cell layer. Symptoms associated with a follicular cyst may include mild to moderate unilateral lower abdominal pain and alteration of the menstrual interval. The latter may be the result of both failed subsequent ovulation and bleeding stimulated by the large amount of estradiol produced in the follicle. This hormonal environment, along with the lack of ovulation, overstimulates the endometrium and causes irregular bleeding. Pelvic examination findings may include unilateral tenderness with a palpable, mobile, cystic adnexal mass.

Pelvic ultrasonography is often warranted in reproductive-age patients who have cysts larger than 5 cm in diameter. Ultrasound characteristics of benign tumors include unilocular simple cyst without evidence of thick septations, soft tissue elements, or evidence of internal or external excrescences (Fig. 46.1). For many patients, however, ultrasound confirmation is not required. Instead, the patient

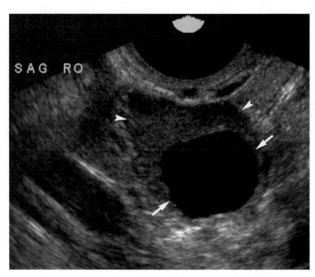

FIGURE 46.1. Sagittal ultrasonographic view of an ovarian cyst (arrows). Normal ovarian tissue (arrowheads) is seen around a portion of the cyst. (From Doubilet PM, Benson CB. *Atlas of Ultrasound in Obstetrics and Gynecology.* Philadelphia, PA: Lippincott Williams & Wilkins; 2003:304.)

may be reassured and followed with a repeat pelvic examination in about 6 weeks, once pregnancy has been ruled out.

Most follicular cysts spontaneously resolve during this time. Alternatively, an estrogen- and progesterone-containing oral contraceptive may be given to suppress gonadotropin stimulation of the cyst. Although this practice has not been shown to "shrink" the existing follicular cyst, it may suppress the development of a new cyst and permit resolution of the existing problem. If the cyst persists despite expectant management, another type of cyst or neoplasm should be suspected and further evaluated by imaging studies and/or surgery.

On occasion, rupture of a follicular cyst may cause acute pelvic pain. Because release of follicular fluid into the peritoneum produces only transient symptoms, surgical intervention is rarely necessary.

*A **corpus luteum cyst** is the other common type of functional ovarian cyst, designated a cyst rather than simply a corpus luteum when its diameter exceeds about 3 cm.* It is related to the postovulatory (i.e., progesterone-dominant) phase of the menstrual cycle. Two variations of corpus luteum cysts are encountered. The first is a slightly enlarged corpus luteum, which may continue to produce progesterone for longer than the usual 14 days. Menstruation is delayed from a few days to several weeks, although it usually occurs within 2 weeks of the missed period. Persistent corpus luteum cysts are often associated with dull lower-quadrant pain. This pain and a missed menstrual period are the most common complaints associated with persistent corpus luteum cysts. Pelvic examination usually discloses an enlarged, tender, cystic, or solid adnexal mass. Because of the triad of missed menstrual period, unilateral lower-quadrant pain, and adnexal enlargement, ectopic pregnancy is often considered in the differential diagnosis. A negative pregnancy test eliminates this possibility, whereas a positive pregnancy test mandates further evaluation regarding the location of the pregnancy. Patients with recurrent persistent corpus luteum cysts may benefit from cyclic oral contraceptive therapy.

The second less-common type of corpus luteum cyst is the rapidly enlarging **luteal-phase cyst** into which there is spontaneous hemorrhage. Sometimes called the **corpus hemorrhagicum,** this hemorrhagic corpus luteum cyst may rupture late in the luteal phase, resulting in the following clinical picture: a patient not using oral contraceptives, with regular periods, who presents with acute pain late in the luteal phase. Some patients present with evidence of hemoperitoneum as well as hypovolemia and require surgical resection of the bleeding cyst. In others, the acute pain and blood loss are self-limited. These patients may be managed with mild analgesics and reassurance. Patients at risk for repetitive hemorrhagic corpus luteum cysts include those who are taking anticoagulation medication and those who have inherent bleeding disorders. This process may be the hallmark to initiate an investigation for an inherent bleeding disorder.

The least common functional cyst is the **theca lutein cyst,** associated with pregnancy and usually bilateral. They are more common in multiple gestations, trophoblastic disease, and also with ovulation induction with clomiphene and human menopausal gonadotropin/human chorionic gonadotropin (hCG). They may become large and are multicystic, but also regress spontaneously in most cases without intervention.

## BENIGN OVARIAN NEOPLASMS

*Although most ovarian enlargements in the reproductive-age group are functional cysts, about 25% prove to be **nonfunctional ovarian neoplasms.*** In the reproductive-age group, 90% of these neoplasms are benign, whereas the risk of malignancy rises to approximately 25% when postmenopausal patients are also included. Thus, ovarian masses in older patients and in reproductive patients who show no response to oral contraceptive treatment are of special concern. Unfortunately, unless the mass is particularly large or becomes symptomatic, these masses may remain undetected for some time. Many ovarian neoplasms are first discovered at the time of routine pelvic examination.

Ovarian neoplasms are usually categorized by the cell type of origin:

* **Epithelial cell tumors,** the largest class of ovarian neoplasm
* **Germ cell tumors,** which include the most common ovarian neoplasm in reproductive-age women, the benign cystic teratoma or dermoid
* **Stromal cell tumors**

The classification of ovarian tumors by cell line of origin is presented in Box 46.1.

### Benign Epithelial Cell Neoplasms

*The exact cell source for the development of **epithelial cell tumors** of the ovary is unclear; however, the cells are characteristic of typical glandular epithelial cells.* Evidence exists to suggest that these cells are derived from mesothelial cells lining the peritoneal cavity. Because the müllerian duct-derived tissue becomes the female genital tract by differentiation of the mesothelium from the gonadal ridge, it is hypothesized that these tissues are also capable of differentiating into glandular tissue. The more common epithelial tumors of the ovary are grouped into serous, mucinous, and endometrioid neoplasms, as shown in Box 46.2.

The most common epithelial cell neoplasm is the **serous cystadenoma** (Fig. 46.2). Seventy percent of serous tumors are benign; approximately 10% have intraepithelial cellular characteristics, which suggest that they are of low malignant potential; and the remaining 20% are frankly malignant by both histologic criteria and clinical behavior.

Treatment of serous tumors is surgical, because of the relatively high rate of malignancy. In the younger patient with smaller tumors, an attempt can be made to perform an ovarian cystectomy to try to minimize the amount of ovarian tissue removed. For large, unilateral serous tumors in

---

**BOX 46.1**

### Histologic Classification of All Ovarian Neoplasms

From coelomic epithelium (epithelial)
  Serous
  Mucinous
  Endometrioid
  Brenner
From gonadal stroma
  Granulosa theca
  Sertoli–Leydig (arrhenoblastoma)
  Lipid cell fibroma
From germ cell
  Dysgerminoma
  Teratoma
  Endodermal sinus (yolk sac)
  Choriocarcinoma
Miscellaneous cell line sources
  Lymphoma
  Sarcoma
  Metastatic
    Colorectal
    Breast
    Endometrial

young patients, unilateral oophorectomy with preservation of the contralateral ovary is indicated to maintain fertility. In patients past reproductive age, bilateral oophorectomy along with hysterectomy may be indicated, not only because of the chance of future malignancy, but because of the increased risk of a similar occurrence in the contralateral ovary.

The **mucinous cystadenoma** is the second most common epithelial cell tumor of the ovary. The malignancy rate of 15% is lower than that for serous tumors. These cystic tumors can become large, sometimes filling the entire pelvis and extending into the abdominal cavity

(Fig. 46.3). Ultrasound assessment will often reveal multilocular septations. Surgery is the treatment of choice.

A third type of benign epithelial neoplasm is the **endometrioid tumor.** Most benign endometrioid tumors take the form of endometriomas, which are cysts lined by well-differentiated, endometrial-like glandular tissue. For further discussion of this neoplasm, see "Malignant Ovarian Neoplasms," later in the chapter.

The **Brenner cell tumor** is an uncommon benign epithelial cell tumor of the ovary. This tumor is usually described as a solid ovarian tumor because of the large amount of stroma and fibrotic tissue that surrounds the epithelial cells. It is more common in older women, and occasionally occurs in association with mucinous tumors of the ovary. When discovered as an isolated tumor of the ovary, it is relatively small compared with the large size often attained by the serous and especially by the mucinous cystadenomas. It is rarely malignant.

## Benign Germ Cell Neoplasms

*Germ cell tumors are derived from the primary germ cells.* The tumors arise in the ovary and may contain relatively differentiated structures, such as hair or bone. The most common tumor found in women of all ages is the **benign cystic teratoma,** also called a **dermoid cyst** or **dermoid** (Fig. 46.4). Eighty percent occur during the reproductive years, with a median age of occurrence of 30 years. However, in children and adolescents, mature cystic teratomas account for about one-half of benign ovarian neoplasms. Dermoids may contain differentiated tissue from all three embryonic germ layers (ectoderm, mesoderm, and endoderm). The most common elements found are of ectodermal origin, primarily squamous cell tissue such as skin appendages (sweat, sebaceous glands) with associated hair follicles and sebum. It is because of this predominance of dermoid derivatives that the term "dermoid" is used. Other constituents of dermoids include central nervous system tissue, cartilage, bone, teeth, and intestinal glandular elements, most of which are found in well-differentiated form. One unusual variant is the struma ovarii, in which functioning thyroid tissue is found.

A dermoid cyst is frequently encountered as an asymptomatic, unilateral cystic adnexal mass that is mobile and

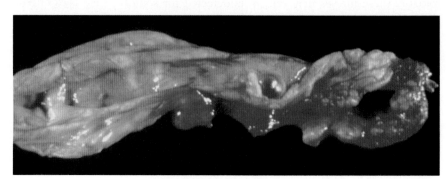

FIGURE 46.2. Serous cystadenoma of the ovary. This unilocular cyst has a smooth lining, microscopically resembling the fallopian tube epithelium. (Berek JS, Hacker NH. *Practical Gynecologic Oncology.* 4th ed. Philadelphia, PA: Lippincott Williams & Wilkins; 2005: Fig. 6.51.)

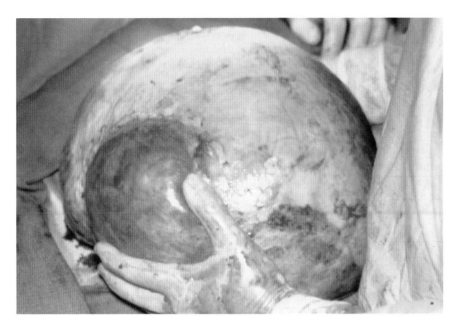

FIGURE 46.3. Mucinous cystadenoma. This cyst is extremely large and fills the entire pelvic cavity. (Berek JS, Hacker NH. *Practical Gynecologic Oncology*. 4th ed. Philadelphia, PA: Lippincott Williams & Wilkins; 2005: Fig. 6.55.)

nontender. This tumor often has a high fat content that makes it more readily identified by computer tomography (CT) evaluation, as well as giving it a more buoyant tendency in the pelvis, resulting in a relatively high rate of ovarian torsion (15%), in comparison with other types of neoplasms.

Treatment of benign cystic teratomas is necessarily surgical, even though the rate of malignancy is <1%. Surgical removal is required because of the possibility of ovarian torsion and rupture, resulting in intense chemical peritonitis and a potential surgical emergency. Between 10% and 20% of these cysts are bilateral, underscoring the need for examination of the contralateral ovary at the time of surgery.

## Benign Stromal Cell Neoplasms

*Stromal cell tumors of the ovary are usually considered solid tumors and are derived from specialized sex cord stroma of the developing gonad.* These tumors may develop along a primarily female cell type into **granulosa theca cell tumors,** or into a primarily male gonadal type of tissue, known as **Sertoli–Leydig cell tumors.** Both of these tumors are referred to as functioning tumors because of their hormone production. *Granulosa theca cell tumors primarily produce estrogenic components and may be manifest in patients through feminizing characteristics, and Sertoli–Leydig cell tumors produce androgenic components, which may contribute to hirsutism or virilizing symptoms.* These neoplasms occur with approximately

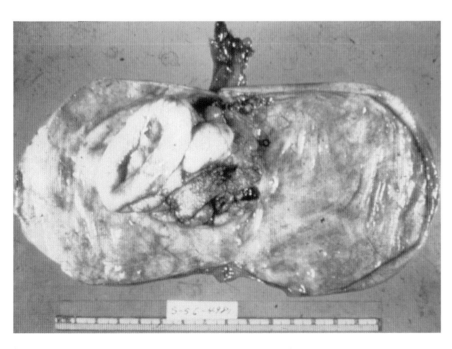

FIGURE 46.4. Dermoid cyst. This cyst contains hair and sebaceous material. The solid white area represents mature cartilage. (Berek JS, Hacker NH. *Practical Gynecologic Oncology*. 4th ed. Philadelphia, PA: Lippincott Williams & Wilkins; 2005: Fig. 5.64.)

equal frequency in all age groups, including pediatric patients. When the granulosa cell tumor occurs in the pediatric age group, it may contribute to signs and symptoms of precocious puberty, including precocious thelarche and vaginal bleeding. Vaginal bleeding may also occur when this tumor develops in the postmenopausal years. Both the granulosa cell tumor and the Sertoli–Leydig cell tumor have malignant potential, as discussed later.

The **ovarian fibroma** is the result of collagen production by spindle cells. These tumors account for 4% of ovarian tumors and are most common during middle age. It is unlike other stromal cell tumors in that it does not secrete sex steroids. It is usually a small, solid tumor with a smooth surface and occasionally is clinically misleading because ascites are present. The combination of benign ovarian fibroma coupled with ascites and right pleural effusion has historically been referred to as **Meigs syndrome.**

The following are the key points that can be made regarding benign ovarian neoplasms:

- They are more common than malignant tumors of the ovary in all age groups.
- The risk for malignant transformation increases with increasing age.
- They warrant surgical treatment because of their potential for malignancy or torsion.
- Preoperative assessment may be assisted by the use of pelvic imaging techniques such as ultrasound.
- Surgical treatment may be conservative for benign tumors, especially if future reproduction is desired.

## MALIGNANT OVARIAN NEOPLASMS

*Ovarian cancer is the fifth most common of all cancers in women in the United States and the most common cause of gynecologic cancer. The mortality rate of this disease is the highest of all the gynecologic malignancies,* primarily because of the difficulty in detecting the disease before widespread dissemination. Of the estimated 25,000 new cases of ovarian cancer yearly, approximately 60% will die within 5 years. Sixty-five to seventy percent are diagnosed at an advanced state when the 5-year survival rate is 20–30%.

## Risk Factors and Early Symptoms

*Ovarian cancer presents most commonly in the fifth and sixth decades of life.* The incidence of ovarian cancer in Western European countries and in the United States is higher, with a five- to sevenfold greater incidence than age-matched populations in East Asia. Whites are 50% more likely to develop ovarian cancer than blacks living in the United States.

Symptoms of ovarian cancer are often confused with benign conditions or interpreted as part of the aging process, with the final diagnosis often delayed.

*The most common symptoms in order from highest percentage to lowest are abdominal fullness or distension, abdominal or back pain, decreased energy or lethargy, and urinary frequency.*

Because no clinically applicable screening test is available, approximately two-thirds of patients with ovarian cancer have advanced disease at the time of diagnosis.

*The risk of a woman developing ovarian cancer during her lifetime is approximately 1 in 70.* The risk increases with age until approximately age 70. In addition to age, the epidemiologic factors associated with development of ovarian cancer include nulliparity, primary infertility, and endometriosis. Approximately 8% to 13% of cases of ovarian cancer are caused by inherited mutations in the cancer-susceptibility genes *BRCA-1* and *BRCA-2*. Additionally, women affected with hereditary nonpolyposis colorectal cancer (HNPCC; formerly called Lynch syndrome) have approximately a 13-fold greater risk of developing ovarian cancer than the general population.

*Long-term suppression of ovulation may protect against the development of ovarian cancer,* at least for epithelial cell tumors. It has been suggested that so-called incessant ovulation may predispose to neoplastic transformation of the epithelial cell surfaces of the ovary. Oral contraceptives that prevent ovulation appear to provide significant protection against the occurrence of ovarian cancer. Five years' cumulative use of oral contraceptives decreases the lifetime risk by one-half. No evidence exists to implicate the use of postmenopausal hormone replacement therapy in the development of ovarian cancer.

## Pathogenesis and Diagnosis

*Malignant ovarian epithelial cell tumors spread primarily by direct extension within the peritoneal cavity as a result of direct cell sloughing from the ovarian surface.* This process explains widespread peritoneal dissemination at the time of diagnosis, even with relatively small primary ovarian lesions. Although epithelial cell ovarian cancers also spread by lymphatic and blood-borne routes, their direct extension into the virtually unlimited space of the peritoneal cavity is the primary basis for their late clinical presentation.

Currently, it appears that the best way to detect early ovarian cancer is for both the patient and her clinician to be aware of early warning signs (Box 46.3). These signs should not be ignored in postmenopausal women (median age, approximately 60 years).

*The early diagnosis of ovarian cancer is made even more difficult by the lack of effective screening tests.* CA-125 should not be routinely used to screen for ovarian cancer, but, instead, should be used to follow response to therapy and evaluate for recurrent disease. CA-125 can also be used to evaluate the presence of ovarian cancer in selected cases:

## BOX 46.3
### Early Warning Signs of Ovarian Cancer

Increase in abdominal size
Abdominal bloating
Fatigue
Abdominal pain
Indigestion
Inability to eat normally
Urinary frequency
Constipation
Back pain
Urinary incontinence of recent onset
Unexplained weight loss

- In premenopausal women with symptoms, a CA-125 measurement has not been shown to be useful in most circumstances, because elevated levels of CA-125 are associated with a variety of common benign conditions, including uterine leiomyomata, pelvic inflammatory disease, endometriosis, adenomyosis, pregnancy, and even menstruation.
- In postmenopausal women with a pelvic mass, a CA-125 measurement may be helpful in predicting a higher likelihood of a malignant tumor than a benign tumor. However, a normal CA-125 measurement alone does not rule out ovarian cancer, because up to 50% of early-stage cancers and 20% to 25% of advanced cancers are associated with normal values.

### HISTOLOGIC CLASSIFICATION

*The cell type of origin, similar to their benign counterparts, usually categorizes malignant ovarian neoplasms:* **malignant epithelial cell tumors,** which are the most common type; malignant **germ cell tumors;** and malignant **stromal cell tumors** (see Box 46.1). Most malignant ovarian tumors have histologically similar but benign counterparts. The relationship between a benign ovarian neoplasm and its malignant counterpart is clinically important. If the benign counterpart is found in a patient, removal of both ovaries is considered, because there is a possibility of future malignant transformation in the remaining ovary. The decision regarding removal of one or both ovaries, however, must be individualized based on age, type of tumor, desire for future fertility, genetic predisposition for malignancy, and the patient's concern regarding future risks.

### STAGING

The staging of ovarian carcinoma is based on extent of spread of tumor and histologic evaluation of the tumor. The International Federation of Gynecology and Obste-

trics (FIGO) classification of ovarian cancer is presented in Table 46.1.

### Borderline Ovarian Tumors

*Approximately 10% of seemingly benign epithelial cell tumors may contain histologic evidence of intraepithelial neoplasia, commonly referred to as borderline malignancies, or "tumors of low malignant potential."* These tumors generally remain confined to the ovary, are more common in premenopausal women (30 to 50 years of age), and have good prognoses. About 20% of such tumors show spread beyond the ovary. They require carefully individualized therapy following the initial surgical resection of the primary tumor. If frozen section pathology demonstrates borderline histology, unilateral oophorectomy with a staging procedure and follow-up is appropriate, assuming the woman wishes to retain ovarian function and/or fertility and understands the risks of such conservative management.

### Epithelial Cell Ovarian Carcinoma

*Approximately 90% of all ovarian malignancies are of the epithelial cell type, derived from mesothelial cells.* The ovary contains these cells as part of an ovarian capsule just overlying the actual stroma of the ovary. When these mesothelial cell elements are situated over developing follicles, they go through metaplastic transformation whenever ovulation occurs. Repeated ovulation is, therefore, associated with the histologic change in these cells derived from coelomic epithelium.

**Malignant epithelial serous tumors** (serous cystadenocarcinoma) are the most common malignant epithelial cell tumors. Approximately 50% of these cancers are thought to be derived from their benign precursors (serous cystadenoma), and as many as 30% of these tumors are bilateral at the time of clinical presentation. They are typically multiloculated and often have external excrescences on an otherwise smooth capsular surface. Calcified, laminated structures, **psammoma bodies,** are found in more than one-half of serous carcinomas.

Another epithelial cell variant that contains cells reminiscent of endocervical glandular mucous-secreting cells is the **malignant mucinous epithelial tumor (mucinous cystadenocarcinoma).** They make up approximately one-third of all epithelial tumors, the majority of which are benign or of low malignant potential; only 5% are cancerous. These tumors have a lower rate of bilaterality and can be among the largest of ovarian tumors, often measuring more than 20 cm. They may be associated with widespread peritoneal extension with thick, mucinous ascites, termed **pseudomyxomatous peritonei.**

Although most epithelial carcinomas occur sporadically, a small percentage (5% to 10%) occurs in familial or hereditary patterns involving first- or second-degree

| TABLE 46.1 | International Federation of Gynecology and Obstetrics (FIGO) Staging for Primary Carcinoma of the Ovary |
|---|---|
| **Stage** | **Description** |
| I | Growth limited to the ovaries |
| Ia | Growth limited to one ovary; no ascites containing malignant cells; no tumor on the external surface; capsule intact |
| Ib | Growth limited to both ovaries; no ascites containing malignant cells; no tumor on the external surface; capsule intact |
| Ic | Tumor either stage Ia or Ib but with tumor on the surface of one or both ovaries; or with capsule ruptured, or with ascites present containing malignant cells, or with positive peritoneal washings |
| II | Growth involving one or both ovaries with pelvic extension |
| IIa | Extension and/or metastases to the uterus and/or tubes |
| IIb | Extension to other pelvic tissues |
| IIc | Tumor either stage IIa or IIb but with tumor on the surface of one or both ovaries; or with capsule(s) ruptured, or with ascites present containing malignant cells, or with positive peritoneal washings |
| III | Tumor involving one or both ovaries with peritoneal implants outside the pelvis and/or positive retroperitoneal or inguinal nodes; superficial liver metastasis equals stage III; tumor is limited to the true pelvis, but histologically proven malignant extension is to small bowel or omentum |
| IIIa | Tumor grossly limited to the true pelvis with negative nodes but with histologically confirmed microscopic seeding of abdominal peritoneal surfaces |
| IIIb | Tumor of one or both ovaries with histologically confirmed implants of abdominal peritoneal surface; none exceeding 2 cm wide; nodes negative |
| IIIc | Abdominal implants 2 cm wide and/or positive retroperitoneal or inguinal nodes |
| IV | Growth involving one or both ovaries with distant metastasis; if pleural effusion is present, positive cytologic test results must deem a case stage IV; parenchymal liver metastasis equals stage IV |

Heintz Ap, Odicino F, Maisonneuave P, Wuinn MA, Benedet JL, Creasman WT, et al. Carcinoma of the ovary: International Federation of Gynecology and Obstetrics (FIGO) annual report on the results of treatment in gynecological cancer. *Int J Gynec Obstetr.* 2006;95(Supplement):S161–S192.

relatives with a history of epithelial ovarian cancer. Having a first-degree relative (i.e., mother, sister, daughter) with an epithelial carcinoma gives a 5% lifetime risk for ovarian cancer, whereas having two first-degree relatives increases this risk to 20% to 30%. Such hereditary ovarian cancers generally occur earlier than nonhereditary tumors.

Women with **breast/ovarian familial cancer syndrome,** a combination of epithelial ovarian and breast cancers in first- and second-degree family members, are at two to three times the risk of these cancers as the general population. Women with this syndrome have an increased risk of bilaterality of breast cancer and developing ovarian tumors at a younger age. This syndrome has been associated with the *BRCA-1* gene. Women with this gene mutation have a cumulative lifetime risk of 85% to 90% for breast cancer and 50% for ovarian cancer. Women of Ashkenazi Jewish ancestry have a 1% chance of carrying this gene, a 10-fold risk over the general population.

**HNPCC** occurs in families with first- and second-degree members with combinations of colon, ovarian, endometrial, and breast cancers. Women in families with this syndrome may have a threefold increased risk of cancer over the general population. Women in families with these syndromes should have more frequent screening tests and may benefit from risk-reducing salpingo-oophorectomy.

## ENDOMETRIOID TUMORS

Most **endometrioid tumors** are malignant. These tumors contain histologic features similar to those of endometrial carcinoma, and are commonly found in association with endometriosis or are coincident with endometrial cancer of the uterus.

## OTHER EPITHELIAL CELL OVARIAN CARCINOMAS

Of the remaining epithelial cell carcinomas of the ovary, clear cell carcinomas are thought to arise from mesonephric elements, and Brenner tumors are thought to arise rarely from their benign counterpart. Brenner tumors may occur in the same ovary that contains mucinous cystadenoma; the reason for this is unclear.

## Germ Cell Tumors

*Germ cell tumors are the most common ovarian cancers in women younger than 20 years of age.* Germ cell tumors may be functional, producing hCG or α-fetoprotein (AFP), both of which can be used as tumor markers. The most common germ cell malignancies are dysgerminoma and immature teratoma. Other tumors are recognized as mixed germ cell tumors, endodermal sinus tumors, and embryonal tumors. Improved chemotherapeutic and radiation protocols have resulted in greatly improved 5-year survival rates.

*Dysgerminomas* *are usually unilateral and are the most common type of germ cell tumor seen in patients with gonadal dysgenesis* (Fig. 46.5). These tumors often arise in benign counterparts, called the gonadoblastoma. The tumors are particularly radiosensitive and chemosensitive.

Because of the young age of patients with dysgerminomas, removing only the involved ovary while preserving the uterus and contralateral tube and ovary may be considered if the tumor is less than approximately 10 cm and if no evidence of extraovarian spread is found. Unlike the epithelial cell tumors, these malignancies are more likely to spread by lymphatic channels, and therefore the pelvic and periaortic lymph nodes must be sampled at the time of surgery. If disease has spread outside the ovaries, conventional hysterectomy and bilateral salpingo-oophorectomy are necessary, usually followed by cisplatin-based chemotherapy that is used in combination with bleomycin and etoposide. The prognosis of these tumors is generally excellent. The overall 5-year survival rate for patients with dysgerminoma is 90% to 95% when the disease is limited to one ovary.

**Immature teratomas** are the malignant counterpart of benign cystic teratomas (dermoids). *These tumors are the second most common germ cell cancer and are most often found in women younger than 25 years of age.* They are usually unilateral, although on occasion a benign counterpart may be found in the contralateral ovary. Because these tumors are rapidly growing, they may produce painful symptomatology relatively early, due to hemorrhage and necrosis. The disease is therefore diagnosed when it is limited to one ovary in two-thirds of patients. As with dysgerminoma, if an immature teratoma is limited to one ovary, unilateral oophorectomy is sufficient. Treatment with chemotherapeutic agents provides a good prognosis.

## Rare Germ Cell Tumors

**Endodermal sinus tumors** and **embryonal cell carcinomas** are uncommon malignant ovarian tumors that have had a remarkable improvement in cure rate. Until about 10 years ago, these tumors were almost uniformly fatal. New chemotherapeutic protocols have resulted in an overall 5-year survival rate of more than 60%. These tumors typically occur in childhood and adolescence, with the primary treatment being surgical resection of the involved ovary followed by combination chemotherapy. The endodermal sinus tumor produces AFP, whereas the embryonal cell carcinoma produces both AFP and β-hCG.

## Gonadal Stromal Cell Tumors

The gonadal stromal cell tumors make up an unusual group of tumors characterized by hormone production; hence, these tumors are called **functioning tumors.** The hormonal output from these tumors is usually in the form of female or male sex steroids, or on occasion, adrenal steroid hormones.

The **granulosa cell tumor** is the most common in this group. These tumors occur in all ages, although in older patients they are more likely to be benign. *Granulosa cell tumors may secrete large amounts of estrogen, which in some older women may cause endometrial hyperplasia or endometrial carcinoma.* Thus, endometrial sampling is especially important when ovarian tumors such as the granulosa tumor are estrogen-producing. Surgical treatment should include removal of the uterus and both ovaries in postmenopausal women as well as in women of reproductive age who no longer wish to remain fertile. In a young woman with the lesion limited to one ovary with an intact capsule, unilateral oophorectomy with careful surgical staging may be adequate. This tumor may demonstrate recurrences up to

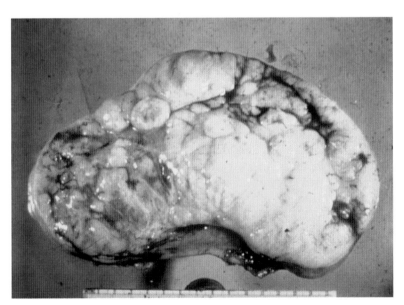

FIGURE 46.5. Dysgerminoma. This solid tumor has a gray, fleshy, and lobulated cut surface. (Berek JS, Hacker NH. *Practical Gynecologic Oncology.* 4th ed. Philadelphia, PA: Lippincott Williams & Wilkins; 2005: Fig. 5.62.)

10 years later. This is especially true with large tumors, which have a 20% to 30% chance of late recurrence.

*Sertoli–Leydig cell tumors (arrhenoblastoma) are the rare, testosterone-secreting counterparts to granulosa cell tumors.* They usually occur in older patients and should be suspected in the differential diagnosis of perimenopausal or postmenopausal patients with hirsutism or virilization and an adnexal mass. Treatment of these tumors is similar to that for other ovarian malignancies in this age group, and is based on extirpation of uterus and ovaries.

Other stromal cell tumors include **fibromas** and **thecomas,** which rarely demonstrate malignant potential, and their malignant counterparts, the **fibrosarcoma** and **malignant thecoma.**

### Other Ovarian Cancers

Rarely, the ovary may be the site of initial manifestation of lymphoma. These tumors are usually found in association with lymphoma elsewhere, although cases have been reported of primary ovarian lymphoma. Once diagnosed, their management is similar to that for lymphoma of other origin.

**Malignant mesodermal sarcomas** (carcinosarcomas) are another rare type of ovarian tumor that usually show aggressive behavior and are diagnosed at late stages. The survival rate is poor, and clinical experience with these tumors is limited.

### Cancer Metastatic to the Ovary

Classically, the term **Krukenberg tumor** describes an ovarian tumor that is metastatic from other sites such as the gastrointestinal tract and breast. Between 5% and 10% of women thought to have a primary ovarian malignancy ultimately will receive the diagnosis of a nongenital tract malignancy. Most of these tumors are characterized as infiltrative, mucinous carcinoma of predominantly signet-ring cell type and as bilateral and associated with widespread metastatic disease. On occasion, these tumors are associated with abnormal uterine bleeding or virilization, leading to the supposition that some may produce estrogens or androgens. Breast cancer metastatic to the ovary is common, with autopsy data suggesting ovarian metastasis in one quarter of cases.

In approximately 10% of patients with cancer metastatic to the ovary, an extraovarian primary site cannot be demonstrated. In this regard, it is important to consider ovarian preservation versus prophylactic oophorectomy at the time of hysterectomy in patients who have a strong family history (first-degree relatives) of epithelial ovarian cancer, primary gastrointestinal tract cancer, or breast cancer. In patients previously treated for breast or gastrointestinal cancer, consideration should be given to the incidental removal of the ovaries at the time of hysterectomy, because

these patients have a high predilection for development of ovarian cancer. The prognosis for most patients with carcinoma metastatic to the ovary is generally poor.

## FALLOPIAN TUBE DISEASE

*Normal fallopian tubes cannot be palpated and usually are not considered in the differential diagnosis of adnexal disease in the asymptomatic patient.* Common problems involving the fallopian tubes include ectopic pregnancy, salpingitis/hydrosalpinx/ tubo-ovarian abscess, and endometriosis (which can present as masses or be symptomatic). These conditions are discussed in other chapters.

### Benign Disease of the Fallopian Tube and Mesosalpinx

**Paraovarian cysts** develop in the mesosalpinx from vestigial Wolffian duct structures, tubal epithelium, and peritoneum inclusions. These are differentiated from paratubal cysts, which are found near the fimbriated end of the fallopian tube, are common, and are called **hydatid cysts of Morgagni.** Both are usually small and symptomatic, although, rarely, they can reach large proportions.

### Carcinoma of the Fallopian Tube

**Primary fallopian tube carcinoma** is usually an adenocarcinoma, although other cell types, including adenosquamous carcinoma and sarcoma, are rarely reported. About two-thirds of patients with this rare gynecologic cancer (<1% of gynecologic cancers) are postmenopausal. Grossly, these tumors are often rather large, resembling a hydrosalpinx, and unilateral. Microscopically, most are typical papillary serous cystadenocarcinomas of the ovary. The symptoms of this tumor are so slight that the tumor is often advanced before a problem is recognized. The most common complaint associated with fallopian tube carcinoma is postmenopausal bleeding, followed by abnormal vaginal discharge. Profuse serosanguineous discharge, called **hydrotubae profluens,** is sometimes considered diagnostic of this tumor; however, other findings are watery vaginal discharge, pain, and pelvic mass. Staging is surgical, similar to that for ovarian carcinoma (Table 46.2); progression is similar to that of ovarian carcinoma, with intraperitoneal metastases and ascites. Because the fallopian tubes are richly permeated with lymphatic channels, para-aortic and pelvic lymph node spread often occurs. Seventy percent of fallopian tube cancers present as stage I or II disease. The overall 5-year survival rate is 35% to 45%, with stage I having the most favorable rate. Too few data are available to ascertain whether adjunctive therapy is useful, and this management must be made on a case-by-case basis; however, initial management with staging and debulking is the same as for ovarian cancer treatment.

| TABLE 46.2 | International Federation of Gynecology and Obstetrics (FIGO) Staging for Primary Tubal Carcinoma |
|---|---|

| Stage | Description |
|---|---|
| 0 | Carcinoma in situ (limited to tubal mucosa) |
| I | Growth limited to the fallopian tubes |
| IA | Growth limited to one tube, with extension into the submucosa, or muscularis, or both but not penetrating the serosal surface; no ascites |
| IB | Growth limited to both tubes, with extension into the submucosa, or muscularis, or both but not penetrating the serosal surface; no ascites |
| IC | Tumor either stage IA or IB but with tumor extension through or onto tubal serosa, or with ascites present containing malignant cells, or with positive peritoneal washings |
| II | Growth involving one or both fallopian tubes with pelvic extension |
| IIA | Extension, or metastasis, or both to the uterus, or ovaries, or both |
| IIB | Extension to other pelvic tissues |
| IIC | Tumor either stage IIA or IIB and with ascites present containing malignant cells or with positive peritoneal washings |
| III | Tumor involves one or both fallopian tubes, with peritoneal implants outside the pelvis, or positive retroperitoneal nodes, or inguinal nodes, or all; superficial liver metastases equals stage III; tumor appears limited to the true pelvis, but with histologically proven malignant extension to the small bowel or omentum |
| IIIA | Tumor grossly limited to the true pelvis, with negative nodes, but with histologically confirmed microscopic seeding of abdominal peritoneal surfaces |
| IIIB | Tumor involving one or both tubes, with histologically confirmed implants of abdominal peritoneal surfaces, none exceeding 2 cm in diameter; lymph nodes are negative |
| IIIC | Abdominal implants greater than 2 cm in diameter, or positive retroperitoneal nodes, or inguinal nodes, or all |
| IV | Growth involving one or both fallopian tubes with distant metastases; if pleural effusion is present, there must be positive cytologic findings to be stage IV; parenchymal liver metastases equals stage IV |

Heintz Ap, Odicino F, Maisonneuave P, Wuinn MA, Benedet JL, Creasman WT, et al. Carcinoma of the ovary: International Federation of Gynecology and Obstetrics (FIGO) annual report on the results of treatment in gynecological cancer. *Int J Gynec Obstetr.* 2006; 95(Supplement):S145–160.

**Carcinoma metastatic to the fallopian tube,** coming mainly from the uterus and ovary, is far more common than primary fallopian tube carcinoma. Other rare tumors of the fallopian tube include malignant mixed müllerian tumors, primary choriocarcinoma, fibroma, and adenomatoid tumors.

## SURGICAL MANAGEMENT OF OVARIAN AND FALLOPIAN TUBE CANCERS

Primary surgical therapy is indicated in most of the ovarian malignancies, using the principle of **cytoreductive surgery, or "tumor debulking."** The rationale for cytoreductive surgery is that adjunctive radiation therapy and chemotherapy are more effective when all tumor masses are reduced to less than 1 cm in size (see Chapter 41, Gestational Trophoblastic Neoplasia). Because direct peritoneal seeding is the primary method of intraperitoneal spread, multiple adjacent structures commonly contain tumor, resulting in cytoreductive procedures that are often extensive. Each procedure includes the following:

1. Peritoneal cytology is obtained on entering the abdomen to assess microscopic spread of tumor. Gross ascites is aspirated and submitted for cytologic analysis or, if no ascites are found, saline irrigation is used to "wash" the peritoneal cavity in an attempt to find microscopic disease.
2. Inspection and palpation of the entire peritoneal cavity is done to determine the extent of disease. This includes the pelvis, pericolic gutters, omentum, and upper abdomen, including the liver, spleen, and undersurface of the diaphragm.
3. Partial omentectomy is usually performed, whether or not tumor involvement is evident.
4. Sampling of the pelvic and periaortic lymph nodes is performed. Without gross disease, biopsies are obtained from the anterior and posterior cul-de-sac, right and left pelvic sidewalls, right and left pericolic gutters, and diaphragm.

Because most ovarian cancer presents at an advanced stage, adjunctive treatment using chemotherapy is usually necessary. First-line chemotherapy is with **paclitaxel (Taxol)** combined with **carboplatin.**

With recurrence of disease, other chemotherapeutic agents may be used, including ifosfamide, hexamethylmelamine, doxorubicin, topotecan, gemcitabine, etoposide, vinorelbine, and tamoxifen. **Radiation therapy** has only a limited role in the management of ovarian cancer.

**Follow-up** consists of clinical history and examination, various imaging studies (ultrasound and/or CT), and in epithelial cell tumors, the use of serum tumor markers such as CA-125.

## SUGGESTED READINGS

American College of Obstetricians and Gynecologists. *Guidelines for Women's Health Care: A Resource Manual.* 3rd ed. Washington, D.C.: ACOG; 2007.

American College of Obstetricians and Gynecologists. Management of endometrial cancer. ACOG Practice Bulletin No. 65. *Obstet Gynecol.* 2005;106(2):413–425.

American College of Obstetricians and Gynecologists. Management of adnexal masses. ACOG Practice Bulletin No. 83. *Obstet Gynecol.* 200;110(1):201–214.

American College of Obstetricians and Gynecologists. Medical management of endometriosis. ACOG Practice Bulletin No. 11. *Obstet Gynecol.* 1999;94(6):1–14.

American College of Obstetricians and Gynecologists. The role of the generalist obstetrician–gynecologist in the early detection of ovarian cancer. ACOG Committee Opinion No. 280. *Obstet Gynecol.* 2002;100(6):1413–1416.

American College of Obstetricians and Gynecologists. *Precis: Gynecology.* 3rd ed. Washington, DC: American College of Obstetricians and Gynecologists; 2006:113–116.

# 47 Human Sexuality

**Topic 57:** Sexuality and Modes of Sexual Expression

Students should be able to describe the female human sexual response and its variability and explain how emotional, societal, and physiologic influences affect sexuality during various stages in the female life cycle. Students should also be able to describe both the traditional model and the intimacy-based model of human female sexual response and some patterns of sexual dysfunction. Students should be aware that there are diverse sexual behavior patterns, including heterosexual, homosexual, bisexual, and transgender lifestyles. They should be able to demonstrate awareness of the influence of the physician's behaviors and attitudes on interactions with patients and to describe appropriate physician behavior.

An estimated 35% to 45% of women perceive they have some type of sexual problem—most commonly low sexual desire. Illness, medical and surgical treatment, lack of knowledge to manage this life experience, and emotional and physical stresses contribute to the frequency and severity of sexual problems. Physicians should be able to identify sexual disorders and know whether to offer treatment or refer patients to a specialist.

Determinants of healthy sexuality are complex and multifactorial. Intrapersonal factors include the sense of one's self as a sexual being, one's overall health status, a general perception of well-being, and the quality of an individual's previous sexual experiences. For partnered individuals, this same list applies to the partner. Interpersonal aspects include the duration and overall quality of the relationship, communication styles, and the number and type of ongoing life events and stressors. Examples of generally "positive" life events which nevertheless can contribute to sexual dysfunctions include the birth of a child and retirement.

Sexuality involves a broad range of expressions of intimacy and is fundamental to self-identification, with strong cultural, biologic, and psychological components. The obstetrician-gynecologist has an important role in assessing sexual function, because many women view their sexuality as an important quality-of-life issue. Moreover, gynecologic disease processes and therapeutic interventions

have the potential to affect sexual response. The clinician should not make assumptions or judgments about the woman's behavior and, when counseling patients, should keep in mind the possibility of cultural and personal variation in sexual practices.

## SEXUAL IDENTITY

At the most basic level, the experience of sexuality begins with an individual's genotype and phenotype. From this basic biologic underpinning, children develop a gender identity during early childhood. Eventually, each individual develops a sense of self as a sexual being and a sexual orientation. Each of these latter components is fluid and can vary over time and with particular circumstances. For example, many individuals who consider themselves heterosexual periodically engage in sexual encounters with same-sex partners.

## HUMAN SEXUAL RESPONSE

In evaluating sexual problems, it is useful to consider the mechanisms of sexual response in women. Sexual function and dysfunction are perhaps the supreme examples of a necessary blending of mind and body. This interaction is crucial to the understanding of the assessment and management of sexual problems. The dualistic approach common to more traditional models of sexual response limits the understanding of female sexuality insofar as it suggests that dysfunction is either psychologic or biologic or psychologic plus biologic. Newer approaches are more holistic in their representations of female sexual response.

## Traditional Model

The traditional Masters and Johnson and Kaplan models of the human sexual response cycle are being replaced by intimacy-based sexual response models that take other factors into consideration. The traditional cycle depicts a linear sequence of events: desire, arousal, plateau of constant high arousal, peak intensity arousal and release (orgasm), possible repeated orgasms, and then resolution (Fig. 47.1). However, the sexual response cycle in women is complex and events do not always occur in a predictable sequence, as they usually do in men.

Neither the stimuli to which the response occurs nor the nature of the "cyclicity" is evident in the traditional model. The usefulness of this model for depicting women's sexuality is limited by the following considerations:

- Women are sexual for many reasons—sexual desire, as in sexual thinking and fantasizing, may be absent initially.
- Sexual stimuli are integral to women's sexual responses.
- The phases of women's desire and arousal overlap.
- Nongenital sensations and a number of emotions frequently overshadow genital sensations in terms of importance.
- Arousal and orgasm are not separate phenomena.
- The intensity of arousal (even if orgasm occurs) is highly variable from one occasion to another.
- Orgasm may not be necessary for satisfaction.

- The outcome of the experience strongly influences the motivation to repeat it.
- Dysfunctions may overlap (e.g., desire and arousal disorders, orgasm and arousal disorders).

## Intimacy-based Model

An alternative sexual response model depicts an intimacy-based motivation, integral sexual stimuli, and the psychological and biologic factors that govern the processing of those stimuli (i.e., determining the woman's arousability) (Fig. 47.2).

A woman's primary motivation for sexual response often is to be closer to her partner. If sexual arousal is experienced, the stimuli continue, the woman remains focused, and the sexual arousal is enjoyed, she may then sense sexual desire to continue the experience for the sake of the sexual sensations. A psychologic and physically positive outcome heightens emotional intimacy with her partner, thereby strengthening the motivation. Any spontaneous desire (i.e., sexual thinking, conscious sexual wanting, and fantasizing) may augment the intimacy-based cycle. Spontaneous desire is particularly common early in relationships or when partners have been apart, is sometimes related to the menstrual cycle, and is extremely variable among women.

## Physiology of Female Sexual Response

Systemically, the physiologic components of the female sexual response (Box 47.1) are mediated by increased activity of the autonomic nervous system and include tachycardia, skin flushing, and vaginal lubrication. Several neurotransmitters have been linked to the sexual response cycle. Norepinephrine, dopamine, oxytocin, and serotonin via

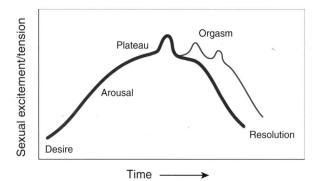

FIGURE 47.1. Traditional sexual response cycle of Masters, Johnson, and Kaplan. (From Basson R. Female sexual response: the role of drugs in the management of sexual dysfunction. *Obstet Gynecol.* 2001;98(2):350–353.)

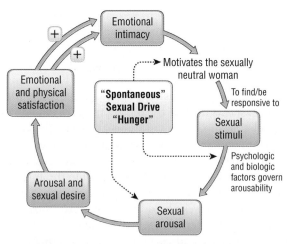

FIGURE 47.2. Negative and positive feedback loops of sexual function. (From Basson R. Female sexual response: the role of drugs in the management of sexual dysfunction. *Obstet Gynecol.* 2001;98(2):350–353.)

## BOX 47.1
### Components of Subjective Sexual Arousal in Women

- Mental sexual excitement—proportional to how exciting the woman finds the sexual stimulus and context
- Vulvar congestion—direct awareness (tingling, throbbing) is highly variable
- Pleasure from stimulating the engorging vulva
- Vaginal congestion—the woman's direct awareness is highly variable
- Pleasure from stimulating congested anterior vaginal walls and Halban's fascia
- Increased and modified lubrication—wetness usually is not directly arousing to the woman
- Vaginal nonvascular smooth muscle relaxation—the woman usually is not aware of this
- Pleasure from stimulating nongenital areas of the body
- Other somatic changes—blood pressure level, heart rate, muscle tone, respiratory rate, temperature

5-hydroxytryptamine 1A and 2C are thought to have positive sexual effects; serotonin via most other receptors, prolactin, and gamma-amino butyric acid are thought to affect the cycle negatively.

Throbbing and tingling and feelings of urgency for more genital contact and vaginal entry are far less consistent for sexually healthy women than are the equivalent sensations in men. Sexually healthy women typically experience this confirmatory sexual stimuli indirectly by the enjoyment of manual or oral stimulation or genital stimulation with a vibrator, which are enhanced when there is vulvar engorgement.

The measurement most commonly used for vaginal congestion is the vaginal pulse amplitude. The upper portion of the vagina dilates via a mechanism that is poorly understood. Figure 47.3 demonstrates some of the physiologic changes seen in sexual response phases. The duration of each phase varies with each individual and for a given individual at different times in her life, and phases also can overlap. Moreover, the state of subjective arousal is itself cognitively appraised. Women consider the appropriateness of being sexual in a particular situation and evaluate their safety. This moment-to-moment emotional and cognitive feedback modulates the experience of arousal. The value of the phases depicted, then, lies in their use in identifying the physiologic events that occur during intimate encounters leading to climax. Clinically, the provider can inquire, during the initial interview and in the course of ongoing therapy, about whether or not these responses exist.

## SEXUAL DYSFUNCTION

There is uncertainty as to what exactly constitutes a sexual disorder. The definition of "sexual disorder" is made more complex because what is considered "disordered" varies with time and culture. The World Health Organization's *International Statistical Classification of Diseases and Related Problems* (ICD-10) suggests that sexual dysfunctions are "the various ways in which an individual is unable to participate in a sexual relationship the way he or she would wish." Table 47.1 lists the categories of sexual dysfunction as recognized by both the *Diagnostic and Statistical Manual of Mental Disorders: DSM-IV-TR*, which limits its definitions to mental disorders, and the 1998 consensus committee sponsored by the American Foundation of Urological Disease, which is also limited insofar as it conceptualizes sexual response in women as discrete linear experiences, as in the formerly accepted model of female sexual response already discussed. These definitions will continue to be revised and updated to address contextual and other factors.

## FACTORS AFFECTING SEXUALITY

The relationship between an overall sense of personal well-being and sexual function is complex. Approximately one-third of women presenting with sexual dysfunction are clinically depressed. Among individuals in whom depression has already been diagnosed, the type and progress of ongoing therapy and prescribed medication should be noted.

The commonly prescribed selective serotonin-reuptake inhibitors, such as fluoxetine, paroxetine, sertraline, and escitalopram, can be associated with decreased sexual desire. The clinical observation that is helpful when evaluating the contribution of medications to female sexual dysfunction is that antidepressants that activate dopaminergic, (central) noradrenergic, and 5-hydroxytriptamine (5-HT) 1A and 5-HT2C receptors may augment sexual response, whereas those that activate other 5-HT receptors, prolactin, and gamma-amino-butyric acid reduce sexual response. The medications least likely to interfere with sexual response are nefazodone, mirtazapine, bupropion, venlafaxine, and buspirone.

Further complicating this picture is that depression itself causes a decrease in sexual desire. Other medications that can be associated with female sexual dysfunction are included in Box 47.2.

Medical conditions that affect energy and well-being may indirectly affect sexual desire and response, particularly those that are associated with the loss of estrogen and/or androgen production (Box 47.3). Estrogen is thought to have both a direct effect (by producing vulval and vaginal congestion) and an indirect effect (by influencing mood) on female sexual response. There is likewise a strong consensus that androgens are needed for sexual response in women, though the limitations of widely available laboratory assays have made it difficult to establish a direct correlation between specific androgen levels and women's sexual desire.

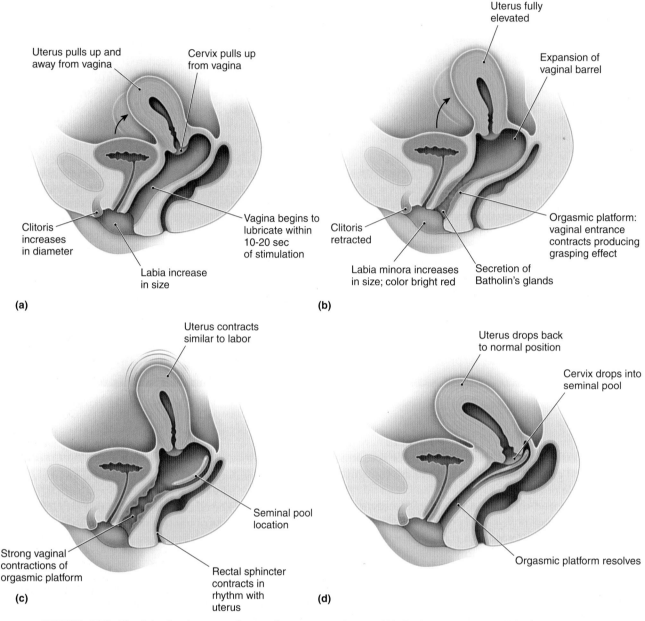

FIGURE 47.3. Physiologic changes of sexual response phases. (A) Excitement stage. (B) Plateau stage. (C) Orgasm stage. (D) Resolution stage.

Psychologic factors commonly affect sexual response in women as well (Box 47.4). These factors continuously modulate any arousal experienced from sexual stimuli and influence the woman's motivation to seek or respond to those sexual stimuli—compounding any negative effects from biologic factors.

## MANAGEMENT

A woman's sexuality is influenced by her health and emotional well-being; likewise, healthy sexual functioning promotes physical and emotional well-being. However, studies suggest that fewer than one-half of patients' sexual concerns are recognized by their physicians. The obstetrician-gynecologist has a paramount role in assessing sexual function and managing sexual dysfunction to ensure the well-being of his or her patients. Beginning with screening a patient for sexual dysfunction, taking her history, and assessing sexual dysfunction risk factors, the physician establishes a diagnosis if dysfunction is present and treats the patient or refers her for treatment, as appropriate.

### Screening for Sexual Dysfunction

Questioning patients about their sexual desire, especially about responsive desire and the components of arousal, can point to management options about which patients and

| TABLE 47.1 | Categories of Sexual Dysfunction | | |

| Disorder | Diagnostic and Statistical Manual of Mental Disorders | American Foundation of Urological Disease | Commentary |
|---|---|---|---|
| Hypoactive sexual desire disorder | Persistently or recurrently deficient (or absent) sexual fantasies and desire for sexual activity. The disturbance causes marked distress or interpersonal difficulty. | The persistent or recurrent deficiency or absence of sexual fantasies, thoughts, and/or desire for, or receptivity to sexual activity, which causes personal distress. | In addition, a caveat should be added, "Any loss of sexual thinking, fantasizing, or yearning for sex is judged to be other than the normal lessening with the relationship duration" |
| Female sexual arousal disorder | Persistent or recurrent inability to attain, or to maintain until completion of the sexual activity, an adequate lubrication-swelling response of sexual excitement. The disturbance causes marked distress or interpersonal difficulty. | The persistent or recurrent inability to attain or maintain sufficient sexual excitement, causing personal distress. This may be expressed as a lack of subjective excitement, or genital (lubrication/swelling) or other somatic responses. | It is necessary to distinguish between women with genital arousal dysfunction who are still aroused mentally by non-genital stimuli from those who are not aroused by any type of stimuli. |
| Female orgasmic disorder | Persistent or recurrent delay in, or absence of, orgasm following a normal excitement phase. The disturbance causes marked distress or interpersonal difficulty. | The persistent or recurrent difficulty, delay in, or absence of attaining orgasm following sufficient sexual stimulation arousal, which causes personal distress. | The clinical usefulness of these definitions is limited for the following reasons:<br>• Women with female orgasmic disorder often have female sexual arousal disorder.<br>• It often is the intensity of orgasm that has markedly diminished and is causing distress—especially with women who have neurologic disorders or sudden premature loss of androgen production. |
| Dyspareunia | Recurrent or persistent genital pain associated with sexual intercourse. The disturbance causes marked distress or interpersonal difficulty. | Dyspareunia is the persistent or recurrent genital pain associated with sexual intercourse. | Penile–vaginal movement of intercourse may be impossible because of the pain caused by partial or complete penile entry. |
| Vaginismus | Recurrent or persistent involuntary spasm of the musculature of the outer third of the vagina that interferes with sexual intercourse. | Vaginismus is the persistent or recurrent involuntary spasm of the musculature of the outer third of the vagina that interferes with vaginal penetration, which causes personal distress. | Muscular "spasm" has never been documented. Reflexive muscle tightening, fear of vaginal entry, and pain with its attempt are characteristic. |
| Noncoital sexual pain disorder | — | Persistent or recurrent genital pain associated with noncoital sexual stimulation. | — |

Data from American Psychiatric Association. Diagnostic and statistical manual of mental disorders: DSM-IV-TR. 4th ed. rev. Washington, DC: APA; 2000; Basson R. Are our definitions of women's desire, arousal and sexual pain disorders too broad and our definition of orgasm too narrow? *J Sex Marital Ther.* 2002;28(4):289–300; and Basson R, Berman J, Burnett A, Derogatis L, Ferguson D, Fourcroy J, Goldstein I, Graziottin A, Heiman J, Laan E, Leiblum S, Padma-Nathan H, Rosen R, Segraves K, Segraves RT, Shabsigh R, Sipski M, Wagner G, Whipple B. Report of the international consensus development conference on female sexual dysfunction: definitions and classifications. *J Urol.* 2000;163(3):888–893.

their partners can be counseled. Simply providing information, confirming that many women have the same concerns, and explaining how one aspect of dysfunction leads to another can be therapeutic.

Discussions of sexuality are accomplished best in a confidential and supportive setting. Mutual trust and respect in the patient–clinician relationship will allow appropriate discussion of questions and concerns about sexuality. A nonjudgmental and respectful approach by the clinician, as well as awareness by the clinician of his or her own biases, is essential for effective care.

Patients are more likely to develop trusting relationships with their healthcare practitioners when the issue of confidentiality has been addressed directly. A

## BOX 47.2
### Medications Commonly Affecting Sexual Response

- Codeine-containing analgesics
- Alcohol (chronic abuse)
- Cyproterone acetate
- Medroxyprogesterone (high doses)
- Some β-blockers used for hypertension or migraine prevention
- Anticonvulsants taken for epilepsy (but not necessarily for other conditions)
- Oral contraceptives
- Selective estrogen receptor modulators (such as raloxifene, tamoxifen, and phytoestrogens)

## BOX 47.4
### Psychologic Factors Commonly Affecting Sexual Response

- Past negative sexual experiences, including abuse
- Knowledge of a likely unsatisfactory or painful outcome
- Decreasing self-image (e.g., from chronic infertility)
- Potent nonsexual distractions
- Lack of physical privacy
- Feelings of shame, naiveté, or embarrassment
- Partner sexual dysfunction
- Lack of safety from pregnancy and sexually transmitted diseases
- Orientation concerns
- Fear of physical safety

## BOX 47.3
### Conditions Commonly Affecting Sexual Response

Conditions associated with loss of adrenal androgen production and/or loss of estrogen production
- Bilateral salpingo-oophorectomy
- Chemotherapy-induced menopause
- Gonadotropin–releasing hormone-induced menopausal symptoms
- Premature ovarian failure
- Oral estrogen therapy (may cause androgen insufficiency)
- Oral contraceptives (may cause androgen insufficiency)
- Addison disease
- Hypopituitary states
- Hypothalamic amenorrhea

Chronic renal failure
Chronic cardiac failure
Chronic neurologic conditions
Chronic renal disease
Arthritis
Hyperprolactinemia
Hypothyroid and hyperthyroid states
Conditions interfering with autonomic function
+/− somatic genital nerve function
- Diabetes mellitus
- Multiple sclerosis
- Spinal cord injury
- Radical pelvic surgery
- Post Guillain-Barré syndrome

confidential relationship, in turn, can facilitate the open disclosure of health histories and behaviors. The use of broad, open-ended questions in a routine history gathering can help disclose problems that require further exploration. Inquiry about the partner's sexual function and level of satisfaction may elicit more specific information and give an indication of the couple's level of communication.

The following are examples of basic questions, posed in a gender-neutral fashion:

- "Are you sexually active?"
- "Are you sexually satisfied?"
- "Do you think your partner is satisfied?"
- "Do you have questions or concerns about sexual functioning?"

The clinician should not make assumptions about the woman's choice of partner. Although most women report that their sexual partners are men, some women only have sex with other women, and others may have partners of both sexes. The use of terms such as *partner* instead of *husband* and *sexual activity* instead of *intercourse* and an understanding of nonheterosexual sexuality—including that of lesbians, bisexual women, and transgendered individuals—will assist in open communication and assessment of the patient's problem.

## History

The patient's history is the crucial part of an assessment for sexual dysfunction. The duration of the dysfunction and how long it has evolved over months or years should be clarified. Lifelong problems are particularly difficult to evaluate and manage, and a concomitant in-depth psychological assessment may be needed. The context of the patient's life when the dysfunction began is needed, addressing psychologic, biologic, and relationship factors. Her medical history and past sexual experiences are recorded, including medications and any substance abuse. The woman's developmental history also may be needed, particularly if her dysfunction is lifelong.

Deliberate inquiries should be made to assess the quality of the interpersonal relationship between the patient and her partner, including mutual satisfaction with their sexual relationship. The perceived importance of physical intimacy for a given couple depends largely on whether or not they are satisfied with that aspect of their relationship. Among couples who are not experiencing sexual dysfunctions, each partner will estimate that the sexual component of their relationship accounts for approximately 10% of their overall happiness. In couples experiencing sexual difficulties, however, the sexual aspects are estimated as accounting for approximately 60% of the overall relationship quality. This dramatic shift in perception underscores the importance that physical intimacy holds within the context of the overall relationship.

## Risk Factors

Sexual disorders often are disclosed by women during visits for routine gynecologic care. Some patients present with a complaint involving a sexual issue or of a specific sexual dysfunction. Other patients neither express a sexually related complaint nor have a medical problem with a commonly associated sexual issue. Still other patients have a medical problem or have or have had a medical or surgical therapy that is known to be associated with sexual issues or problems (Box 47.5).

In addition, sexual function may be affected by biologic and psychologic aspects of reproduction and the life cycle (Box 47.6). The mechanisms governing the interplay

---

> **BOX 47.6**
> ### Biologic and Psychologic Risk Factors for Sexual Disorders
>
> - Healthy pregnancy
> - Complicated pregnancy where intercourse and orgasm are precluded
> - Postpartum considerations
> - Recurrent miscarriage
> - Therapeutic abortion
> - Infertility
> - Perimenopause
> - Natural menopause
> - Premature menopause (idiopathic and iatrogenic)
> - Use of oral contraceptives

between psychologic responses to reproductive events and the biologic changes themselves are not well-understood. However, women's past sexual experiences, self-image, support from and attraction to their sexual partners, sufficiency of their knowledge of sexuality, and sense of control are all typically important factors.

## Establishing a Diagnosis

For all of the various dysfunctions, it is important to establish whether it is lifelong or acquired and to distinguish between dysfunctions that are situational and those that are global or generalized (Fig. 47.4). If the woman's sexual response is healthy in some circumstances, physical organic factors are not involved in a dysfunction. It is therefore important to ask patients about their sexual response with masturbation, with viewing or reading erotica, and with being with individuals other than their regular partners—even if this activity does not involve physical sexual interaction.

## Treatment

*Some sexual problems can be managed by the primary physician, whereas others are best referred to a sex therapist.* A detailed, sensitive, and respectful assessment will help establish a dialogue with the patient. It is difficult to distinguish between assessment and treatment, because the physician often provides information during the assessment that is therapeutic. Treatment may be within the scope of the obstetrician-gynecologic practice, or a referral may be appropriate, depending on the nature and the extent of the problem. Box 47.7 shows interventions that commonly occur in gynecologic offices. Largely, the decision should be based on whether or not the physician

---

> **BOX 47.5**
> ### Medical Risk Factors for Sexual Disorders
>
> - Depression, with or without antidepressants
> - Breast cancer that required chemotherapy
> - Radical hysterectomy for cancer of the cervix
> - Multiple sclerosis
> - Hypertension
> - Diabetes
> - Sexual abuse

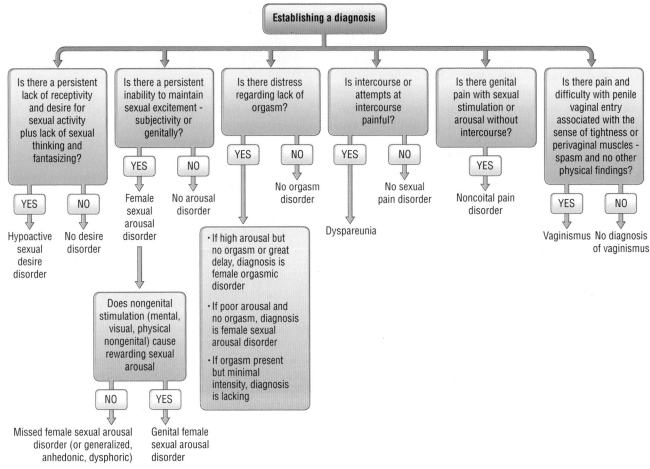

FIGURE 47.4. Algorithm for establishing a diagnosis of female sexual dysfunction. (From Basson R. *Clinical Updates in Women's Health Care: Sexuality and Sexual Disorders.* Vol. II, 2. Washington, DC: American College of Obstetricians and Gynecologists; 2003:36.)

## BOX 47.7
### Primary Care Treatments for Sexual Dysfunction

- Giving nonjudgmental and respectful information (e.g., of women's sexual response cycles)
- Normalizing nonpenetrative sex to both partners
- Screening for depression and sexual side effects of antidepressants
- Screening for medication-associated female sexual dysfunction and advising alternative medications
- Replacing estrogen locally or systemically
- Replacing testosterone (formulations for women currently are being developed)

- Treating hyperprolactinemia, hypothyroidism, or hyperthyroidism
- Possibly using vasoactive drugs for genital arousal disorder in the future
- Applying the model of women's responsive desire to the individual patient experiencing low desire, empowering her and her partner to make the necessary changes

---

**BOX 47.8**
**Primary Care Treatments for Sexual Dysfunction**

The decision to refer a patient depends on a number of factors, including:
- Expertise of the obstetrician-gynecologist
- Complexity of the sexual dysfunction
- Presence or absence of partner sexual dysfunction
- Availability of a psychologist, psychiatrist, or sex therapist
- Motivation of the patient (and partner) to undergo more detailed assessment before therapeutic interventions

More detailed assessments and management may be available from:
- Physicians with extra training and expertise in sexuality—psychiatrists, family practitioners, gynecologists, urologists
- Psychologists
- Sex therapists and abuse counselors
- Physiotherapists (regarding hypertonic pelvic-muscle-associated dyspareunia)
- Relationship counselors
- Support groups (e.g., for women with past histories of breast cancer, women with vulvar-vestibulitis-syndrome-associated chronic dyspareunia, women with interstitial-cystitis-associated dyspareunia)

---

has adequate resources to approach sexual dysfunction from an integrated perspective, rather than merely a biological one. Psychology, pharmacology, partner intimacy, and alternative therapies are some of the other factors that must be addressed in treating sexual dysfunction. Referrals to mental health practitioners, marriage or relationship counselors, or sex therapists may be appropriate. Box 47.8 shows when and why to refer patients.

## SUGGESTED READINGS

Basson R. *Clinical Updates in Women's Health Care: Sexuality and Sexual Disorders.* Washington, DC: American College of Obstetricians and Gynecologists; 2007:II;2.

Nolan TE, Ettinger BB, Johnson SR, Levine RU, Phelan ST, Poindexter AN, Snyder TE, Barbieri RL, Basson R, Berenson AB, eds. *Precis: Primary and Preventive Care*, 3rd ed. American College of Obstetricians and Gynecologists; 2007:108–116.

# 48

# Sexual Assault and Domestic Violence

Topic 57:  Sexual Assault

Topic 58:  Domestic Violence

Students should be able to define sexual assault in adults and children and describe the evaluation and management of each, including age-appropriate sexual assault history and physical examination and forensic examination, as well as crisis, immediate, and long-term counseling. Students should also be able to describe the types of violence against women in domestic situations, their evaluation and management, and the psychosocial issues that they engender.

S exual assault and domestic violence pose obvious immediate and often enduring long-term health and emotional risks. The compassionate and thoughtful care of victims and their families is an important goal of everyone involved in healthcare.

## SEXUAL ASSAULT

*Sexual assault is defined legally as involving any genital, oral, or anal penetration by a part of the accused's body or by an object, using force or without consent.* Criminal sexual assault, or rape, often is further characterized to include acquaintance rape, date rape, "statutory rape," child sexual abuse, and incest. These terms generally relate to the age of the victim and her relationship to the abuser.

Each year, some 365,000 women in the United States experience sexual assault, rape, or attempted rape. An estimated 1 in 6 women have experienced sexual assault in their lifetimes. However, most do not file a complaint or report and, thus, its true prevalence is unknown. In the years between 1992 and 2000, 63% percent of completed rapes, 65% of attempted rapes, and 74% of completed and attempted sexual assaults against females were not reported to the police. Because of the complex problems caused by sexual assault, treatment is best managed by a multidisciplinary team that fulfills the following roles:

- **Care for the victim's emotional needs,** acute and (if possible within the constraints of the healthcare system) long-term
- **Evaluation and treatment of medical needs,** acute and follow-up

- **Collection of forensic specimens** and preparation of a record acceptable for healthcare and in the legal process

## Definitions and Types of Sexual Assault

Sexual assault occurs in all age, racial, and socioeconomic groups; the very young, handicapped, and the very old are particularly susceptible. Although the act may be committed by a stranger, in many cases it is committed by an acquaintance.

Some situations have been defined as variants of sexual assault. **Marital rape** is defined as forced coitus or related sexual acts within a marital relationship without the consent of a partner; it often occurs in conjunction with and as part of physical abuse in cases of domestic or intimate-partner violence.

**Date rape** or **acquaintance rape** is another manifestation of intimate-partner violence. In this situation, a woman may voluntarily participate in sexual play, but coitus occurs, often forcibly, without her consent. Date rape often goes unreported, because the woman may think that she contributed to the act by participating up to a point or that she will not be believed. Lack of consent also may occur in situations where cognitive function is impaired by flunitrazepam, alcohol, or other drugs; sleep; injury with unconsciousness; or developmental delay.

All states have statutory rape statutes criminalizing sexual intercourse with a girl younger than a specific age, because she is defined, by statute, as being incapable of consenting. Many states also have laws addressing **aggravated criminal sexual assault,** which has the following attributes: weapons are used, lives are endangered, or physical violence is inflicted; the act is committed in relationship to another felony; or the woman is older than 60 years, physically handicapped, or mentally retarded.

## Management

The medical and health consequences of sexual assault are both short- and long-term. Clinicians should be aware that their practices will include women with a history of sexual assault, and they should be familiar with both the short- and long-term sequelae. All patients should be screened for a history of sexual assault. Most women with a history of sexual assault will not have reported it to a nonpsychiatric physician. Yet, women with a history of assault are more likely to present with chronic pelvic pain, dysmenorrhea, menstrual cycle disturbances, and sexual dysfunction than are women without such a history.

Clinicians evaluating women in the acute phase who have experienced sexual assault have a number of responsibilities, both medical and legal (Table 48.1). They should be familiar with state rape and assault laws, and comply with any legal requirements regarding reporting and the collection of evidence. They also must be aware that every state and the District of Columbia require physicians to report child abuse, including sexual assault against children and adolescents. Physicians should be familiar with any state laws regarding the reporting of statutory rape. Additionally, physicians should be aware of local protocols regarding the use of specially trained sexual assault forensic examiners or

| TABLE 48.1 | Physician's Role in Evaluation of Sexual Assault Patients | |
|---|---|
| **Medical Issues** | **Legal Issues\*** |
| Ensure that informed consent is obtained from patient. | Provide accurate recording of events. |
| Assess and treat physical injuries or triage and refer. | Document injuries. |
| Obtain pertinent past gynecologic history. | Collect samples (pubic hair, fingernail scrapings, vaginal secretion and discharge samples, saliva, blood-stained clothing or other personal articles) as indicated by local protocol or regulation. |
| Perform physical examination, including pelvic examination (with appropriate chaperone or support person present). | Identify the presence or absence of sperm in the vaginal fluids and make appropriate slides. |
| Obtain appropriate specimens for sexually transmitted disease testing. | Report to authorities as required. |
| Obtain baseline serologic tests for hepatitis B virus, human immunodeficiency virus, and syphilis. | Ensure security of chain of evidence. |
| Provide appropriate infectious disease prophylaxis as indicated. | |
| Provide or arrange for provision of emergency contraception as indicated. | |
| Provide counseling regarding findings, recommendations, and prognosis. | |
| Arrange follow-up medical care and referrals for psychosocial needs. | |

\*Many jurisdictions have prepackaged "rape kits" for the initial forensic examination that provide specific containers and instructions for the collection of physical evidence and for written and pictorial documentation of the victim's subjective and objective findings. Hospital emergency rooms or the police themselves may supply the kits when called to respond or when bringing a patient to the hospital. Most often the emergency physician or specially trained nurse response team will perform the examination, but all physicians should be familiar with the forensic examination procedure. If called to perform this examination and the physician has no or limited experience, it may be judicious to call for assistance because any break in the technique in collecting evidence, or break in the chain of custody of evidence, including improper handling of samples or mislabeling, will virtually eliminate any effort to prosecute in the future.

sexual assault nurse examiners. Specific responsibilities are determined by the patient's needs and by state law.

The clinician should provide medical and counseling services, inform the patient of her rights, refer her to legal assistance, and help her develop prevention strategies to avoid future assault. Many jurisdictions and several clinics have developed a sexual assault assessment kit, which lists the steps necessary and the items to be obtained so that as much information as possible can be prepared for forensic purposes. Many clinics have nurses who are trained to collect needed samples and information. If these individuals are available, it is appropriate to request their assistance. Rape crisis counselors and centers also can provide valuable support. In addition, the clinician must assess and treat all injuries, perform sexually transmitted disease (STD) screening, and provide prophylaxis against infectious diseases and unintended pregnancy.

## INITIAL CARE

*When a woman who has experienced sexual assault communicates with the physician's office, emergency room, or clinic before presenting for evaluation, she should be encouraged to come immediately to a medical facility and be advised not to bathe, douche, urinate, defecate, wash out her mouth, clean her fingernails, smoke, eat, or drink.*

In recent years, there has been a trend toward the implementation of hospital-based programs to provide acute medical and evidentiary examinations by sexual assault nurse examiners or sexual assault forensic examiners. Physicians play a role in the policy and procedure development and implementation of these programs, and serve as sources for referral, consultation, and follow-up. In some parts of the country, however, obstetrician–gynecologists will still be the first point of contact for evaluation and care in the acute aftermath of a sexual assault. In addition, virtually all obstetrician–gynecologists will be called on to perform evaluations and, if conducting screening for history of sexual assault, will realize the utility of this information to the conduct of primary-care and specialty-care practice.

In an optimal situation, the woman is able to seek care in a facility where there is a trained multidisciplinary team. A team member should remain with the patient to help provide a sense of safety and security and, thereby, begin the therapeutic process, including, specifically, assurance of the patient's lack of guilt. *The patient should be encouraged, in a supportive, nonjudgmental manner, to talk about the assault and her feelings.* Treatment for life-threatening trauma needs to begin immediately. Such trauma is uncommon, although minor trauma is seen in one-fourth of victims. Even in life-threatening situations, any sense of control that can be given the patient is helpful. Obtaining consent for treatment is not only a legal requirement, but also an important aspect of the emotional care of the patient, by helping her participate in regaining control of her body and her circumstances.

Although patients are commonly reluctant to do so, they should be gently encouraged to work with the police, because such cooperation is clearly associated with improved emotional outcomes for victims.

History taking about a sexual assault is necessary to gain medical and forensic information, and is as well an important therapeutic activity. Recalling the details of the assault in the supportive environment of the healthcare setting allows the victim to begin to gain an understanding of what has happened and to start emotional healing (see Box 48.1.).

Victims of sexual assault should be given a complete general physical examination, including a pelvic examination. Forensic specimens should be collected, and cultures for STDs should be obtained. When collecting forensic specimens, it is critical that the clinician follow the directions on the forensic specimens kit. These specimens are kept in a health professional's possession or control until turned over to an appropriate legal representative. This "protective custody" of the specimens ensures that the correct specimen reaches the forensic laboratory and is called the **"chain of evidence."**

Initial laboratory tests should include cultures from the vagina, anus, and pharynx for STDs. Collection of serum for rapid plasma reagin (RPR) for syphilis, hepatitis antigens, and human immunodeficiency virus (HIV) are needed. Urinalysis, culture and sensitivity, as well as a pregnancy test for menstrual-age women (regardless of contraceptive status) are collected. **Antibiotic prophylaxis** should be offered to all adult patients. **Emergency**

---

### BOX 48.1
### Documenting Patient History after Assault

**Gynecologic History**
- Menstrual history
- Method of contraception
- Date of last consensual sexual experience
- Obstetric history
- Gynecologic history, including infections
- Activities (e.g., bathing, douching, eating, or drinking since the assault) that could affect forensic evidence gathered

**Details of Sexual Assault**
- Location, timing, and nature of the sexual assault
- Use of force, weapons, or any substances that would impair the mental status of the victim
- Loss of consciousness
- Information about the assailant, including ejaculation and use of a condom, contraceptive, or lubricant

**contraception** should be offered and is described in Chapter 27 on contraception (see Table 48.2).

*Within 24 to 48 hours of disclosure and initial treatment, victims should be contacted by phone or seen for an immediate post-treatment evaluation.* At this time, emotional or physical problems are managed and follow-up appointments arranged. Potentially serious problems, such as suicidal ideation, rectal bleeding, or evidence of pelvic infection, may go unrecognized by the victim during this time because of fear or continued cognitive dysfunction. Specific questions must be asked to ensure that such problems have not arisen.

## SUBSEQUENT CARE

At the 1-week follow-up visit, a general review of the patient's progress is made and any specific new problems ad-

dressed. The next routine visit is at 6 weeks, when a complete evaluation, including physical examination, repeat cultures for sexually transmitted diseases, and a repeat RPR is performed. Another visit at 12 to 18 weeks may be indicated for repeat HIV titers, although the current understanding of HIV infection does not allow an estimate of the risk of exposure for sexual assault victims. Each victim should receive as much counseling and support as is necessary, with referral to a long-term counseling program if needed.

If the physician is not directly involved in the acute care of the victim, it is helpful for him or her to obtain records of the patient's emergency evaluation. These enable the physician to be certain that all appropriate testing was performed and to provide the patient with full results. Patients may be disturbed to learn that the results of their forensic

**TABLE 48.2    Testing and Medical Prophylaxis for Sexual Assault Patients**

| Sexually Transmitted Disease Infections | Prophylaxis |
|---|---|
| Gonococcal infection<br>*Chlamydia trachomatis* infection<br>Trichomoniasis | Ceftriaxone, 125 mg intramuscularly in a single dose<br>PLUS |
| Bacterial vaginosis | Metronidazole, 2 g orally in a single dose<br>PLUS<br>Azithromycin, 1 g orally single dose<br>OR<br>Doxycycline, 100 mg twice daily orally for 7 days<br>(Testing for gonorrhea, chlamydia, and *Trichomonas vaginalis* should be done at initial examination. If vaginal discharge, malodor, and itching are present, examination for bacterial vaginosis and candidiasis should be conducted.) |
| Syphilis | Routine prophylaxis is not currently recommended. (Serologic tests should be conducted at initial evaluation, and repeated 6, 12, and 24 weeks after the assault.) |
| Hepatitis B | Postexposure hepatitis B vaccination (without hepatitis B immune globulin) administered at time of initial examination if not previously vaccinated. Follow-up doses should be administered at 1–2 months and 4–6 months after first dose. (Serologic tests should be conducted at initial evaluation.) |
| Human immunodeficiency virus infection (HIV) | <72 hours postexposure with an individual known to have HIV, 28-day course of highly active retroviral therapy (HAART). Consultation with an HIV specialist is recommended. (Serologic tests should be conducted at initial evaluation, and repeated 6, 12, and 24 weeks after the assault.) 72 hours postexposure to an individual of unknown HIV status, or >72 hours postexposure, individualized assessment |
| Herpes simplex virus infection | Routine prophylaxis is not currently recommended but should be individualized if there is a report of a genital lesion on assailant. A 7–10-day course of acyclovir, famcyclovir, or valacyclovir may be offered. However, there are no data on the efficacy of this treatment. |
| Human papillomavirus infection | There is no preventive treatment recommended at this time. |
| Pregnancy | Emergency contraception. First dose should be given within 72 hours of the assault. |
| Injuries | Tetanus toxoid booster, 0.5 mL intramuscularly, if more than 10 years since last immunization. |

Adapted from Workowski KA, Levine WC; Centers for Disease Control and Prevention. Sexually transmitted diseases treatment guidelines 2002. *MMWR Recomm Rep.* 2002;51(RR-6):1–8; Smith OK, Grohskopf LA, Black RJ, Auerbach JD, Veronese F, Struble KA, et al. Antiretroviral postexposure prophylaxis after sexual, injection-drug use, or other nonoccupational exposure to HIV in the United States: recommendations from the U.S. Department of Health and Human Services. *MMWR Recomm Rep.* 2005;54(RR-2):1–20; and Holmes M. Sexually transmitted infections in female rape victims. *AIDS Patient Care STDS.* 1999;13(12):703–708.

evaluation are usually not provided to their physician. In this situation, it is helpful to refer the patient to local legal or police authorities, who can also be helpful in answering patients' questions about the health status of the assailant and whether the assailant was apprehended.

## Emotional Issues

A woman who is sexually assaulted loses control over her life during the period of the assault. Her integrity, and sometimes her life, is threatened. She may experience intense anxiety, anger, or fear. After the assault, a "rape-trauma" syndrome commonly occurs, comprising two phases:

**ACUTE PHASE** (IMMEDIATE RESPONSE)
- May last for hours or days
- Characterized by distortion or paralysis of the individual's coping mechanisms
- Outward responses vary from complete loss of emotional control to an apparently well-controlled behavior pattern.
- Signs may include generalized pain throughout the body; headache; eating and sleep disturbances; and emotional symptoms, such as depression, anxiety, and mood swings.

**DELAYED (OR ORGANIZATION) PHASE**
- Characterized by flashbacks, nightmares, and phobias as well as somatic and gynecologic symptoms
- Often occurs months or years after the event, and may involve major life adjustments

This rape-trauma syndrome is similar to a grief reaction in many respects. As such, it can only be resolved when the victim has emotionally worked through the trauma and personal loss related to the event and replaced it with other life experiences. *An inability to think clearly or remember things such as her past medical history, termed "cognitive dysfunction," is a particularly distressing aspect of the syndrome.* The involuntary loss of cognition may raise fears of "being crazy" or of being perceived as "crazy" by others. It is also frustrating for the healthcare team, unless it is recognized that this is an involuntary, temporary, and understandable reaction to the emotionally intolerable nature of the sexual assault and not a willful action.

Those who have experienced physical and sexual assault also are at great risk of developing posttraumatic stress disorder. Clusters of symptoms may not appear for months or even years after a traumatic experience. These clusters are typical symptom categories associated with posttraumatic stress disorder, including:

- Reliving the event
- Experiencing flashbacks, recurring nightmares, and, more specifically, intrusive images that appear at any time

- Extreme emotional or physical reactions, including shaking, chills, palpitations, or panic reactions, often accompany vivid recollections of the attack.

Avoiding reminders of the event constitutes another symptom cluster in posttraumatic stress disorder. These women become emotionally numb, withdrawing from friends and family and losing interest in everyday activities. There may be an even deeper reaction of denial of awareness that the event actually happened.

Symptoms such as easy startling, being hypervigilant, irritability, sleep disturbances, and lack of concentration are part of a third symptom cluster known as **hyper-arousal.** These women often will have a number of co-occurring conditions, such as depression, dissociative disorders (losing conscious awareness of the present, or "zoning out"), addictive disorders, and many physical symptoms.

## CHILD SEXUAL ASSAULT

**Ninety percent (90%) of child victimization is by parents, family members, or family friends;** "stranger rape" is relatively uncommon in children. It is extremely important to know who the perpetrator is and how the child sustained the injury, so that the child can be removed from an unsafe environment. Box 48.2 shows behavioral and physical signs and symptoms commonly associated with child sexual abuse.

## Assessment/Examination

Because the assessment of a child for sexual abuse involves specific skills and has the potential for legal challenge, the

---

**BOX 48.2**
**Signs of Child Sexual Assault**

- Night terrors
- Changes in sleeping habits
- Clinging
- Sexual acting out
- Aggression
- Regression
- Eating disturbances
- Recurrent somatic complaints of abdominal pain
- Headaches
- Vaginal pain
- Dysuria
- Encopresis
- Enuresis
- Hematochezia
- Vaginal erythema
- Vaginal discharge or bleeding

individual who undertakes this evaluation should have significant experience in this area. This assessment usually is done by pediatricians and is beyond the skills of most general gynecologists. Awareness of and sensitivity to the issues, special needs, and circumstances of the child are important for obstetrician–gynecologists who are consulted to treat an injury to the pelvic floor. In many cities, a child abuse team consisting of trained experts and including physicians, social workers, and counselors is available to perform the assessment.

The sexual abuse evaluation begins with an interview of the caretaker and the child. Unless the child refuses to leave the caretaker, the child should be interviewed privately to obtain specific details of the abuse. Questioning should be nondirect to elicit spontaneous responses such as time and location of the abuse, description of the scene, name and description of the perpetrator, and type of sexual acts. The child's statements should be recorded verbatim; electronic interviews are helpful so that the child does not have to describe the abuse repeatedly. Good documentation of the interview is critical in the prosecution of sexual abuse cases because, in many instances, the patient's statement is the only evidence that the abuse occurred. Documentation of the specific names the child uses for her genitalia is recommended to help others understand the context of her statements.

The urgency of an evaluation of sexual abuse depends on how soon after the event the child is brought in for care. If the child presents within 72 hours of the last episode of abuse, the physician should immediately arrange for evaluation of the child and focus on collection of forensic evidence. However, fewer than 10% of child sexual abuse cases are reported within 72 hours. In cases that are reported after 72 hours, the patient should be referred to the nearest sexual abuse center, where more resources are available to conduct the evaluation.

### Management

In the treatment of a child who is the victim of sexual abuse, management should focus (as applicable) on repair of injuries, treatment of STDs, prevention of pregnancy, protection against further abuse, and psychologic support for the patient and her family. Superficial injuries (e.g., bruises, edema, local irritation) resolve within a few days and require only meticulous perineal hygiene. In some patients with extensive skin abrasions, broad-spectrum antibiotics should be given as prophylaxis. Small vulvar hematomas usually can be controlled by pressure with an ice pack, and even massive swelling of the vulva usually subsides promptly when cold packs and external pressure are applied. Injuries to the vagina or rectum may present surgical difficulties because of the small size of the organs involved. More extensive penetrative vaginal and anal injuries require thorough radiographic and anesthetic examination to rule out intraabdominal penetration.

## DOMESTIC VIOLENCE

Domestic violence is reported by over 25% of women at some time during their lives and is a significant source of illness and injury to women.

### Definition

**Domestic violence** refers to violence perpetrated within the context of family or intimate relationships. Family members include parents, siblings, and other blood relatives, as well as legal relatives such as stepparents, in-laws, and guardians. Violence that occurs between current or former partners is referred to as **intimate-partner violence** and includes male abuse by female partners and violence between partners in lesbian, gay, bisexual, and transgendered relationships.

*Domestic violence may involve one or more of three presentations.* **Physical abuse** such as hitting, slapping, kicking, and choking, is the most obvious presentation. It is suspected with evidence of trauma, especially to the head and neck or trunk associated with a history of violence, or when an explanation of the trauma doesn't seem appropriate (Table 48.3). Unfortunately, pregnancy appears to be a period of greater risk for such episodes. **Sexual abuse** is another presentation of domestic violence. The third presentation is **emotional, financial, or psychological abuse, neglect, or threat,** and is often traumatic and/or long-standing. Examples include undermining of self-worth, deprivation of sleep or emotional support, repetitive unpredictability of response to life situations, threats, destruction of personal property or the killing of pets, lies, manipulation of friends, and interference in the workplace. Domestic violence is usually cyclic and repetitive, with periods of calm alternating with periods of rapidly in-

| TABLE 48.3 | Indicators of Physical Abuse in Domestic Violence |
|---|---|
| **Area of Injury** | **Descriptions** |
| Head and neck | Bruises, abrasions, strangle marks, black eye, broken nose, orbital ridge, or jaw, pulled hair, permanent hearing loss, facial lacerations |
| Trunk | Evidence of blunt trauma, including bruises (especially breasts and abdomen), fractured collarbones and ribs |
| Skin | Multiple lesions in various stages of healing, "rug rash" abrasions, burns (cigarette, lighter, liquid splash), bites |
| Extremities | Evidence of restraint, including muscle strains, spiral fractures, rope or restraint burns, "crescent moon"-shape fingernail marks or bruises in the shape of a hand or blunt instrument |

---

**BOX 48.3**
## Identifying the Abused Woman

**No true stereotype exists, but certain risk factors are found among victims:**
- Younger women, especially those in long, difficult relationships
- History of violence or dysfunctional family of origin
- Dysfunctional past relationships
- Pregnancy, especially if unintended
- Relationships in transitions (i.e., separation, divorce)
- Any situation where the partner is overly attentive, especially if he repeatedly answers for her
- Sexually transmitted diseases
- Substance abuse

**Clinical clues that the patient is or has been abused:**
- Unexplained, multiple, and recurring injuries
- Elusive pain and other somatic complaints
- Specific problems in pregnancy
- Poor compliance, hostility, passivity, minimal response

- Psychologic changes, especially depression, anxiety, panic attacks, sleep and eating disorders
- Compulsive sexual behaviors, seductive behavior with examiners (not sexual, but to gain attention)
- Self-destructive, high-risk behaviors (poor self-care, substance abuse, self-neglect and self-injury, suicidal ideation)
- Increased use of prescription narcotics and tranquilizers
- Frequent visits and increased use of the health-care system
- Extensive medical records documenting unresolved problems
- Unusual disclosure style (too detailed, not credible, cannot explain injuries in a satisfactory way, cannot explain why instructions have not been followed)
- Difficulty in tolerating examination
- Difficulty tolerating other medical situations that recreate traumatic experiences (isolation, injection of medications, restraints and immobilization, surgery)

---

creasing tensions or violence, the latter often increasing in severity with each iteration of the cycle.

## Screening: Risk Factors

*Recognition is the first, most important, and most often a missed issue.* When domestic violence is suspected, compassionate and thoughtful discussion with the possible victim, as well as attention to any physical injury, is requisite. All patients should be asked about violence in their lives as part of the routine health history. Although all women are at risk for abuse, certain life experiences and circumstances may place some women at greater risk (Box 48.3).

The clinician's role is 1) to know the signs and symptoms of intimate-partner violence, 2) to ask all patients about past or present exposure to violence, 3) to intervene and refer as appropriate, and 4) to assess the patient's risk of danger (Box 48.4).

## Counseling

If the patient will be returning to an unsafe home, safety planning should be conducted, and referrals to service agencies in the community should be provided. Women can be encouraged to call a woman's shelter for more help

---

**BOX 48.4**
## The RADAR Model of the Physician's Approach to Domestic Violence

R: **Remember** to ask routinely about partner violence in your own practice
A: **Ask directly** about violence with such questions as, "At any time, has a partner hit, kicked, or otherwise hurt or frightened you?" Interview your patient in private at all times.
D: **Document** information about "suspected domestic violence" or "intimate-partner violence" in the patient's chart, and file reports when required by law.
A: **Assess** your patient's safety. Is it safe to return home? Find out if any weapons are kept in the house, if the children are in danger, and if the violence is escalating.
R: **Review** options with your patients. Know about the types of referral options (e.g., shelters, support groups, legal advocates).

Massachusetts Medical Society. Partner violence: how to recognize and treat victims of abuse. 4th ed. Waltham, MA: Massachusetts Medical Society; 2004.

---

**BOX 48.5**
**Making an Exit Plan to Leave an Abusive Relationship**

- Pack a bag in advance and leave it at a neighbor's or friend's house. Include cash or credit cards and extra clothes for yourself and your children. Take each child's favorite toy or plaything.
- Hide an extra set of car and house keys outside of the house in case you have to leave quickly.
- Take important papers, such as the following:
  - Birth certificate (including children's)
  - Health insurance cards and medicine
- Deed or lease to the house or apartment
- Checkbook and extra checks
- Social Security number or green card/work permit
- Court papers or orders
- Driver's license or photo identification
- Pay stubs

Modified from American College of Obstetricians and Gynecologists. Intimate partner violence. In: *Special issues in women's health.* Washington, DC: ACOG; 2005:169–188.

---

with a safety plan, and be assured that such calls would be anonymous. Box 48.5 details suggested steps for patients when they are ready to leave an abusive situation.

## SUGGESTED READINGS

American College of Obstetricians and Gynecologists. *Guidelines for Women's Health Care: A Resource Manual.* 3rd ed. Washington, D.C.: ACOG; 2007:276–281.

Intimate partner violence. In: *Special Issues In Women's Health.* Washington, DC: American College of Obstetricians and Gynecologists; 2005:169–188.

Violence against women. In: *Precis: Primary and Preventive Care.* 3rd ed. Washington, DC: American College of Obstetricians and Gynecologists; 2007:116–133.

# APPENDIX A

# ACOG Woman's Health Record

 **ACOG WOMAN'S HEALTH RECORD**

## HOW TO USE THE ACOG WOMAN'S HEALTH RECORD

The ACOG Woman's Health Record is intended to serve as a complete record for a woman's gynecologic care. It allows documentation of both preventive services and services directed to a chief complaint. This record has been specifically designed to aid in documentation and correct coding of women's health services.

The recommendations contained in the ACOG Woman's Health Record may be subject to change by subsequently released ACOGguidelines. The ACOG Woman's Health Record includes:

Form A—Physician History

Form B—Patient Intake History

Form C—Problem List/Immunization Record/Routine and High-Risk Screening Records

### Form A—Physician History includes:

**Physician History:** The Physician History can be used to record the history for every type of outpatient encounter, including consultations. A new Physician History should becompleted by the physician at each visit when clinically indicated.

**Physical Examination:** The Physical Examination section should be completed by the physician each time a physical examination is provided. The form offers prompts to aidin documenting the services that are provided. This form is based on the 1997 CMS (formerly, HCFA) guidelines for the female genitourinary system examination and can be used to document any level of examination.

**Medical Decision Making:** The Medical Decision Making section provides space to document minutes counseled, total encounter time, and other services needed to determine the correct level of medical decision making.

**Form B—Patient Intake History** is anoptional form giving practices the flexibility to have patients complete their own history at or before the visit. It uses language that a patient is likely to understand and includes ample

space for physician notes. Space at the end of the form allows physicians to review the history and sign off for 4 years. At year 5, the patient should be asked to complete a new Patient Intake History.

### Form C includes:

### Problem List and Immunization Record:

The Problem List captures problems, allergies, family history, and current medication use. The Immunization Record lists immunization services recommended by ACOG for either routine use or in high-risk patients, as defined in the enclosed table of high-risk factors. Ample space for listing problems and immunization services allows the same form to be used for years.

### Routine and High-Risk Screening Records:

The Routine and High-Risk Screening Records provide ample space to document laboratory and other screening services. The Routine Screening Record includes those screening tests recommended by ACOG for routine use and provides reminders for recommended frequency of services. The High-Risk Screening Record includes those screening tests recommended by ACOG on the basis of the risk factors defined in the enclosed table of high-risk factors.

The ACOG Woman's Health Record also includes helpful reference information (one each per package):

**Coding Tips:** This sheet includes all the reminders a physicianneeds to code correctly the history, physical examination, and medical decision making provided during the visit. Once these elements have been coded correctly, the summary tables can be used to select the appropriate code for the visit.

**Table of High-Risk Factors:** The table (see back of this card) lists in one place the risk factors that should prompt recommended interventions, laboratory tests, and immunizations. It is to be used in completing the Immunization Record and the Routine and High-Risk Screening Records.

Patient Addressograph

PATIENT NAME:_____

BIRTH DATE:_____

ID NO.:_____

DATE:_____

# PHYSICIAN HISTORY

☐ NEW PATIENT          ☐ ESTABLISHED PATIENT          ☐ CONSULTATION          ☐ REPORT SENT:    /    /

PRIMARY CARE PHYSICIAN:                              WHO SENT PATIENT:

OTHER PHYSICIAN(S):

**CHIEF COMPLAINT (CC) (REQUIRED FOR ALL VISITS EXCEPTPREVENTIVE):**     CURRENT PRESCRIPTIONMEDICATIONS: ☐ NONE

HISTORY OF PRESENT ILLNESS (HPI):     CURRENT NONPRESCRIPTION, COMPLEMENTARY, ANDALTERNATIVEMEDICATIONS: ☐ NONE

| CHANGES SINCE LAST VISIT | YES | NO | NOTES |
|---|---|---|---|
| ILLNESSES | ☐ | ☐ | |
| SURGERY | ☐ | ☐ | |
| NEW MEDICATIONS | ☐ | ☐ | |
| CHANGE IN FAMILY HISTORY | ☐ | ☐ | |
| NEW ALLERGIES | ☐ | ☐ | |
| CHANGE IN GYNECOLOGIC HISTORY | ☐ | ☐ | |
| CHANGE IN OBSTETRIC HISTORY | ☐ | ☐ | |

ALLERGIES (DESCRIBE REACTION): ☐ NONE

LAST CERVICALCANCERSCREENING: ☐ CYTOLOGY   /   /   ☐ HPV TEST   /   /

LAST MAMMOGRAM:   /   /

LAST COLORECTAL SCREENING:   /   /

## GYNECOLOGIC HISTORY (PH)

LMP:   /   /     AGE AT MENARCHE:_____   LENGTH OF FLOW:_____   INTERVAL BETWEEN PERIODS:_____   RECENT CHANGES:_____

SEXUALLY ACTIVE ☐ YES ☐ NO     EVER HAD SEX ☐ YES ☐ NO     NUMBER OF PARTNERS (LIFETIME):_____

PARTNERS ARE: ☐ MEN   ☐ WOMEN   ☐ BOTH

CURRENT METHOD OF CONTRACEPTION:          PAST CONTRACEPTIVE HISTORY:

## OBSTETRIC HISTORY (PH)

| | NUMBER | | NUMBER | | NUMBER |
|---|---|---|---|---|---|
| PREGNANCIES | | ABORTIONS | | MISCARRIAGES | |
| PREMATURE BIRTHS (<37 WEEKS) | | LIVE BIRTHS | | LIVING CHILDREN | |

| NO. | BIRTH DATE | WEIGHT AT BIRTH | BABY'S SEX | WEEKS PREGNANT | TYPE OF DELIVERY (VAGINAL, CESAREAN, ETC.) | PHYSICIAN'S NOTES |
|---|---|---|---|---|---|---|
| 1. | | | | | | |
| 2. | | | | | | |
| 3. | | | | | | |
| 4. | | | | | | |

ANY PREGNANCY COMPLICATIONS?

☐ DIABETES   ☐ HYPERTENSION/HIGH BLOOD PRESSURE   ☐ PREECLAMPSIA/TOXEMIA   ☐ OTHER

ANY HISTORY OF DEPRESSION BEFORE OR AFTER PREGNANCY? ☐ NO   ☐ YES, HOW TREATED

## PAST HISTORY (PH)

☐ NONCONTRIBUTORY  ☐ NO INTERVAL CHANGE SINCE:   /   /

SURGERIES:

ILLNESSES (PHYSICALANDMENTAL):

INJURIES:

IMMUNIZATIONS/TUBERCULOSIS TEST:

ACOG WOMAN'S HEALTH RECORD (FORM A—PHYSICIAN HISTORY) PAGE 1 OF 4

## PHYSICIAN HISTORY *(Continued)*

| PATIENT NAME: | BIRTH DATE:  /  / | ID NO.: | DATE:  /  / |
|---|---|---|---|

### FAMILY HISTORY (FH)

☐ NONCONTRIBUTORY  ☐ NO INTERVAL CHANGE SINCE:  /  /

MOTHER: ☐ LIVING  ☐ DECEASED—CAUSE: _____ AGE: ___  FATHER: ☐ LIVING  ☐ DECEASED—CAUSE: _____ AGE: ___

SIBLINGS: NUMBER LIVING: _____ NUMBER DECEASED: _____ CAUSE(S)/AGE(S): _____

CHILDREN: NUMBER LIVING: _____ NUMBER DECEASED: _____ CAUSE(S)/AGE(S): _____

(IF YES, INDICATE WHOM AND AGE AT DIAGNOSIS)

| | | |
|---|---|---|
| ☐ DIABETES | ☐ HEART DISEASE | ☐ HYPERLIPIDEMIA |
| ☐ CANCER | ☐ HYPERTENSION | ☐ DEEP VENOUS THROMBOEMBOLISM/PULMONARY EMBOLISM |
| ☐ OSTEOPOROSIS | ☐ OTHER ILLNESSES | |

### SOCIAL HISTORY (SH)

☐ NONCONTRIBUTORY  ☐ NO INTERVAL CHANGE SINCE:  /  /

| | YES | NO | NOTES | | YES | NO | NOTES |
|---|---|---|---|---|---|---|---|
| TOBACCO USE | ☐ | ☐ | | DIET DISCUSSED | ☐ | ☐ | |
| ALCOHOL USE—SPECIFY AMOUNT AND TYPE (12 OZ BEER = 5 OZ WINE = 1½ OZ LIQUOR) | ☐ | ☐ | | FOLIC ACID INTAKE | ☐ | ☐ | |
| | | | | CALCIUM INTAKE | ☐ | ☐ | |
| ILLEGAL/STREET DRUG USE | ☐ | ☐ | | REGULAR EXERCISE | ☐ | ☐ | |
| MISUSE OF PRESCRIPTION DRUGS | ☐ | ☐ | | CAFFEINE INTAKE | ☐ | ☐ | |
| INTIMATE PARTNER VIOLENCE | ☐ | ☐ | | ADVANCE DIRECTIVE (LIVING WILL) | ☐ | ☐ | |
| SEXUAL ABUSE | ☐ | ☐ | | ORGAN DONATION | ☐ | ☐ | |
| HEALTH HAZARDS AT HOME/WORK | ☐ | ☐ | | OTHER | | | |
| SEAT BELT USE | ☐ | ☐ | | ☐ NO CHANGES SINCE:  /  / | | | |

### REVIEW OF SYSTEMS (ROS)

| 1. CONSTITUTIONAL | ☐ NEGATIVE  ☐ FEVER | ☐ WEIGHT LOSS  ☐ FATIGUE | ☐ WEIGHT GAIN  ☐ OTHER |  TALLEST HEIGHT_____ |
|---|---|---|---|---|
| 2. EYES | ☐ NEGATIVE  ☐ OTHER | ☐ VISION CHANGE | ☐ GLASSES/CONTACTS | |
| 3. EAR, NOSE, AND THROAT | ☐ NEGATIVE  ☐ HEADACHE | ☐ ULCERS  ☐ HEARING LOSS | ☐ SINUSITIS  ☐ OTHER | |
| 4. CARDIOVASCULAR | ☐ NEGATIVE  ☐ EDEMA | ☐ ORTHOPNEA  ☐ PALPITATION | ☐ CHEST PAIN  ☐ OTHER | ☐ DIFFICULTY BREATHING ON EXERTION |
| 5. RESPIRATORY | ☐ NEGATIVE  ☐ SHORTNESS OF BREATH | ☐ WHEEZING | ☐ HEMOPTYSIS  ☐ COUGH | ☐ OTHER |
| 6. GASTROINTESTINAL | ☐ NEGATIVE  ☐ CONSTIPATION | ☐ DIARRHEA  ☐ FLATULENCE | ☐ BLOODY STOOL  ☐ PAIN | ☐ NAUSEA/VOMITING/INDIGESTION  ☐ FECAL INCONTINENCE  ☐ OTHER |
| 7. GENITOURINARY | ☐ NEGATIVE  ☐ FREQUENCY  ☐ DYSPAREUNIA  ☐ ABNORMAL VAGINAL BLEEDING | ☐ HEMATURIA  ☐ INCOMPLETE EMPTYING  ☐ ABNORMAL OR PAINFUL PERIODS | ☐ DYSURIA  ☐ ABNORMAL VAGINAL DISCHARGE | ☐ URGENCY  ☐ INCONTINENCE  ☐ PMS  ☐ OTHER |
| 8. MUSCULOSKELETAL | ☐ NEGATIVE  ☐ MUSCLE OR JOINT PAIN | ☐ MUSCLE WEAKNESS | ☐ OTHER | |
| 9a. SKIN | ☐ NEGATIVE  ☐ DRY SKIN | ☐ RASH  ☐ PIGMENTED LESIONS | ☐ ULCERS  ☐ OTHER | |
| 9b. BREAST | ☐ NEGATIVE  ☐ DISCHARGE | ☐ MASTALGIA  ☐ MASSES | ☐ OTHER | |
| 10. NEUROLOGIC | ☐ NEGATIVE  ☐ TROUBLE WALKING | ☐ SYNCOPE  ☐ SEVERE MEMORY PROBLEMS | ☐ SEIZURES | ☐ NUMBNESS  ☐ OTHER |
| 11. PSYCHIATRIC | ☐ NEGATIVE  ☐ SEVERE ANXIETY | ☐ DEPRESSION  ☐ OTHER | ☐ CRYING | |
| 12. ENDOCRINE | ☐ NEGATIVE  ☐ HOT FLASHES | ☐ DIABETES  ☐ HAIR LOSS | ☐ HYPOTHYROID  ☐ HEAT/COLD INTOLERANCE | ☐ HYPERTHYROID  ☐ OTHER |
| 13. HEMATOLOGIC/LYMPHATIC | ☐ NEGATIVE  ☐ BLEEDING | ☐ BRUISES  ☐ ADENOPATHY | ☐ OTHER | |
| 14. ALLERGIC/IMMUNOLOGIC | (SEE FIRST PAGE) | | | |

ACOG WOMAN'S HEALTH RECORD (FORM A—PHYSICIAN HISTORY) PAGE 2 OF 4

# PHYSICAL EXAMINATION

| PATIENT NAME: | BIRTH DATE:  /  / | ID NO.: | DATE:  /  / |

## CONSTITUTIONAL

• VITAL SIGNS (RECORD ≥ 3 VITAL SIGNS):

HEIGHT: _____ WEIGHT: _____ BMI: _____ BLOOD PRESSURE (SITTING): _____ TEMPERATURE: _____ PULSE: _____ RESPIRATION: _____

• GENERAL APPEARANCE (NOTE ALL THAT APPLY):

☐ WELL-DEVELOPED  ☐ OTHER                      ☐ NO DEFORMITIES  ☐ OTHER
☐ WELL-NOURISHED  ☐ OTHER                      ☐ WELL-GROOMED  ☐ OTHER
☐ NORMAL HABITUS  ☐ OBESE  ☐ OTHER

## NECK

• NECK  ☐ NORMAL  ☐ ABNORMAL  _____
• THYROID  ☐ NORMAL  ☐ ABNORMAL  _____

## RESPIRATORY

• RESPIRATORY EFFORT  ☐ NORMAL  ☐ ABNORMAL  _____
• AUSCULTATED LUNGS  ☐ NORMAL  ☐ ABNORMAL  _____

## CARDIOVASCULAR

• AUSCULTATED HEART
    SOUNDS  ☐ NORMAL  ☐ ABNORMAL  _____
    MURMURS  ☐ NORMAL  ☐ ABNORMAL  _____
• PERIPHERAL VASCULAR  ☐ NORMAL  ☐ ABNORMAL  _____

## GASTROINTESTINAL

• ABDOMEN  ☐ NORMAL  ☐ ABNORMAL  _____
• HERNIA  ☐ NONE  ☐ PRESENT  _____
• LIVER/SPLEEN
    LIVER  ☐ NORMAL  ☐ ABNORMAL  _____
    SPLEEN  ☐ NORMAL  ☐ ABNORMAL  _____
• STOOL GUAIAC, IF INDICATED  ☐ POSITIVE  ☐ NEGATIVE

## LYMPHATIC

• PALPATION OF NODES (CHOOSE ALL THAT ARE APPLICABLE)
    NECK  ☐ NORMAL  ☐ ABNORMAL  _____
    AXILLA  ☐ NORMAL  ☐ ABNORMAL  _____
    GROIN  ☐ NORMAL  ☐ ABNORMAL  _____
    OTHER SITE  ☐ NORMAL  ☐ ABNORMAL  _____

## SKIN

• INSPECTED/PALPATED  ☐ NORMAL  ☐ ABNORMAL

## NEUROLOGIC/PSYCHIATRIC

• ORIENTATION  ☐ TIME  ☐ PLACE  ☐ PERSON  ☐ COMMENTS
• MOOD AND AFFECT  ☐ NORMAL  ☐ DEPRESSED  ☐ ANXIOUS  ☐ AGITATED  ☐ OTHER

## GYNECOLOGIC (AT LEAST 7)

• BREASTS  ☐ NORMAL  ☐ ABNORMAL  _____
• EXTERNAL GENITALIA  ☐ NORMAL  ☐ ABNORMAL  _____
• URETHRAL MEATUS  ☐ NORMAL  ☐ ABNORMAL  _____
• URETHRA  ☐ NORMAL  ☐ ABNORMAL  _____
• BLADDER  ☐ NORMAL  ☐ ABNORMAL  _____
• VAGINA/PELVIC SUPPORT  ☐ NORMAL  ☐ ABNORMAL  _____
• CERVIX  ☐ NORMAL  ☐ ABNORMAL  _____
• UTERUS  ☐ NORMAL  ☐ ABNORMAL  _____
• ADNEXA/PARAMETRIA  ☐ NORMAL  ☐ ABNORMAL  _____
• ANUS/PERINEUM  ☐ NORMAL  ☐ ABNORMAL  _____
• RECTAL  ☐ NORMAL  ☐ ABNORMAL  _____

(SEE ALSO "STOOL GUAIAC" ABOVE)

• TOTAL NUMBER OF BULLETED (•) ELEMENTS EXAMINED: _____

American College of Obstetricians and Gynecologists

Copyright © 2005  (AA322)  12345/98765

ACOG WOMAN'S HEALTH RECORD (FORM A—PHYSICIAN HISTORY) PAGE 3 OF 4

# MEDICAL DECISION MAKING

| PATIENT NAME: | BIRTH DATE:  /  / | ID NO.: | DATE:  /  / |
|---|---|---|---|

## AMOUNT AND COMPLEXITY OF DATA REVIEWED

**TEST(S) ORDERED:**

☐ LABORATORY
   —CERVICAL CYTOLOGY
   —HPV TEST
   —WET MOUNT
   —CHLAMYDIA
   —GONORRHEA
   —OTHER: _____
☐ RADIOLOGY/ULTRASOUND
   —MAMMOGRAM
   —OTHER: _____

**REVIEW OF RECORDS:**

☐ PREVIOUS TEST RESULTS:_____
☐ DISCUSSION OF TEST RESULTS WITH PERFORMING PHYSICIAN:_____
☐ OLD RECORDS REVIEWED AND SUMMARIZED: _____
☐ HISTORY OBTAINED FROM OTHER SOURCE: _____
☐ INDEPENDENT REVIEW OF IMAGE/SPECIMEN: _____

## DIAGNOSES/MANAGEMENT OPTIONS

☐ ESTABLISHED PROBLEM    ☐ NEW PROBLEM

**ASSESSMENT AND PLAN:**

RISK OF COMPLICATIONS AND/OR MORBIDITY/MORTALITY:

   ☐ MINIMAL (EG, COLD, ACHES AND PAINS, OVER-THE-COUNTER MEDICATIONS)

   ☐ LOW (EG, CYSTITIS, VAGINITIS, PRESCRIPTION RENEWAL, MINOR SURGERY WITHOUT RISK FACTORS)

   ☐ MODERATE (EG, BREAST MASS, IRREGULAR BLEEDING, HEADACHES, MINOR SURGERY WITH RISK FACTORS, MAJOR SURGERY WITHOUT RISK FACTORS, NEW PRESCRIPTION)

   ☐ HIGH (EG, PELVIC PAIN, RECTAL BLEEDING, MULTIPLE COMPLAINTS, MAJOR SURGERY WITH RISK FACTORS, CHEMOTHERAPY, EMERGENCY SURGERY)

| **PATIENT COUNSELED ABOUT:** | ☐ SMOKING CESSATION | ☐ CONTRACEPTION |
|---|---|---|
| | ☐ WEIGHT MANAGEMENT | ☐ SAFE SEX |
| | ☐ EXERCISE | ☐ OTHER |

☐ **PATIENT EDUCATION MATERIALS PROVIDED**

| **MINUTES COUNSELED:** | **TOTAL ENCOUNTER TIME:** |
|---|---|

| **SIGNATURE:** | **DATE:**  /  / |
|---|---|

American College of Obstetricians and Gynecologists        Copyright © 2005  (AA322)  12345/98765

Patient Addressograph

# PATIENT INTAKE HISTORY

| PATIENT NAME: | BIRTH DATE:  /   / | ID NO.: | DATE:  /   / |
|---|---|---|---|

ADDRESS:

| CITY: | STATE/ZIP: |
|---|---|
| HOME TELEPHONE: (        ) | WORK TELEPHONE: (        ) |
| EMPLOYER: | INSURANCE: | POLICY NO.: |
| NAME YOU WOULD LIKE US TO USE: | PRIMARY LANGUAGE: |

| NAME OF SPOUSE/PARTNER: | EMERGENCY CONTACT: |
|---|---|
| | RELATIONSHIP: |
| | HOME TELEPHONE: (        ) | WORK TELEPHONE: (        ) |

REFERRED BY:

WHY HAVE YOU COME TO THE OFFICE TODAY?

IF YOU ARE HERE FOR AN ANNUAL EXAMINATION IS THIS A  ☐ PRIMARY CARE VISIT OR  ☐ GYNECOLOGY ONLY

IS THIS A NEW PROBLEM?

PLEASE DESCRIBE YOUR PROBLEM, INCLUDING WHERE IT IS, HOW SEVERE IT IS, AND HOW LONG IT HAS LASTED.

**If you are uncomfortable answering any questions, leave them blank; you can discuss them with your doctor or nurse.**

## GYNECOLOGIC HISTORY

| | PHYSICIAN'S NOTES |
|---|---|
| LAST NORMAL MENSTRUAL PERIOD (FIRST DAY):   /   / | |
| AGE PERIODS BEGAN: | |
| LENGTH OF PERIODS (NUMBER OF DAYS OF BLEEDING): | |
| NUMBER OF DAYS BETWEEN PERIODS: | |
| ANY RECENT CHANGES IN PERIODS? | |
| ARE YOU CURRENTLY SEXUALLY ACTIVE? | |
| HAVE YOU EVER HAD SEX? | |
| NUMBER OF SEXUAL PARTNERS (LIFETIME): | |
| SEXUAL PARTNERS ARE ☐ MEN ☐ WOMEN ☐ BOTH | |
| PRESENT METHOD OF BIRTH CONTROL: | |
| HAVE YOU EVER USED AN INTRAUTERINE DEVICE (IUD) OR BIRTH CONTROL PILLS? | |
| IF YES, FOR HOW LONG? | |
| WHEN WAS YOUR LAST PAP TEST? | |
| WHAT WAS THE RESULT? | |
| HAVE YOU EVER HAD AN ABNORMAL PAP TEST? | |
| DO YOU DO BREAST SELF-EXAMINATIONS? | |
| HAVE YOU BEEN EXPOSED TO DIETHYLSTILBESTROL (DES)? | |

ACOG WOMAN'S HEALTH RECORD (FORM B—PATIENT INTAKE HISTORY) PAGE 1 OF 6

## PATIENT INTAKE HISTORY *(Continued)*

| PATIENT NAME: | BIRTH DATE: / / | ID NO.: | DATE: / / |
|---|---|---|---|

### OBSTETRIC HISTORY

| | NUMBER | | NUMBER | | NUMBER |
|---|---|---|---|---|---|
| PREGNANCIES | | ABORTIONS | | MISCARRIAGES | |
| PREMATURE BIRTHS (<37 WEEKS) | | LIVE BIRTHS | | LIVING CHILDREN | |

| NO. | BIRTH DATE | WEIGHT AT BIRTH | BABY'S SEX | WEEKS PREGNANT | TYPE OF DELIVERY (VAGINAL, CESAREAN, ETC.) | PHYSICIAN'S NOTES |
|---|---|---|---|---|---|---|
| 1. | | | | | | |
| 2. | | | | | | |
| 3. | | | | | | |
| 4. | | | | | | |

ANY PREGNANCY COMPLICATIONS?

☐ DIABETES  ☐ HYPERTENSION/HIGH BLOOD PRESSURE  ☐ PREECLAMPSIA/TOXEMIA  ☐ OTHER

ANY HISTORY OF DEPRESSION BEFORE OR AFTER PREGNANCY? ☐ NO  ☐ YES, HOW TREATED

### CURRENT MEDICATIONS
**(Including hormones, vitamins, herbs, nonprescription medications)**

| DRUG NAME | DOSAGE | WHO PRESCRIBED | DRUG NAME | DOSAGE | WHO PRESCRIBED |
|---|---|---|---|---|---|
| | | | | | |
| | | | | | |
| | | | | | |
| | | | | | |

### FAMILY HISTORY

MOTHER: ☐ LIVING  ☐ DECEASED—CAUSE:          AGE:        FATHER: ☐ LIVING  ☐ DECEASED—CAUSE:          AGE:

SIBLINGS: NUMBER LIVING:          NUMBER DECEASED:          CAUSE(S)/AGE(S):

CHILDREN: NUMBER LIVING:          NUMBER DECEASED:          CAUSE(S)/AGE(S):

| ILLNESS | YES | WHICH RELATIVE(S) AND AGE OF ONSET | PHYSICIAN'S NOTES |
|---|---|---|---|
| DIABETES | ☐ | | |
| STROKE | ☐ | | |
| HEART DISEASE | ☐ | | |
| BLOOD CLOTS IN LUNGS OR LEGS | ☐ | | |
| HIGH BLOOD PRESSURE | ☐ | | |
| HIGH CHOLESTEROL | ☐ | | |
| OSTEOPOROSIS (WEAK BONES) | ☐ | | |
| HEPATITIS | ☐ | | |
| HIV/AIDS | ☐ | | |
| TUBERCULOSIS | ☐ | | |
| BIRTH DEFECTS | ☐ | | |
| ALCOHOL OR DRUG PROBLEMS | ☐ | | |
| BREAST CANCER | ☐ | | |
| COLON CANCER | ☐ | | |
| OVARIAN CANCER | ☐ | | |
| UTERINE CANCER | ☐ | | |
| MENTAL ILLNESS/DEPRESSION | ☐ | | |
| ALZHEIMER'S DISEASE | ☐ | | |
| OTHER | ☐ | | |

ACOG WOMAN'S HEALTH RECORD (FORM B—PATIENT INTAKE HISTORY) PAGE 2 OF 6

## PATIENT INTAKE HISTORY *(Continued)*

| PATIENT NAME: | BIRTH DATE:   /   / | ID NO.: | DATE:   /   / |
|---|---|---|---|

### SOCIAL HISTORY

| | YES | NO | PHYSICIAN'S NOTES |
|---|---|---|---|
| EVER SMOKED? CURRENT SMOKING: PACKS PER DAY:          YEARS: | ☐ | ☐ | |
| ALCOHOL: DRINKS PER DAY:     DRINKS PER WEEK:     TYPE OF DRINK: | ☐ | ☐ | |
| DRUG USE | ☐ | ☐ | |
| SEAT BELT USE | ☐ | ☐ | |
| REGULAR EXERCISE: HOW LONG AND HOW OFTEN? | ☐ | ☐ | |
| DAIRY PRODUCT INTAKE AND/OR CALCIUM SUPPLEMENTS: DAILY INTAKE: | ☐ | ☐ | |
| HEALTH HAZARDS AT HOME OR WORK? | ☐ | ☐ | |
| HAVE YOU BEEN SEXUALLY ABUSED, THREATENED, OR HURT BY ANYONE? | ☐ | ☐ | |
| DO YOU HAVE AN ADVANCE DIRECTIVE (LIVING WILL)? | ☐ | ☐ | |
| ARE YOU AN ORGAN DONOR? | ☐ | ☐ | |

### PERSONAL PROFILE

SEXUAL ORIENTATION: ☐ HETEROSEXUAL  ☐ HOMOSEXUAL  ☐ BISEXUAL

MARITAL STATUS: ☐ MARRIED  ☐ LIVING WITH PARTNER  ☐ SINGLE  ☐ WIDOWED  ☐ DIVORCED

NUMBER OF LIVING CHILDREN:

NUMBER OF PEOPLE IN HOUSEHOLD:

SCHOOL COMPLETED: ☐ HIGH SCHOOL  ☐ SOME COLLEGE/AA DEGREE  ☐ COLLEGE  ☐ GRADUATE DEGREE  ☐ OTHER

CURRENT OR MOST RECENT JOB:

TRAVEL OUTSIDE THE UNITED STATES?                    LOCATION(S):

### PERSONAL PAST HISTORY OF ILLNESSES

| MAJOR ILLNESSES | YES (DATE) | NO | NOT SURE | PHYSICIAN'S NOTES |
|---|---|---|---|---|
| ASTHMA | | | | |
| PNEUMONIA/LUNG DISEASE | | | | |
| KIDNEY INFECTIONS/STONES | | | | |
| TUBERCULOSIS | | | | |
| FIBROIDS | | | | |
| SEXUALLY TRANSMITTED DISEASE/CHLAMYDIA | | | | |
| INFERTILITY | | | | |
| HIV/AIDS | | | | |
| HEART ATTACK/DISEASE | | | | |
| DIABETES | | | | |
| HIGH BLOOD PRESSURE | | | | |
| STROKE | | | | |
| RHEUMATIC FEVER | | | | |
| BLOOD CLOTS IN LUNGS OR LEGS | | | | |
| EATING DISORDERS | | | | |
| AUTOIMMUNE DISEASE (LUPUS) | | | | |
| CHICKENPOX | | | | |
| CANCER | | | | |
| REFLUX/HIATAL HERNIA/ULCERS | | | | |
| DEPRESSION/ANXIETY | | | | |
| ANEMIA | | | | |
| BLOOD TRANSFUSIONS | | | | |
| SEIZURES/CONVULSIONS/EPILEPSY | | | | |
| BOWEL PROBLEMS | | | | |
| GLAUCOMA | | | | |
| CATARACTS | | | | |
| ARTHRITIS/JOINT PAIN/BACK PROBLEMS | | | | |
| BROKEN BONES | | | | |
| HEPATITIS/YELLOW JAUNDICE/LIVER DISEASE | | | | |
| THYROID DISEASE | | | | |

American College of Obstetricians and Gynecologists

ACOG WOMAN'S HEALTH RECORD (FORM B—PATIENT INTAKE HISTORY) PAGE 3 OF 6

## PATIENT INTAKE HISTORY *(Continued)*

| PATIENT NAME: | BIRTH DATE:  /  / | ID NO.: | DATE:  /  / |
|---|---|---|---|

### PERSONAL PAST HISTORY OF ILLNESSES *(Continued)*

| MAJOR ILLNESSES | YES (DATE) | NO | NOT SURE | PHYSICIAN'S NOTES |
|---|---|---|---|---|
| GALLBLADDER DISEASE | | | | |
| HEADACHES | | | | |
| DES EXPOSURE | | | | |
| INFERTILITY | | | | |
| BLEEDING DISORDERS | | | | |
| OTHER | | | | |
| | | | | |
| | | | | |
| | | | | |

### OPERATIONS/HOSPITALIZATIONS

| REASON | DATE | HOSPITAL |
|---|---|---|
| | | |
| | | |
| | | |
| | | |
| | | |
| | | |

### INJURIES/ILLNESSES

| TYPE | DATE | TYPE | DATE |
|---|---|---|---|
| | | | |
| | | | |
| | | | |
| | | | |
| | | | |

### IMMUNIZATIONS/TEST

| | DATE | | DATE |
|---|---|---|---|
| TETANUS–DIPHTHERIA BOOSTER | | INFLUENZA VACCINE (FLU SHOT) | |
| HEPATITIS A VACCINE | | HEPATITIS B VACCINE | |
| VARICELLA (CHICKENPOX) VACCINE | | PNEUMOCOCCAL (PNEUMONIA) VACCINE | |
| MEASLES–MUMPS–RUBELLA (MMR) VACCINE | | TUBERCULOSIS (TB) SKIN TEST:    RESULT: | |

**PHYSICIAN'S NOTES:**

### REVIEW OF SYSTEMS
**Please check (x) if any of the following symptoms apply to you now or since adulthood**

| | NOW | PAST | NOT SURE | PHYSICIAN'S NOTES |
|---|---|---|---|---|
| **1. CONSTITUTIONAL** | | | | |
| WEIGHT LOSS | ☐ | ☐ | ☐ | |
| WEIGHT GAIN | ☐ | ☐ | ☐ | |
| FEVER | ☐ | ☐ | ☐ | |
| FATIGUE | ☐ | ☐ | ☐ | |
| CHANGE IN HEIGHT | ☐ | ☐ | ☐ | |

ACOG WOMAN'S HEALTH RECORD (FORM B—PATIENT INTAKE HISTORY) PAGE 4 OF 6

## PATIENT INTAKE HISTORY *(Continued)*

| PATIENT NAME: | BIRTH DATE:   /   / | ID NO.: | DATE:   /   / |
|---|---|---|---|

## REVIEW OF SYSTEMS *(Continued)*

| | NOW | PAST | NOT SURE | PHYSICIAN'S NOTES |
|---|---|---|---|---|
| **2. EYES** | | | | |
| DOUBLE VISION | ☐ | ☐ | ☐ | |
| SPOTS BEFORE EYES | ☐ | ☐ | ☐ | |
| VISION CHANGES | ☐ | ☐ | ☐ | |
| GLASSES/CONTACTS | ☐ | ☐ | ☐ | |
| **3. EAR, NOSE, AND THROAT** | | | | |
| EARACHES | ☐ | ☐ | ☐ | |
| RINGING IN EARS | ☐ | ☐ | ☐ | |
| HEARING PROBLEMS | ☐ | ☐ | ☐ | |
| SINUS PROBLEMS | ☐ | ☐ | ☐ | |
| SORE THROAT | ☐ | ☐ | ☐ | |
| MOUTH SORES | ☐ | ☐ | ☐ | |
| DENTAL PROBLEMS | ☐ | ☐ | ☐ | |
| **4. CARDIOVASCULAR** | | | | |
| CHEST PAIN OR PRESSURE | ☐ | ☐ | ☐ | |
| DIFFICULTY BREATHING ON EXERTION | ☐ | ☐ | ☐ | |
| SWELLING OF LEGS | ☐ | ☐ | ☐ | |
| RAPID OR IRREGULAR HEARTBEAT | ☐ | ☐ | ☐ | |
| **5. RESPIRATORY** | | | | |
| PAINFUL BREATHING | ☐ | ☐ | ☐ | |
| WHEEZING | ☐ | ☐ | ☐ | |
| SPITTING UP BLOOD | ☐ | ☐ | ☐ | |
| SHORTNESS OF BREATH | ☐ | ☐ | ☐ | |
| CHRONIC COUGH | ☐ | ☐ | ☐ | |
| **6. GASTROINTESTINAL** | | | | |
| FREQUENT DIARRHEA | ☐ | ☐ | ☐ | |
| BLOODY STOOL | ☐ | ☐ | ☐ | |
| NAUSEA/VOMITING/INDIGESTION | ☐ | ☐ | ☐ | |
| CONSTIPATION | ☐ | ☐ | ☐ | |
| INVOLUNTARY LOSS OF GAS OR STOOL | ☐ | ☐ | ☐ | |
| **7. GENITOURINARY** | | | | |
| BLOOD IN URINE | ☐ | ☐ | ☐ | |
| PAIN WITH URINATION | ☐ | ☐ | ☐ | |
| STRONG URGENCY TO URINATE | ☐ | ☐ | ☐ | |
| FREQUENT URINATION | ☐ | ☐ | ☐ | |
| INCOMPLETE EMPTYING | ☐ | ☐ | ☐ | |
| INVOLUNTARY/UNINTENDED URINE LOSS | ☐ | ☐ | ☐ | |
| URINE LOSS WHEN COUGHING OR LIFTING | ☐ | ☐ | ☐ | |
| ABNORMAL BLEEDING | ☐ | ☐ | ☐ | |
| PAINFUL PERIODS | ☐ | ☐ | ☐ | |
| PREMENSTRUAL SYNDROME (PMS) | ☐ | ☐ | ☐ | |
| PAINFUL INTERCOURSE | ☐ | ☐ | ☐ | |
| ABNORMAL VAGINAL DISCHARGE | ☐ | ☐ | ☐ | |
| **8. MUSCULOSKELETAL** | | | | |
| MUSCLE WEAKNESS | ☐ | ☐ | ☐ | |

## PATIENT INTAKE HISTORY *(Continued)*

| PATIENT NAME: | | | | BIRTH DATE:  /  / | ID NO.: | DATE:  /  / |

### REVIEW OF SYSTEMS *(Continued)*

| | NOW | PAST | NOT SURE | PHYSICIAN'S NOTES |
|---|---|---|---|---|
| **8. MUSCULOSKELETAL** *(Continued)* | | | | |
| MUSCLE OR JOINT PAIN | ☐ | ☐ | ☐ | |
| **9a. SKIN** | | | | |
| RASH | ☐ | ☐ | ☐ | |
| SORES | ☐ | ☐ | ☐ | |
| DRY SKIN | ☐ | ☐ | ☐ | |
| MOLES (GROWTH OR CHANGES) | ☐ | ☐ | ☐ | |
| **9b. BREASTS** | | | | |
| PAIN IN BREAST | ☐ | ☐ | ☐ | |
| NIPPLE DISCHARGE | ☐ | ☐ | ☐ | |
| LUMPS | ☐ | ☐ | ☐ | |
| **10. NEUROLOGIC** | | | | |
| DIZZINESS | ☐ | ☐ | ☐ | |
| SEIZURES | ☐ | ☐ | ☐ | |
| NUMBNESS | ☐ | ☐ | ☐ | |
| TROUBLE WALKING | ☐ | ☐ | ☐ | |
| MEMORY PROBLEMS | ☐ | ☐ | ☐ | |
| FREQUENT HEADACHES | ☐ | ☐ | ☐ | |
| **11. PSYCHIATRIC** | | | | |
| DEPRESSION OR FREQUENT CRYING | ☐ | ☐ | ☐ | |
| ANXIETY | ☐ | ☐ | ☐ | |
| **12. ENDOCRINE** | | | | |
| HAIR LOSS | ☐ | ☐ | ☐ | |
| HEAT/COLD INTOLERANCE | ☐ | ☐ | ☐ | |
| ABNORMAL THIRST | ☐ | ☐ | ☐ | |
| HOT FLASHES | ☐ | ☐ | ☐ | |
| **13. HEMATOLOGIC/LYMPHATIC** | | | | |
| FREQUENT BRUISES | ☐ | ☐ | ☐ | |
| CUTS DO NOT STOP BLEEDING | ☐ | ☐ | ☐ | |
| ENLARGED LYMPH NODES (GLANDS) | ☐ | ☐ | ☐ | |
| **14. ALLERGIC/IMMUNOLOGIC** | | | | |
| MEDICATION ALLERGIES | ☐ | ☐ | ☐ | |
| IF ANY, PLEASE LIST ALLERGY AND TYPE OF REACTION: | | | | |
| LATEX ALLERGY | ☐ | ☐ | ☐ | |
| OTHER ALLERGIES | ☐ | ☐ | ☐ | |
| PLEASE LIST ALLERGY AND TYPE OF REACTION: | | | | |

| FORM COMPLETED BY: ☐ PATIENT  ☐ OFFICE NURSE  ☐ PHYSICIAN  ☐ OTHER: |
|---|

| SIGNATURE OF PATIENT: |
|---|

| DATE REVIEWED BY PHYSICIAN WITH PATIENT:  /  / | PHYSICIAN SIGNATURE: |
|---|---|

| **ANNUAL REVIEW OF HISTORY** | |
|---|---|
| DATE REVIEWED:  /  / | PHYSICIAN SIGNATURE: |
| DATE REVIEWED:  /  / | PHYSICIAN SIGNATURE: |
| DATE REVIEWED:  /  / | PHYSICIAN SIGNATURE: |
| DATE REVIEWED:  /  / | PHYSICIAN SIGNATURE: |
| DATE REVIEWED:  /  / | PHYSICIAN SIGNATURE: |

ACOG WOMAN'S HEALTH RECORD (FORM B—PATIENT INTAKE HISTORY)  PAGE 6 OF 6

Patient Addressograph

PATIENT NAME:_____

BIRTH DATE:_____

ID NO.:_____

DATE:_____

# PROBLEM LIST

| HIGH RISK: | FAMILY HISTORY: |
|---|---|
| | |
| | |
| | |
| | |
| **DRUG/LATEX/TRANSFUSION/ALLERGIC REACTIONS:** | **CURRENT MEDICATIONS:** |
| | |
| | |
| | |
| | |
| | |
| | |

| NO. | ENTRY DATE | PROBLEM/RESOLUTION | ONSET AGE AND DATE | RESOLUTION DATE |
|---|---|---|---|---|
| 1 | | | | |
| 2 | | | | |
| 3 | | | | |
| 4 | | | | |
| 5 | | | | |
| 6 | | | | |
| 7 | | | | |
| 8 | | | | |
| 9 | | | | |
| 10 | | | | |
| 11 | | | | |
| 12 | | | | |
| 13 | | | | |
| 14 | | | | |
| 15 | | | | |
| 16 | | | | |
| 17 | | | | |
| 18 | | | | |
| 19 | | | | |
| 20 | | | | |
| 21 | | | | |
| 22 | | | | |
| 23 | | | | |
| 24 | | | | |
| 25 | | | | |

ACOG WOMAN'S HEALTH RECORD (FORM C—PROBLEM LIST/IMMUNIZATIONS/SCREENING RECORD) PAGE 1 OF 4

American College of Obstetricians and Gynecologists

ACOG WOMAN'S HEALTH RECORD (FORM C—PROBLEM LIST/IMMUNIZATIONS/SCREENING RECORD) PAGE 2 OF 4

## IMMUNIZATION RECORD*

PATIENT NAME:     BIRTH DATE:  / /     ID NO.:

| AGE | TETANUS–DIPHTHERIA BOOSTER | INFLUENZA VACCINE | PNEUMOCOCCAL VACCINE | MMR VACCINE | HEPATITIS B VACCINE | HEPATITIS A VACCINE | VARICELLA VACCINE |
|---|---|---|---|---|---|---|---|
| 13–18 | ONCE BETWEEN AGES 11–16 | BASED ON RISK | BASED ON RISK | BASED ON RISK | ONE SERIES FOR THOSE NOT PREVIOUSLY IMMUNIZED | BASED ON RISK | BASED ON RISK |
| 19–39 | EVERY 10 YEARS | BASED ON RISK | BASED ON RISK | BASED ON RISK | BASED ON RISK | BASED ON RISK | BASED ON RISK |
| 40–64 | EVERY 10 YEARS | ANNUALLY BEGINNING AT AGE 50 YEARS | BASED ON RISK | BASED ON RISK | BASED ON RISK | BASED ON RISK | BASED ON RISK |
| 65 AND OLDER | EVERY 10 YEARS | ANNUALLY | ONCE | | BASED ON RISK | BASED ON RISK | BASED ON RISK |

| DATE | | | | | | | |
|---|---|---|---|---|---|---|---|
| DATE | | | | | | | |
| DATE | | | | | | | |
| DATE | | | | | | | |
| DATE | | | | | | | |
| DATE | | | | | | | |
| DATE | | | | | | | |
| DATE | | | | | | | |
| DATE | | | | | | | |
| DATE | | | | | | | |
| DATE | | | | | | | |
| DATE | | | | | | | |
| DATE | | | | | | | |
| DATE | | | | | | | |
| DATE | | | | | | | |
| DATE | | | | | | | |
| DATE | | | | | | | |
| DATE | | | | | | | |
| DATE | | | | | | | |

*For immunizations based on risk refer to the Table of High-Risk Factors.

American College of Obstetricians and Gynecologists

**ROUTINE SCREENING RECORD**

PATIENT NAME: _____    BIRTH DATE: __/__/__    ID NO.: _____

| AGE | CERVICAL CYTOLOGY | LIPID PROFILE ASSESSMENT* | MAMMOGRAPHY* | COLORECTAL CANCER SCREENING* | BONE DENSITY SCREENING* | CHLAMYDIA SCREENING* | GONORRHEA SCREENING* | URINALYSIS | FASTING GLUCOSE TEST* | THYROID STIMULATING HORMONE SCREENING* |
|---|---|---|---|---|---|---|---|---|---|---|
| 13–18 | ANNUALLY BEGINNING APPROXIMATELY 3 YEARS AFTER INITIATION OF SEXUAL INTERCOURSE | | | | | SEXUALLY ACTIVE WOMEN UNDER AGE 25 | SEXUALLY ACTIVE ADOLESCENTS | | | |
| 19–39 | ANNUALLY BEGINNING NO LATER THAN AGE 21 YEARS | | | | | SEXUALLY ACTIVE WOMEN UNDER AGE 25 | | | | |
| 40–64 | EVERY 2–3 YEARS AFTER 3 CONSECUTIVE NEGATIVE TEST RESULTS IF NO HISTORY OF CIN 2 OR 3, IMMUNOSUPPRESSION, HIV INFECTION, OR DES EXPOSURE IN UTERO | EVERY 5 YEARS BEGINNING AT AGE 45 | EVERY 1–2 YEARS UNTIL AGE 50; YEARLY BEGINNING AT AGE 50 | BEGINNING AT AGE 50 YEARLY FOBT OR FLEXIBLE SIGMOIDOSCOPY EVERY 5 YEARS OR YEARLY FOBT PLUS FLEXIBLE SIGMOIDOSCOPY EVERY 5 YEARS OR DCBE EVERY 5 YEARS OR COLONOSCOPY EVERY 10 YEARS | | | | | EVERY 3 YEARS AFTER AGE 45 | EVERY 5 YEARS BEGINNING AT AGE 50 |
| 65 AND OLDER | EVERY 2–3 YEARS AFTER 3 CONSECUTIVE NEGATIVE TEST RESULTS IF NO HISTORY OF CIN 2 OR 3, IMMUNOSUPPRESSION, HIV INFECTION, OR DES EXPOSURE IN UTERO | EVERY 5 YEARS | YEARLY OR AS APPROPRIATE | YEARLY FOBT OR FLEXIBLE SIGMOIDOSCOPY EVERY 5 YEARS OR YEARLY FOBT PLUS FLEXIBLE SIGMOIDOSCOPY EVERY 5 YEARS OR DCBE EVERY 5 YEARS OR COLONOSCOPY EVERY 10 YEARS | IN THE ABSENCE OF NEW RISK FACTORS, SUBSEQUENT SCREENING NOT MORE FREQUENTLY THAN EVERY 2 YEARS | | | YEARLY OR AS APPROPRIATE | EVERY 3 YEARS | EVERY 5 YEARS |

| | | | | | | | | | | |
|---|---|---|---|---|---|---|---|---|---|---|
| DATE: | | | | | | | | | | |
| RESULT: | | | | | | | | | | |
| DATE: | | | | | | | | | | |
| RESULT: | | | | | | | | | | |
| DATE: | | | | | | | | | | |
| RESULT: | | | | | | | | | | |
| DATE: | | | | | | | | | | |
| RESULT: | | | | | | | | | | |
| DATE: | | | | | | | | | | |
| RESULT: | | | | | | | | | | |
| DATE: | | | | | | | | | | |
| RESULT: | | | | | | | | | | |
| DATE: | | | | | | | | | | |
| RESULT: | | | | | | | | | | |
| DATE: | | | | | | | | | | |
| RESULT: | | | | | | | | | | |
| DATE: | | | | | | | | | | |
| RESULT | | | | | | | | | | |

*This test may be appropriate for other patients based on risk (see High-Risk Laboratory Record and Table of High-Risk Factors)

American College of Obstetricians and Gynecologists

**ACOG WOMAN'S HEALTH RECORD** (FORM C—PROBLEM LIST/IMMUNIZATIONS/SCREENING RECORD) PAGE 3 OF 4

ACOG WOMAN'S HEALTH RECORD (FORM C—PROBLEM LIST/IMMUNIZATIONS/SCREENING RECORD) PAGE 4 OF 4

## HIGH-RISK SCREENING RECORD*

PATIENT NAME: _____  BIRTH DATE: ___/___/___  ID NO.: _____

| | HEMOGLOBIN TEST | BONE DENSITY SCREENING | BACTERIURIA TEST | STD TESTING | HIV TEST** | GENETIC TESTING | RUBELLA TITER | TB SKIN TEST | LIPID PROFILE ASSESSMENT | MAMMOGRAPHY | FASTING GLUCOSE TEST | TSH TEST | COLORECTAL CANCER SCREENING | HEPATITIS C VIRUS TEST |
|---|---|---|---|---|---|---|---|---|---|---|---|---|---|---|
| DATE: | | | | | | | | | | | | | | |
| RESULT: | | | | | | | | | | | | | | |
| DATE: | | | | | | | | | | | | | | |
| RESULT: | | | | | | | | | | | | | | |
| DATE: | | | | | | | | | | | | | | |
| RESULT: | | | | | | | | | | | | | | |
| DATE: | | | | | | | | | | | | | | |
| RESULT: | | | | | | | | | | | | | | |
| DATE: | | | | | | | | | | | | | | |
| RESULT: | | | | | | | | | | | | | | |
| DATE: | | | | | | | | | | | | | | |
| RESULT: | | | | | | | | | | | | | | |
| DATE: | | | | | | | | | | | | | | |
| RESULT: | | | | | | | | | | | | | | |
| DATE: | | | | | | | | | | | | | | |
| RESULT: | | | | | | | | | | | | | | |
| DATE: | | | | | | | | | | | | | | |
| RESULT: | | | | | | | | | | | | | | |
| DATE: | | | | | | | | | | | | | | |
| RESULT: | | | | | | | | | | | | | | |

*See Table of High-Risk Factors.

**Check state requirements before recording results.

American College of Obstetricians and Gynecologists

## ACOG WOMAN'S HEALTH RECORD

# CODING TIPS*

## HISTORY

### CHIEF COMPLAINT (CC)

REQUIRED FOR ALL VISITS EXCEPT PREVENTIVE VISITS

### HISTORY OF PRESENT ILLNESS (HPI)

BRIEF = 1–3 ELEMENTS                    EXTENDED = 4+ ELEMENTS OR STATUS OF 3+ CHRONIC/INACTIVE CONDITIONS

FACTORS TO BE CONSIDERED INCLUDE:

LOCATION, QUALITY, SEVERITY, DURATION, TIMING, CONTEXT, MODIFYING FACTORS, ASSOCIATED SIGNS AND SYMPTOMS

### PAST, FAMILY, AND SOCIAL HISTORY (PFSH)

PERTINENT PFSH =    1 SPECIFIC ITEM FROM EITHER PAST, FAMILY, OR SOCIAL HISTORY

COMPLETE PFSH =    NEW PATIENT: 1 SPECIFIC ITEM FROM EACH HISTORY TYPE (PAST, FAMILY, OR SOCIAL HISTORY)

    ESTABLISHED PATIENT: 1 SPECIFIC ITEM FROM 2 OF THE 3 HISTORY TYPES (PAST, FAMILY, OR SOCIAL HISTORY)

### REVIEW OF SYSTEMS (ROS)

PROBLEM PERTINENT ROS = POSITIVE AND PERTINENT NEGATIVE RESPONSES RELATED TO PROBLEM

EXTENDED ROS = POSITIVE AND PERTINENT NEGATIVE RESPONSES FOR 2–9 SYSTEMS

COMPLETE ROS = POSITIVE AND PERTINENT NEGATIVE RESPONSES FOR AT LEAST 10 SYSTEMS

### LEVEL OF HISTORY

(All three elements must be met for a given level of history, eg, brief HPI, problem pertinent ROS, and pertinent PFSH is an Expanded Problem Focused history)

| CC | HPI | ROS | PFSH | LEVEL OF HISTORY |
|---|---|---|---|---|
| REQUIRED | BRIEF (1–3 ELEMENTS) | NONE REQUIRED | NONE REQUIRED | PROBLEM FOCUSED |
| REQUIRED | BRIEF (1–3 ELEMENTS) | PROBLEM PERTINENT | NONE REQUIRED | EXPANDED PROBLEM FOCUSED |
| REQUIRED | EXTENDED (4+ ELEMENTS OR STATUS OF 3+ CHRONIC/INACTIVE CONDITIONS) | EXTENDED (2–9 SYSTEMS) | PERTINENT (1 OF 3) | DETAILED |
| REQUIRED | EXTENDED (4+ ELEMENTS OR STATUS OF 3+ CHRONIC/INACTIVE CONDITIONS) | COMPLETE (10+ SYSTEMS) | COMPLETE (NEW PATIENT: 3 OF 3; ESTABLISHED PATIENT: 2 OF 3) | COMPREHENSIVE |

## PHYSICAL EXAMINATION

1997 CMS Guidelines, Female Genitourinary System Examination

The female genitourinary examination template includes 9 organ systems/body areas with 3 shaded boxes and 6 unshaded boxes. The shading only becomes important when a comprehensive examination is performed. For all other levels of examination, the total number of bulleted elements documented in the medical record will determine the level that can be reported.

| LEVEL OF EXAMINATION | PERFORM AND DOCUMENT |
|---|---|
| PROBLEM FOCUSED | 1–5 ELEMENTS IDENTIFIED BY A BULLET |
| EXPANDED PROBLEM FOCUSED | 6–11 ELEMENTS IDENTIFIED BY A BULLET |
| DETAILED | 12 OR MORE ELEMENTS IDENTIFIED BY A BULLET |
| COMPREHENSIVE | ALL ELEMENTS IDENTIFIED BY A BULLET IN CONSTITUTIONAL AND GASTROINTESTINAL, ANY 7 BULLETS IN GYNECOLOGIC, AT LEAST 1 BULLET IN ALL OTHER SYSTEMS |

## MEDICAL DECISION MAKING

### AMOUNT AND COMPLEXITY OF DATA REVIEWED

MINIMAL/NONE = 1 BOX    LIMITED = 2 BOXES    MODERATE = 3 BOXES    EXTENSIVE = 4+ BOXES

THE FOLLOWING ITEMS (IF CHECKED) COUNT AS 2 BOXES:
• OLD RECORDS REVIEWED AND SUMMARIZED
• HISTORY OBTAINED FROM OTHER SOURCE
• INDEPENDENT REVIEW OF IMAGE/SPECIMEN

## CODING TIPS* *(Continued)*

## MEDICAL DECISION MAKING *(Continued)*

**DIAGNOSES/MANAGEMENT OPTIONS**

**MINIMAL** = MINOR PROBLEM; ESTABLISHED PROBLEM, STABLE/IMPROVED

**MULTIPLE** = NEW PROBLEM, NO ADDITIONAL WORKUP PLANNED

**LIMITED** = ESTABLISHED PROBLEM, WORSENING

**EXTENSIVE** = NEW PROBLEM, ADDITIONAL WORKUP PLANNED

**RISK OF COMPLICATIONS AND/OR MORBIDITY/MORTALITY FROM DIAGNOSES, DIAGNOSTIC PROCEDURES, AND MANAGEMENT CHOICES:**

**MINIMAL** (EG, COLD, ACHES AND PAINS, OVER-THE-COUNTER MEDICATIONS)

**MODERATE** (EG, BREAST MASS, IRREGULAR BLEEDING, HEADACHES, BIOPSY, MINOR SURGERY WITH RISK FACTORS, MAJOR SURGERY WITHOUT RISK FACTORS, NEW PRESCRIPTION)

**LOW** (EG, CYSTITIS, VAGINITIS, PRESCRIPTION RENEWAL, MINOR SURGERY WITHOUT RISK FACTORS)

**HIGH** (EG, PELVIC PAIN, RECTAL BLEEDING, MULTIPLE COMPLAINTS, MAJOR SURGERY WITH RISK FACTORS, CHEMOTHERAPY, EMERGENCY SURGERY)

**2 of the 3 elements must be met or exceeded to qualify for a given type of medical decision making**

| AMOUNT/COMPLEXITY OF DATA | DIAGNOSES/MANAGEMENT OPTIONS | RISK OF COMPLICATIONS | TYPE OF DECISION MAKING |
|---|---|---|---|
| MINIMAL/NONE | MINIMAL | MINIMAL | STRAIGHTFORWARD |
| LIMITED | LIMITED | LOW | LOW COMPLEXITY |
| MODERATE | MULTIPLE | MODERATE | MODERATE COMPLEXITY |
| EXTENSIVE | EXTENSIVE | HIGH | HIGH COMPLEXITY |

## CODING SUMMARY

### Office or Other Outpatient Services, New Patient

| KEY COMPONENTS | 99201 | 99202 | 99203 | 99204 | 99205 |
|---|---|---|---|---|---|
| HISTORY | PROBLEM FOCUSED | EXPANDED PROBLEM FOCUSED | DETAILED | COMPREHENSIVE | COMPREHENSIVE |
| EXAMINATION | PROBLEM FOCUSED | EXPANDED PROBLEM FOCUSED | DETAILED | COMPREHENSIVE | COMPREHENSIVE |
| MEDICAL DECISION MAKING | STRAIGHTFORWARD | STRAIGHTFORWARD | LOW COMPLEXITY | MODERATE COMPLEXITY | HIGH COMPLEXITY |
| NO. OF KEY COMPONENTS REQUIRED | ALL 3 | ALL 3 | ALL 3 | ALL 3 | ALL 3 |
| TYPICAL FACE-TO-FACE TIME (MIN) | 10 | 20 | 30 | 45 | 60 |

### Office or Other Outpatient Services, Established Patient

| KEY COMPONENTS | 99211 | 99212 | 99213 | 99214 | 99215 |
|---|---|---|---|---|---|
| HISTORY | NOT REQUIRED | PROBLEM FOCUSED | EXPANDED PROBLEM FOCUSED | DETAILED | COMPREHENSIVE |
| EXAMINATION | NOT REQUIRED | PROBLEM FOCUSED | EXPANDED PROBLEM FOCUSED | DETAILED | COMPREHENSIVE |
| MEDICAL DECISION MAKING | NOT REQUIRED | STRAIGHTFORWARD | LOW COMPLEXITY | MODERATE COMPLEXITY | HIGH COMPLEXITY |
| NO. OF KEY COMPONENTS REQUIRED | NOT REQUIRED | 2 OF 3 | 2 OF 3 | 2 OF 3 | 2 OF 3 |
| TYPICAL FACE-TO-FACE TIME (MIN) | 5 | 10 | 15 | 25 | 40 |

### Office or Other Outpatient Consultations, New or Established Patient

| KEY COMPONENTS | 99241 | 99242 | 99243 | 99244 | 99245 |
|---|---|---|---|---|---|
| HISTORY | PROBLEM FOCUSED | EXPANDED PROBLEM FOCUSED | DETAILED | COMPREHENSIVE | COMPREHENSIVE |
| EXAMINATION | PROBLEM FOCUSED | EXPANDED PROBLEM FOCUSED | DETAILED | COMPREHENSIVE | COMPREHENSIVE |
| MEDICAL DECISION MAKING | STRAIGHTFORWARD | STRAIGHTFORWARD | LOW COMPLEXITY | MODERATE COMPLEXITY | HIGH COMPLEXITY |
| NO. OF KEY COMPONENTS REQUIRED | ALL 3 | ALL 3 | ALL 3 | ALL 3 | ALL 3 |
| TYPICAL FACE-TO-FACE TIME (MIN) | 15 | 30 | 40 | 60 | 80 |

# Primary and Preventive Care: Periodic Assessments

*ABSTRACT: Periodic assessments offer an excellent opportunity for obstetricians and gynecologists to provide preventive screening, evaluation, and counseling. This Committee Opinion provides the recommendations of the American College of Obstetricians and Gynecologists' Committee on Gynecologic Practice for routine assessments in primary and preventive care for women based on age and risk factors.*

The following charts are updated versions of those previously published by the American College of Obstetricians and Gynecologists (ACOG) in Committee Opinion No. 292. This version replaces the pervious version. The policies and recommendations of ACOG committees regarding specific aspects of the health care of women have been incorporated; they may differ from the recommendations of other groups. Although there will be differences of opinion regarding some specific recommendations, the major benefit to be derived should not be lost in debating those issues. The American College of Obstetricians and Gynecologists recommends that the first visit to the obstetrician–gynecologist for screening and the provision of preventive health care services and guidance take place between the ages of 13 and 15 years.

Periodic assessments provide an excellent opportunity to counsel patients about preventive care. These assessments, yearly or as appropriate, should include screening, evaluation, and counseling based on age and risk factors. Personal behavioral characteristics are important aspects of a woman's health. Positive behaviors, such as exercise, should be reinforced, and negative ones, such as smoking, should be discouraged. The following guidelines indicate routine assessments for nonpregnant women based on age groups and risk factors (see Table 1) and list leading causes of death and morbidity for each age group identified by various sources (see box). It is recognized that variations may be required to adjust to the needs of a specific individual. For example, certain risk factors may influence additional assessments and interventions. Physicians should be alert to high-risk factors (indicated by an asterisk and further elucidated in Table 1). During evaluation, the patient should be made aware of high-risk conditions that require targeted screening or treatment.

## Periodic Assessment
## Ages 13–18 Years

### Screening

#### History

Reason for visit

Health status: medical, menstrual, surgical, family

Dietary/nutrition assessment

Physical activity

Use of complementary and alternative medicine

Tobacco, alcohol, other drug use

Abuse/neglect

Sexual practices

#### Physical Examination

Height

Weight

Body mass index

Blood pressure

Secondary sexual characteristics (Tanner staging)

Pelvic examination (when indicated by the medical history)

Skin*

#### Laboratory Testing

Periodic

Cervical cytology (annually beginning at approximately 3 years after initiation of sexual intercourse)

Chlamydia and gonorrhea testing (if sexually active)

High-Risk Groups*

Hemoglobin level assessment

Bacteriuria testing

Sexually transmitted disease testing

Human immunodeficiency virus (HIV) testing

Genetic testing/counseling

Rubella titer assessment

Tuberculosis skin testing

Lipid profile assessment

Fasting glucose testing

Hepatitis C virus testing

Colorectal cancer screening[†]

### Evaluation and Counseling

#### Sexuality

Development

High-risk behaviors

Preventing unwanted/unintended pregnancy

——Postponing sexual involvement

——Contraceptive options, including emergency contraception Sexually transmitted diseases

——Partner selection

——Barrier protection

#### Fitness and Nutrition

Dietary/nutrition assessment (including eating disorders) Exercise: discussion of program

Folic acid supplementation (0.4 mg/d)

Calcium intake

#### Psychosocial Evaluation

Suicide: depressive symptoms

Interpersonal/family relationships

Sexual identity

Personal goal development

Behavioral/learning disorders

Abuse/neglect

Satisfactory school experience

Peer relationships

Date rape prevention

#### Cardiovascular Risk Factors

Family history

Hypertension

Dyslipidemia

Obesity

Diabetes mellitus

#### Health/Risk Behaviors

Hygiene (including dental), fluoride supplementation*

Injury prevention

——Safety belts and helmets

——Recreational hazards

——Firearms

——Hearing

——Occupational hazards

——School hazards

——Exercise and sports involvement

Skin exposure to ultraviolet rays

Tobacco, alcohol, other drug use

### Immunizations

#### Periodic

Tetanus–diphtheria–pertussis booster (once between ages 11 years and 16 years)

Hepatitis B vaccine (1 series for those not previously immunized)

Human papillomavirus vaccine (1 series for those not previously immunized)

Meningococcal conjugate vaccine (before entry into high school for those not previously immunized)

#### High-Risk Groups*

Influenza vaccine

Hepatitis A vaccine

Pneumococcal vaccine

Measles–mumps–rubella vaccine

Varicella vaccine

---

**Leading Causes of Death[‡]**

1. Accidents
2. Malignant neoplasms
3. Homicide
4. Suicide
5. Congenital anomalies
6. Diseases of the heart
7. Chronic lower respiratory diseases
8. Influenza and pneumonia
9. Septicemia
10. Pregnancy, childbirth, and puerperium

---

**Leading Causes of Morbidity[‡]**

Acne

Asthma

Chlamydia

Headache

Mental disorders, including affective and neurotic disorders

Nose, throat, ear, and upper respiratory infections

Obesity

Sexual assault

Sexually transmitted diseases

Urinary tract infections

Vaginitis

---

*See Table 1.

[†]Only for those with a family history of familial adenomatous polyposis or 8 years after the start of pancolitis. For a more detailed discussion of colorectal cancer screening, see Smith RA, von Eschenbach AC, Wender R, Levin B, Byers T, Rothenberger D, et al. ACS American Cancer Society guidelines for the early detection of cancer: update of early detection guidelines for prostate, colorectal, and endometrial cancers. Also: update 2001—testing for early lung cancer detection. Prostate Cancer Advisory Committee, ACS Colorectal Cancer Advisory Committee, ACS Endometrial Cancer Advisory Committee [published erratum appears in CA Cancer J Clin 2001;51:150]. CA Cancer J Clin 2001;51:38-75; quiz 77–80.

[‡]See box.

**Periodic Assessment**
**Ages 19–39 Years**

## Screening

### History

Reason for visit

Health status: medical, surgical, family

Dietary/nutrition assessment

Physical activity

Use of complementary and alternative medicine

Tobacco, alcohol, other drug use

Abuse/neglect

Sexual practices

Urinary and fecal incontinence

### Physical Examination

Height

Weight

Body mass index

Blood pressure

Neck: adenopathy, thyroid

Breasts

Abdomen

Pelvic examination

Skin*

### Laboratory Testing

#### Periodic

Cervical cytology (annually beginning no later than age 21 years; every 2–3 years after three consecutive negative test results if age 30 years or older with no history of cervical intraepithelial neoplasia 2 or 3, immunosuppression, human immunodeficiency virus [HIV] infection, or diethylstilbestrol exposure in utero)†

Chlamydia testing (if ≤aged 25 years or older and sexually active)

#### High-Risk Groups*

Hemoglobin level assessment

Bacteriuria testing

Mammography

Fasting glucose testing

Sexually transmitted disease testing

Human Immunodeficiency virus (HIV) testing

Genetic testing/counseling

Rubella titer assessment

Tuberculosis skin testing

Lipid profile assessment

Thyroid-stimulating hormone testing

Hepatitis C virus testing

Colorectal cancer screening

Bone density screening

## Evaluation and Counseling

### Sexuality and Reproductive Planning

High-risk behaviors

Discussion of a reproductive health plan‡

Contraceptive options for prevention of unwanted pregnancy, including emergency contraception

Preconception and genetic counseling

Sexually transmitted diseases

—Partner selection

—Barrier protection

Sexual function

### Fitness and Nutrition

Dietary/nutrition assessment

Exercise: discussion of program

Folic acid supplementation (0.4 mg/d)

Calcium intake

### Psychosocial Evaluation

Interpersonal/family relationships

Intimate partner violence

Work satisfaction

Lifestyle/stress

Sleep disorders

### Cardiovascular Risk Factors

Family history

Hypertension

Dyslipidemia

Obesity

Diabetes mellitus

Lifestyle

### Health/Risk Behaviors

Hygiene (including dental)

Injury prevention

—Safety belts and helmets

—Occupational hazards

—Recreational hazards

—Firearms

—Hearing

—Exercise and sports involvement

Breast self-examination§

Chemoprophylaxis for breast cancer (for high-risk women aged 35 years or older)‖

Skin exposure to ultraviolet rays

Suicide: depressive symptoms

Tobacco, alcohol, other drug use

### Immunizations

#### Periodic

Human papillomavirus vaccine (one series for those aged 26 years or less and not previously immunized)

Tetanus–diphtheria–pertussis booster (every 10 years)

#### High-Risk Groups*

Measles–mumps–rubella vaccine

Hepatitis A vaccine

Hepatitis B vaccine

Influenza vaccine

Meningococcal vaccine

Pneumococcal vaccine

Varicella vaccine

### Leading Causes of Death‖

1. Malignant neoplasms
2. Accidents
3. Diseases of the heart
4. Suicide
5. Human immunodeficiency virus (HIV) disease
6. Homicide
7. Cerebrovascular diseases
8. Diabetes mellitus
9. Chronic liver diseases and cirrhosis
10. Chronic lower respiratory diseases

### Leading Causes of Morbidity‖

Acne

Arthritis

Asthma

Back symptoms

Cancer

Chlamydia

Depression

Diabetes mellitus

Gynecologic disorders

Headache/migraine

Hypertension

Joint disorders

Menstrual disorders

Mental disorders, including affective and neurotic disorders

Nose, throat, ear, and upper respiratory infections

Obesity

Sexual assault/domestic violence

Sexually transmitted diseases

Substance abuse

Urinary tract infections

---

*See Table 1.

†For a more detailed discussion of cervical cytology screening, including the use of human papillomavirus DNA testing and screening after hysterectomy, see Cervical cytology screening. ACOG Practice Bulletin No. 99. American College of Obstetricians and Gynecologists. Obstet Gynecol 2008;112:1419–44.

‡For a more detailed discussion of the reproductive health plan, see The importance of preconception care in the continuum of women's health care. ACOG Committee Opinion No. 313. American College of Obstetricians and Gynecologists. Obstet Gynecol 2005;106:665–6.

§Despite a lack of definite data for or against breast self-examination, breast self-examination has the potential to detect palpable breast cancer and can be recommended.

‖For a more detailed discussion of risk assessment and chemoprevention therapy, see Selective estrogen receptor modulators. ACOG Practice Bulletin No. 39. American College of Obstetricians and Gynecologists. Obstet Gynecol 2002;100:835-43.

¶See box.

## Periodic Assessment
## Ages 40–64 Years

### Screening

#### History

Reason for visit

Health status: medical, surgical, family

Dietary/nutrition assessment

Physical activity

Use of complementary and alternative medicine

Tobacco, alcohol, other drug use

Abuse/neglect

Sexual practices

Urinary and fecal incontinence

#### Physical Examination

Height

Weight

Body mass index

Blood pressure

Oral cavity

Neck: adenopathy, thyroid

Breasts, axillae

Abdomen

Pelvic examination

Skin*

#### Laboratory Testing

##### Periodic

Cervical cytology (every 2–3 years after three consecutive negative test results if no history of cervical intraepithelial neoplasia 2 or 3, immunosuppression, human immunodeficiency virus [HIV] infection, or diethylstilbestrol exposure in utero)†

Mammography (every 1–2 years beginning at age 40 years, yearly beginning at age 50 years)

Lipid profile assessment (every 5 years beginning at age 45 years)

Colorectal cancer screening (beginning at age 50 years), using one of the following options:

1. Yearly patient-collected fecal occult blood testing‡

2. flexible sigmoidoscopy every 5 years

3. yearly patient-collected fecal occult blood testing‡ plus flexible sigmoidoscopy every 5 years

4. double contrast barium enema every 5 years

5. colonoscopy every 10 years

Fasting glucose testing (every 3 years after age 45 years)

Thyroid-stimulating hormone screening (every 5 years beginning at age 50 years)

##### High-Risk Groups*

Hemoglobin level assessment

Bacteriuria testing

Fasting glucose testing

Sexually transmitted disease testing

Human immunodeficiency virus (HIV) testing

Tuberculosis skin testing

Lipid profile assessment

Thyroid-stimulating hormone testing

Hepatitis C virus testing

Colorectal cancer screening

### Evaluation and Counseling

#### Sexuality§

High-risk behaviors

Contraceptive options for prevention of unwanted pregnancy, including emergency contraception

Sexually transmitted diseases

——Partner selection

——Barrier protection

Sexual function

#### Fitness and Nutrition

Dietary/nutrition assessment

Exercise: discussion of program

Folic acid supplementation (0.4 mg/d before age 50 years)

Calcium intake

#### Psychosocial Evaluation

Family relationships

Intimate partner violence

Work satisfaction

Retirement planning

Lifestyle/stress

Sleep disorders

#### Cardiovascular Risk Factors

Family history

Hypertension

Dyslipidemia

Obesity

Diabetes mellitus

Lifestyle

#### Health/Risk Behaviors

Hygiene (including dental)

Hormone therapy

Injury prevention

——Safety belts and helmets

——Occupational hazards

——Recreational hazards

——Exercise and sports involvement

——Firearms

——Hearing

Breast self-examinationǁ

Chemoprophylaxis for breast cancer (for high-risk women)¶

Skin exposure to ultraviolet rays

Suicide: depressive symptoms

Tobacco, alcohol, other drug use

### Immunizations

#### Periodic

Influenza vaccine (annually beginning at age 50 years)

Tetanus-diphtheria-pertussis booster (every 10 years)

#### High-Risk Groups*

Measles–mumps–rubella vaccine

Hepatitis A vaccine

Hepatitis B vaccine

Influenza vaccine

Meningococcal vaccine

Pneumococcal vaccine

Varicella vaccine

#### Leading Causes of Death*

1. Malignant neoplasms
2. Diseases of the heart
3. Cerebrovascular diseases
4. Chronic lower respiratory diseases
5. Accidents
6. Diabetes mellitus
7. Chronic liver disease and cirrhosis
8. Septicemia
9. Suicide
10. Human immunodeficiency virus (HIV) disease

#### Leading Causes of Morbidity**

Arthritis/osteoarthritis

Asthma

Cancer

Cardiovascular disease

Depression

Diabetes mellitus

Disorders of the urinary tract

Headache/migraine

Hypertension

Menopause

Mental disorders, including affective and neurotic disorders

Musculoskeletal symptoms

Nose, throat, ear, and upper respiratory infections

Obesity

Sexually transmitted diseases

Ulcers

Vision impairment

*See Table 1.

†For a more detailed discussion of cervical cytology screening, including the use of human papillomavirus DNA testing and screening after hysterectomy, see Cervical Cytology screening. ACOG Practice Bulletin No. 99. American College of Obstetricians and Gynecologists. Obstet Gynecol 2008;112:1419–44.

‡Fecal occult blood testing (FOBT) requires two or three samples of stool collected by the patient at home and returned for analysis. A single stool sample for FOBT obtained by digital rectal examination is not adequate for the detection of colorectal cancer.

§Preconception and genetic counseling is appropriate for certain women in this age group.

ǁDespite a lack of definitive data for or against breast self-examination, breast self-examination has the potential to detect palpable breast cancer and can be recommended.

¶For a more detailed discussion of risk assessment and chemoprevention therapy, see Selective estrogen receptor modulators. ACOG Practice Bulletin No. 39. American College of Obstetricians and Gynecologists. Obstet Gynecol 2002;100:835–43.

**See box.

## Periodic Assessment
## Ages 65 Years and Older

### Screening

*History*

Reason for visit

Health status: medical, surgical, family

Dietary/nutrition assessment

Physical activity

Use of complementary and alternative medicine

Tobacco, alcohol, other drug use, and concurrent medication use

Abuse/neglect

Sexual practices

Urinary and fecal incontinence

Physical Examination

Height

Weight

Body mass index

Blood pressure

Oral cavity

Neck: adenopathy, thyroid

Breasts, axillae

Abdomen

Pelvic examination

Skin*

*Laboratory Testing*

Periodic

Cervical cytology (every 2–3 years after three consecutive negative test results if no history of cervical intraepithelial neoplasia 2 or 3, immunosuppression, human immunodeficiency virus [HIV] infection, or diethylstilbestrol exposure in utero)[†]

Urinalysis

Mammography

Lipid profile assessment (every 5 years)

Colorectal cancer screening using one of the following methods:

1. yearly patient-collected fecal occult blood testing[‡]

2. flexible sigmoidoscopy every 5 years

3. yearly patient-collected fecal occult blood testing[‡] plus flexible sigmoidoscopy every 5 years

4. double contrast barium enema every 5 years

5. colonoscopy every 10 years

Fasting glucose testing (every 3 years)

Bone density screening[§]

Thyroid-stimulating hormone screening (every 5 years)

*High-Risk Groups**

Hemoglobin level assessment

Sexually transmitted disease testing

Human immunodeficiency virus (HIV) testing

Tuberculosis skin testing

Thyroid-stimulating hormone screening

Hepatitis C virus testing

Colorectal cancer screening

### Evaluation and Counseling

*Sexuality*

Sexual function

Sexual behaviors

Sexually transmitted diseases

——Partner selection

——Barrier protection

*Fitness and Nutrition*

Dietary/nutrition assessment

Exercise: discussion of program

Calcium intake

*Psychosocial Evaluation*

Neglect/abuse

Lifestyle/stress

Depression/sleep disorders

Family relationships

Work/retirement satisfaction

*Cardiovascular Risk Factors*

Hypertension

Dyslipidemia

Obesity

Diabetes mellitus

Sedentary Lifestyle

*Health/Risk Behaviors*

Hygiene (including dental)

Hormone therapy

Injury prevention

——Safety belts and helmets

——Prevention of falls

——Occupational hazards

——Recreational hazards

——Exercise and sports involvement

——Firearms

Visual acuity/glaucoma

Hearing

Breast self-examination‖

Chemoprophylaxis for breast cancer (for high-risk women)

Skin exposure to ultraviolet rays

Suicide: depressive symptoms

Tobacco, alcohol, other drug use

### Immunizations

*Periodic*

Tetanus-diphtheria booster (every 10 years)

Influenza vaccine (annually)

Pneumococcal vaccine (once)

*High-Risk Groups**

Hepatitis A vaccine

Hepatitis B vaccine

Meningococcal vaccine

Varicella vaccine

---

*Leading Causes of Death***

1. Diseases of the heart
2. Malignant neoplasms
3. Cerebrovascular diseases
4. Chronic lower respiratory diseases
5. Alzheimer's disease
6. Influenza and pneumonia
7. Diabetes mellitus
8. Nephritis, nephrotic syndrome, and nephrosis
8. Septicemia
9. Accidents
10. Septicemia

---

*Leading Causes of Morbidity***

Arthritis/Osteoarthritis

Asthma

Cancer

Cardiovascular disease

Chronic obstructive pulmonary diseases

Diabetes mellitus

Diseases of the nervous system and sense organs

Hearing and vision impairment

Hypertension

Mental disorders

Musculoskeletal symptoms

Nose, throat, ear, and upper respiratory infections

Obesity

Osteoporosis

Pneumonia

Ulcers

Urinary incontinence

Urinary tract infections

Vertigo

---

*See Table 1.

[†]For a more detailed discussion of cervical cytology screening, including the use of human papillomavirus DNA testing and screening after hysterectomy, see Cervical Cytology screening. ACOG Practice Bulletin No. 99. American College of Obstetricians and Gynecologists. Obstet Gynecol 2008;112:1419–44.

[‡]Fecal occult blood testing (FOBT) requires two or three samples of stool collected by the patient at home and returned for analysis. A single stool sample for FOBT obtained by digital rectal examination is not adequate for detection of colorectal cancer.

[§]In the absence of new risk factors, subsequent bone density screening should not be performed more frequently than every 2 years.

‖Despite a lack of definitive data for or against breast self-examination, breast self-examination has the potential to detect palpable breast cancer and can be recommended.

¶For a more detailed discussion of risk assessment and chemoprevention therapy, See Selective estrogen receptor modulators. ACOG Practice Bulletin No. 39. American College of Obstetricians and Gynecologists. Obstet Gynecol 2002;100:835–43.

**See box.

**Table 1.** High-Risk Factors

| Intervention | High-Risk Factor |
|---|---|
| Bacteriuria testing | Diabetes mellitus |
| Bone density screening* | Postmenopausal women younger than 65 years: history of prior fracture as an adult; family history of osteoporosis; Caucasian; dementia; poor nutrition; smoking; low weight and BMI; estrogen deficiency caused by early (age younger than 45 years) menopause, bilateral oophorectomy or prolonged (longer than 1 year) premenopausal amenorrhea; low lifelong calcium intake; alcoholism; impaired eyesight despite adequate correction; history of falls; inadequate physical activity<br><br>All women: certain diseases or medical conditions and those who take certain drugs associated with an increased risk of osteoporosis |
| Colorectal cancer screening† | Colorectal cancer or adenomatous polyps in first-degree relative younger than 60 years or in two or more first-degree relatives of any ages; family history of familial adenomatous polyposis or hereditary nonpolyposis colon cancer; history of colorectal cancer, adenomatous polyps, inflammatory bowel disease, chronic ulcerative colitis, or Crohn's disease |
| Fasting glucose testing | Overweight (BMI greater than or equal to 25); family history of diabetes mellitus; habitual physical inactivity; high-risk race/ethnicity (eg, African American, Hispanic, Native American, Asian, Pacific Islander); have given birth to a newborn weighing more than 9 lb or have a history of gestational diabetes mellitus; hypertension; high-density lipoprotein cholesterol level less than or equal to 35 mg/dL; triglyceride level greater than or equal to 250 mg/dL; history of impaired glucose tolerance or impaired fasting glucose; polycystic ovary syndrome; history of vascular disease |
| Fluoride supplementation | Live in area with inadequate water fluoridation (less than 0.7 ppm) |
| Genetic testing/counseling | Considering pregnancy and: patient, partner, or family member with history of genetic disorder or birth defect; exposure to teratogens; or African, Cajun, Caucasian, European, Eastern European (Ashkenazi) Jewish, French Canadian, Mediterranean, or Southeast Asian ancestry |
| Hemoglobin level assessment | Caribbean, Latin American, Asian, Mediterranean, or African ancestry; history of excessive menstrual flow |
| HAV vaccination | Chronic liver disease, clotting factor disorders, illegal drug users, individuals who work with HAV-infected nonhuman primates or with HAV in a research laboratory setting, individuals traveling to or working in countries that have high or intermediate endemicity of hepatitis A |
| HBV vaccination | Hemodialysis patients; patients who receive clotting factor concentrates; health care workers and public safety workers who have exposure to blood in the workplace; individuals in training in schools of medicine, dentistry, nursing, laboratory technology, and other allied health professions; injecting drug users; individuals with more than one sexual partner in the previous 6 months; individuals with a recently acquired STD; all clients in STD clinics; household contacts and sexual partners of individuals with chronic HBV infection; clients and staff of institutions for the developmentally disabled; international travelers who will be in countries with high or intermediate prevalence of chronic HBV infection for more than 6 months; inmates of correctional facilities |
| HCV testing | History of injecting illegal drugs; recipients of clotting factor concentrates before 1987; chronic (long-term) hemodialysis; persistently abnormal alanine aminotransferase levels; recipients of blood from donors who later tested positive for HCV infection; recipients of blood or blood-component transfusion or organ transplant before July 1992; occupational percutaneous or mucosal exposure to HCV-positive blood |
| HIV testing | More than one sexual partner since most recent HIV test or a sex partner with more than one sexual partner since most recent HIV test, seeking treatment for STDs, drug use by injection, history of prostitution, past or present sexual partner who is HIV positive or bisexual or injects drugs, long-term residence or birth in an area with high prevalence of HIV infection, history of transfusion from 1978 to 1985, invasive cervical cancer, adolescents who are or ever have been sexually active, adolescents entering detention facilities. Offer to women seeking preconception evaluation. |

*(continued)*

**Table 1.** High-Risk Factors *(continued)*

| Intervention | High-Risk Factor |
| --- | --- |
| Influenza vaccination | Anyone who wishes to reduce the chance of becoming ill with influenza; chronic cardiovascular or pulmonary disorders, including asthma; chronic metabolic diseases, including diabetes mellitus, renal dysfunction, hemoglobinopathies, and immunosuppression (including immunosuppression caused by medications or by HIV); residents and employees of nursing homes and other long-term care facilities; individuals likely to transmit influenza to high-risk individuals (eg, household members and caregivers of the elderly, children aged from birth to 59 months, and adults with high-risk conditions); those with any condition (eg, cognitive dysfunction, spinal cord injury, seizure or other neuromuscular disorder) that compromises respiratory function or the handling of respiratory secretions, or that increases the risk of aspiration; health care workers |
| Lipid profile assessment | Family history suggestive of familial hyperlipidemia; family history of premature (age younger than 50 years for men, age younger than 60 years for women) cardiovascular disease; diabetes mellitus; multiple coronary heart disease risk factors (eg, tobacco use, hypertension) |
| Mammography | Women who have had breast cancer or who have a first-degree relative (ie, mother, sister, or daughter) or multiple other relatives who have a history of premenopausal breast or breast and ovarian cancer |
| Meningococcal vaccination | Adults with anatomic or functional asplenia or terminal complement component deficiencies, first-year college students living in dormitories, microbiologists routinely exposed to *Neisseria meningitidis* isolates, military recruits, travel to hyperendemic or epidemic areas |
| MMR vaccination | Adults born in 1957 or later should be offered vaccination (one dose of MMR) if there is no proof of immunity or documentation of a dose given after first birthday; individuals vaccinated in 1963–1967 should be offered revaccination (two doses); health care workers, students entering college, international travelers, and rubella-negative postpartum patients should be offered a second dose. |
| Pneumococcal vaccination | Chronic illness, such as cardiovascular disease, pulmonary disease, diabetes mellitus, alcoholism, chronic liver disease, cerebrospinal fluid leaks, functional asplenia (eg, sickle cell disease) or splenectomy; exposure to an environment where pneumococcal outbreaks have occurred; immuno-compromised patients (eg, HIV infection, hematologic or solid malignancies, chemotherapy, steroid therapy). Revaccination after 5 years may be appropriate for certain high-risk groups. |
| Rubella titer assessment | Childbearing age and no evidence of immunity |
| STD testing | History of multiple sexual partners or a sexual partner with multiple contacts, sexual contact with individuals with culture-proven STD, history of repeated episodes of STDs, attendance at clinics for STDs, women with developmental disabilities; routine screening for chlamydial infection for all sexually active women aged 25 years or younger and other asymptomatic women at high risk for infection; routine screening for gonorrheal infection for all sexually active adolescents and other asymptomatic women at high risk for infection; sexually active adolescents who exchange sex for drugs or money, use intravenous drugs, are entering a detention facility, or live in a high prevalence area should also be tested for syphilis. |
| Skin examination | Increased recreational or occupational exposure to sunlight; family or personal history of skin cancer; clinical evidence of precursor lesions |
| Thyroid-stimulating hormone testing | Strong family history of thyroid disease; autoimmune disease (evidence of subclinical hypothyroidism may be related to unfavorable lipid profiles) |
| Tuberculosis skin testing | HIV infection; close contact with individuals known or suspected to have tuberculosis; medical risk factors known to increase risk of disease if infected; born in country with high tuberculosis prevalence; medically underserved; low income; alcoholism; intravenous drug use; resident of long-term care facility (eg, correctional institutions, mental institutions, nursing homes and facilities); health professional working in high-risk health care facilities |
| Varicella vaccination | All susceptible adults and adolescents, including health care workers; household contacts of immunocompromised individuals; teachers; daycare workers; residents and staff of institutional settings, colleges, prisons, or military installations; adolescents and adults living in households with children; international travelers; nonpregnant women of childbearing age |

Abbreviations: BMI, body mass index; HAV, hepatitis A virus; HBV, hepatitis B virus; HCV, hepatitis C virus; HIV, human immunodeficiency virus; MMR, measles–mumps–rubella; STD, sexually transmitted disease.

*For a more detailed discussion of bone density screening, see Osteoporosis. ACOG Practice Bulletin 50. American College of Obstetricians and Gynecologists. Obstet Gynecol 2004;103:203–16.

†For a more detailed discussion of colorectal cancer screening, see Smith RA, von Eschenbach AC, Wender R, Levin B, Byers T, Rothenberger D, et al. American Cancer Society guidelines for the early detection of cancer: update of early detection guidelines for prostate, colorectal, and endometrial cancers. Also: update 2001—testing for early lung cancer detection. Prostate Cancer Advisory Committee, ACS Colorectal Cancer Advisory Committee, ACS Endometrial Cancer Advisory Committee [published erratum appears in CA Cancer J Clin 2001;51:150]. CA Cancer J Clin 2001;51:38–75; quiz 77–80.

### Sources of Leading Causes of Mortality and Morbidity

Leading causes of mortality are provided by the Mortality Statistics Branch at the National Center for Health Statistics. Data are from 2002, the most recent year for which final data are available. The causes are ranked.

Leading causes of morbidity are unranked estimates based on information from the following sources:
- National Health Interview Survey, 2004
- National Ambulatory Medical Care Survey, 2004
- National Health and Nutrition Examination Survey, 2003–2004
- National Hospital Discharge Survey, 2004
- National Nursing Home Survey, 1999
- U.S. Department of Justice National Violence Against Women Survey, 2006
- U.S. Centers for Disease Control and Prevention Sexually Transmitted Disease Surveillance, 2004
- U.S. Centers for Disease Control and Prevention HIV/AIDS Surveillance Report, 2004

# ACOG Antepartum Record and Postpartum Form

Patient Addressograph

DATE _____

NAME _____
      LAST                        FIRST                      MIDDLE

ID # _____ HOSPITAL OF DELIVERY _____

NEWBORN'S PHYSICIAN _____ REFERRED BY _____

PRIMARY PROVIDER/GROUP _____

| FINAL EDD _____ | ADDRESS _____ |

| BIRTH DATE     AGE     RACE     MARITAL STATUS<br>MONTH DAY YEAR                  SMWD     SEP | ADDRESS |
|---|---|
| OCCUPATION          EDUCATION<br>               (LAST GRADE COMPLETED) | ZIP     PHONE          (H)          (O) |
| LANGUAGE          ETHNICITY | INSURANCE CARRIER/MEDICAID # |
| HUSBAND/DOMESTIC PARTNER          PHONE | POLICY # |
| FATHER OF BABY          PHONE | EMERGENCY CONTACT          PHONE |

| TOTAL PREG | FULL TERM | PREMATURE | AB, INDUCED | AB, SPONTANEOUS | ECTOPICS | MULTIPLE BIRTHS | LIVING |
|---|---|---|---|---|---|---|---|

## MENSTRUAL HISTORY

LMP ☐ DEFINITE   ☐ APPROXIMATE (MONTH KNOWN)     MENSES MONTHLY ☐ YES ☐ NO    FREQUENCY: Q _____ DAYS     MENARCHE _____ (AGE ONSET)

      ☐ UNKNOWN   ☐ NORMAL AMOUNT/DURATION     PRIOR MENSES _____ DATE    ON BCP AT CONCEPT ☐ YES ☐ NO     hCG + ____/____/____

      ☐ FINAL _____

## PAST PREGNANCIES (LAST SIX)

| DATE<br>MONTH/<br>YEAR | GA<br>WEEKS | LENGTH<br>OF<br>LABOR | BIRTH<br>WEIGHT | SEX<br>M/F | TYPE<br>DELIVERY | ANES. | PLACE OF<br>DELIVERY | PRETERM<br>LABOR<br>YES/NO | COMMENTS/<br>COMPLICATIONS |
|---|---|---|---|---|---|---|---|---|---|
| | | | | | | | | | |
| | | | | | | | | | |
| | | | | | | | | | |
| | | | | | | | | | |
| | | | | | | | | | |

## MEDICAL HISTORY

| | ○ Neg.<br>+ Pos. | DETAIL POSITIVE REMARKS<br>INCLUDE DATE & TREATMENT | | ○ Neg.<br>+ Pos. | DETAIL POSITIVE REMARKS<br>INCLUDE DATE & TREATMENT |
|---|---|---|---|---|---|
| 1. DIABETES | | | 17. D (Rh) SENSITIZED | | |
| 2. HYPERTENSION | | | 18. PULMONARY (TB, ASTHMA) | | |
| 3. HEART DISEASE | | | 19. SEASONAL ALLERGIES | | |
| 4. AUTOIMMUNE DISORDER | | | 20. DRUG/LATEX ALLERGIES/<br>REACTIONS | | |
| 5. KIDNEY DISEASE/UTI | | | | | |
| 6. NEUROLOGIC/EPILEPSY | | | 21. BREAST | | |
| 7. PSYCHIATRIC | | | 22. GYN SURGERY | | |
| 8. DEPRESSION/POSTPARTUM<br>DEPRESSION | | | 23. OPERATIONS/<br>HOSPITALIZATIONS<br>(YEAR & REASON) | | |
| 9. HEPATITIS/LIVER DISEASE | | | | | |
| 10. VARICOSITIES/PHLEBITIS | | | 24. ANESTHETIC COMPLICATIONS | | |
| 11. THYROID DYSFUNCTION | | | 25. HISTORY OF ABNORMAL PAP | | |
| 12. TRAUMA/VIOLENCE | | | 26. UTERINE ANOMALY/DES | | |
| 13. HISTORY OF BLOOD TRANSFUS. | | | 27. INFERTILITY | | |

| | AMT/DAY<br>PREPREG | AMT/DAY<br>PREG | # YEARS<br>USE | |
|---|---|---|---|---|
| 14. TOBACCO | | | | 28. ART TREATMENT |
| 15. ALCOHOL | | | | 29. RELEVANT FAMILY HISTORY |
| 16. ILLICIT/RECREATIONAL DRUGS | | | | 30. OTHER |

COMMENTS _____

_____

Version 6. Copyright © 2007 The American College of Obstetricians and Gynecologists, 409 12th Street, SW, PO Box 96920, Washington, DC 20090-6920     AA128     12345/10987

ACOG ANTEPARTUM RECORD (FORM A)

Patient Addressograph

| SYMPTOMS SINCE LMP |
| --- |
| |
| |
| |
| |

## GENETIC SCREENING/TERATOLOGY COUNSELING
### INCLUDES PATIENT, BABY'S FATHER, OR ANYONE IN EITHER FAMILY WITH:

| | YES | NO | | YES | NO |
| --- | --- | --- | --- | --- | --- |
| 1. PATIENT'S AGE 35 YEARS OR OLDER AS OF ESTIMATED DATE OF DELIVERY | | | 13. HUNTINGTON'S CHOREA | | |
| 2. THALASSEMIA (ITALIAN, GREEK, MEDITERRANEAN, OR ASIAN BACKGROUND): MCV LESS THAN 80 | | | 14. MENTAL RETARDATION/AUTISM | | |
| | | | IF YES, WAS PERSON TESTED FOR FRAGILE X? | | |
| 3. NEURAL TUBE DEFECT (MENINGOMYELOCELE, SPINA BIFIDA, OR ANENCEPHALY) | | | 15. OTHER INHERITED GENETIC OR CHROMOSOMAL DISORDER | | |
| 4. CONGENITAL HEART DEFECT | | | 16. MATERNAL METABOLIC DISORDER (EG, TYPE 1 DIABETES, PKU) | | |
| 5. DOWN SYNDROME | | | 17. PATIENT OR BABY'S FATHER HAD A CHILD WITH BIRTH DEFECTS NOT LISTED ABOVE | | |
| 6. TAY–SACHS (ASHKENAZI JEWISH, CAJUN, FRENCH CANADIAN) | | | 18. RECURRENT PREGNANCY LOSS, OR A STILLBIRTH | | |
| 7. CANAVAN DISEASE (ASHKENAZI JEWISH) | | | 19. MEDICATIONS (INCLUDING SUPPLEMENTS, VITAMINS, HERBS OR OTC DRUGS)/ILLICIT/RECREATIONAL DRUGS/ALCOHOL SINCE LAST MENSTRUAL PERIOD | | |
| 8. FAMILIAL DYSAUTONOMIA (ASHKENAZI JEWISH) | | | IF YES, AGENT(S) AND STRENGTH/DOSAGE | | |
| 9. SICKLE CELL DISEASE OR TRAIT (AFRICAN) | | | | | |
| 10. HEMOPHILIA OR OTHER BLOOD DISORDERS | | | 20. ANY OTHER | | |
| 11. MUSCULAR DYSTROPHY | | | | | |
| 12. CYSTIC FIBROSIS | | | | | |

**COMMENTS/COUNSELING** _____

_____

| INFECTION HISTORY | YES | NO | | |
| --- | --- | --- | --- | --- |
| 1. LIVE WITH SOMEONE WITH TB OR EXPOSED TO TB | | | 4. HEPATITIS B, C          YES ☐   NO ☐ | |
| 2. PATIENT OR PARTNER HAS HISTORY OF GENITAL HERPES | | | 5. HISTORY OF STD, GONORRHEA, CHLAMYDIA, HPV, HIV, SYPHILIS (CIRCLE ALL THAT APPLY) | |
| 3. RASH OR VIRAL ILLNESS SINCE LAST MENSTRUAL PERIOD | | | 6. OTHER (SEE COMMENTS) | |

**COMMENTS** _____

_____  **INTERVIEWER'S SIGNATURE** _____

## INITIAL PHYSICAL EXAMINATION

DATE _____ / _____ / _____     WEIGHT _____     HEIGHT _____     BMI _____     BP_____

| 1. HEENT | ☐ NORMAL | ☐ ABNORMAL | 12. VULVA | ☐ NORMAL | ☐ CONDYLOMA | ☐ LESIONS |
| --- | --- | --- | --- | --- | --- | --- |
| 2. FUNDI | ☐ NORMAL | ☐ ABNORMAL | 13. VAGINA | ☐ NORMAL | ☐ INFLAMMATION | ☐ DISCHARGE |
| 3. TEETH | ☐ NORMAL | ☐ ABNORMAL | 14. CERVIX | ☐ NORMAL | ☐ INFLAMMATION | ☐ LESIONS |
| 4. THYROID | ☐ NORMAL | ☐ ABNORMAL | 15. UTERUS SIZE | _____ WEEKS | | ☐ FIBROIDS |
| 5. BREASTS | ☐ NORMAL | ☐ ABNORMAL | 16. ADNEXA | ☐ NORMAL | ☐ MASS | |
| 6. LUNGS | ☐ NORMAL | ☐ ABNORMAL | 17. RECTUM | ☐ NORMAL | ☐ ABNORMAL | |
| 7. HEART | ☐ NORMAL | ☐ ABNORMAL | 18. DIAGONAL CONJUGATE | ☐ REACHED | ☐ NO | _____ CM |
| 8. ABDOMEN | ☐ NORMAL | ☐ ABNORMAL | 19. SPINES | ☐ AVERAGE | ☐ PROMINENT | ☐ BLUNT |
| 9. EXTREMITIES | ☐ NORMAL | ☐ ABNORMAL | 20. SACRUM | ☐ CONCAVE | ☐ STRAIGHT | ☐ ANTERIOR |
| 10. SKIN | ☐ NORMAL | ☐ ABNORMAL | 21. SUBPUBIC ARCH | ☐ NORMAL | ☐ WIDE | ☐ NARROW |
| 11. LYMPH NODES | ☐ NORMAL | ☐ ABNORMAL | 22. GYNECOID PELVIC TYPE | ☐ YES | ☐ NO | |

**COMMENTS** (Number and explain abnormals) _____

_____

_____  **EXAM BY** _____

ACOG ANTEPARTUM RECORD (FORM B)

Patient Addressograph

NAME ____________________________________________
LAST FIRST MIDDLE

| | |
|---|---|
| DRUG ALLERGY________________________ | LATEX ALLERGY ☐ YES ☐ NO |
| IS BLOOD TRANSFUSION ACCEPTABLE? ☐ YES ☐ NO | ANTEPARTUM ANESTHESIA CONSULT PLANNED ☐ YES ☐ NO |

| PROBLEMS/PLANS | MEDICATION LIST (Include Dosage) | Start date | Stop date |
|---|---|---|---|
| 1. | 1. | ___/___/___ | ___/___/___ |
| 2. | 2. | ___/___/___ | ___/___/___ |
| 3. | 3. | ___/___/___ | ___/___/___ |
| 4. | 4. | ___/___/___ | ___/___/___ |
| 5. | 5. | ___/___/___ | ___/___/___ |
| 6. | 6. | ___/___/___ | ___/___/___ |

**EDD CONFIRMATION**

INITIAL EDD

| | | | |
|---|---|---|---|
| LMP | ___/___/___ | = | EDD ___/___/___ |
| INITIAL EXAM | ___/___/___ | = ___ WKS = | EDD ___/___/___ |
| ULTRASOUND | ___/___/___ | = ___ WKS = | EDD ___/___/___ |
| INITIAL EDD | ___/___/___ | | INITIALED BY ____________ |

**18–20-WEEK EDD UPDATE**

| | | | |
|---|---|---|---|
| QUICKENING | ___/___/___ | +22 WKS = | ___/___/___ |
| FUNDAL HT. AT UMBIL. | ___/___/___ | +20 WKS = | ___/___/___ |
| ULTRASOUND | ___/___/___ | = ___ WKS = | ___/___/___ |
| FINAL EDD | ___/___/___ | | INITIALED BY ____________ |

**PREPREGNANCY WEIGHT**

__________

| | WEEKS GEST. (BEST EST.) | FUNDAL HEIGHT (CM) | PRESENTATION | FHR | FETAL MOVEMENT | PRETERM LABOR SIGNS/SYMPTOMS: +=PRESENT o=ABSENT | CERVIX EXAM (DIL/EFF/STA.) ULTRASOUND LENGTH | BLOOD PRESSURE | WEIGHT | URINE (ALBUMIN/GLUCOSE) | EDEMA | PAIN SCALE* (0-10) | NEXT APPOINTMENT | PROVIDER (INITIALS) |
|---|---|---|---|---|---|---|---|---|---|---|---|---|---|---|
| | | | | | | | | | | | | | | |
| | | | | | | | | | | | | | | |
| | | | | | | | | | | | | | | |
| | | | | | | | | | | | | | | |
| | | | | | | | | | | | | | | |
| | | | | | | | | | | | | | | |
| | | | | | | | | | | | | | | |
| | | | | | | | | | | | | | | |
| | | | | | | | | | | | | | | |
| | | | | | | | | | | | | | | |
| | | | | | | | | | | | | | | |
| | | | | | | | | | | | | | | |
| | | | | | | | | | | | | | | |
| | | | | | | | | | | | | | | |
| | | | | | | | | | | | | | | |

**COMMENTS**

**PROBLEMS** ____________________________________________

**COMMENTS** ____________________________________________

*Describe the intensity of discomfort ranging from 0 (no pain) to 10 (worst possible pain).

**ACOG ANTEPARTUM RECORD** (FORM C)

Patient Addressograph

## LABORATORY AND EDUCATION

| INITIAL LABS | DATE | RESULT | REVIEWED |
|---|---|---|---|
| BLOOD TYPE | / / | A     B     AB     O | |
| D (Rh) TYPE | / / | | |
| ANTIBODY SCREEN | / / | | |
| HCT/HGB/MCV | / / | _____ % _____ g/dL | |
| PAP TEST | / / | NORMAL/ABNORMAL/_____ | |
| VARICELLA | / / | | |
| RUBELLA | / / | | |
| VDRL | / / | | |
| URINE CULTURE/SCREEN | / / | | |
| HBsAg | / / | | |
| HIV COUNSELING/TESTING* | / / | POS.     NEG.     DECLINED | |

| OPTIONAL LABS | DATE | RESULT | |
|---|---|---|---|
| HEMOGLOBIN ELECTROPHORESIS | / / | AA  AS  SS  AC  SC  AF  ↑A$_2$<br>POS.     NEG.     DECLINED | |
| PPD | / / | | |
| CHLAMYDIA | / / | | |
| GONORRHEA | / / | | |
| CYSTIC FIBROSIS | / / | POS.     NEG.     DECLINED | |
| TAY-SACHS | / / | POS.     NEG.     DECLINED | |
| FAMILIAL DYSAUTONOMIA | / / | POS.     NEG.     DECLINED | |
| HEMOGLOBIN | | | |
| GENETIC SCREENING TESTS (SEE FORM B) | / / | | |
| OTHER | | | |

| 8–20-WEEK LABS (WHEN INDICATED/ELECTED) | DATE | RESULT | |
|---|---|---|---|
| ULTRASOUND | / / | | |
| 1ST TRIMESTER ANEUPLOIDY RISK ASSESSMENT | / / | POS.     NEG.     DECLINED | |
| MSAFP/MULTIPLE MARKERS | / / | POS.     NEG.     DECLINED | |
| 2ND TRIMESTER SERUM SCREENING | / / | POS.     NEG.     DECLINED | |
| AMNIO/CVS | / / | | |
| KARYOTYPE | / / | 46,XX  OR  46,XY/OTHER_____ | |
| AMNIOTIC FLUID (AFP) | / / | NORMAL_____  ABNORMAL_____ | |
| ANTI-D IMMUNE GLOBULIN (RHIG) | / / | | |

**COMMENTS/ADDITIONAL LABS**

*Check state requirements before recording results.

*(CONTINUED)*

PROVIDER SIGNATURE (AS REQUIRED)_____

ACOG ANTEPARTUM RECORD (FORM D)

## LABORATORY AND EDUCATION (continued)

| 24–28-WEEK LABS (WHEN INDICATED) | DATE | RESULT | | COMMENTS/ADDITIONAL LABS |
|---|---|---|---|---|
| HCT/HGB/MCV | / / | _____ % _____ g/dL | | |
| DIABETES SCREEN | / / | 1 HOUR_____ | | |
| GTT (IF SCREEN ABNORMAL) | / / | ____FBS ____1 HOUR ____2 HOUR ____3 HOUR | | |
| D (Rh) ANTIBODY SCREEN | / / | | | |
| ANTI-D IMMUNE GLOBULIN (RhIG) GIVEN (28 WKS OR GREATER) | / / | SIGNATURE _____ | | |

| 32–36-WEEK LABS | DATE | RESULT | | |
|---|---|---|---|---|
| HCT/HGB | / / | _____ % _____ g/dL | | |
| ULTRASOUND (WHEN INDICATED) | / / | | | |
| HIV (WHEN INDICATED)* | | | | |
| VDRL (WHEN INDICATED) | / / | | | |
| GONORRHEA (WHEN INDICATED) | / / | | | |
| CHLAMYDIA (WHEN INDICATED) | / / | | | |
| GROUP B STREP | / / | | | |

*Check state requirements before recording results.

**COMMENTS**

_____
_____
_____
_____
_____
_____
_____

PROVIDER SIGNATURE (AS REQUIRED)_____

ACOG ANTEPARTUM RECORD (FORM D, *continued*)

Patient Addressograph

NAME _____

LAST                    FIRST                    MIDDLE

**PLANS/EDUCATION**
(COUNSELED ☐)—BY TRIMESTER. INITIAL AND DATE WHEN DISCUSSED.

| FIRST TRIMESTER | COMPLETED | NEED FOR FURTHER DISCUSSION |
|---|---|---|
| ☐ HIV AND OTHER ROUTINE PRENATAL TESTS | | ☐ FOLLOW-UP IN 3RD TRIMESTER, IF NEEDED |
| ☐ RISK FACTORS IDENTIFIED BY PRENATAL HISTORY | | |
| ☐ ANTICIPATED COURSE OF PRENATAL CARE | | |
| ☐ NUTRITION AND WEIGHT GAIN COUNSELING; SPECIAL DIET | | |
| ☐ TOXOPLASMOSIS PRECAUTIONS (CATS/RAW MEAT) | | |
| ☐ SEXUAL ACTIVITY | | |
| ☐ EXERCISE | | |
| ☐ INFLUENZA VACCINE | | |
| ☐ SMOKING COUNSELING | | |
| ☐ ENVIRONMENTAL/WORK HAZARDS | | |
| ☐ TRAVEL | | |
| ☐ TOBACCO (ASK, ADVISE, ASSESS, ASSIST, AND ARRANGE) | | |
| ☐ ALCOHOL | | |
| ☐ ILLICIT/RECREATIONAL DRUGS | | |
| ☐ USE OF ANY MEDICATIONS (INCLUDING SUPPLEMENTS, VITAMINS, HERBS, OR OTC DRUGS) | | |
| ☐ INDICATIONS FOR ULTRASOUND | | |
| ☐ DOMESTIC VIOLENCE | | |
| ☐ SEAT BELT USE | | |
| ☐ CHILDBIRTH CLASSES/HOSPITAL FACILITIES | | |
| **SECOND TRIMESTER** | | |
| ☐ SIGNS AND SYMPTOMS OF PRETERM LABOR | | |
| ☐ ABNORMAL LAB VALUES | | |
| ☐ INFLUENZA VACCINE | | |
| ☐ SELECTING A NEWBORN CARE PROVIDER | | |
| ☐ SMOKING COUNSELING | | |
| ☐ DOMESTIC VIOLENCE | | |
| ☐ POSTPARTUM FAMILY PLANNING/TUBAL STERILIZATION | | |

*(CONTINUED)*

**COMMENTS**
_____
_____
_____
_____
_____

ACOG ANTEPARTUM RECORD (FORM E)

Patient Addressograph

**PLANS/EDUCATION** *(continued)*
(COUNSELED ☐)—BY TRIMESTER. INITIAL AND DATE WHEN DISCUSSED.

| THIRD TRIMESTER | COMPLETED | NEED FOR FURTHER DISCUSSION |
|---|---|---|
| ☐ ANESTHESIA/ANALGESIA PLANS | | |
| ☐ FETAL MOVEMENT MONITORING | | |
| ☐ LABOR SIGNS | | |
| ☐ VBAC COUNSELING | | |
| ☐ SIGNS AND SYMPTOMS OF PREGNANCY-INDUCED HYPERTENSION | | |
| ☐ POSTTERM COUNSELING | | |
| ☐ CIRCUMCISION | | |
| ☐ BREAST OR BOTTLE FEEDING | | |
| ☐ POSTPARTUM DEPRESSION | | |
| ☐ INFLUENZA VACCINE | | |
| ☐ SMOKING COUNSELING | | |
| ☐ DOMESTIC VIOLENCE | | |
| ☐ NEWBORN EDUCATION (NEWBORN SCREENING, JAUNDICE, SIDS, CAR SEAT) | | |
| ☐ FAMILY MEDICAL LEAVE OR DISABILITY FORMS | | |

REQUESTS

TUBAL STERILIZATION CONSENT SIGNED               DATE               INITIALS
                                        ___/___/___        _____

HISTORY AND PHYSICAL HAVE BEEN SENT TO HOSPITAL, IF APPLICABLE.     DATE               INITIALS
                                        ___/___/___        _____

COMMENTS

ACOG ANTEPARTUM RECORD (FORM E, *continued*)

## Plans/Education Notes

_____
_____
_____
_____
_____
_____
_____
_____
_____
_____
_____
_____
_____
_____
_____
_____
_____
_____
_____
_____
_____
_____
_____
_____
_____
_____
_____
_____
_____
_____

ACOG ANTEPARTUM RECORD (FORM E, *continued*)

Patient Addressograph

NAME _____
      LAST           FIRST          MIDDLE

ID # _____

EDD _____

## Supplemental Visits

PREPREGNANCY WEIGHT

_____

Column headers (rotated): WEEKS GEST. (BEST EST.) | FUNDAL HEIGHT (CM) | PRESENTATION | FHR | FETAL MOVEMENT | PRETERM LABOR SIGNS/SYMPTOMS: +=PRESENT o=ABSENT | CERVIX EXAM (DIL./EFF./STA.) ULTRASOUND LENGTH | BLOOD PRESSURE | WEIGHT | URINE (ALBUMIN/GLUCOSE) | EDEMA | PAIN SCALE* (0-10) | NEXT APPOINTMENT | PROVIDER (INITIALS)

COMMENTS

*Describe the intensity of discomfort ranging from 0 (no pain) to 10 (worst possible pain).

## Progress Notes

PROVIDER SIGNATURE (AS REQUIRED) _____

**ACOG ANTEPARTUM RECORD** (FORM F)

Patient Addressograph

NAME ______________________________________________
LAST FIRST MIDDLE

ID # ______________________________________________

EDD ______________________________

## Supplemental Visits

PREPREGNANCY WEIGHT ____________

| | WEEKS GEST. (BEST EST.) | FUNDAL HEIGHT (CM) | PRESENTATION | FHR | FETAL MOVEMENT | PRETERM LABOR SIGNS/SYMPTOMS: +=PRESENT o=ABSENT | CERVIX EXAM (DIL./EFF./STA.) ULTRASOUND LENGTH | BLOOD PRESSURE | WEIGHT | URINE (ALBUMIN/GLUCOSE) | EDEMA | PAIN SCALE* (0-10) | NEXT APPOINTMENT | PROVIDER (INITIALS) |
|---|---|---|---|---|---|---|---|---|---|---|---|---|---|---|
| | | | | | | | | | | | | | | |
| | | | | | | | | | | | | | | |
| | | | | | | | | | | | | | | |
| | | | | | | | | | | | | | | |
| | | | | | | | | | | | | | | |
| | | | | | | | | | | | | | | |
| | | | | | | | | | | | | | | |
| | | | | | | | | | | | | | | |
| | | | | | | | | | | | | | | |
| | | | | | | | | | | | | | | |
| | | | | | | | | | | | | | | |
| | | | | | | | | | | | | | | |
| | | | | | | | | | | | | | | |
| | | | | | | | | | | | | | | |
| | | | | | | | | | | | | | | |

**COMMENTS**

*Describe the intensity of discomfort ranging from 0 (no pain) to 10 (worst possible pain).

## Progress Notes

PROVIDER SIGNATURE (AS REQUIRED) ______________________________________________

**ACOG ANTEPARTUM RECORD** (FORM F, *continued*)

NAME _____
　　　LAST　　　　　　　　FIRST　　　　　　　MIDDLE

ID # _____

# Progress Notes

_____
_____
_____
_____
_____
_____
_____
_____
_____
_____
_____
_____
_____
_____
_____
_____
_____
_____
_____
_____
_____
_____
_____
_____
_____
_____
_____
_____
_____
_____
_____

PROVIDER SIGNATURE (AS REQUIRED)_____

**ACOG ANTEPARTUM RECORD** (FORM G)

NAME _____
      LAST                FIRST           MIDDLE

ID # _____

## Progress Notes

_____

_____

_____

_____

_____

_____

_____

_____

_____

_____

_____

_____

_____

_____

_____

_____

_____

_____

_____

_____

_____

_____

_____

_____

_____

_____

_____

_____

_____

PROVIDER SIGNATURE (AS REQUIRED)_____

**ACOG ANTEPARTUM RECORD** (FORM G, continued)

Patient Addressograph

## DISCHARGE/POSTPARTUM FORM

DELIVERY DATE _____    HOSPITAL _____

DISCHARGE DATE _____

### DELIVERY INFORMATION

**DELIVERY AT_____WEEKS**

☐ VAGINAL ☐ CESAREAN    TUBAL STERILIZATION ☐ YES ☐ NO
  ☐ SVD ☐ PRIMARY (For_____ )    NOTES _____
  ☐ VACUUM ☐ REPEAT - ELECTIVE    _____
  ☐ FORCEPS ☐ REPEAT - UNSUCCESSFUL VBAC    _____
  ☐ EPISIOTOMY ☐ INCISION    _____
  ☐ LACERATIONS ☐ LOW TRANSVERSE    _____
  ☐ VBAC ☐ LOW VERTICAL    _____
  ☐ CLASSICAL    DELIVERED BY_____

LABOR
  ☐ NONE
  ☐ SPONTANEOUS
  ☐ INDUCED
  ☐ AUGMENTED

ANESTHESIA
  ☐ NONE
  ☐ LOCAL/PUDENDAL
  ☐ EPIDURAL
  ☐ SPINAL
  ☐ GENERAL
  ☐ OTHER

### POSTPARTUM INFORMATION

**COMPLICATIONS**

☐ NONE    ☐ HEMORRHAGE    ☐ INFECTION    ☐ HYPERTENSION    ☐ OTHER _____

### DISCHARGE INFORMATION

**NEONATAL INFORMATION**

NAME OF BABY _____

SEX
  ☐ FEMALE    ☐ MALE
    CIRCUMCISION
      ☐ YES    ☐ NO

BIRTH WEIGHT _____

DISPOSITION
  ☐ HOME WITH MOTHER ☐ IN HOSPITAL
  ☐ TRANSFER ☐ NEONATAL DEATH
  ☐ STILLBIRTH ☐ OTHER

COMPLICATIONS/ANOMALIES _____
_____
_____
_____

PEDIATRICIAN _____

**MATERNAL INFORMATION**

HGB/HCT LEVEL _____

MEDICATIONS _____
_____

FEEDING METHOD    ☐ BREAST    ☐ BOTTLE

CONTRACEPTIVE METHOD (IF APPLICABLE) _____
_____

DIAGNOSTIC STUDIES PENDING _____
_____
_____
_____

SECONDARY DIAGNOSIS/PREEXISTING CONDITIONS
  ☐ ASTHMA    ☐ HYPERTENSION
  ☐ DIABETES    ☐ OTHER _____

IMMUNIZATIONS GIVEN
  ☐ ANTI-D IMMUNE GLOBULIN
  ☐ RUBELLA
  ☐ OTHER _____
  _____

FOLLOW-UP APPT
  DATE _____
  LOCATION _____
  OTHER _____
  _____
  _____
  _____

### INTERIM CONTACTS

| DATE | COMMENT |
|------|---------|
| _____ | _____ |
| _____ | _____ |
| _____ | _____ |
| _____ | _____ |
| _____ | _____ |
| _____ | _____ |
| _____ | _____ |
| _____ | _____ |
| _____ | _____ |
| _____ | _____ |
| _____ | _____ |
| _____ | _____ |

PROVIDER SIGNATURE (AS REQUIRED)_____

## POSTPARTUM VISIT

DATE _____

LAB STUDIES REQUESTED _____

_____

HGB/HCT _____ LAST PAP TEST _____

FEEDING METHOD _____

CONTRACEPTIVE METHOD _____

POSTPARTUM DEPRESSION SCREENING _____

INTIMATE PARTNER VIOLENCE SCREENING _____

**INTERIM HISTORY**

_____

_____

_____

_____

**PHYSICAL EXAM**

BP _____        WT _____

BREASTS              ☐ NORMAL _____

ABDOMEN              ☐ NORMAL _____

EXTERNAL GENITALS    ☐ NORMAL _____

VAGINA               ☐ NORMAL _____

CERVIX               ☐ NORMAL _____

UTERUS               ☐ NORMAL _____

ADNEXA               ☐ NORMAL _____

RECTAL-VAGINAL       ☐ NORMAL _____

PAP TEST        ☐ YES   ☐ NO

**COMMENT**

_____

_____

_____

_____

_____

_____

_____

_____

_____

_____

_____

_____

_____

_____

_____

_____

_____

_____

_____

_____

_____

_____

_____

ALLERGIES _____

MEDICATIONS/CONTRACEPTION _____

_____

☐ DISPENSED

**INTERVAL CARE RECOMMENDATIONS**

FOR GENERAL HEALTH PROMOTION _____

_____

_____

_____

_____

_____

_____

_____

FOR REPRODUCTIVE HEALTH PROMOTION _____

_____

_____

_____

_____

_____

RETURN VISIT _____

REFERRALS _____

_____

EXAMINED BY _____

PROVIDER SIGNATURE (AS REQUIRED) _____

Page numbers in *italics* denote figures; those followed by a 't' denote tables; those followed by a *b* denote boxes.